Veterinary Oral Diagnostic Imaging

Veterinary Oral Diagnostic Imaging

Edited by

Brenda L. Mulherin, DVM, DAVDC
Iowa State University
College of Veterinary Medicine
Ames, IA, USA

WILEY Blackwell

Published by John Wiley & Sons, Inc., Hoboken, New Jersey.
Published simultaneously in Canada.

For general information on our other products and services or for technical support, please contact our Customer Care Department within the United States at (800) 762-2974, outside the United States at (317) 572-3993 or fax (317) 572-4002.

Wiley also publishes its books in a variety of electronic formats. Some content that appears in print may not be available in electronic formats. For more information about Wiley products, visit our website at www.wiley.com.

Library of Congress Cataloging-in-Publication Data Applied for

LCCN No: 2023023184
Hardback ISBN: 9781119780502
ePDF: 9781119780519
ePUB: 9781119780540
oBook: 9781119780571

Cover Design: Wiley
Cover Images: Courtesy of Author

Set in 9.5/12.5pt STIXTwoText by Straive, Pondicherry, India

Printed in Singapore
M114788_140923

Contents

List of Contributors

Michael Congiusta
Veterinary Dentistry and Oromaxillofacial Surgery
School of Veterinary Medicine
University of Wisconsin-Madison
Madison, WI, USA

Kara Frerichs
Lloyd Veterinary Medical Center
Iowa State University College of Veterinary Medicine
Ames, IA, USA

Stephanie Goldschmidt
Department of Surgical and Radiologic Sciences
University of California-Davis School
of Veterinary Medicine
Davis, CA, USA

Joan Howard
Lloyd Veterinary Medical Center
Iowa State University College of Veterinary Medicine
Ames, IA, USA

Chad Lothamer
College of Veterinary Medicine
University of Tennessee
Knoxville, TN, USA

Megan Mickelson
University of Missouri Veterinary Health Center
Columbia, MO, USA

Chanda Miles
Veterinary Dentistry Specialists
Katy, TX, USA

Brenda L. Mulherin
Lloyd Veterinary Medical Center
Iowa State University College of Veterinary Medicine
Ames, IA, USA

June Olds
Lloyd Veterinary Medical Center
Iowa State University College of Veterinary Medicine
Ames, IA, USA

Molly Rice
Midwest Veterinary Dental Services
Elkhorn, WI, USA

Beatrice Sponseller
Lloyd Veterinary Medical Center
Iowa State University College of Veterinary Medicine
Ames, IA, USA

Preface

Most veterinarians will need to perform dentistry and oral surgery procedures on the various patients they see during their career. Dental radiography has become a mainstay of general practice and specialty practices throughout the country. Dental radiography has become a standard of care and according to the 2013 and 2019 AAHA Dental Care Guidelines for Dogs and Cats, dental imaging of the oral cavity in some fashion is the only way in which an accurate treatment plan can be made for dogs and cats. Imaging of the oral cavity establishes a baseline for the patient as well as allows the practitioner to monitor progression of disease. It is common for general practitioners to use what they see clinically to evaluate whether they should initiate treatment for both small animal, equine, and exotic and zoo patients. Additional information can be gained relating to the health of the oral cavity by evaluating the structures below the surface.

Education relating to imaging of the oral cavity in the veterinary curriculum is minimal at best. Many veterinary schools have little to no education related to the art of veterinary dentistry and oral surgery and even less related to diagnostic imaging of the oral cavity. Fortunately for small animal, equine, and exotic and zoo animals, diagnostic imaging is becoming more common, and the utility of its use is being appreciated by general practitioners and specialists alike. Unfortunately, many veterinarians invest in the equipment to procure diagnostic images but are unsure how to collect diagnostic images or interpret them appropriately.

The goal of this textbook is to provide a quick reference for those individuals looking to understand the different diagnostic imaging modalities and how to interpret the images that are collected. It is focused on the fundamentals of dental radiographic imaging, interpretation, and its application to the oral cavity for a multitude of species. The emphasis is heavily photographic and figure based and attempts to incorporate the most common dental pathology associated with canines, felines, zoo/exotic animal species, and equine patients. It is meant to be an easy read and a reference for help in procuring and interpreting diagnostic images within the oral cavity.

Acknowledgements

The authors would like to give a special acknowledgement to Kristina Miles, DVM, DACVR and Robin White, DVM, DACVR for assistance in interpretation of several diagnostic images in the Interpretation of Uncommon Pathology in the Canine and Feline Patient chapter.

The author would like to give a special acknowledgement to Elizabeth Riedesel DVM, DACVR for assistance in interpretation of several diagnostic images and editing of figure legends within the Diagnostic Imaging of Exotic Pet Mammals and Zoo Animals chapter.

The authors would like to give a special acknowledgment to Wolfgang Weber for assistance in providing skull specimens and ideas for their presentation in the Diagnostic Imaging and Interpretation of the Equine Patient chapter.

1

History, Physiology, Modality Options, and Safety for Diagnostic Imaging of the Oral Cavity

Brenda L. Mulherin

Lloyd Veterinary Medical Center, Iowa State University College of Veterinary Medicine, Ames, IA, USA

CONTENTS

History of Diagnostic Imaging

Discovery of X-rays

8 November 1895 was the extraordinary discovery of Roentgen rays, otherwise known as X-rays [1, 2]. X-rays were discovered by a German physicist named Wilhelm Conrad Roentgen (Figure 1.1). Roentgen published a paper regarding this unique discovery entitled "On a new kind of rays" in *Sitzungsberichte der Wurzburger Physik. -Medic. -Gesellschaft.* on 28 December 1895 [1, 2]. This date is now considered the true discovery of X-rays [2]. In Roentgen's research, his wife Bertha Roentgen assisted in acquiring the first radiographic image of the human body [3]. She placed her hand on the photographic plate, and the X-ray beam was applied to her hand. This experiment yielded the first X-ray image of the bones and soft tissue of Bertha's hand and her wedding ring [3] (Figure 1.2). Interestingly, during the days of research in his laboratory, Roentgen did not know what kind of radiation he was experimenting with, so he referred to the waves as X-rays, which is how they are still known today [2]. Early in the discovery of radiology, most of the radiographic images produced were taken and created by photographers, or medical experts who had interest in photography [4].

Developing of Safety Measures

Following the discovery of X-rays, Nikola Tesla tried to develop a protection shield from what he perceived the harm that could come from X-ray exposure [2]. Tesla suggested that by placing an aluminum plate between the object of interest and the X-rays, there would be a reduction in the amount of X-ray energy received, hence the concept of the inverse square law [2].

Shortening of Exposure Time

Historically, X-ray energy was continuously emitted to the object of interest anywhere from 15 to 60 minutes at a time. In 1896, Professor Mihajo Idvorski Pupin from Columbia University, also known as Michael Pupin, tried to find a

Veterinary Oral Diagnostic Imaging, First Edition. Edited by Brenda L. Mulherin.
© 2024 John Wiley & Sons, Inc. Published 2024 by John Wiley & Sons, Inc.

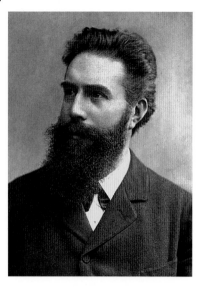

Figure 1.1   William Conrad Roentgen, the German physicist who first discovered X-rays. *Source:* Courtesy of John Wiley & Sons.

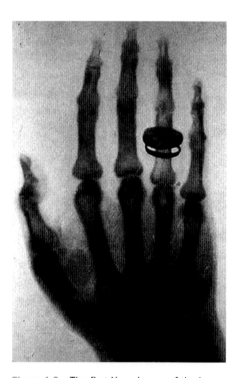

Figure 1.2   The first X-ray image of the bones and soft tissue of the hand of Bertha Roentgen. *Source:* Courtesy of John Wiley & Sons.

way to shorten the exposure time required to acquire an image [2, 4]. He placed a photographic plate behind a fluorescent screen and then applied the X-ray energy to the object of interest to create an image on the film [2, 4]. This was found to reduce the exposure time to only a few seconds [2, 4].

Glass Plates to Film

In 1896, Carl Schleusner manufactured the first glass plates to be used for radiographic image creation [4]. At the time, radiographs that were taken on glass plates were thought to be superior to those taken on film [4]. In 1914, during World War I, glass plates needed to be replaced with film as the glass needed to create the radiographic plates was manufactured in Belgium [4]. Due to the war, the supply of glass decreased, while the demand for radiographic images increased. In 1918, the first radiographic film was produced with high-speed emulsion on both sides, reducing radiation exposure and exposure times [4]. By the 1940s, non-screen radiograph film was introduced, and automatic film processors were becoming available [4].

Progression to Digital

Since the 1980s, digital radiography (DR) has slowly been replacing film in many hospitals and practices [5]. DR was quickly accepted into the veterinary profession as the speed of digital acquisition and ability to read images at computer terminals throughout the hospital allow for efficient interpretation and maximization of patient care.

The main difference between using conventional radiographic film and a digital system is in the viewing of the images. Digital radiographic images are electronically captured and viewed at a computer terminal, whereas conventional radiographic film is viewed with an illuminated view box. Transitioning to digital has significant benefits for diagnostic evaluation compared to conventional radiography. Digital systems allow a radiologist, specialist, or practitioner to evaluate images remotely. It allows for simpler storage, organization, and an easier way to compare images. Many advanced imaging methods including computed tomography (CT), magnetic resonance imaging (MRI), ultrasound, and cone beam computed tomography (CBCT) allow imaging of the body in such detail that 3D reconstructions of organs can be made. This helps to prepare the surgeon in advance for a procedure. Over the years, the application of radiation for visualization within a patient's body without surgical exploration has changed the field of medicine. These different imaging modalities have revolutionized the diagnostic field of medicine [2].

Philosophy of Diagnostic Imaging

Choosing the Appropriate Modality

It is the responsibility of the clinician to choose the imaging modality appropriate to gather the most information possible bearing in mind modality availability, ability for swift interpretation, patient stability, and any financial considerations an owner may have. Ideally, a clinician will choose the imaging modality that is the most cost-effective and readily available yet yielding the necessary information to make a diagnosis. Radiographic imaging is of no use if the images created cannot be accurately interpreted by the clinician or at the very least, quickly distributed to an outside source that can interpret the images in an expedited manner.

Ability to Interpret Findings

The ability to interpret diagnostic images is based on the ability to interpret shadows. A comprehensive grasp of anatomy and the interaction of radiation with different structure densities is imperative to be able to evaluate areas of the body for disease conditions. Unfortunately, not everything is black and white when attempting to interpret radiographic images. Variations in patient confirmation and ranges of normal within the same species can lead the interpreter to difficulties of identifying normal from abnormal even within the same patient.

Diagnostic imaging can allow the clinician to survey an organ system, assess trauma, explore an area for a suspected neoplastic process, or allow for patient follow-up in monitoring disease progression or therapeutic effectiveness. There are many different imaging modalities that can be used to create a diagnostic picture of a specific area of interest. Each modality has its own advantages and disadvantages to their use. It is up to the clinician to decide which imaging modality is best suited to provide the diagnostic picture of what question they would like to answer. Regardless of the modality used to acquire diagnostic images, any findings should be interpreted based on a thorough examination of the patient and how those findings relate to an anesthetized oral examination and the patient's presenting complaint.

Radiographic Indications

Documentation of Disease

Dental radiographic imaging can document the amount of disease that is present within the oral cavity. It can be used to estimate the amount of bone loss that has occurred, evaluate for evidence of endodontic disease and any embedded teeth, or retained tooth roots that may be present, among other things [6].

Value of Full-Mouth Radiography

Taking full-mouth radiographs of canine and feline patients is included in the American Animal Hospital Association Guidelines regarding the dental care for dogs and cats [7]. Full-mouth radiography is defined as a series of images taken of the teeth and bone of the jaw, both dentulous and edentulous portions [6]. The main reason full-mouth radiographs are taken is to establish a baseline to monitor for disease progression as well as determine if there is any existing disease or abnormalities present within the mouth prior to treatment.

American Animal Hospital Association Guidelines Regarding Dental Radiography

According to the most recent American Animal Hospital Association Guidelines relating to dental radiography, a person evaluating the oral cavity can underestimate the presence of disease when only examining a conscious patient compared to when intraoral radiographs are taken [7]. When intraoral radiographs are taken and combined with the oral examination findings, the examiner can only then assess the full extent of disease or any oral pathology present within an oral cavity [7]. While the ability to take intraoral radiographs is important, what is more imperative is that the practitioner has gained the knowledge and skills to interpret the radiographic findings associated with the radiographs. The American Animal Hospital Association Guidelines recommend that all dental patients receive full-mouth intraoral dental radiographs [7].

Intraoral Dental Radiographic Equipment

Generators

Dental generators come in a variety of forms. There are wall-mounted units, handheld units, and rolling units. The main difference between a dental X-ray unit and a standard radiographic unit is that the standard radiograph unit, milliamperes, kilovolts, and exposure time can be adjusted in any combination to create a diagnostic image. In a dental X-ray unit, the milliamperes and kilovolts are usually preset and are not able to be adjusted. Generally, the kilovoltage is fixed at 70–90 kVp, and the milliampere is fixed at 10–15 mA. The only adjustment available is exposure time. Exposure time is usually displayed in impulses or seconds on the unit. Some units are designed to be preprogrammed according to the type of tooth to be radiographed or based on the size of the patient that is being radiographed: small, medium, or large.

Viewing a radiographic image depends on the size of the tube head and focal spot of the generator, in essence, the amount of radiation collimation. The smaller the focal spot, the better the image detail [8]. The distance the area of interest is from the focal spot created by the generator is directly related to the magnification and detail of the image [8]. The closer the area of interest is to the film, the more improved image clarity as well as a lesser amount of distortion and magnification [8]. The area of interest should be as close to the film as possible to create the best image [8].

Wall-Mounted Units

Wall-mounted units are the most frequently used generators for procuring dental radiographs. Units attached to a stationary surface allow the arm to be positioned and left to procure the image without the operator being near the radiographic beam. These radiographic tube heads can be easily positioned. Frequently, they can be purchased secondhand from human dental operatories. Wall-mounted units have less drift of the positioning arm allowing for better image quality. A unit that is attached to the wall does have the limitation of being stationary and unable to be transported to a separate room if needed. For many dental procedures, there is a dedicated wet table associated with a wall-mounted unit to have the patient in proximity of the radiographic generator (Figure 1.3).

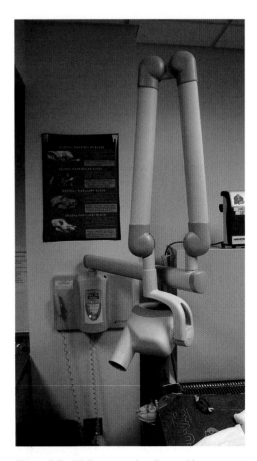

Figure 1.3   Wall-mounted radiographic generator.

Handheld Units

Handheld X-ray generators are battery-powered units that produce intraoral radiographs that can be easily transported between multiple rooms. They are compatible with digital sensors, standard film, and phosphor plates. Handheld units have an internal shielding from radiation and a scatter shield to protect the operator from direct and scattered radiation. Procuring images from a handheld unit takes practice as the positioning is based on the height, strength, and stability of the operator. Many of these units can weigh 8–10 pounds. This can cause fatigue of the operator as they are holding the unit for radiographic acquisition. When images need to be repeated, it may be difficult to reposition the unit to acquire a similar or improved image (Figure 1.4a and b).

Mobile Units/Castor-Mounted Units

Generators that are moveable can be of great benefit to the operator. These units can be moved from room to room. These units have the structure of a wall-mounted unit, with the freedom to move the generator to a different room. Depending on the unit, issues with stability have occurred with the units being disproportionally weighted, leaving them in danger of toppling over. Difficulty in being able to position the unit close enough to the patient to acquire an image may be encountered depending on the arrangement of the room and table. This is because the base of the unit needs to be positioned near or under a table to have appropriate access and positioning to the patient. This type of generator can be cumbersome and potentially a safety threat as the stabilization legs can be a tripping hazard (Figure 1.5).

Film

A dental generator needs to have some form of film to be able to release the photons against. There are three main types of film: standard film, indirect plates, and direct plates. As shown in Table 1.1, there are various film sizes that can be used which are adapted from human patients. Each type of film has specific sizes that are available to use with the generator. The flexibility of standard physical film and indirect plates allows them to be easily placed within the oral cavity of the patient to take an image. Direct plates are rigid and cannot be easily manipulated. Most commonly, intraoral radiographs for canine and feline patients use a Size 2 film. This size appears to be adequate for most small animal veterinary patients. A Size 4 film is helpful in larger breed dogs as it allows the operator to image more than one to two teeth at a time. It also allows the operator to procure an image of the whole tooth in one image rather than in multiple images for larger teeth, such as the canine tooth.

(a)

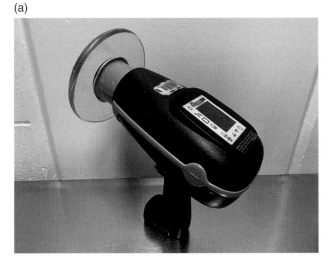

(b)

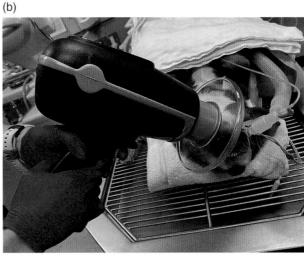

Figure 1.4 (a) Handheld radiographic generator. (b) A handheld radiographic generator has an internal radiation shielding and a scatter shield to protect the operator from radiation exposure. *Source:* Courtesy of Christopher J. Snyder, DVM, DAVDC, Founding Fellow, AVDC Oral and Maxillofacial Surgery, University of Wisconsin-Madison, School of Veterinary Medicine.

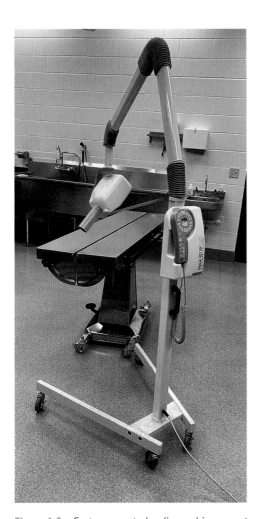

Figure 1.5 Castor-mounted radiographic generator.
Source: Courtesy of Christopher J. Snyder, DVM, DAVDC, Founding Fellow, AVDC Oral and Maxillofacial Surgery, University of Wisconsin-Madison, School of Veterinary Medicine.

Standard Film

Standard film is tightly wrapped to avoid exposing the film itself to moisture or light. The sheet of unexposed film is wrapped in a black paper envelope. There is a lead foil sheet that protects the film from secondary radiation exposure. It is placed on the side of the film that is positioned farthest away from the generator (Figure 1.6). Since standard dental film is too small to be able to mark patient identity and medical record information, there is a "dimple" in the corner of the film to help the interpreter with orientation once the film has been exposed. The "dimple" has a concave or convex surface, depending on how you are looking at it. A concave shape curves inward, while a convex shape curves outward (Figure 1.7a and b). For proper orientation, the convex surface of the dimple should always be positioned toward the dental generator during exposure. Standard intraoral film comes in five sizes: 0, 1, 2, 3, and 4. Most commonly in veterinary patients, Sizes 0, 2, and 4 are employed for procuring oral diagnostic images [9].

Standard radiographic film can be developed either manually or with an automatic processor. Dental film can be attached to a larger film and run through an automatic processor or can be developed using a chairside developer. Automatic processors have been created to process dental film that is fully fixed and air-dried. When film is hand-processed, it is performed in four steps: developing, rinsing, fixing, and washing (Figure 1.8a and b). Using rapid processing solutions will allow the radiographic film to be processed within 90 seconds. Traditional light boxes can be used to view the films after they are processed. Due to the decreased size of the film compared to standard

Table 1.1 Table depicting the differences between the three most common types of radiographic film: standard, computed radiography (indirect) and direct digital radiography (direct) plates.

Type of film	Sizes	Chemicals	Speed of processing	Plate rigidity	Cost of replacement	Ease of retake image acquisition
Standard	0, 1, 2, 3, 4	Yes	5 min	Flexible	$	Moderate
Computed radiography (indirect plate)	0, 1, 2, 3, 4	No	1–2 min	Flexible	$$	Moderate
Direct digital radiography (direct plate)	0, 2	No	3–5 seconds	Rigid	$$$	Easiest

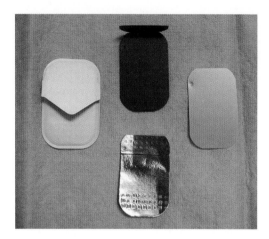

Figure 1.6 Image of standard radiographic film opened to expose the contents. Standard film is wrapped to avoid exposure to moisture and light. The sheet of unexposed film is wrapped in a black paper envelope. There is a lead foil sheet that protects the film from secondary exposure.

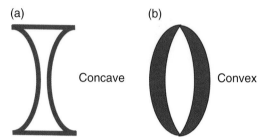

(a) Concave (b) Convex

Figure 1.7 (a) An indentation, or "dimple," is present on standard radiographic film to help the reader interpret orientation of the image. If the "dimple" is positioned so that it has an inward curve, the reader is looking at the concave surface. (b) If the "dimple" is positioned so that the surface curves outward, the reader is looking at the convex surface. The convex surface should always be positioned toward the generator during exposure, point to point.

radiographs, smaller viewers are utilized in most practices. Due to the nuances and limitations of this type of film, its use in veterinary medicine is obsolete and rarely used.

Digital Image Acquisition

There are two main types of digital radiographic acquisition systems: computed radiography (CR) and direct digital radiography (DDR) systems. Conventional radiographic generators or specific dental radiographic generators can be used with either system. The main difference between the two different acquisition systems lies in the film that is used. The CR system uses a physical flexible imaging plate, and the DDR system uses a rigid sensor or radiographic recording device. Digital acquisition systems should produce an image of diagnostic quality and have similar or less radiation exposure as to what is needed for standard dental film [10]. They should also be compatible with most conventional X-ray generators, have their information processed like any other formatted digital imaging and communications in medicine (DICOM) image, and be able to be processed in a timely manner [10].

Computed Radiography (CR) Photostimulable Phosphor (PSP) Plates (Indirect Plates)

This method of obtaining an intraoral radiograph involves taking the image on a phosphor plate and then transferring the image to a computer to be interpreted. Older photostimulable plates must be erased before taking an additional image, or the operator risks superimposition of multiple images on the same plate. Most photostimulable phosphor (PSP) plate systems now automatically erase the image from the system after transferring the previous image to the computer. The time from radiation exposure to digital image interpretation for the PSP systems can range from a few seconds to a few minutes depending on the system. There are five common phosphor plate sizes used for dental radiographic procurement: 0, 1, 2, 3, and 4. When cared for properly, most PSP plate systems can be used hundreds of times before they need to be replaced. The plates are thin and flexible and act like standard film, but with the benefit of being able to manipulate and store images digitally on a computer and reuse them multiple times (Figure 1.9). The main disadvantage of the CR system includes the increased anesthetic time required for retaking radiographic images due to the need to remove

(a)

(b)

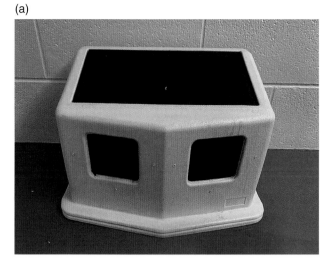 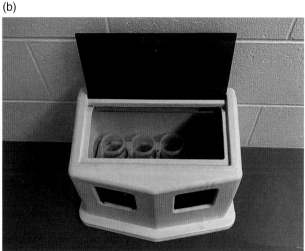

Figure 1.8 (a) Image depicts a hand processing unit with the lid closed, protecting the processing fluids. (b) Image depicts the open hand processing unit showing the containers for the different solutions: developer, rinse, fixer, and rinse solutions. *Source:* Courtesy of Jill Medenwaldt, CVT, VTS-D, University of Wisconsin-Madison, School of Veterinary Medicine.

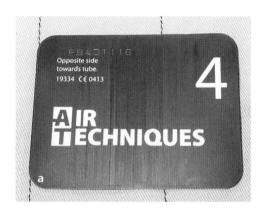

Figure 1.9 Computed radiography (CR) Size 4 image sensor: indirect plate. *Source:* Courtesy of Chad Lothamer, DVM, DAVDC, University of Tennessee College of Veterinary Medicine.

the plate from the oral cavity to process the image. Advantages of this system include the cost to replace the plate if it becomes damaged and the increased selection of plate sizes compared to the DR system.

Digital Radiography (DR) Image Sensors (Direct Plates)

Most direct digital sensors consist of either a charge-coupled device (CCD) or a complementary metal oxide semiconductor (CMOS) which is sensitive to light [9]. These sensors also have a scintillator layer which converts X-ray energy into light to create an image [9]. The sensors are directly connected to a computer to process the information to create an image within a few seconds (Figure 1.10a and b). This type of radiographic plate requires less radiation and is the most efficient of the intraoral dental radiography imaging modalities to acquire the images. Positioning is easier with these units because the sensor does not need to leave the oral cavity to acquire and process an image. The main disadvantages of a direct system are the sensor size and its durability. The largest size currently available for a digital sensor is a Size 2. Direct plates are rigid and directly attached to the computer. If they are dropped, bitten, or bent, this will adversely affect the sensor and the radiographic image, potentially necessitating replacement of the sensor, which can be costly (Figure 1.11a and b). The benefits of a direct system are the speed of image acquisition and easier ability to retake images if there are positional alterations that need to be made or artifacts appearing on the image.

Similarities of Indirect and Direct Plates

Both direct and indirect digital plate images can be altered on the computer for underexposure or overexposure. Images from both systems can be manipulated to magnify an area of interest. The images are also easily transferred digitally to another clinician for interpretation or to the clients through a computer.

Radiographic Imaging

Basic Unit of an X-ray

The basic component of an X-ray is composed of photon energy [11]. This is expressed as a unit of energy called the electron volt (eV). X-rays are a form of radiant energy that has a short wavelength and is capable of penetrating hard

(a)   (b)

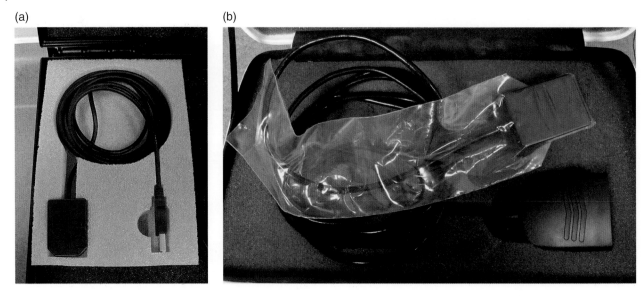

Figure 1.10 (a) Image depicts the DR system (direct radiography) plate which is attached directly to the computer. (b) A Size 2 sensor wrapped in its storage container. This sensor is in a sleeve which is changed out between uses to keep the sensor clean and to avoid cross-contamination of saliva and other fluids between patients.

(a)   (b)

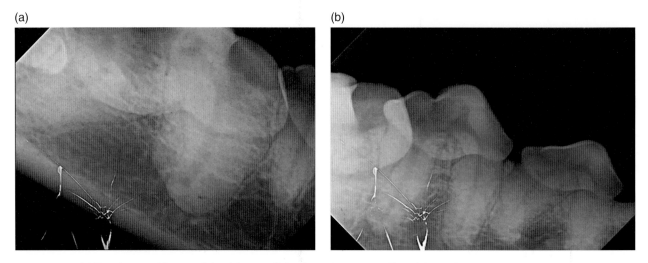

Figure 1.11 (a) Foreshortened image of the right mandible of a canine patient. The white spiderweb appearance on the sensor is damage to the direct plate. (b) Foreshortened image of the right mandible of the same patient. The radiographic image also depicts not including at least 2 mm of the apex of the root, for a diagnostic image. The white spiderweb appearance depicts damage to the sensor, making it difficult to interpret the radiographic findings.

and soft tissues alike [8]. Photons are either absorbed through tissues or pass through the tissues with minimal interference to expose an X-ray film. An X-ray is produced when electrons moving at a high rate of speed interact with a suitable material. During the interaction, as the electrons hit the material, they are either slowed down, change their direction, or are completely absorbed by the material. The energy is converted into heat and X-rays to produce an image. The radiographic tube head, or generator, is designed to direct these interactions and control this process.

Milliamperes (mA), Kilovoltage Peak (kVp), and Exposure Time

When looking at a standard X-ray generator, there are usually three controls that can be adjusted: mA, kVp, and exposure time (Figure 1.12).

mA control stands for milliamperes of energy released. This controls the number of electrons that are freed from the filament and ultimately the number of X-rays that are produced and measured per second. The number of X-rays

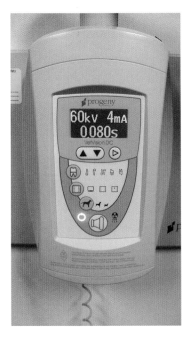

Figure 1.12 Image of a standard radiographic generator. There are three controls that can be adjusted: milliamperes (mA), kilovoltage peak (kVp), and exposure time.

produced is directly proportional to the number of electrons released. Therefore, the higher the mA, the larger the number of electrons released. Milliamperage-second controls the quantity of X-rays that are emitted.

kVp or kilovoltage peak is the amount of voltage that is applied across the radiographic tube head. It is referred to as the speed at which the electrons travel to the target. The higher the kVp, the more rapid the travel of the electrons and the more kinetic energy or heat is created. kVp controls the quality of the X-ray beam (wavelength).

Exposure time controls the duration of time at which radiation is being emitted. The duration of exposure is directly correlated with the number of X-rays produced.

There is also a direct correlation between the mA and seconds in that the result of the mA and the exposure time is equivalent to the number of X-rays that are produced:

$$mA\big(\#/\,seconds\big)\times time\big(seconds\big)$$
$$= mAs\big(total\ number\ of\ X-rays\big)$$

Radiographic Densities

When describing radiographic density, the interpreter needs to be able to describe the degree of opacity of the tissues. There are five different radiographic opacities that can be observed based on the density of the material [8]. The materials that produce different opacities are gas, fat, muscle, bone, and mineral [8] (Figure 1.13). The density of air allows most of the radiographic electrons to pass freely to the film causing an increased exposure, therefore increasing the blackness of a film [8]. Alternatively, the density of bone and mineral will absorb more electrons creating a further radiopaque shadow on the film [8]. Overall, thicker tissues will reduce the number of X-rays that ultimately reach the film compared to thinner tissues.

Radiopaque

Radiopaque is used to describe the degree of whiteness on a radiographic image. The degree of whiteness depends on the density of the area of interest. The denser the area, the more the X-ray beams are absorbed. The terms increased or decreased opacity can also be used to describe the degree of opaqueness of the material. The degree of opacity should be used to describe the organ or structure in relation to what the structure should look like under normal circumstances (Figure 1.14).

Figure 1.13 Illustration of radiographic densities. Gas allows the majority of radiographic electrons to pass freely to the film, followed by fat and then muscle. Bone and mineral will absorb more electrons creating a radiopaque shadow on the film.

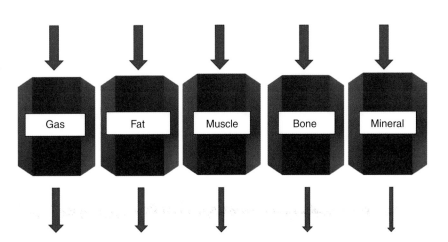

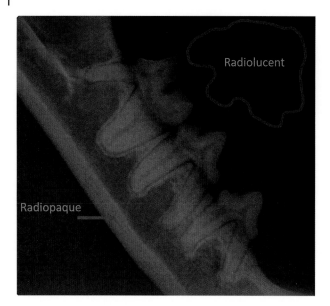

Figure 1.14 Radiograph of a normal right mandible of a feline patient. Radiopaque is used to describe the degree of whiteness of an image, and radiolucent is used to describe the degree of blackness of an image. The denser the area, the more radiopaque or white the structure is on the radiograph, the less dense the area, the more radiolucent or black the structure is.

Radiolucent

Radiolucent is used to describe the degree of blackness on a radiographic image. The degree of blackness depends on the lack of density of the area. Radiolucent objects do not absorb a significant amount of radiographic energy, rather the beams of radiation pass through the object unrestricted. Again, a change in the radiolucency of an object should be interpreted in relation to what the organ or structure should look like under normal circumstances.

Tissues that have a greater thickness will absorb more photons than thinner tissues. The greater the tissue absorption, the fewer the number of photons that expose the film and hence the more radiopaque the image is created on the film (see Figure 1.13).

Digital Image Creation

Creation of a Digital Image

The creation of a digital radiographic images involves three steps: a measurement of the transmission of the pattern of radiation emitted to the patient, converting the measurement into a digital format, and viewing the processed digital information with a computer [10].

Digital Imaging and Communications in Medicine Format (DICOM)

A digital file used in medical imaging is a DICOM file. This stands for Digital Imaging and Communications in Medicine format. Most DICOM files are in a standard format to allow different computer hardware and programs to be able to create and produce an image [10]. DICOM images can be transferred outside of the generating clinic for interpretation by sending through a web-based program [10]. The interpreter usually downloads the program along with the digital image information to allow the viewer to see and interpret the images [10]. DICOM files can be stored within an electronic repository to help manage all radiographic imaging modalities. When digital storage systems are utilized with a picture archiving system (PACS), transferring information between practitioners can be seamless.

Pixels

A digital image is composed of pixels. Radiographic imaging is an exercise in interpreting shades of gray. Each pixel is attached to a specific shade of gray. The greater the number of pixels, the larger the file size. The size of the pixel relates to the spatial resolution of an image [10]. This relates to the clarity and detail of an image. The computer program and hardware system determine the size of pixels as it arranges and assigns them to the digital radiographic image [10]. As a general statement, the more pixels an image has, the better the image quality, but at some point, the quality cannot be improved by increasing the number of pixels.

Advanced Imaging Modalities

Computed Tomography

The imaging modality of CT (Figure 1.15) is commonly used for the evaluation of the brain, sinus and nasal cavities, orbit, mediastinum, lung, liver, adrenal glands, elbow joint, and spine [12]. This imaging modality creates a cross-sectional reconstruction of the area of interest through ionizing radiation from an X-ray tube. A fan-shaped collimated beam of radiation is generated on one side of a patient, and multiple detectors on the opposite side of the patient measure the amount of radiation transmission through the tissue slice from the patient [12]. The density of the tissue depicts how much radiation is passed through the tissue compared to how much the radiation is absorbed. For example, gas allows radiation to pass through unobstructed. The amount of radiation passing through gas at

Figure 1.15   Computed tomography unit.

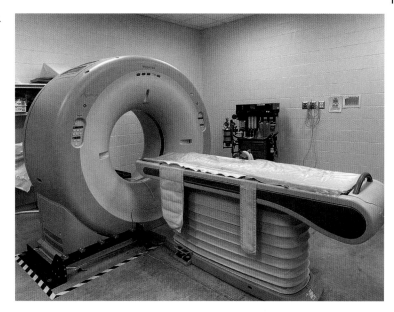

Figure 1.16   Illustration of the information gathering capacity of a multislice computed tomography unit. Increasing the number of slices a computed tomography unit can collect will increase the amount of information gathered to create a more detained reconstruction.

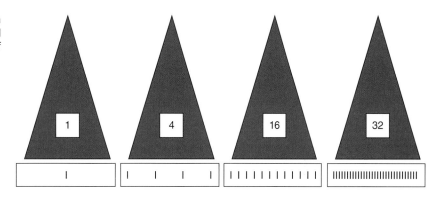

the beginning is similar to the amount of radiation at the end of the emission. In contrast, if the same beam of radiation passes through mineral or bone, the density of these materials is far greater than gas. Therefore, more radiation is absorbed by these structures, and the amount of radiation present at the end of the emission is far less than when radiation was first emitted.

Increasing the number of slices a CT unit can collect will increase the amount of information gathered about an area of interest. The more information gathered can help create more detail of the reconstructed area (Figure 1.16). It is thought that with an increased slice thickness, there is a reduced diagnostic quality of the images created and there is an increased amount of image noise which can lead to distortion of the image [13]. The more the slices collected, hence the smaller the slice thickness, the better the detail of the area of interest as more information can be gathered with multiple slices. Currently, tissue thickness can be from 0.5 to 10 mm and usually takes only a few seconds to acquire an image. Currently, a 3-mm slice

thickness is thought to produce the best diagnostic quality and as well as the least amount of image distortion [13]. As the unit rotates around the patient, multiple measurements are taken from various directions to create a reconstructed image of the area of interest. The massive amount of data collected from the multiple images recreates the desired area of interest. The smaller the slice thickness, the larger the volume of data collected. There is significantly superior differentiation of soft and hard tissues within the images, and the ability to produce images without superimposition of the overlying structures makes this a very good imaging modality.

Commonly, intravenous contrast agents are injected to help differentiate between lesions and the normal parenchyma of a tissue [12]. Contrast media can also aid in the vascular anatomy and patency of vessels within the area of interest [12]. Using a contrast agent can assist in visualizing defects in an area including hemorrhage and infection, as well as accumulation of the agent in abnormal tissues, potentially indicating neoplasia.

Spatial resolution is the ability of an imaging modality to differentiate between adjacent objects or structures. Spatial resolution for a CT image is dependent on the number of projections and the number of detectors [14]. The resolution of areas with low contrast is highly determined by the filtering ability of the X-ray beam [14]. When the X-ray beam is less filtered, the beam releases more radiation due to the tissues absorbing more radiation, producing a higher contrast image [14]. When the beam is more filtered, it reduces the radiation exposure but also results in images that are lower in contrast [14].

Cone Beam Computed Tomography (CBCT)

Advancement of dental radiographic imaging modalities has progressed to the use of CBCT (Figure 1.17a and b). The ability to generate a three-dimensional image to create a complete diagnostic picture is vital to a clinician's ability to treat a patient. Using a CBCT unit has shown superior image quality while still allowing for three-dimensional reconstruction of the structures within the orofacial region. A CBCT unit employs a radiographic source, image detector, computer, and a monitor to display the images created. It differs from a conventional CT unit by using cone beam geometry rather than a collimated beam. The detectors within the standard CT unit are arranged in rows while in CBCT flat panels or image intensifiers are used. The CBCT

rotates around the patient only once, collecting its volume of information on the flat panel detectors. The radiation source of the CBCT unit rotates synchronously to acquire a 360° depiction of the area of interest [15]. The standard CT unit rotates around the area of interest multiple times and collects information with multiple scans, while a CBCT rotates once, thus reducing the radiation exposure to the patient. The volume of raw data acquired by the CBCT unit is processed and reconstructed by computer software to be viewed on a display unit, similar to a conventional CT unit. Compared to a conventional multidetector unit, cone beam images have superior diagnostic quality in assessing anatomical structures [15]. CBCT technology allows for better spatial resolution allowing the interpreter to better differentiate subtle differences between objects that are next to each other, such as teeth and bone. Electrical requirements for these units are standard, and the investment costs for a CBCT unit are less than a conventional CT unit. CBCT technology offers three-dimensional imaging and superior image creation of the dentoalveolar structures at a lower cost than a conventional CT unit [15]. It also uses a similar radiation exposure to intraoral radiography, making it a very viable option for the clinician to use for diagnostic imaging of the oral cavity. CBCT is an excellent imaging modality for evaluating bone and teeth, but not soft tissues or potential neoplastic conditions. The contrast resolution of this modality makes it difficult to differentiate between

(a)

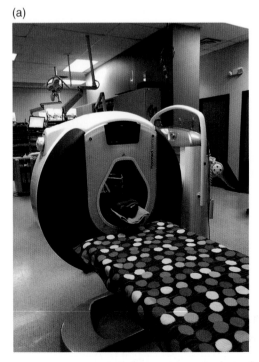

(b)

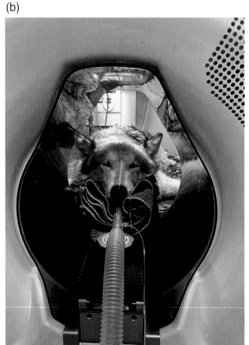

Figure 1.17 (a) Cone beam computed tomography unit. Photo courtesy of Scott MacGee, DVM, DAVDC, Companion Animal Dentistry of Kansas City. (b) Cone beam tomography unit with a canidae species in the scanner. *Source:* Courtesy of Scott MacGee, DVM, DAVDC, Companion Animal Dentistry of Kansas City.

slight changes in soft tissue structures, therefore making it a less desirable modality for evaluating neoplastic conditions. CBCT is an excellent imaging modality for evaluating periodontal disease, endodontic disease, and for tooth resorption in both canine and feline patients. It is also a good modality to evaluate maxillofacial trauma. CBCT has been shown to have superior diagnostic quality in comparison with dental radiographs for the evaluation of periodontal disease in brachycephalic breed dogs [16]. Using CBCT has also been shown to be very effective in evaluating patients for furcation exposure and intrabony defects [17]. Compared to intraoral radiographs, CBCT has been shown to be effective in the detection of apical lucencies as well, making it an excellent imaging modality for cases with suspected endodontic disease [18].

Magnetic Resonance Imaging

MRI is a diagnostic modality that uses magnetic fields and radio waves to create an image [12] (Figure 1.18). An MRI utilizes a high and low magnetic field and a coil to detect the frequency and signal created by changes in the cellular composition within an organ to produce an image which is viewed on a computer. Tissues within the body absorb and release energy in different ways and levels [12]. Water produces a high MR signal, while bone and collagenous tissues produce a low MR signal [12]. An MRI produces exceptional contrast and differentiation of the soft tissues of the body. This type of imaging modality does not use ionizing radiation.

When using this imaging modality, care needs to be taken to identify patients or operators who have ferromagnetic implants, foreign bodies, or other metallic devices or objects on or within their bodies. Examples of such items include bullets, vascular staples, shrapnel, or other objects containing metal. These items may travel through soft and hard tissues leading to additional injury. Items may also become potential projectiles within the MRI unit or the room due to the intense magnetic field that is created during the use of this imaging modality (Figure 1.19). More information regarding the use of MRI can be found in Chapter 10.

Definitions Relating to Imaging Modalities

Sagittal Plane

Sagittal plane divides the area of interest in a vertical plane. A sagittal plane divides the area into left and right halves. For veterinary patients, this is in a lengthwise plane from the tip of the nose to the tip of the tail from the right side to the left side (Figure 1.20). This plane is also called vertical plane parallel to the median plane.

Transverse Plane

Transverse plane divides the area of interest in a horizontal plane. A transverse plane divides the area into a top and bottom half for human patients. For veterinary patients,

Figure 1.18 Magnetic resonance imaging unit.

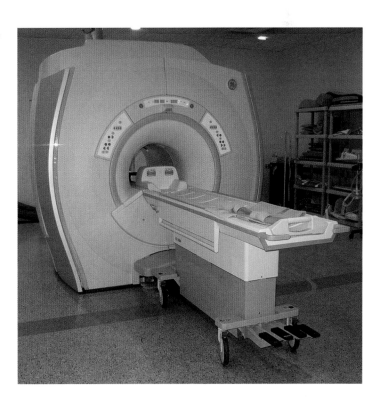

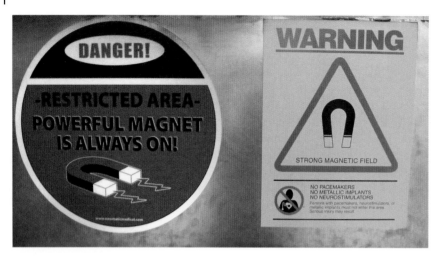

Figure 1.19 Image depicts warnings frequently found outside of a magnetic resonance imaging unit. Metallic objects can become projectiles within the unit due to the magnetic field created by this imaging modality.

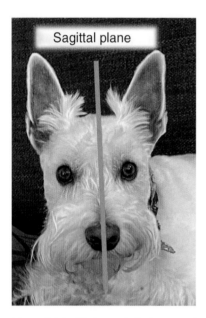

Figure 1.20 Photograph depicts a sagittal plane. A sagittal plane divides the area of interest into right and left halves.

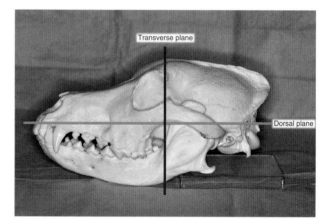

Figure 1.21 Photograph depicts the transverse and dorsal planes. A transverse plane divides the area of interest into a top and bottom half. A dorsal plane divides the area of interest parallel to the spine.

this is in a plane from the tip of the nose to the tip of the tail from the front to the back, like slicing a loaf of bread lengthwise (Figure 1.21). This plane is also called the axial plane.

Dorsal Plane

Dorsal plane divides the area of interest parallel to the spine. A dorsal plane divides the area parallel with the long axis of the body. This divides the body from the top of the skull lengthwise to the bottom of the toes, from top to bottom (see Figure 1.21). This plane is perpendicular to the sagittal and the transverse planes.

Computed Tomography Window Width and Window Level

CT images can be viewed by standard settings set by the computer program. How a study is viewed is dependent on the information collected from the CT unit and how it is windowed. Windowing is the process by which the different shades of gray are contrast-enhanced to produce an image. The different windows change the appearance of an image to highlight specific areas within the chosen location to feature particular structures. Proper windowing of a CT study can significantly impact the ability of a clinician to interpret the normal anatomy as well as any pathology that may be present. Therefore, prior to interpretation, the most appropriate window for the area of interest should be chosen.

Window Width

Window width measures the range of CT numbers. A CT number is directly related to the intensity of an X-ray beam as it travels through hard and soft tissues and its grayscale value. A grayscale value is assigned based on its brightness of a three-dimensional element or voxel, relative to water [19]. The range of CT numbers is displayed on the image as it is being interpreted. CT numbers are measured in Hounsfield units (HU). Images can be displayed with HU on a scale from −1000 to +3000 HU, for over 4000 different shades of gray [20] (Table 1.2). The HU value is based on the density of a tissue to absorb radiation from the X-ray beam. The scale is arbitrarily based on the premise that water is defined as being zero HU and air is defined as −1000 HU [21]. The higher the HU value, the denser the area. A HU that falls below the lowest value of the window width will show as black, and any value of window width above the highest HU value on the image will show white [19]. The human eye can only discern about 40 different shades of gray [21]; thus, using the most appropriate window for viewing the images is of utmost importance.

The wider the window width, the more CT numbers will be displayed causing the transition from dark to light to occur over a larger transitional field. As the window width increases, a larger change in the density of the tissues will be needed to alter the change in HU or shade of gray. This will decrease the contrast of an image, and structures will be more likely to be viewed similarly, despite having different densities. Therefore, a larger window width will cause the interpreter to have difficulty discerning the different attenuations between similar density tissues, such as soft tissue.

A wide window width, e.g. >+1500, is better for evaluating areas with significantly different attenuating values, such as the lungs where air-filled structures are closely associated with fluid or blood-filled structures. A wide window width is also an excellent choice for evaluating bone.

A narrow window width, e.g. <+800 HU, is excellent when evaluating areas of similar attenuation, such as soft tissues. Decreasing the window width will create a greater increase in the contrast of an area. As the window width decreases, a significantly smaller change in a tissue's density will result in a change in the grayscale color on the image. This narrowing of the window width will allow similarly dense structures to have more obvious shades of white to gray to black assigned to allow the interpreter to visualize subtle differences in similarly dense tissues.

Table 1.2 Illustration of the grayscale value assigned to common gas and material densities related to their Hounsfield units assigned based on the gas or tissue's ability to absorb radiation.

Tissue type	Hounsfield unit
Bone	+400 to +1000 or higher
Soft tissue	+40 to +80
Water	0
Fat	−60 to −100
Lung	−400 to −600
Air	−1000

Window Level

The window level is often referred to as the window center. The window level is related to the midpoint of the CT numbers displayed on the image. It refers to the brightness and darkness of an image. Decreasing a window level will cause the image to be brighter and increasing the window level will cause the image to be darker (Figure 1.22). As the window level is increased, a higher HU value will be needed for a tissue density to be brighter or white, whereas decreasing the window level will require less HU for a tissue density to be displayed as bright or white.

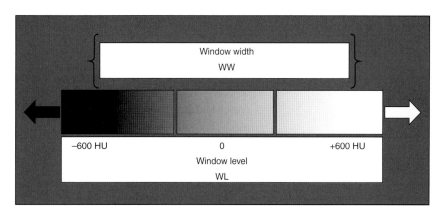

Figure 1.22 Illustration of window width and window level. The window width determines the shades of gray or Hounsfield units of an image. The window level is related to the midpoint of the shades of gray. Window level refers to the brightness and darkness of an image.

Other Common Viewing Windows

Bone Window

A bone window is best used to view bone in detail and when trying to differentiate from the cortex and the medulla. It is usually set at a window width of 2000–3000 HU and a window level of around 1000 HU. A bone window helps to visualize subtle details within the bone [22]. Soft tissue structure detail is much less obvious due to the lack of density in these tissues [22]; therefore, the other modality windows should be considered when evaluating soft tissue structures. Evaluation of fine details such as mineralized areas or bony structures is better visualized with a bone window [22].

Soft Tissue Window

A soft tissue window is used to evaluate most organs. It is usually set at a window width of around 200–400 HU and a window level of 20–60 HU. However, it is not a good window for evaluating lung parenchyma, due to the density of this tissue being air-filled.

Radiation Safety

Radiation Safety Apparel

It has been found through the advancement of diagnostic imaging modalities that there is indeed some risk associated with exposing patients to ionizing radiation and intravenous contrast agents [23]. The development of radiation safety procedures began in the 1930s with the invention of lead aprons (Figure 1.23) and lead gloves [23] (Figure 1.24). In the years and decades that followed, advancement and production of thyroid shields (Figure 1.25) and leaded protective eyewear (Figure 1.26) have attempted to make using these radiation imaging modalities safer to the radiology technician [23].

Collimation

Utilizing columniation instruments to narrow the X-ray beams to reduce scatter radiation and increasing the speed of exposure were found to reduce excessive radiation exposure [23]. An X-ray beam is restricted by the amount of collimation that the radiographic tube head creates. Not focusing the collimation beam on the area of interest only will allow for more radiation to be released and expose the patient to unnecessary radiation. Most dental units have a very narrow beam of radiation released and do not have the ability to be collimated as the beam is already as narrow as possible to create a diagnostic image relating to the film size.

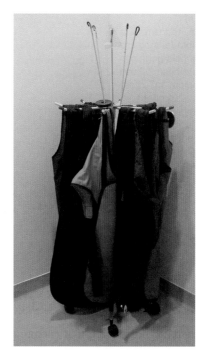

Figure 1.23 Lead aprons can be used to prevent scattered radiation exposure.

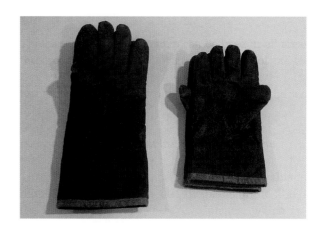

Figure 1.24 Lead gloves can be worn to prevent scattered radiation exposure to the extremities.

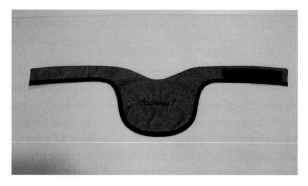

Figure 1.25 Thyroid shields can be worn to prevent scattered radiation exposure.

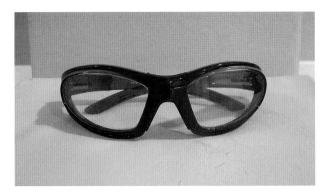

Figure 1.26 Lead glasses can be worn as part of the personal protective equipment to protect the radiology technician's eyes.

As Low As Reasonably Achievable (ALARA)

Exposure to ionizing radiation in any amount could induce side effects of radiation exposure. Minimizing the amount of radiation that a patient or operator is exposed to is imperative to avoid potentially fatal side effects (Figure 1.27). The guiding principle of radiation safety is to act in accordance with the principle of as low as reasonably achievable (ALARA) [24]. This principle is to create an environment in which the radiation exposure is ALARA [24]. It is extremely important to increase the education and awareness of the effects of ionizing radiation to the patient and choose a diagnostic imaging modality that minimizes the amount of radiation exposure to all involved [24].

Time, Distance, and Shielding

There are three basic measures that you can apply to achieve the lowest amount of radiation delivered to the user as well as the patient. These measures include time, distance, and shielding [25].

Time

Minimizing the amount of time that is spent near a radiation source is imperative to help reduce radiation exposure. Time and exposure can be reduced with the use of sedation or anesthesia for better precision in positioning, as well as improved positioning for uncooperative patients. This reduces the need for retakes based on poor positioning. Fortunately, this is not usually an issue in dental radiographic procurement in veterinary patients as sedation or general anesthesia is required to generate the images.

Distance

Maximizing the amount of distance from the radiation source will thereby reduce the dose of radiation received. Distance and dose are inversely related, therefore increasing the distance from the radiation source will reduce the dosage of radiation received. The operator should try to stand at least 6 ft away from the radiographic tube head and at a 90–135° angle from the primary beam [7, 9].

Shielding

Placing something between the radiation source and the object being irradiated will reduce the radiation received by the object. Effective shielding is dependent on the source of radiation. Lead doors, shields, and tabletop barriers are available to help shield the operator from radiation exposure (Figure 1.28a and b).

Radiation Safety Equipment Inspection

Protective Apparel

The reduction in radiation exposure begins with the radiology technician wearing radiation protective equipment. Personal protective equipment such as lead aprons, lead shields, thyroid shields, radiation dosimeter, and lead gloves can be utilized to avoid scattered radiation exposure [7] (Figure 1.29).

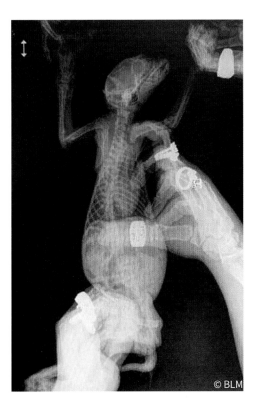

© BLM

Figure 1.27 Image depicts poor radiation safety of the radiology technician. Minimizing the amount of radiation exposure to the patient and the operator is important to avoid potentially fatal side effects.

(a)

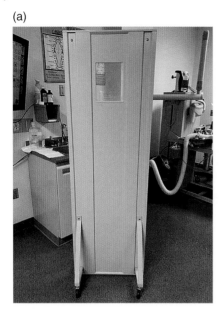

(b)

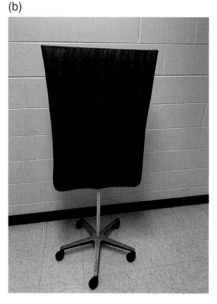

Figure 1.28 (a) Lead doors can be used as protection against radiation exposure. Placing a shield between the radiation source and the radiology technician will help to reduce scatter radiation. This can be used in addition to personal protective equipment. (b) Lead shields can also be used for radiation protection.

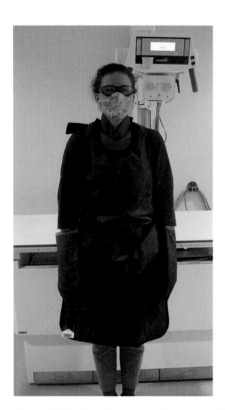

Figure 1.29 Model demonstrating appropriate personal protective equipment: wearing a lead apron, thyroid shield, lead glasses, and lead gloves.

The operator needs to be protected from three sources of radiation: the primary beam, secondary radiation emitted from the patient, and finally leakage of radiation from the machine housing unit or radiographic tube head [7].

Contrary to popular belief, the use of lead shields and aprons is not to protect the patient or the operator from the primary beam of radiation. Their purpose is to prevent scattered radiation exposure. Personal protective equipment used for shielding against radiation exposure should be evaluated at least annually for signs of visible cracks, tears, and areas of wear [11, 26]. Radiation protective equipment can be damaged when stored inappropriately. All protective equipment should be stored properly to prevent cracks in the lead shielding, therefore decreasing its protectiveness [26] (Figure 1.30). Improperly stored equipment can lead to deterioration of the lead-impregnated vinyl [27]. Inspections of the radiation protective equipment are necessary for the health and safety of the radiology technicians as well as the patients, depending on what type of protection is being used [27]. The protective apparel should also be radiographed in any area that appears to have physical damage to reduce unexpected radiation exposure and verify the lead within the apparel is not damaged [26] (Figure 1.31). Monitoring parameters are also available to observe the levels of radiation in a specific area over time or a specific person over time (Figure 1.32a and b).

Care of Radiation Safety Equipment

Radiation protection equipment should be inspected before each use for signs of defects, tears, or creases in the lead. Lead aprons should be properly hung by the shoulders on a rack when not in use and not folded or crumpled on the floor [27]. All equipment should be kept clean and dry, attempting to keep it free of blood and other body fluids as well as away from sources of heat [27]. If the protective equipment becomes soiled, refrain from cleaning with chemicals or putting the equipment in the laundry. It should only be spot-cleaned or hand-washed with mild soap and left to hang dry. If any equipment is found to be defective, it should be removed from service until it can be inspected for safety for continued use.

Radiation Safety Inspection Protocol

A radiation safety inspection protocol should be made for clinics utilizing any form of radiation. An individual or group of individuals should be identified to be responsible for the regular visual and radiographic inspection of all protective equipment. Protocols for conducting safety equipment inventory and inspection of the equipment should be done on a regular basis. Criteria for the replacement of any damaged equipment should be clear. Radiation protection equipment should be supplied for all staff members in appropriate numbers and sizes to fit the needs of all individuals at the clinic with potential exposure to radiation [27]. Individuals utilizing the protective equipment should have a contact person to notify them if there appears to be an issue with the fit or integrity of the equipment [27]. Radiation protective equipment should be marked with a unique identification system to refer to when evaluating

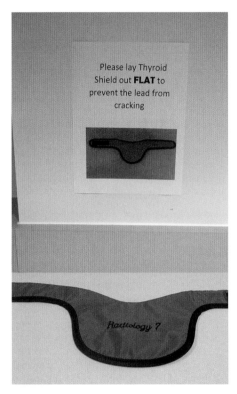

Figure 1.30 Image depicting appropriate storage of thyroid shields to prevent damage to the lead lining.

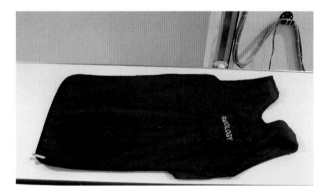

Figure 1.31 Lead aprons should be radiographed to evaluate for any cracks in the lead shielding and to verify there is no unexpected radiation exposure.

(a)

(b)

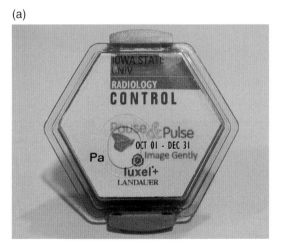
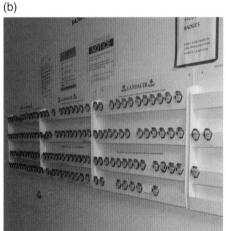

Figure 1.32 (a) Dosimeters are used to assess the amount of radiation for a given area or a specific person. This image depicts a single dosimeter for a given area. (b) Wall of dosimeters of individuals who may be exposed to radiation within a clinic setting.

(a)

(b)

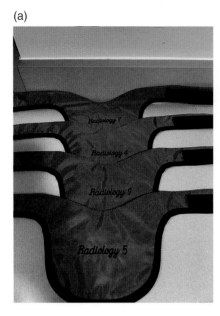 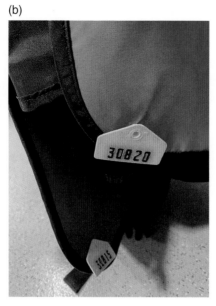

Figure 1.33 (a) Personal protection equipment should be marked with individual identifiers when evaluating the protective equipment for its integrity. For example, unique identifiers can be stitched on the thyroid shields help to identify each shield. (b) A cattle identification marker was used to uniquely identify the lead aprons individually.

the integrity of the equipment [27] (Figure 1.33a and b). Different criteria can be used to identify whether the protective equipment may be defective or have decreased integrity. Some clinics may choose to examine their equipment with radiography or fluoroscopy, while others may only perform the initial visual inspection of the equipment for any obvious defective areas. They are then again evaluated only when suspected to be defective. A written or computerized log of defects and need for replacement should be kept. Further guidance on radiation safety guidelines can be found by contacting the Joint Commission on Accreditation of Healthcare Organizations.

References

1 Roentgen, W.C. (1896). On a new kind of rays. *Nature* 53 (1369): 274–276.

2 Babic, R.R., Babic, G.S., Babic, S.R., and Babic, N.R. (2016). 120 years since the discovery of X-rays. *Med. Pregl.* 69 (9–10): 323–330.

3 Hubar, J.S. (2017). Part one: fundamentals: history: discovery of X-rays. In: *Fundamentals of Oral and Maxillofacial Radiology* (ed. J.S. Hubar), 32–42. New Jersey: Wiley.

4 Haus, A.G. and Cullinan, J.E. (1989). Screen film processing systems for medical radiography: a historical review. *RadioGraphics* 9 (6): 1203–1224.

5 Mattoon, J.S. (2006). Digital radiography. *Vet. Comp. Orthop. Traumatol.* 19: 123–132.

6 Verstraete, F.J., Kass, P.H., and Terpak, C.H. (1998). Diagnostic value of full mouth radiography in dogs. *Am. J. Vet. Res.* 59: 686–691.

7 Bellows, J., Berg, M.L., Dennis, S. et al. (2019). 2019 AAHA dental care guidelines for dogs and cats. *J. Am. Anim. Hosp. Assoc.* 55: 49–69.

8 Owens, J.M. and Biery, D.N. (1999). Principles of radiographic interpretation. In: *Radiographic Interpretation for the Small Animal Clinician*, 9–13. Baltimore: Williams & Wilkins.

9 Roy, C.G. (2018). Canine and feline dental radiographic technique. In: *Textbook of Veterinary Diagnostic Radiology*, 7e (ed. D.E. Thrall), 39–57. St. Louis: Elsevier.

10 Robertson, I.D. and Thrall, D.E. (2018). Digital radiographic imaging. In: *Textbook of Veterinary Diagnostic Radiology*, 7e (ed. D.E. Thrall), 23–38. St. Louis: Elsevier.

11 Thrall, D.E. and Widmer, W.R. (1998). Radiation physics, radiation protection, and darkroom theory. In: *Textbook of Veterinary Diagnostic Radiology*, 3e (ed. D.E. Thrall), 1–19. Philadelphia: W.B. Saunders.

12 Owens, J.M. and Biery, D.N. (1999). The scope of diagnostic imaging in small animal practice. In: *Radiographic Interpretation for the Small Animal Clinician*, 1–8. Baltimore: Williams & Wilkins.

13 Alshipli, M. and Kabir, N.A. (2017). Effect of slice thickness on image noise and diagnostic content of single-source-dual energy computed tomography. *J. Phys. Conf. Ser.* 851 (1): 1–6. https://doi.org/10.1088/1742-6596/851/1/012005.

14 Rogella, P., Kloeters, C., and Hein, P.A. (2009). CT technology overview: 64-slice and beyond. *Radiol. Clin. N. Am.* 47: 1–11. https://doi.org/10.1016/j.rcl.2008.10.004.

15 Soukup, J.S., Drees, R., Koenig, L.J. et al. (2015). Comparison of the diagnostic image quality of the canine maxillary dentoalveolar structures obtained by cone beam computed tomography and 64-multidetector row computed tomography. *J. Vet. Dent.* 32 (2): 80–86.

16 Doring, S., Arzi, B., Kass, P.H., and Verstraete, F.J. (2018). Evaluation of the diagnostic yield of dental radiography and cone-beam computed tomography for the identification of dental disorders in small to medium sized brachycephalic dogs. *Am. J. Vet. Res.* 79: 62–72.

17 Eshragi, V.T., Malloy, K.A., and Tahmasbi, M. (2019). Role of cone-beam computed tomography in the management of periodontal disease. *Dent. J.* 7 (57): 1–9. https://doi.org/10.3390/dj7020057.

18 de Paula-Silva, F.W.G., Santamaria, M., Leonardo, M.R. et al. (2009). Cone-beam computerized tomographic, radiographic, and histologic evaluation of periapical repair in dogs' post-endodontic treatment. *Oral Surg. Oral Med. Oral Pathol. Oral Radiol. Endod.* 108: 796–805.

19 Barnes, J.E. (1992). Characteristics and control of contrast in CT. *RadioGraphics* 12: 825–837.

20 d'Anjou, M.A. (2018). Principles of computed tomography and magnetic resonance imaging. In: *Textbook of Veterinary Diagnostic Radiology*, 7e (ed. D.E. Thrall), 71–95. St. Louis: Elsevier.

21 Frederiksen, N.L., White, S.C., and Pharoah, M.J. (2009). Advanced imaging. In: *Oral Radiology Principles and Interpretation*, 6e (ed. S.C. White and M.J. Pharoah), 207–224. St. Louis: Elsevier.

22 Xue, Z., Antani, S., Long, L.R. et al. (2012). Window classification of brain CT images in biomedical articles. In: *AMIA Annual Symposium Proceedings*, 1023–1029. National Library of Medicine, National Center for Biotechnology Information Epub 3 November 2012.

23 Scatliff, J.H. and Morris, P.J. (2014). From rontgen to magnetic resonance imaging: the history of medical imaging. *N. C. Med. J.* 75 (2): 111–113.

24 Atci, I.B., Yilmaz, H., Antar, V. et al. (2017). What do we know about ALARA? Is our knowledge sufficient about radiation safety? *J. Neurosurg.* 61: 597–602.

25 Cheon, B.K., Kim, C.L., Kim, K.R. et al. (2018). Radiation safety: a focus on lead aprons and thyroid shields in interventional pain management. *Korean J. Pain* 31 (4): 244–252.

26 Matsuda, M. and Suzuki, T. (2016). Evaluation of lead aprons and their maintenance and management at our hospital. *J. Anesth.* 30: 518–521.

27 Michel, R. and Zorn, M.J. (2002). Implementation of an X-ray radiation protective equipment inspection program. *Health Phys.* 82 (2 Suppl): 51–53.

2

Digital Dental Radiographic Positioning and Image Labeling

Brenda L. Mulherin[1] and Chad Lothamer[2]

[1] *Lloyd Veterinary Medical Center, Iowa State University College of Veterinary Medicine, Ames, IA, USA*
[2] *College of Veterinary Medicine, University of Tennessee, Knoxville, TN, USA*

CONTENTS

Benefits to Proper Positioning

The ability to properly interpret dental radiographs is based on the interpreter's personal knowledge of normal and abnormal anatomy and the diagnostic quality of the image. An image of high quality will enable the viewer to maximally assess the area being viewed by providing as close of a representation of the actual anatomy as possible. Proper positioning will create an image with minimal distortion of the anatomical targets. An understanding of proper radiographic image positioning techniques and the ability to correctly implement the techniques into practice will maximize the information gathered on the images produced. This will limit the number of radiographs required to assess an area, resulting in less time under anesthesia for the patient and less radiation exposure to the patient and the positioner. As with any skill, time and practice are required to become adept at radiographic positioning of the oral cavity.

Practicing Techniques

Dental radiographs are acquired using similar equipment as other diagnostic imaging modalities. Practicing the acquisition of diagnostic intraoral radiographs should be performed on cadaveric specimens or skulls [1]. This will help to minimize the stress on the radiographer and the patient [1]. An anesthetized patient adds a level of stress as the patient needs to be monitored while the radiographer is learning a new technique [1]. Practicing techniques on a model or skull will reduce the anxiety of learning something new. The radiographer will feel more comfortable once they learn the technique on a model and then transfer those skills to a live patient. When learning radiographic techniques, the ability to learn how to change an image after an error has been made can help the radiographer understand how to avoid the error on future images. Taking the time to understand positioning techniques on a model will help the technician acquire diagnostic images on the live patient more effectively and efficiently.

Use of Position Indicating Device (PID)

X-rays are produced by a generator. The X-rays are directed at a specific area of anatomy with the use of a collimator or position indicating device (PID) [2]. On the other side of an anatomic target is either a film, sensor, or phosphor plate that is exposed to the X-rays after it has passed through the target area [2]. The tissues of the anatomic target will block some of the X-rays from being transmitted to the sensor creating different levels of exposure due to the different densities of an object. This in effect creates a shadow of the anatomic target. With standard radiographs, the area of interest is placed parallel to the sensor. The X-ray generator and PID are positioned so that the X-rays will hit the target and the sensor in a perpendicular orientation. This positioning creates an image with minimal distortion from the actual size and shape of the target anatomy. Dental radiography places the sensor so that each quadrant of the oral cavity and each individual tooth can be viewed radiographically without superimposition from the contralateral quadrant or tooth. The anatomy of the mouth makes acquisition of images more difficult than standard radiographs as positioning of the sensor parallel to the anatomic target is not always possible. Multiple views may be necessary to acquire the diagnostic information to assess if disease is present within the mouth. If there is an area that appears to have radiographic evidence of disease, multiple views of that area may need to be taken. Therefore, a comprehension of the different positioning techniques that can be employed to accurately image the teeth is necessary. For the average canine patient, 12–18 images may be needed to acquire a full-mouth radiographic series [3]. The variation in number is dependent on the size of the patient and the size of the sensor. A Size 2 sensor will not accommodate as many teeth as a Size 4 sensor. For a full-mouth radiographic series for a feline patient, 8–10 images may be needed [3]. Several techniques have been developed for different areas of the mouth to ensure a high-quality image can be obtained despite the limitations of sensor placement due to anatomical structures. These techniques include parallel techniques, bisecting angle techniques, and extraoral techniques [2, 4, 5].

Positioning Techniques

Patient Positioning

Ideally each patient should be positioned the same way when a diagnostic image is to be obtained. This will help build the muscle memory of the operator. It will also allow the radiographer to use an already calculated bisecting angle and apply it to the different-sized patients on the table. Before the PID or sensor is placed near the oral cavity to obtain an image, the patient needs to be positioned appropriately to facilitate access to the desired anatomical targets. The most frequent options are to position the patient in sternal, dorsal, or left and right lateral recumbencies (Figure 2.1a–c). Factors such as personal preference and final position for cleaning and treatment will play a role in the way the person obtaining the radiographs chooses to position the patient. Regardless of preference, the target area to be radiographed needs to be accessible to place the sensor in the mouth on the palatal/lingual side of the tooth for intraoral radiographs with the PID on the facial side of the tooth, outside of the oral cavity. Therefore, the target area needs to be assessable to the radiographic generator. For example, radiographic imaging of the maxilla is easiest when the patient is in sternal or lateral recumbency. If a maxillary tooth needs to be radiographed while the patient is in dorsal recumbency, the head will need to be tilted and potentially elevated from the table so that the table does not prevent appropriate positioning of the PID (Figure 2.2). For mandibular radiographs, the patient can be in dorsal or lateral recumbency (Figure 2.3).

(a)   (b)   (c)

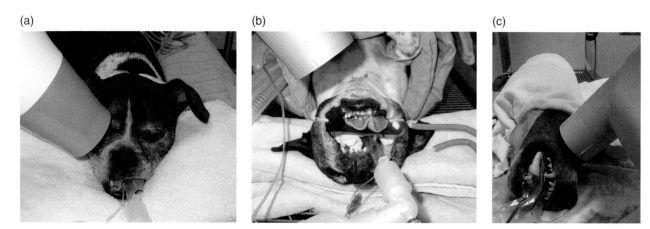

Figure 2.1   (a) Canine patient in STERNAL recumbency with a radiographic plate/sensor placed intraorally and the PID (generator) positioned for the bisecting angle technique to acquire diagnostic images of the right maxillary teeth. (b) Canine patient in DORSAL recumbency with a radiographic plate/sensor placed intraorally and the PID (generator) positioned for the bisecting angle technique to acquire diagnostic images of the left mandibular premolar teeth. (c) Canine patient in LATERAL recumbency with a radiographic plate/sensor placed intraorally and the PID (generator) positioned for the bisecting angle technique to acquire diagnostic images of the right maxillary arcade.

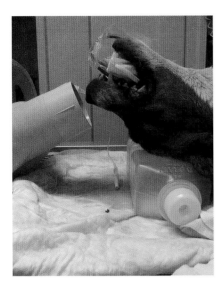

Figure 2.2 Image depicting a canine patient positioned in dorsal recumbency with the head of the patient elevated from the table. This positioning allows the target area to be exposed to the PID. The patient can remain in dorsal recumbency for the entire procedure if the head can be elevated from the table. Elevation of the head allows for radiographic procurement of the right and left maxillary arcades. If the head cannot be elevated from the table when the patient is positioned in dorsal recumbency, acquiring diagnostic images of the maxillary arcade is difficult, if not impossible. This is because the table blocks the ability of the PID to penetrate the desired teeth. The patient's head should not remain elevated during the entire procedure, only during diagnostic image procurement of the right and left maxillary arcades.

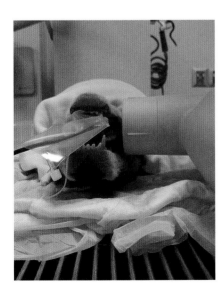

Figure 2.3 Image depicts positioning of a canine patient for radiographic procurement of the mandibular teeth. The patient is in dorsal recumbency. The head does not need to be elevated from the table for acquiring diagnostic images of the mandibular teeth in canine or feline patients when the patient is in dorsal or lateral recumbency.

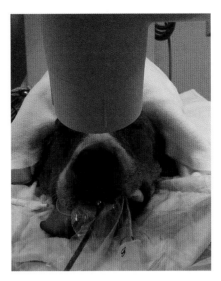

Figure 2.4 Image depicts a Size 2 radiographic sensor in the oral cavity of a dog in sternal recumbency positioned for radiographic images of the maxillary incisors.

Sternal Recumbency

The benefit of using sternal recumbency for radiographic imaging of the maxilla and dorsal recumbency for imaging of the mandible is the conceptualization of the bisecting angle technique. The bisecting angle technique is generally easier to understand and put into practice for someone with less experience or comfort when patients are positioned in dorsal or sternal recumbency. This is due to the surface of the sensor being parallel to the floor, while the long axis of the tooth is in a vertical orientation, and the PID and generator are oriented above the patient (Figure 2.4). The patient is often already in sternal recumbency when anesthesia is initiated, making this an opportune time to acquire maxillary radiographs of both the left and right sides (Figure 2.5a and b). Once the maxilla has been radiographed, the patient can be put into dorsal recumbency and the mandibular teeth can be radiographed for both the left and right sides (Figure 2.6a and b).

Dorsal Recumbency

Dorsal recumbency positioning is especially useful when ultrasonic scaling, hand scaling, polishing, and oral surgery treatments are necessary. When the patient is in dorsal recumbency, this positioning minimizes the number of times the patient needs to be moved for other procedures or diagnostics. It allows the anesthetic equipment to be placed with minimal need for disconnecting and reconnecting the anesthetic monitoring devices.

Lateral Recumbency

When using lateral recumbency positioning for intraoral radiographs, the right maxillary arcade and the right mandibular arcade are radiographed when the patient is in left

(a)

(b)

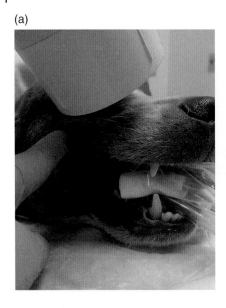
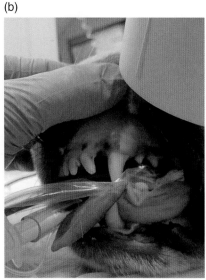

Figure 2.5 (a) Image depicts a Size 2 radiographic sensor in the oral cavity of a dog in sternal recumbency positioned for radiographic images of the right maxillary arcade. (b) Image depicts a Size 2 radiographic sensor in the oral cavity of a dog in sternal recumbency positioned for radiographic images of the left maxillary arcade.

(a)

(b)

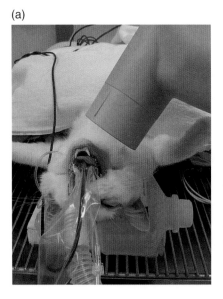
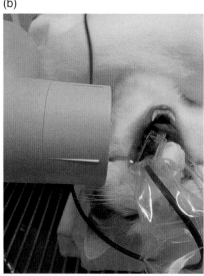

Figure 2.6 (a) Image depicts a Size 2 radiographic sensor in the oral cavity of a cat in dorsal recumbency positioned for radiographic images of the right mandibular arcade. (b) Image depicts a Size 2 radiographic sensor in the oral cavity of a cat in dorsal recumbency positioned for radiographic images of the left mandibular arcade.

lateral recumbency, and the left arcades are radiographed with the patient in right lateral recumbency (Figure 2.7a and b). When obtaining radiographs in lateral recumbency, the patient's hard palate should be perpendicular to the table. The benefit of this patient positioning is that in practices without oral suction or an alternative way to keep water out of the oropharynx, lateral recumbency positioning is usually the positioning used for ultrasonic and hand scaling, polishing, and any necessary treatments. The disadvantage to lateral recumbency positioning is that the patient will need to be repositioned to radiographically acquire images or perform treatments on the contralateral side.

There is no singular positioning technique that will work for all patients. A combination of techniques can be used.

In general, it is ideal to minimize movement of the patient to decrease the chances of iatrogenic tracheal injury and anesthesia complications [6]. Positioning props may be needed to help stabilize the head while images are being acquired. Props such as rolled towels, blankets, and water bottles are commonly used to help position the head for radiographic procurement (Figure 2.8a and b).

See Table 2.1 for patient positioning.

Sensor/Phosphor Plate/Film Placement

To obtain a radiograph, the X-rays are generated and aimed with a positioning indicating device (PID) at a target object and toward a device that will absorb the X-rays which are converted into a diagnostic image. The device may either

Figure 2.7 (a) Image depicts a Size 2 radiographic sensor in the oral cavity of a dog in right lateral recumbency positioned for radiographic imaging of the left maxillary arcade. (b) Image depicts a Size 2 radiographic sensor in the oral cavity of a dog in left lateral recumbency positioned for radiographic imaging of the right maxillary arcade.

(a)

(b)

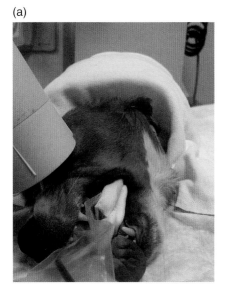
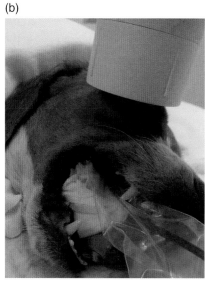

Figure 2.8 (a) Image depicts a canine patient positioned in dorsal recumbency for dental radiographic images of the maxillary incisor teeth. A positioning prop (empty sterile saline bottle) was utilized for adequate accessibility of the PID to the targeted area of interest. (b) Image depicts a feline patient positioned in lateral recumbency with the head elevated from the table with a positioning prop (empty sterile saline bottle) placed for adequate accessibility of the PID to the targeted area of interest, in this case the left maxillary arcade.

(a)

(b)

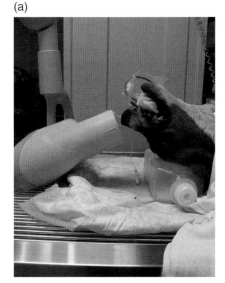
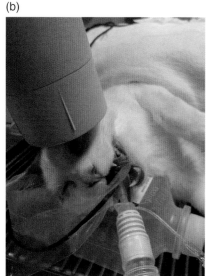

be a standard film for traditionally developed radiographs, a sensor for a DR system (Figure 2.9a), or a phosphor plate for a CR system [2, 7] (Figure 2.9b) (see Chapter 1, for more information regarding the different systems). For simplicity, we will refer to any of these options as a sensor for the remainder of the text.

Basic Positioning of Sensor

To obtain a high-quality radiograph, proper placement of the sensor is just as important as positioning of the PID in relation to the target area being imaged. When utilizing an intraoral technique, all techniques position the sensor within the oral cavity. Make sure that the correct side of the sensor or the portion of the sensor that absorbs

the X-rays is facing the target object and the PID (Figure 2.10a and b). For the DR sensor, the correct surface of the sensor is the flat surface. This portion of the sensor should be positioned so that the flat surface is facing the target area. The correct surface has the associated cord connecting into the back of the sensor on the side away from the target area. For film there will be a convex dot in the corner of the film and an indicator on the outside packaging. For the phosphor plates, there is usually a white or blue surface of the plate that is to be radiographed, compared to the black surface on the opposite side which is not to be radiographed. These plates generally display language indicating which side is the correct side to expose.

Table 2.1 Patient positioning.

Position	Pros	Cons	Image
Sternal recumbency	• Maxilla easily accessible • Bisecting angle easier to visualize	• Access to the mandible is difficult, may need to elevate the head from the table	
Dorsal recumbency	• Mandible easily accessible • Bisecting angle easier to visualize • Cleaning and necessary treatments can be performed on any arcade with the patient in this positioning • Reduced need for readjustment of anesthetic monitoring devices	• Access to the maxilla is difficult, may need to elevate head from the table • Need to have suction available during the procedure to prevent water accumulation within the oropharynx	
Left or right lateral recumbency	• Maxilla and mandible of one side are accessible • Cleaning and necessary treatment can be performed on the accessible side	• Need to reposition patient for acquiring images of the other side • Harder to visualize the bisecting angle	

The table describes the pros and cons of positioning the patient in either sternal, dorsal, or lateral recumbencies. Sternal recumbency is where the patient is positioned with its sternum contacting the table. Dorsal recumbency is where the patient is positioned with its back contacting the table. Lateral recumbency is where the patient is lying with either its right or left side contacting the table.

Figure 2.9 (a) Image depicts a Size 2 DR (direct digital radiography) sensor. (b) Image of Sizes 0, 2, and 4 CR (computed radiography) phosphor plates. Size 0 plates are commonly used for exotic species as well as small dogs and cats. The Size 2 sensor is the most universal plate as it can be used in both dogs and cats to acquire most images. The Size 4 plate is used in larger canine patients or to acquire diagnostic images of larger teeth. For example, the maxillary and mandibular canine teeth and mandibular first molar teeth. The Size 4 plate has the surface area to accommodate the crown and root of these larger teeth to allow for more efficient diagnostic interpretation. The Size 4 plate can also accommodate the acquisition of more teeth on a singular image than the Size 2 plate.

(a)

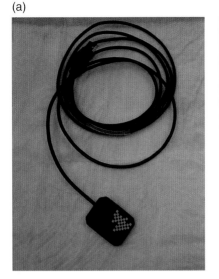

(b)

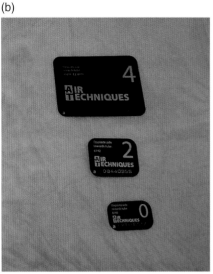

Figure 2.10 (a) Image of the back side of a Size 2 sensor from a DR system. The back side of the sensor generally has a small protuberance where the DR cord connects the sensor to the computer.
(b) Radiographic image of the back side of a Size 2 sensor from a DR system. The digital image that is created does not have any diagnostic information concerning the patient. The image created is a digitized representation of the contents of the sensor itself.

(a)

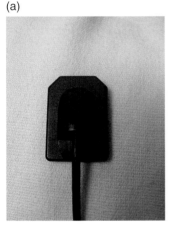

(b)

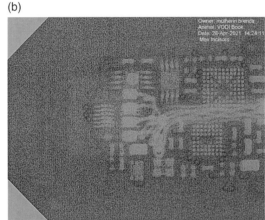

Eliminating Unused Film Space

Radiographs are in essence, a shadow that is cast by an object onto a sensor from the generated beam of radiation. When placing the sensor, it is ideal to have the sensor as close as possible to the target object [8]. This will minimize distortion of the size and shape of the targeted object in the image [8]. To capture as much of the area of interest as possible on the sensor, position the sensor so that the cusp of the desired tooth/teeth is only a few millimeters from the edge of the sensor (Figure 2.11). This will eliminate any unused space on the sensor, commonly referred to as dead space. If there is a single target, such as one tooth, position the sensor so that the radiograph created has the target in the center of the sensor.

Visualization of the Crown and Space Apical to Root

Ideally a minimum of 2–4 mm of tissue should be visible around the desired tooth [3, 9]. Positioning that allows for

a minimum of 2–4 mm of space apical to the root apex will allow for the periodontal structures to be accurately evaluated. When using a Size 2 sensor for imaging larger teeth, such as the canine tooth in a German Shepherd Dog, multiple radiographs will need to be obtained to be able to evaluate the crown, body, and root of the tooth as well as the surrounding periapical tissue (Figure 2.12a–c). The images will then need to be assimilated for diagnostic interpretation. If there is a large amount of unused (black) space around the crowns of the teeth on the sensor, the apex of the tooth root is not visualized, or if there is not enough periapical tissue visible, the image can be altered by positioning the sensor deeper into the mouth while the PID potentially stays in the same position (Figure 2.13). Opposite positioning of the sensor can be elected if there is not enough crown visible on the image or if teeth from the contralateral arcade are visible on the radiograph. In both situations, the sensor placement can be adjusted so that it

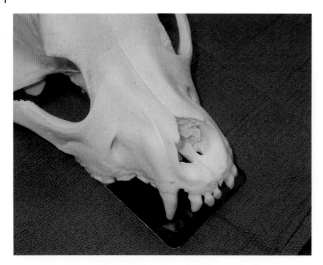

Figure 2.11 Correct positioning of the Size 4 CR plate for a maxillary canine tooth to minimize dead space on the radiograph while capturing all the canine tooth within the image. Using this plate positioning and size of plate will maximize the diagnostic information acquired.

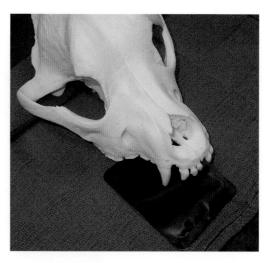

Figure 2.13 Incorrect positioning of the Size 4 CR plate for a maxillary canine tooth. Positioning the plate in this manner will not acquire a diagnostic image. This plate positioning will not show the entire tooth structure of the canine tooth as only a small amount of the film is positioned within the oral cavity. It will include a significant amount of dead space and display minimal diagnostic information as most of the film is positioned outside of the oral cavity.

(a) (b) (c)

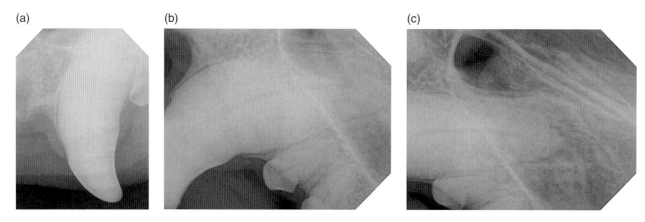

Figure 2.12 (a) Three images may be necessary to evaluate the entire canine tooth of a large breed dog. Radiographic image of the crown of the left maxillary canine tooth (204) in a large dog. (b) Radiographic image of the body of the left maxillary canine tooth (204) in a large dog. (c) Radiographic image of the root and periapical area of the left maxillary canine tooth (204) in a large dog.

is positioned either further outside of the oral cavity or further inside the oral cavity while the PID remains static. For mesial to distal adjustments of the target tooth within the image, the targeted tooth will move in the opposite direction that the sensor is moved. With the PID static, if the sensor is moved more mesial, then the target will move distal in the new image, and vice versa (Figure 2.14a–d).

Intraoral Parallel Technique

Ideal Radiographic Technique

The parallel technique for radiographic imaging of the oral cavity is similar to techniques used to acquire diagnostic images of most other areas of the body [4, 5, 8, 10]. The sensor is placed parallel to the target and the PID is positioned so that X-rays will hit both the target and the sensor in a perpendicular orientation [4, 5, 8, 10] (Figure 2.15a and b). This technique can only be achieved when acquiring diagnostic images of the mandibular molars and caudal mandibular premolars in most canine and feline patients. This technique is the preferred method as it allows for image acquisition with minimal distortion of the targeted area. The parallel technique is used when there are no hard tissues, such as the hard palate or mandibular symphysis, which will inhibit sensor placement.

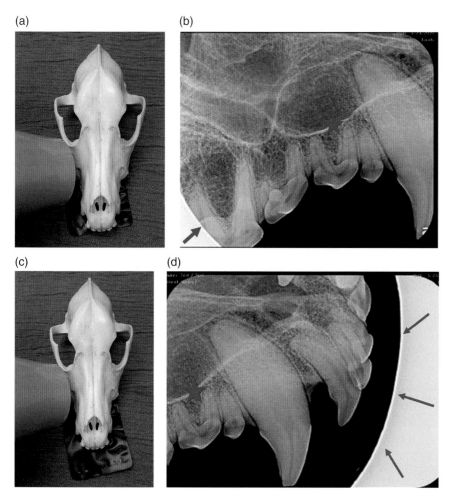

Figure 2.14 (a) Radiographic positioning using a Size 4 CR plate utilizing the bisecting angle technique for acquiring radiographic images of the right maxillary premolar teeth in a dog. (b) Radiographic image of the right maxillary premolar teeth utilizing the bisecting angle technique and a Size 4 CR sensor. Note the position of the right maxillary 2nd premolar (red star), and note the radiographic artifact of cone cutting (arrow). The radiographic image contains some information regarding the right maxillary canine tooth, 1st, 2nd, 3rd, and 4th premolars teeth (104–108). The image is not completely diagnostic for the right maxillary canine tooth (104) or the right maxillary 4th premolar tooth (108). While there is some diagnostic information provided by this image, other images will be needed for full evaluation of these teeth. (c) Radiographic positioning using a Size 4 CR plate utilizing the bisecting angle technique for acquiring diagnostic images of the right maxillary canine tooth in a dog. The Size 4 CR plate has been positioned more rostral in comparison to its placement in Figure (a). (d) Radiographic image of the right maxilla. Note the position of the right maxillary 2nd premolar tooth (red star). This tooth is now positioned more distally within the radiograph. Also note the radiographic artifact of cone cutting in the rostral aspect of the image (arrows). Radiographic image contains information regarding the right maxillary 3rd incisor, canine, 1st and 2nd premolar teeth (103–106). Due to the close association of the right maxillary 2nd premolar (106) to the edge of the film, an additional radiographic image would be needed for complete evaluation of this tooth. The right maxillary 3rd incisor (103) is superimposed on the right maxillary 2nd incisor (102). An additional radiographic image of the 3rd incisor (103) is also needed for complete evaluation of this tooth.

Placement of Sensor for Parallel Technique

The sensor is placed on the lingual surface of the tooth. Generally, the tongue will help hold the sensor in place, but gauze, foam hair curlers, or other objects can be used to help position the sensor as needed (Figure 2.16). The sensor is ideally placed so that the entire crown and roots of the targeted teeth can be viewed with at least 2–4 mm of surrounding alveolar bone.

Size Matters

Depending on the size of the patient or the size of the sensor, a single radiograph may be able to produce an image that allows for viewing of all of the molars [8]. In larger dogs, several images may be needed to be able to see all of the teeth and surrounding tissues [8]. If a DR Size 2 sensor is being used on large patients, multiple images of the mandibular first molar may be needed to capture the entire tooth and surrounding periapical tissues [8].

(a)

(b)

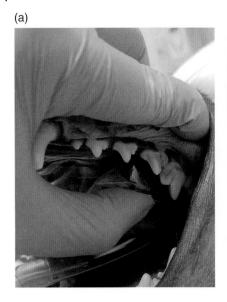
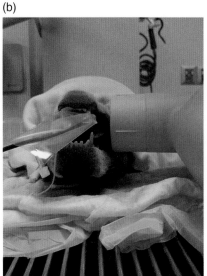

Figure 2.15 (a) Image depicts placement of the radiographic sensor for the parallel radiographic technique for acquiring diagnostic images of the right caudal mandibular premolar and molar teeth. The radiographic sensor is placed parallel to the long axis of the target teeth. (b) Image depicts positioning of the PID perpendicular to the sensor and the long axis of the teeth in this region. This is proper positioning of the PID for the parallel radiographic technique. This technique is utilized for acquiring diagnostic images of the caudal mandibular premolar and molar teeth in the dog and cat.

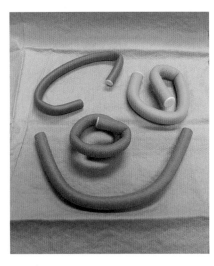

Figure 2.16 Image of a positioning device that can be used to assist in holding a plate or sensor in a proper position. Foam hair curlers can be used to help position the radiographic film and hold it in place.

Alternative Positioning

An alternative positioning technique to accommodate the mandibular first molar tooth on one image is to rotate the sensor vertically within the oral cavity as opposed to horizontally (Figure 2.17a–c). This positioning still maintains the sensor placement parallel to the long axis of the tooth.

Parallel Technique for Cats

In cats, the parallel technique can only be used to image the mandibular first molar and potentially the mandibular 4th premolar (Figure 2.18a and b). The location of the mandibular symphysis will inhibit the placement of the sensor directly parallel with the long axis of the mandibular 3rd

premolar tooth. Depending on the size of the cat, a combination of techniques may be required to image the mandibular molar and premolar teeth.

Intraoral Bisecting Angle Technique

The bisecting angle technique can be used in all areas of the oral cavity to acquire diagnostic images of the teeth. Generally, this technique is used in areas where the parallel technique is not possible due to obstruction of the sensor by anatomic structures within the oral cavity.

Plane of the Tooth, Plane of the Film, and the Angle that Bisects

Three things need to be identified to perform this technique. The plane of the tooth, the plane of the film, and the angle that bisects these two planes, which is the bisecting angle. The PID should be positioned perpendicular to the bisecting angle. The angle should always be bisected inside the animal's mouth. The goal of the bisecting angle technique is to produce an image with as little distortion of the shape and size of the target anatomy as possible.

Shadow Game: Elongation, Foreshortening, and the Bisecting Angle

An analogy to the bisecting angle would be to think about how a shadow looks on a sidewalk during the day [8] (Figure 2.19). At dusk and dawn, when the sun is at a low angle to the sidewalk, a shadow is produced that appears much taller than the target object (Figure 2.20). At midday, when the sun is directly overhead or at a high angle, the shadow produced appears much shorter than the target

(a)

(b)

(c)

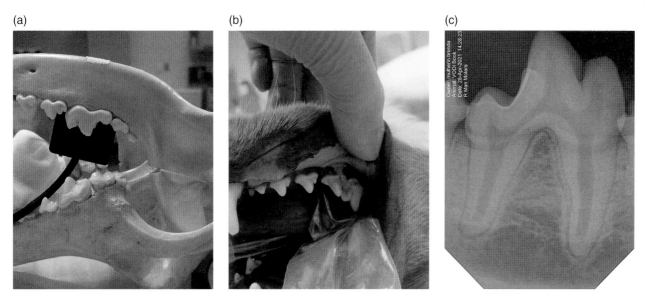

Figure 2.17 (a) Image of an alternative positioning technique of the sensor to acquire a diagnostic image of the right mandibular first molar tooth on the skull of a dog. The sensor is oriented vertically within the oral cavity as opposed to the traditional horizontal orientation. This positioning can accommodate the entire mandibular first molar tooth on one radiographic image, depending on the size of the patient. (b) Image of an alternative positioning technique to acquire a diagnostic image of the right mandibular first molar tooth of a dog. The sensor is oriented vertically within the oral cavity as opposed to the traditional horizontal orientation. This positioning can accommodate the entire mandibular first molar tooth on one radiographic image, depending on the size of the patient. (c) Radiographic image of an alternative positioning technique to acquire a diagnostic image of the right mandibular first molar tooth of a dog (409). The sensor is oriented vertically, allowing the capture of the entire tooth on one radiographic image.

(a)

(b)

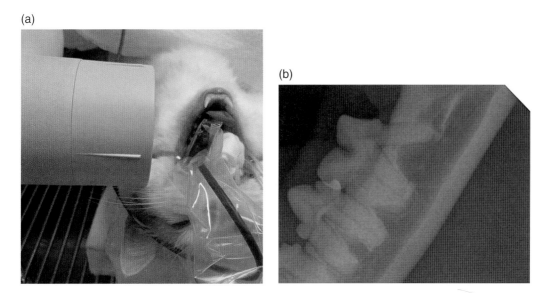

Figure 2.18 (a) Image of the intraoral parallel radiographic technique utilized to acquire diagnostic images of the caudal mandibular premolar and molar teeth of a cat. (b) Radiographic image of the intraoral parallel radiographic technique used to acquire diagnostic images of the caudal mandibular premolar and mandibular molar teeth of the cat (308, 309).

object (Figure 2.21). Between dusk or dawn and midday, the sun will be at an angle to the sidewalk that produces a shadow that is the exact same size as the target object. A shadow without distortion of the size and shape is what the bisecting angle is trying to achieve (Figure 2.22). The bisecting angle technique positions the PID in a position

to the long axis of the tooth and the surface of the sensor to produce an image with minimal distortion.

Axis of the Sensor, the Tooth, and the PID

The bisecting angle technique is first accomplished by placing the sensor in the mouth in a flat or horizontal axis.

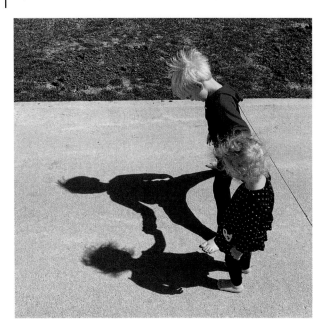

Figure 2.19 Image of the sun creating a shadow on the sidewalk. The sun acts as the PID, the children as the target teeth, and the sidewalk as the sensor.

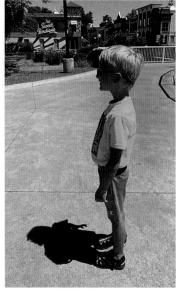

Figure 2.21 Image of the sun creating a shadow on the sidewalk. When the sun or PID is positioned at a high angle to the sidewalk and a target object (the child), the shadow that is produced appears much shorter than the actual height of the object. The image depicts foreshortening of an object.

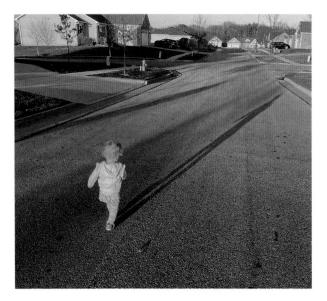

Figure 2.20 Image of the sun creating a shadow on the sidewalk. When the sun or PID is positioned at a low angle to the sidewalk and a target object (the child), the shadow that is produced appears much taller than the actual height of the object. The image depicts elongation of an object.

The vertical axis is the long axis of the target tooth. The long axis of the tooth is created by the line that exists from the point of the crown of the tooth to the tip of the root. The vertical axis of the tooth and the horizontal axis of the sensor create an imaginary angle within the oral cavity (Figure 2.23). This angle is then bisected, or divided,

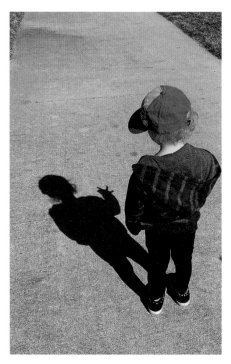

Figure 2.22 Image of the sun creating a shadow on the sidewalk. When the sun or PID is positioned perpendicular to the bisecting angle that is created between the long axis of the object and the sensor, a shadow is created at the same height and size of the target object. A shadow without distortion of the object's shape and size is what the bisecting angle technique depicts.

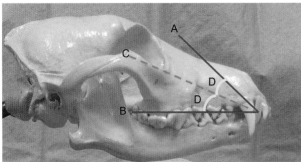

Figure 2.23 Image depicting the application of the bisecting angle technique to the skull of a dog. The bisecting angle technique employs three axes to be applied to the patient to acquire a diagnostic image: the horizontal axis of the sensor, the vertical axis of the tooth and the angle created between these two points, or the bisecting angle. The red axis (A) follows the long axis of the crown and root of the right maxillary canine tooth. The red axis (B) corresponds to the surface of the sensor placed horizontal in the mouth. The blue axis (C) corresponds to the bisected angle between the two planes. The yellow arcs (D) depict an even angle between the bisecting line and both the sensor axis and the axis of the tooth.

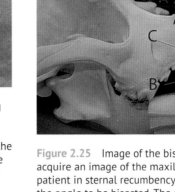

Figure 2.25 Image of the bisecting angle technique applied to acquire an image of the maxillary incisor teeth of a canine patient in sternal recumbency. The red lines are the two axes of the angle to be bisected. The axis (A) follows the long axis of the crowns and roots of the incisor teeth. The axis (B) corresponds to the surface of the plate/sensor. The blue line (C) represents the bisected angle between the long axis of the teeth and the surface of the plate/sensor. The PID is positioned so that the emitted X-rays (green arrow) will be perpendicular to the bisected angle line.

Figure 2.24 Image depicting the application of the bisecting angle technique to the skull of a dog and the positioning of the PID in relation to the bisecting angle. The bisecting angle technique employs three axes to be applied to the patient to acquire a diagnostic image: the horizontal axis of the sensor, the vertical axis of the tooth and the angle created between these two points, or the bisecting angle. The PID is positioned so that radiation generated will transect the bisecting angle in a perpendicular orientation.

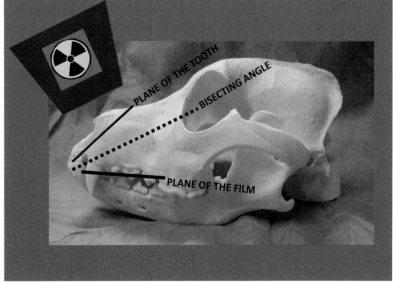

creating the bisecting angle. The PID is then positioned so that the X-rays generated will hit the bisected angle in a perpendicular orientation [4, 5] (Figure 2.24). For the maxillary canine tooth, the sensor is placed in the oral cavity at a 90° angle to the long axis of the canine tooth. This 90° angle is bisected creating an imaginary line at an angle of 45°. The PID is then positioned so that the X-rays will hit perpendicular to this imaginary 45° angle. The bisected angle is viewed from the side of the patient's head for the incisors (Figure 2.25) and from the front of the head for the canines, premolars, and molars (Figure 2.26).

Positioning of the Patient Matters

Knowing the anatomical positioning of roots and their orientation within the oral cavity is important and will help the radiographer correctly calculate the appropriate bisecting angle. Generalizations can be made that will help determine approximate positioning of all the components more efficiently [11]. When the patient is in sternal or dorsal recumbency the long axis of the roots of the canines, premolars, and molars will be in a vertical orientation. If the sensor is placed in a horizontal orientation in relation to the dental arcade, this makes a right angle of 90° between

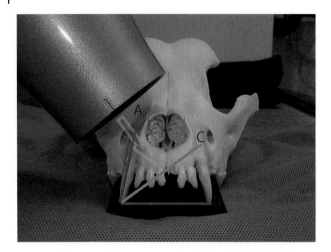

Figure 2.26 Image of the bisecting angle technique applied to the right maxillary canine tooth. The red lines are the two axes of the angle to be bisected. The axis (A) follows the long axis of the crown and root of the right maxillary canine tooth. The axis (B) corresponds to the surface of the plate/sensor. The blue line (C) represents the bisected angle between the long axis of the tooth and the surface of the plate/sensor. The PID is positioned so that the emitted X-rays (green arrow) will be perpendicular to the bisected angle line.

the plane of the sensor and the long axis of the tooth. This creates a bisecting angle of 45° between these two planes. The roots of both the maxillary and mandibular incisors are generally in a less vertical anatomic orientation,

directed palatially or lingually, respectively. This creates a smaller bisecting angle that is closer to 20° from the surface of the sensor if it is in a horizontal plane with respect to the dental arcade.

Anatomical Variations

Anatomical variations will be encountered between the different skull types, breeds, and even individuals. The ability to assess the radiographic positioning and recalculate the bisecting angle if needed based on the first few radiographs will expedite the radiographic procurement process.

Uses of the Bisecting Angle Technique

The bisecting angle is utilized to acquire diagnostic images of the maxillary and mandibular incisors and maxillary premolars and molars in both the dog and the cat. To acquire a diagnostic image of the mandibular 3rd premolar in the cat, the bisecting angle technique is usually required (Figure 2.27a and b). The 1st, 2nd, and 3rd mandibular premolars in the dog also require the use of the bisecting angle.

20–30° Method [12, 13]

Some have described a method that simplifies the bisecting angle technique for procuring diagnostic images of the maxillary and mandibular incisors and canine teeth. The technique is described as placing the sensor in the oral

(a)

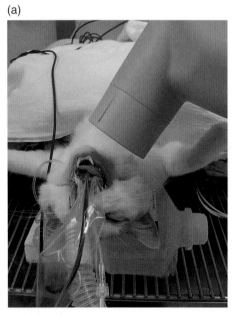

(b)

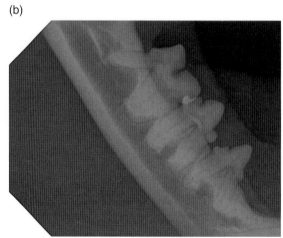

Figure 2.27 (a) Image depicting the bisecting angle technique used for acquiring diagnostic images of the mandibular 3rd premolar in the cat. The PID is positioned perpendicular to the bisecting angle created by the long axis of the tooth and the plane of the sensor or film. (b) Radiographic image of the bisecting angle technique used to acquire diagnostic images of the mandibular 3rd premolar in the cat. Depending on the size of the patient, the bisecting angle technique can be used to acquire diagnostic images of both the mandibular premolar and molar teeth in the cat. The image depicts a diagnostic image of the right mandibular 3rd and 4th premolars and 1st molar teeth (407–409).

cavity in a horizontal plane parallel to the hard palate. The sensor should be placed with the maxillary incisor teeth just inside the edge of the sensor. The PID is first placed directly perpendicular to the sensor on either dorsal or ventral midline of the patient depending on the target area. The PID is then angled 20–30° away from the perpendicular plane so that the beam of radiation is directed caudally [12, 13] (Figure 2.28a–c). This technique is used primarily for the maxillary and mandibular incisor teeth. For the maxillary canine teeth, this technique can also be used. The sensor is placed in the mouth angled slightly toward the targeted canine tooth with the tip of the crown contacting the corner of the sensor, and the remaining portion of the sensor angled toward midline (Figure 2.29a–e). The PID is positioned perpendicular to dorsal surface of the canine tooth. The PID is then angled 20–30° as previously described so that the beam of radiation is directed caudally. An additional 20–30° angulation is made laterally so that the beam of radiation is directed in a caudo-medial direction [12, 13].

Occlusal Radiographic Technique

The occlusal radiographic technique can be used as an adjunctive technique for acquiring additional diagnostic information. It is commonly used for imaging the maxillary teeth and to identify and localize retained tooth roots.

The technique can also be used for gathering additional information for the mandibular teeth [14]. This technique can be used as an adjunct method to verify all tooth roots or root remnants were completely extracted [14]. For this technique, the sensor is placed in the oral cavity in a horizontal plane parallel to the hard palate. The PID is then placed perpendicular to the sensor over the target area (Figure 2.30a–c).

Feline Maxillary Premolar and Molar Teeth

The zygomatic arch of the cat is very pronounced. This anatomical structure routinely becomes an obstacle for acquiring diagnostic images of the feline maxillary premolars and molar. Therefore, additional techniques have been employed to attempt to procure diagnostic images of this area.

Extraoral Technique

The extraoral radiographic technique can be used to acquire diagnostic images of the maxillary premolars and molars in cats when superimposition of the zygomatic arch impedes interpretation of a radiograph obtained with the bisecting angle technique. The extraoral technique requires the sensor to be placed on the table, while the patient's arcade to be imaged is placed on top of the sensor in lateral recumbency [5]. The teeth to be imaged will be closest to

(a)   (b)   (c)

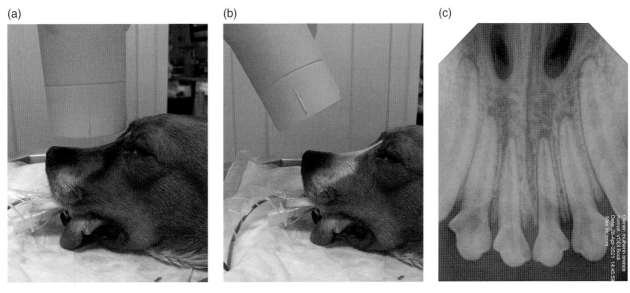

Figure 2.28   (a) Image demonstrating the 20–30° method for acquiring diagnostic images of the maxillary incisor teeth. To utilize this method, the sensor is placed within the oral cavity in a horizontal plane with the occlusal surface of the incisor teeth just inside the edge of the sensor. The PID is then placed directly perpendicular to the sensor. (b) Image demonstrating the 20–30° method for acquiring diagnostic images of the maxillary incisor teeth. After the PID is positioned perpendicular to the sensor, the PID is then angled 20–30° away from the perpendicular plane so the beam of radiation is directed caudally. (c) Radiographic image utilizing the 20–30° method for acquiring images of the maxillary incisor teeth. Diagnostic information is present for the right maxillary 1st, 2nd, and 3rd incisors and the left maxillary 1st, 2nd, and 3rd incisors (101–103, 201–203). Depending on the size of the patient, additional images may need to be taken to fully evaluate the right and left maxillary 3rd incisor teeth (103, 203).

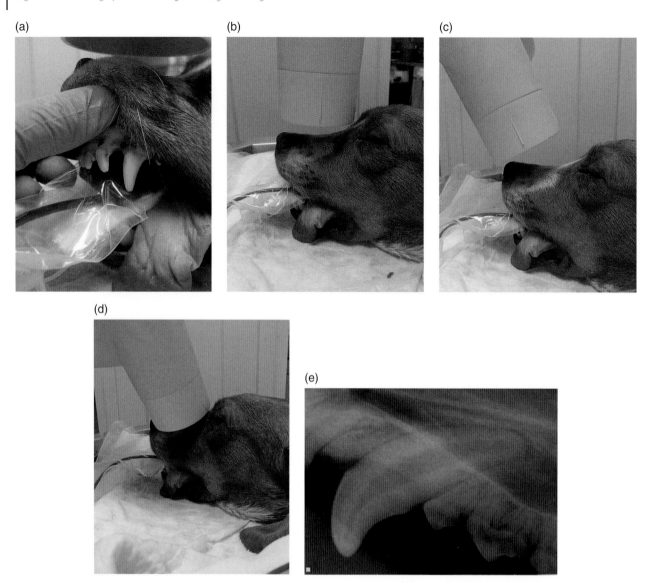

(a)   (b)   (c)

(d)

(e)

Figure 2.29 (a) Image demonstrating the 20–30° method for acquiring diagnostic images of the left maxillary canine tooth (204). To utilize this method, the sensor is placed within the oral cavity in a horizontal plane angled slightly toward the target tooth. The tip of the canine tooth should contact the corner of the sensor and the remaining portion of the sensor should be angled toward midline. (b) Image demonstrating the 20–30° method for acquiring diagnostic images of the left maxillary canine tooth (204). The PID is positioned perpendicular to the dorsal surface of the canine tooth and the sensor. (c) Image demonstrating the 20–30° method for acquiring diagnostic images of the left maxillary canine tooth (204). Following the placement of the PID perpendicular to the dorsal surface of the canine tooth and the sensor, the PID is angled 20–30° caudally so the beam of radiation is directed caudally from the perpendicular plane. (d) Image demonstrating the 20–30° method for acquiring diagnostic images of the left maxillary canine tooth (204). Following the placement of the PID perpendicular to the dorsal surface of the target teeth and angled 20–30° caudally, the PID is then positioned 20–30° laterally so the beam of radiation is angled in a caudo-medial direction. (e) Radiographic image of the maxillary canine tooth utilizing the 20–30° method for acquiring diagnostic images of the left maxillary canine tooth (204).

the sensor. The cusps of the maxillary premolars and molar are positioned so that they are close to the ventral edge of the sensor. This positioning allows the teeth to be radiographed to be in full contact with the sensor. A radiolucent mouth prop is often used to keep the mouth open. The endotracheal tube is positioned along the ventral aspect of the mouth near the tongue. The PID is positioned to bisect the angle of surface of the sensor and the long axis of the teeth. In the cat, this is often 20–30°. The X-ray beam passes through the oral cavity and then hits the palatal surface of the maxillary premolars and molar before hitting the sensor (Figure 2.31a and b). Positioning for the extraoral technique should eliminate the superimposition of the zygomatic arch on the maxillary premolars and molar teeth

(a)

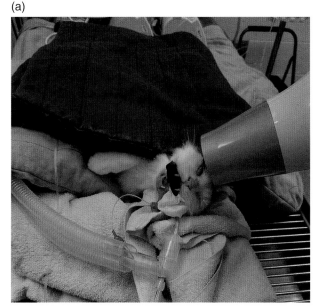

(b)   (c)

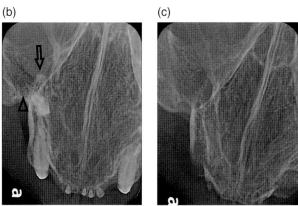

Figure 2.30   (a) The occlusal radiographic technique is commonly used as an adjunctive method for acquiring diagnostic information regarding retained tooth roots. Position the sensor in the oral cavity in a horizontal plane to the hard palate. The PID is placed perpendicular to the sensor over the target area. (b) The occlusal radiographic technique was used to identify retained tooth roots of the right maxillary 4th premolar tooth in the oral cavity of a cat. The arrowhead depicts the empty alveolus of the mesiobuccal root. The arrow depicts the retained tooth root in the area of the mesiopalatal root. (c) The occlusal radiographic technique was used to verify that all three roots of the right maxillary 4th premolar tooth were extracted in the oral cavity of a cat and that there is no evidence of retained tooth roots.

so that the roots are more easily evaluated. The image produced will be a mirror image of an intraoral radiographic technique. This means the image is flipped. Extraoral positioning can lead to confusion on what is the left side and what is the right side. The extraoral radiographic image should be labeled immediately after radiographic procurement so that the viewer knows that it is an extraoral image. The alternative is that the radiographic image is flipped

with viewing software so that image positioning is consistent with an intraoral radiographic technique.

"Almost Parallel" or "Near Parallel" Technique [12–14]

The "almost parallel" or "near parallel" technique has also been described as a means to acquire a diagnostic image of the maxillary premolars and molar teeth when the zygomatic arch is in the way. The technique can be employed when the standard bisecting angle technique is unable to radiographically reposition the zygomatic arch from the periapical area of the premolar and molar teeth in the dog or the cat. For this technique, the sensor is placed within the oral cavity perpendicular to the hard palate, but against the lingual aspect of the contralateral teeth to be imaged [12–14]. The PID is positioned in a dorsoventral direction yet "almost parallel" to the maxillary teeth and the sensor [12–14] (Figure 2.32a and b).

Localization of the Palatal Roots

Superimposition of mesiopalatal and mesiobuccal roots commonly occurs when evaluating the dental radiographs of the maxillary 4th premolar teeth in both canine and feline patients. This can create difficulty when trying to evaluate individual roots for signs of disease (Figure 2.33a and b). The need to identify each root separately is imperative for performing advanced endodontic procedures such as root canal therapy when all three roots of the tooth need to be evaluated and treated (Figure 2.34a and b). To create separation of the mesiopalatal and mesiobuccal roots, a change in the horizontal positioning of the PID can be made [8]. Starting from a lateral radiograph position, in which the mesial roots are superimposed, the PID is positioned to radiograph the roots in either mesial to distal orientation or in a distal to mesial orientation (Figure 2.35a–f). In the mesial to distal orientation, the PID is moved mesial to the tooth and then aimed so that the X-rays will penetrate the mesial-buccal aspect of the tooth first and move in a distal direction. In this case, the separation of the roots that occurs will position the mesiopalatal root in front of or mesial to the mesial-buccal root in a 2D radiographic image. The PID can also be positioned slightly distal to the maxillary 4th premolar and aimed so that the generated beam of radiation will penetrate the distal-buccal aspect of the tooth and move the beams of radiation in a mesial direction. In this case, the separation of the roots that occurs will position the mesial-palatal root behind or distal to the mesial-buccal root in a 2D radiographic image. The technique to localize these roots has been called Clark's rule or the "SLOB" rule [15]. "SLOB" stands for same lingual opposite buccal. The "SLOB" principle explains the palatal root

(a)

(b)

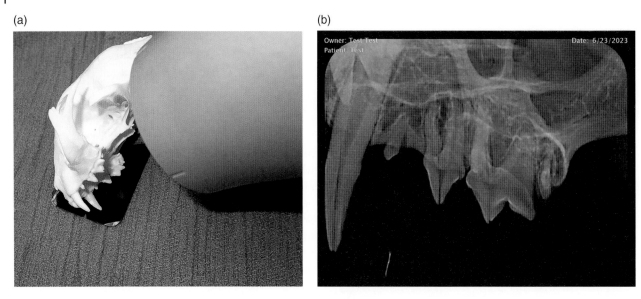

Figure 2.31 (a) Image depicts utilizing the extraoral technique to acquire diagnostic images of the right maxillary premolar and molar teeth in a cat. The sensor is placed outside the oral cavity. The PID is positioned so that the emitted X-rays will cast the shadow of the right maxillary premolar and molar teeth on the sensor, in a modified bisecting angle technique. This technique is used in an attempt to transpose the zygomatic arch off the apex of the roots of these teeth. (b) Radiographic image of the extraoral technique used to acquire a diagnostic image of the right maxillary premolar and molar teeth in a cat. Note this is a radiograph of the right maxillary arcade. The radiograph as viewed with labial mounting technique looks to be the left maxillary arcade. An extraoral radiograph should be flipped from either left to right or right to left as appropriate so it can be interpreted as other intraoral radiographs, or the radiograph needs to have an appropriate label so that the viewer knows this is the right maxillary arcade acquired with an extraoral technique.

(a)

(b)

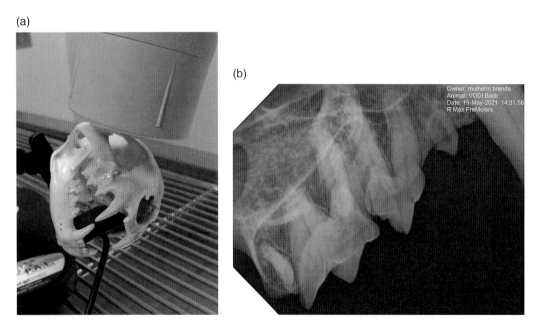

Figure 2.32 (a) The "almost parallel" or "near parallel" radiographic imaging technique can be used to acquire diagnostic images of the maxillary premolars and molar teeth in the dog and cat. The image depicts the placement of the sensor within the oral cavity perpendicular to the hard palate, on the lingual aspect of the contralateral teeth. The PID is positioned in a dorsoventral direction, imitating the "almost parallel" or "near parallel" orientation to the maxillary teeth and the sensor. The image shown is for positioning for radiographic images of the right maxillary premolar and molar teeth. (b) Radiographic image of the "almost parallel" or "near parallel" technique used for acquiring diagnostic images of the maxillary premolar and molar teeth of a cat. This technique allows for imaging of the premolar and molar teeth by repositioning the zygomatic arch away from the periapical area of the target teeth. The image shown provides diagnostic information regarding the right maxillary premolar and molar teeth in a cat (106–109).

(a)

(b)

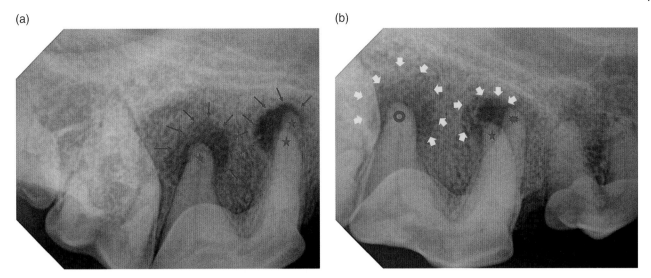

Figure 2.33 (a) Radiographic image of the right maxillary 4th premolar tooth (108) in a dog with endodontic disease. The radiograph shows a lateral projection of the tooth. The three roots of the right maxillary 4th premolar tooth are identified with red stars. There is evidence of periapical disease present in one or both mesial roots (arrows) as well as the distal root (arrows). The lateral projection of the bisecting angle technique makes it difficult for the viewer to identify which of the mesial roots has evidence of periapical disease. The lateral projection of the bisecting angle technique superimposes the mesiobuccal and mesiopalatal roots making it difficult to assess whether there is endodontic disease present in one or both roots. Verification of each root and the extent of disease present in each individual root at the time of treatment is important for postoperative follow-up care if endodontic therapy is pursued. (b) Radiographic image of the same right maxillary 4th premolar tooth (108) in a dog with endodontic disease. The radiograph shows localization of the mesiobuccal and mesiopalatal roots to identify disease present in the mesiobuccal root (star) as well as the distal root (open circle) using the "SLOB" positioning technique. The mesiopalatal root (asterisk) does not show overt evidence of disease. Ideally, additional imaging is needed to verify the mesiopalatal root does not have evidence of disease. The yellow arrowheads outline the periapical lucency noted around the diseased roots.

(a)

(b)

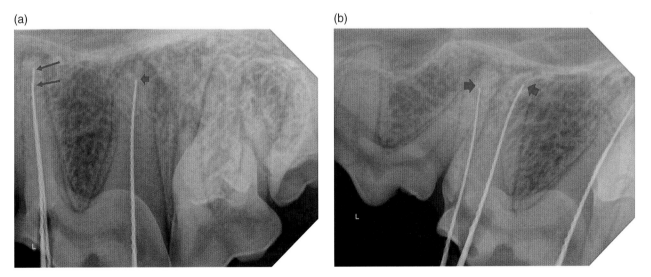

Figure 2.34 (a) Radiographic image of the left maxillary 4th premolar tooth (208) undergoing endodontic therapy. The image depicts the bisecting angle technique to image mesiobuccal, mesiopalatal, and distal roots with an endodontic hand file placed in each of the pulp chambers. Hand files are used to assess working length, or depth/length of the canals. Each canal can have a different measurement, therefore being able to identify whether the file is at the apical extent of the canal is vital to the success of the procedure. Radiographic verification of this measurement is imperative. In this image, it is difficult to evaluate whether both mesiobuccal and mesiopalatal roots have the endodontic file placed at the apical extent of the root. The distal root is the only root that can be evaluated. The arrowhead shows the apical extent of the file of the distal root. The arrows demonstrate the suspected apical extents of the mesiobuccal and mesiopalatal roots. (b) Radiographic image of the left maxillary 4th premolar tooth (208) undergoing endodontic therapy. The image was procured with the PID positioned in a mesial to distal projection compared to Figure 2.34a. The image gives a much more definitive location of the apical extent of the mesiobuccal and mesiopalatal roots (arrowheads) and allows the viewer to verify the working length of the mesiobuccal and mesiopalatal canals. The apical extent of the distal root is unable to be evaluated. The SLOB technique was utilized to separate the mesiopalatal and mesiobuccal roots for appropriate evaluation.

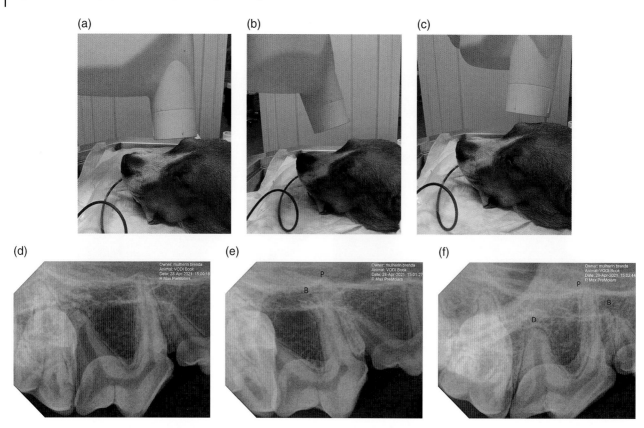

Figure 2.35 (a) Image depicts positioning of the PID for a lateral bisecting angle technique to acquire diagnostic images of the roots of the right maxillary 4th premolar tooth (108). The PID is positioned for a lateral radiographic view of the right maxillary 4th premolar prior to positioning to separate the mesiobuccal and mesiopalatal roots. (b) In this image, the PID is positioned for a mesial to distal radiograph of the right maxillary 4th premolar (108). In this view, the tooth root that moves in the same direction as the PID in comparison to the lateral radiographic image is the mesiopalatal (lingual) root. For this positioning, the mesiopalatal (lingual) root would move mesially in the radiograph. (c) In this image, the PID is positioned for a distal to mesial radiograph of the right maxillary 4th premolar (108). In this view, the tooth root that moves in the same direction as the PID in comparison to the lateral radiographic image is the mesiopalatal (lingual) root. For this positioning, the mesiopalatal (lingual) root would move distally in the radiograph. (d) Radiographic image that corresponds to the images in Figure (a). The radiographic image depicts positioning for a lateral radiograph of the right maxillary 4th premolar tooth (108) with superimposition of the mesiobuccal and mesiopalatal (lingual) roots. (e) Radiographic image that corresponds to the image in Figure (b). The radiographic image depicts mesial to distal positioning of the PID for radiographic procurement of the right maxillary 4th premolar tooth (108). The mesiopalatal (lingual) (P) root is positioned mesial to the mesiobuccal (B) root. (f) Radiographic image that corresponds to the image in Figure (c). The radiographic image depicts positioning of the PID in a distal to mesial orientation for radiographic procurement of the right maxillary 4th premolar tooth (108). The mesiopalatal (lingual) (P) root now appears to be distal to the mesiobuccal (B) root. Note that the distal root (D) also has less superimposition with the first molar depending on the technique used.

positioning in relation to the PID [10]. The terms lingual and palatal are used interchangeably when describing the surface of the maxillary teeth. When applying this "SLOB" acronym to the maxillary 4th premolar tooth, the specific roots that are being evaluated are the mesiobuccal and mesiopalatal roots of the right and left maxillary 4th premolar tooth. When the PID is moved in a mesial direction, the more palatal root of the maxillary 4th premolar tooth will appear more mesial when compared to the original lateral bisecting angle image. The buccal root of the maxillary 4th premolar will appear more distal in its position compared to

the lateral bisecting angle radiographic image. When the PID is moved distal, the palatal root will appear more distal as compared to the original image and the buccal root will move more mesial. When using this technique, it is important to know which way the PID was positioned in the original lateral image as this is the only way to correctly know which root is the mesiopalatal root and which one is mesiobuccal root. This technique can also be used to separate structures in other areas of the dentition when they are oriented in a buccal to palatal/lingual relationship.

See Table 2.2 for summary of radiographic techniques.

Table 2.2   Radiographic techniques.

Technique	Position of the sensor	Position of the PID
Parallel technique	Parallel to the target in a horizontal or vertical plane* *Vertical plane used in mandibular 1st molar teeth	The PID is placed perpendicular to the sensor and the target
Bisecting angle technique	Sensor is placed in a horizontal plane to the long axis of the target	The PID is placed perpendicular to the bisecting angle that is created between the long axis of the target and the horizontal placement of the sensor
20–30° technique	Sensor is placed in a horizontal plane to the long axis of the target or angled slightly toward the tooth* *A slightly angled sensor is used for imaging of the maxillary canine teeth	The PID begins directly perpendicular to the sensor. It is then angled 20–30° caudally for the maxillary and mandibular incisors The PID begins perpendicular to the dorsal surface of the canine tooth, angled 20–30° caudally and 20–30° laterally
Occlusal technique	Sensor is placed in a horizontal plane, parallel to the hard palate	The PID is placed perpendicular to the sensor directly over the target area
Extraoral technique	Sensor is placed extraorally on the table with the arcade to be imaged directly on top of the sensor. The cusps of the premolar and molar teeth should be positioned close to the ventral edge of the sensor* *Extraoral labeling of this image needs to be done immediately or the radiograph needs to be flipped to represent the correct arcade	The PID is placed to bisect the angle of the sensor and the long axis of the teeth (approximately 20–30°). The radiation should penetrate the palatal surface of the maxillary premolars and molars
"Almost parallel" or "near parallel" technique	Sensor is placed perpendicular to the hard palate against the lingual aspect of the contralateral teeth to be imaged	The PID is placed in a dorsoventral or "almost/near parallel" direction to the maxillary premolar and molars
SLOB (same lingual, opposite buccal) technique	Sensor is placed in a horizontal plane to the long axis of the target	The PID is placed perpendicular to the bisecting angle that is created between the long axis of the target and the horizontal placement of the sensor for the first image for a lateral projection of the tooth The PID is then moved from the lateral projection to either a mesiodistal or a distomesial direction for the penetration of the radiation

The table describes the different radiographic techniques used to procure dental radiographs of the patient. The table discusses appropriate positioning of the sensor as well as appropriate positioning of the PID (generator).

Techniques for Imaging Caudal Teeth in Small Patients

Small patients can create difficulty in placing the sensor in the caudal aspect of the oral cavity. This creates a situation in which the sensor can only be positioned mesial to the target tooth due to the size of the oral cavity being imaged. The radiographer is unable to position it farther back into the oral cavity due to anatomic restrictions. When this occurs a combination of techniques will be needed to try to project the X-rays through the target tooth and on to where the sensor can receive the image. Similar to the technique used for localization of the palatal root, the horizontal angle of the PID can be changed to move the projected image of the target on the sensor in a mesial or distal

orientation. For the caudal molars, this generally means that the target is projected in a mesial direction as the hard and soft tissues prevent the placement of the sensor in a parallel technique orientation. Instead, a lateral bisecting angle technique is used. This is accomplished by setting the PID with the standard bisecting angle technique and then moving the PID slightly caudal and aiming it so that the X-rays will travel in a distal to mesial path intersecting the target and where the sensor can be placed. For the mandibular molars, there are patients that do not have enough space in the oral cavity to place the sensor parallel to the teeth. While the bisecting angle technique is commonly used for acquiring images of the maxillary arcade and the rostral mandibular premolars and incisors, it can be used in all areas of the mouth. Utilization of the bisecting angle

(a)

(b)

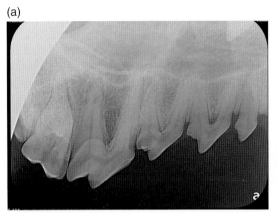 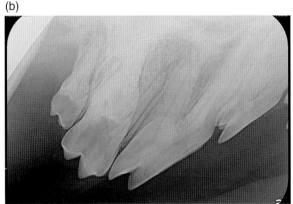

Figure 2.36 (a) Radiographic image of the right maxillary premolars and molars in a dog. With lateral positioning of the PID to the sensor, the positioning cuts off the right maxillary 2nd molar tooth. This image would be diagnostic for the right maxillary 1st, 2nd, 3rd, and 4th premolars (105–108) and the 1st molar (109). The sensor could not be placed in a more caudal position to easily obtain a lateral radiograph of the right maxillary 2nd molar (110); therefore, an additional image is necessary to acquire diagnostic information regarding the right maxillary 2nd molar (110). (b) Radiographic image of the right maxillary premolars and molars in a dog with the same placement of the sensor as in Figure (a), but with the PID positioned from a distal to mesial orientation. This projects the right maxillary 2nd molar (110) mesially on the radiograph. There is an elongation artifact of the radiograph, but the 2nd molar can be more fully evaluated compared to the lateral image in which the tooth is cut off and would be nondiagnostic for this tooth.

technique if the anatomy does not allow placement of the sensor for the parallel technique should be considered for acquiring the needed images. Not all patient anatomy will allow for the perfect radiographic image. It is important to realize that the goal of acquiring more diagnostic information is to procure an image of diagnostic quality, not perfection (Figure 2.36a and b).

Technique Errors

There are three main sources of radiographic positioning errors: the patient, the radiographic beam, and the sensor [1, 3]. If a radiographic error occurs and the image is not of diagnostic quality, identifying the source of the error can help navigate the process of correcting the error. Evaluating whether the patient is properly positioned, if the radiographic generator is positioned appropriately, or if the sensor or film is adequately positioned will help to identify most issues and errors associated with radiographic positioning [3]. Ultimately, identifying and correcting these errors should reduce the number of nondiagnostic radiographic images.

See Table 2.3 for positioning errors.

Foreshortening and Elongation

Distortion of a radiographic image along the long axis of the target object is called foreshortening or elongation. Foreshortening is distortion of an object making it appear shorter than what it actually is in reality or longer than it is (elongation) [8]. Distortion of a radiographic image can

lead to a misinterpretation of the diagnostic findings when interpreting the radiograph. It can result in either an overrepresentation or underrepresentation of true radiographic lesions or normal tissues.

Foreshortening occurs when the PID is positioned so that the X-ray beam is more perpendicular to the surface of the sensor, creating a shallower bisected angle compared to the ideal bisected angle. In our shadow analogy, this occurs when the sun is more directly overhead creating a shadow that is smaller than the object creating the shadow (Figure 2.37a and b). This will generally result in an underrepresentation of the size and changes in tissue seen with pathologic lesions. Correction of this positioning error includes positioning the beam more perpendicular to the bisecting angle. This can also be stated by moving the beam more lateral to the roots or more toward the horizon [13] (Figure 2.38a–d).

Elongation occurs when the generated X-ray beams are more parallel with the surface of the sensor, creating a steeper bisected angle compared to the ideal bisected angle. In the shadow analogy, this occurs at dusk or dawn when the sunrays are coming parallel to the surface of the ground, creating a very tall shadow compared to the actual size of the object (Figure 2.39a and b). This can result in an overrepresentation of the size of object or tissue and overexaggerated changes seen in tissues with pathologic lesions. Correction of this positioning error occurs by positioning the beam more perpendicular to the bisecting angle. This can also be stated by moving the beam more on top of the roots or more toward 12 o'clock (Figure 2.40a–d).

Table 2.3 Positioning errors.

Imaging artifact	Description	Example	Correction
Foreshortening	Radiographic distortion of an object making it shorter than what it should appear		Position the radiographic beam more perpendicular to the bisecting angle. Move the beam more lateral to the roots or more toward the horizon
Elongation	Radiographic distortion of an object making it longer than what it should appear		Position the radiographic beam more perpendicular to the bisecting angle. Move the beam more on top of the tooth roots or more toward a 12 o'clock position
Cone cutting	Radiographic artifact in which a portion of the sensor was not exposed to radiation. A circular-shaped artifact will appear on the image		Move the sensor into the radiographic beam, move the radiographic beam over the sensor, or back the radiographic beam away from the sensor to allow more scattered radiation to penetrate the sensor
Missing the apex	At least 2–4 mm of hard or soft tissue should be present apically to the tooth root. If less than 2–4 mm is present, the apex of the root cannot be fully evaluated		Reposition the sensor more apically within the oral cavity or reposition the radiographic beam to cast the shadow of the apical area on the sensor in a different way. The radiographic beam can also be positioned to foreshorten the target to allow more apical area to be evaluated

The table describes the most common positioning errors that are made when acquiring dental radiographs. It describes the error, gives an example of the error, and describes how to correct for the error.

(a)

(b)

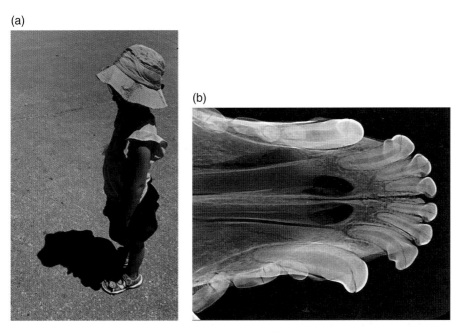

Figure 2.37   (a) The image depicts a foreshortening artifact of the shadow of a child. The sun acting as the radiographic beam is positioned more perpendicular to the sensor (sidewalk) than it is to the target (child), thus creating a shallower bisected angle, compared to the ideal bisected angle. (b) Radiographic image demonstrating foreshortening. Foreshortening creates an image that decreases the length of the target anatomy compared to the actual size of the target. This is a radiograph of the maxillary incisors and right maxillary canine tooth and premolars of a dog. Note the short, squatty appearance of the teeth on the image. The image does not depict the actual size of the teeth as they should appear on a radiographic image, but rather smaller teeth with crowns that appear to slump over the roots.

(a)

(b)

(c)

(d)

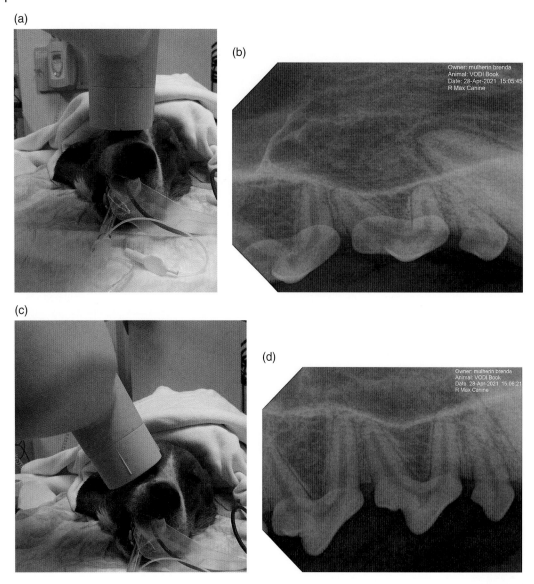

Figure 2.38 (a) Image of the positioning for the right maxillary premolar teeth in a dog. The PID is positioned so that the X-ray beam is more perpendicular to the surface of the sensor, thus creating a shallower bisected angle. Positioning in this manner will create an image that is foreshortened. (b) Corresponding radiographic image for Figure (a). Note the significant foreshortening of the maxillary premolar teeth. While this image may be diagnostic, it does not show a true representation of the teeth and allow for optimal assessment. This is an image of the right maxillary canine tooth, 1st, 2nd premolars, and mesial root of the 3rd premolar (104–107). (c) Image of the positioning for the right maxillary premolars in a dog to correct the foreshortening artifact created in Figure (a) and (b). The X-ray beam is now positioned perpendicular to the bisecting angle creating a better, more diagnostic image to appropriately evaluate the right maxillary arcade. (d) Corresponding radiographic image for Figure (c). Note the foreshortening that was seen in Figure (b) is corrected, creating a more diagnostic image of the maxillary premolar teeth. This radiographic image would be diagnostic for the right maxillary 1st and 2nd premolars and the mesial root of the 3rd premolar (105–107).

To summarize, correction of either positioning error occurs by identifying a distortion of the radiographic image. A change can be made in the angle of the PID to generate X-rays perpendicular to the ideal bisecting angle. In the case of foreshortening, positioning the PID so that a produced X-ray is less perpendicular to the surface of the sensor will correct the distortion. In the case of elongation,

positioning the PID so that a produced X-ray is less parallel to the surface of the sensor will correct the distortion.

Cone Cutting

Cone cutting occurs when the PID is positioned so that not all of the sensor surface is exposed to the generated X-ray beam. This results in an area of dead space, white space, or

(a)

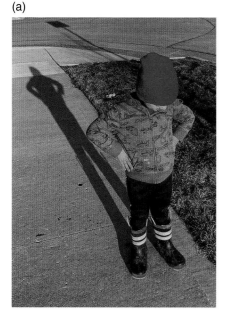

(b)

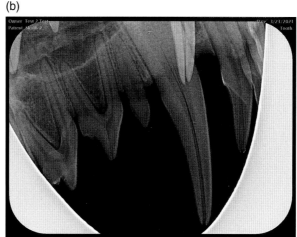

Figure 2.39   (a) The image depicts an elongation artifact of the shadow of a child. The sun acting as the radiographic beam is positioned more perpendicular to target (child) than it is to the sensor (sidewalk), thus creating a steeper bisected angle, compared to the ideal bisected angle. (b) Radiographic image demonstrating elongation. Elongation creates an image that increases the length of the target anatomy compared to the actual size of the target. This is a radiograph of the right maxillary canine tooth and premolars of a dog. The teeth appear longer and more stretched compared to their actual appearance within the patient. This image also demonstrates cone cutting, another radiographic artifact on both the mesial and distal aspects of the radiograph.

wasted potential space on the final radiograph image (Figures 2.39b and 2.41). This can occur when using larger phosphor plates or when the PID is not positioned correctly to generate an X-ray beam over the entire sensor. If the entire surface area of the sensor does not have direct contact with the radiation generated from the X-ray, this area of the sensor or plate will remain unexposed. This unexposed area will appear white on a radiographic image. An image with cone cutting will have a circular-shaped artifact on the radiographic image. This area corresponds to the circular shape of the PID. The rest of the radiographic image outside of this circular area will be white due to lack of radiographic exposure in that area. For larger sensors, such as Size 4 phosphor plates, this can be corrected by positioning the PID away from the surface of the sensor. Using this correction method will reduce the collimation of the X-rays so that they fan out and expose more of the sensor. It is important to note that the further away the PID is from the target area and the sensor, the more power will be needed to penetrate the tissue and transmit the image to the sensor. If the PID is positioned farther away from the sensor and the image appears under exposed, the kVp or mAs can be increased to compensate. The increased surface area of Size 4 sensors can have a degree of cone cutting that still produces a radiographic image of diagnostic quality. Many times, using a larger sized plate

shows the intended target teeth/tissues even if cone cutting is present. If cone cutting appears on the final radiographic image, but the image is still of diagnostic quality for evaluation, correction may not be needed.

Cone cutting on a sensor that is smaller than the aperture of the PID is a positioning error. The alignment of the X-ray beam from the PID to the sensor surface is positioned so that the beam of radiation is not exposing the entire surface of the sensor. The X-ray beams travel in a straight line from the PID to the sensor. Readjusting the position of the PID to accommodate for a straight-line trajectory with the sensor surface will correct the cone cutting artifact. The closer the PID is to the target and the sensor, the easier it is to correct the positioning.

In general, the ability to correct a cone cutting artifact usually involves either moving the sensor into the trajectory of the PID, moving the PID over the sensor, or backing the PID away from the sensor to allow for less collimation of the radiographic beam and more scattered radiation to contact the target.

Missing the Apex

As previously discussed, at least 2–4 mm of hard or soft tissue should be present radiographically, apical to the tooth root for accurate evaluation (Figures 2.40b and 2.44b). If the operator is having difficulty in obtaining the target apex

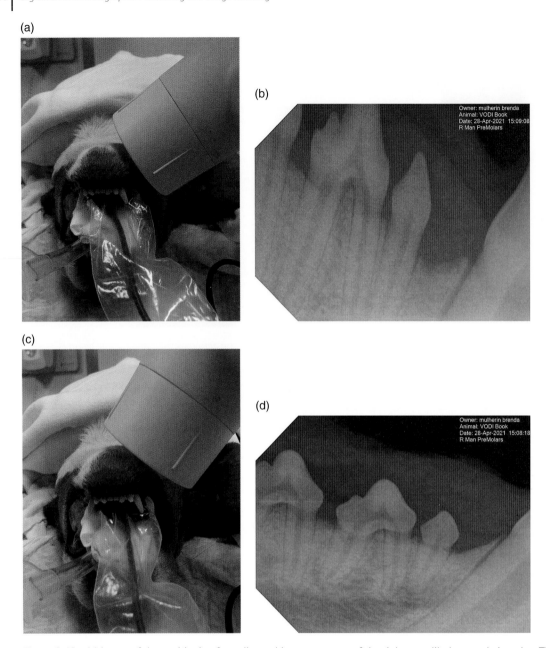

Figure 2.40 (a) Image of the positioning for radiographic procurement of the right mandibular arcade in a dog. The PID is positioned so that the X-ray beam is more parallel to the surface of the sensor. Positioning the PID in this manner will create a steeper bisected angle and thus creates an image that is elongated. (b) Corresponding radiographic image for Figure (a). Note the significant elongation of the right mandibular premolar teeth. The apex of the target teeth is not visualized on the film, making this a nondiagnostic image. (c) Image of the positioning for radiographic procurement of the right mandibular premolar arcade in the dog to correct the elongation artifact created in Figure (a) and (b). The X-ray beam is now positioned perpendicular to the bisecting angle to create a better diagnostic image for evaluating the right mandibular premolar teeth. (d) Corresponding radiographic image for Figure (c). Note the elongation in Figure (b) is corrected, creating a more diagnostic image of the right mandibular premolar teeth. This radiographic image would be diagnostic for the right mandibular 1st and 2nd premolars and the mesial root of the 3rd premolar (405–407).

or periapical area in a radiograph, this area can be captured in a few ways. The sensor can be repositioned more apically to the root or the PID can be repositioned to transmit the apical area on to the sensor. Sometimes a combination of the two approaches is required. To reposition the sensor when using the bisecting angle technique for maxillary and mandibular teeth, move the sensor deeper into the oral cavity, or more toward the patient's midline. For the parallel technique, reposition the sensor more ventral relative to the mandible and the target teeth. To reposition the PID, position the sensor so that it is at a steeper angle to the sensor surface. This in effect decreases the bisected angle or applies foreshortening to the diagnostic image. To state this a bit more simply, position the PID more on top of the tooth when the patient is in sternal or dorsal recumbency. If the target tooth is larger than anticipated, the sensor can be positioned in a vertical plane rather than a horizontal plane in attempt to acquire the entire tooth on one radiographic image (see Figure 2.17a–2.17c).

Overexposed or Underexposed

Exposure of the sensor is based on the power of the X-rays generated. This is controlled by many factors. The kVp setting, the quantity of X-rays generated (mA), length of time the radiation is being released (mAs), the thickness or density of the target object, and the distance of the generator from the sensor all affect sensor exposure [2]. Exposure settings on most digital radiograph generators are preset with

limited ability to make changes to kVp or mA [2]. The main factor that is frequently adjusted is time (mAs). Many radiographic generators come with settings based on the area of the mouth and teeth that are being radiographed. These systems take away the need to set kVp or mAs separately and standardize the power and quantity of X-rays generated. Most modern X-ray machines do not allow for mA adjustment. The mAs (exposure time) is directly related to how light or dark the film is. The longer the exposure time, the more X-ray photons hit the film and the darker the film is. The opposite is true for a shorter exposure time. When the amount of exposure to X-rays is not set correctly, the resulting image will be either underexposed or overexposed. An underexposed image will appear lighter, as less X-rays hit the sensor (Figure 2.42). An overexposed image will appear darker as more X-rays hit the sensor (Figure 2.43). Think of

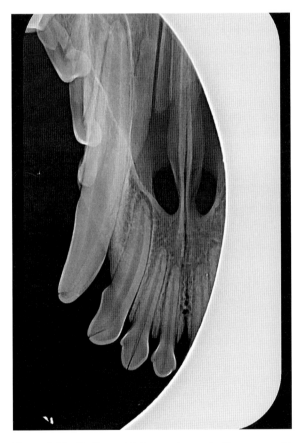

Figure 2.41 Radiographic image demonstrating cone cutting. The image is taken to acquire the right maxillary incisor teeth. There is a large amount of dead space on the radiographic image on the left side of the patient. The PID was positioned too far to the right of the maxilla, allowing for increased areas of the film without any diagnostic information acquired or radiation exposure. This positioning allows for the left maxillary incisors to be "cut" out of the image. Correction of this error would be to move the sensor more to the left side of the mouth and reposition the PID so that the X-rays generated will expose the entire film.

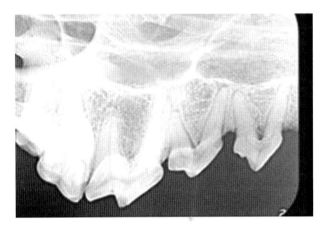

Figure 2.42 Radiographic image of the right maxillary premolars and molars of a dog. The image demonstrates underexposure of an image. Correction of this error would be an in increase in kVp or mAs.

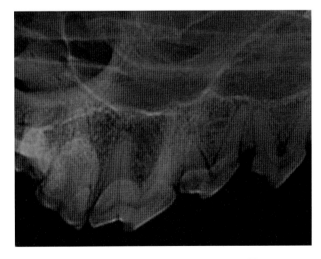

Figure 2.43 Radiographic image of the right maxillary premolars and molars of a dog. The image demonstrates overexposure of an image. Correction of this error would be to decrease the kVp or mAs.

overexposure and underexposure like baking a batch of cookies. If the oven temperature is too high, or you leave the cookies in too long, the cookies will be overbaked and black. This is like increasing the kVp or increasing the mAs. If you have too low of an oven temperature, or do not leave the cookies in long enough, the cookies will be underbaked and light in color. This is like decreasing the kVp or mAs. A proper balance needs to be found to give adequate contrast between the tissues allowing them to be seen and differentiated. For underexposed images, the kVp or mAs should be increased. For overexposed images, the kVp or mAs should be decreased.

See Table 2.4 for technique errors.

Artifacts

Progressing from chemically developed standard radiographic films to digitally exposed radiographs has decreased the number of artifacts that can be encountered due to processing errors. The reduced use of chemicals to develop radiographs has decreased the number of variables that can affect radiographic image quality. Artifacts associated with digital radiographic systems are usually due to contamination of the sensor with an extrinsic source. An extrinsic contamination that absorbs or deflects X-rays can affect the way the processor analyzes and eventually digitizes the radiographic image in CR or DR units. Ensuring that the sensor or plate is clean and that the hardware has not been contaminated will decrease the chances of having an artifact on the final radiographic image. Following recommended cleaning schedules and maintenance will prolong the life and quality of the radiographic equipment. For CR plates, the plate should be fed into the processing machine without exposure to excessive ambient light. This is not an issue for DR sensors as they are not fed through a processor. Intrinsic factors, such as damage to the sensor or plate, can also create artifacts on the image (Figure 2.44a and b). Age of equipment is another factor as phosphor plates will lose image quality over time and need to be replaced. Intrinsic sources of artifacts can come from damage to the equipment from the patient, such as a tooth contacting the surface of the plate or sensor. Scratches and bends to the CR phosphor plates can also create corresponding artifacts on the processed image (Figure 2.45).

Artifacts that can be present on radiographic images that are indirectly related to the sensor itself include endotracheal

Table 2.4 Technique errors.

Technique error	Description	Example	Correction
Underexposure	A technique error causing an image to appear lighter (whiter) in color as less X-rays are reaching the sensor		Increase kVp or mAs
Overexposure	A technique error causing an image to be much darker (blacker) in color as too many X-rays are reaching the sensor		Decrease kVp or mAs

The table describes the two main technique errors of underexposure and overexposure. It gives examples of each error and how to correct for the error.

(a)

(b)

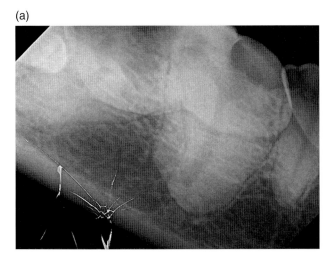
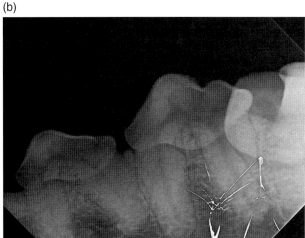

Figure 2.44   (a) Radiographic image of the right mandible of a dog. The image demonstrates an artifact secondary to damage of the sensor. Note the artifact is present on multiple images (b) making it difficult to interpret any radiographic findings. This radiograph also depicts a foreshortening artifact making it difficult to evaluate for any disease present within the right mandibular 1st molar tooth (409). (b) Radiographic image of the left mandible of a dog. The image demonstrated an artifact secondary to damage to the sensor. Note the artifact is present on multiple images (a) making it difficult to interpret any radiographic findings. This radiograph is also nondiagnostic for other reasons as it does not yield any information regarding the periapical area of any of the teeth shown. This is an image of the left mandibular 3rd and 4th premolars with the mesial aspect of the crown of the mandibular 1st molar present (307–309).

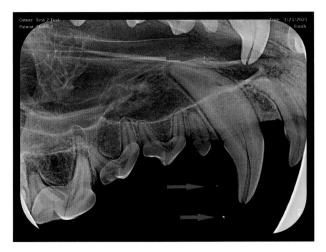

Figure 2.45   Radiographic image of the right maxillary canine and premolar teeth of a dog. The image demonstrates artifacts on a CR plate that are secondary to small scratches or punctures on the plate (red arrows). This image also depicts cone cutting on the right side of the image.

Repeat Radiographs

Frequent causes for repeated radiographs include improper positioning of the PID (elongated, foreshortened, etc.), improper settings of the X-ray generator (over or under exposed), and improper placement of the film (backward, too far out of the oral cavity, too far midline, etc.).

Positioning Assistance

Procuring diagnostic radiographs takes practice to master the concepts of radiographic positioning. There are different aids that can help individuals practice these concepts without the use of an anesthetized patient. Things readily available in a clinic setting include canine and feline skull models. Some companies have even developed models that have canine and feline skulls mounted so to resemble a head attached to a body to practice sternal, lateral, and dorsal positioning without the skulls becoming disarticulated from each other (Figure 2.47a–c).

Other manufactures have created laser devices that can be attached to the PID which will create a laser crosshair that corresponds to the center of the PID target area (Figure 2.48a–c). These devices are used to help improve positioning accuracy and efficiency by reducing anesthetic time for the patient. They are also thought to minimize radiation exposure to the patient and the radiographer. The laser device easily attaches to the PID and moves with the PID. For use of a laser device, the sensor is placed as it normally would be positioned. The PID

tube ties, pumice prophy paste, and positioning devices that are used in attempt to hold the sensor in the proper position (Figure 2.46a and b). Additionally, improper positioning of a DR sensor, including backward placement, can lead to a radiographic artifact and, more importantly, a nondiagnostic image (Figure 2.10b). Being able to identify artifacts on radiographic plates prior to taking a radiographic image will help to reduce the necessity for repeated radiographs.

(a)

(b)

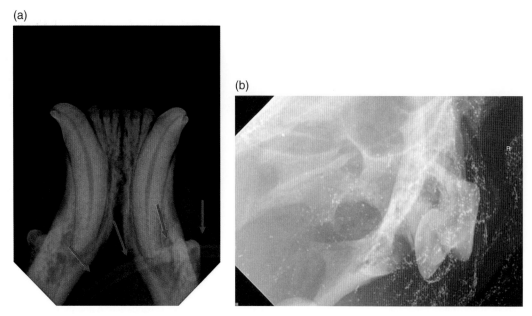

Figure 2.46 (a) Radiographic image of the rostral mandible of a cat. Note the endotracheal tube balloon cuff artifact that is present on the image (arrows). (b) Radiographic image of the maxilla of a dog. Note the dental prophy paste artifact on the sensor causing a snowstorm appearance on the radiographic image. Making sure the oral cavity is rinsed of any debris, including prophy paste will help to provide less artifacts on the radiographic images, making interpretation of the images easier.

(a)　　　　　　　(b)　　　　　　　(c)

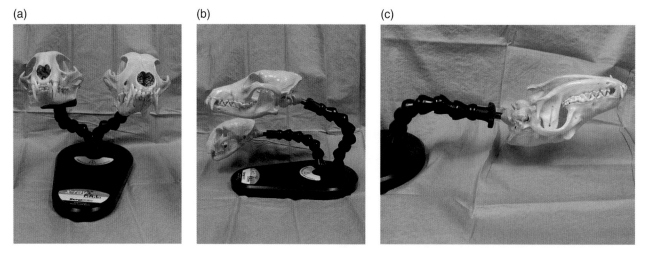

Figure 2.47 (a) Image of a positioning model used to practice radiographic image procurement. The canine and feline skulls are attached to articulating arms to allow for practicing sternal, lateral, and dorsal recumbency positioning. Canine and feline skulls or cadaveric specimens can also be used as models for practicing radiographic positioning. (b) Lateral image of a positioning model used to practice radiographic image procurement. The canine and feline skulls are attached to articulating arms to allow for practicing sternal, lateral, and dorsal recumbency positioning. (c) Image of a positioning model used to practice radiographic image procurement. The canine and feline skulls are attached to articulating arms to allow for practicing sternal, lateral, and dorsal recumbency positioning. Note how the positioning model can be manipulated into a dorsal recumbency position to practice image acquisition.

is then placed so that the crosshairs of the laser device will be associated with the target area. If using these devices, make sure to follow the manufacturer's recommendation for safety procedures including covering the patient's eyes to prevent damage from the laser device. Rubber sheeting or medical tape can be used to help protect the eyes from the laser.

Conclusion

Diagnostic image procurement commonly requires the parallel and bisecting angle techniques or variations of these techniques to be utilized. The proper settings for the radiographic generator are chosen based on the size of patient and target area of interest. Proper positioning and settings

(a) (b) (c)

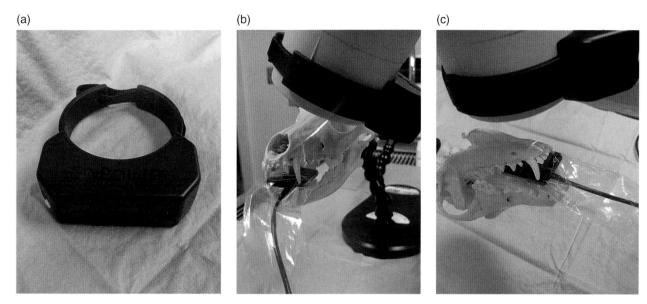

Figure 2.48 (a) Image of a laser positioning device. The device attaches to the PID to create a red laser crosshair to help identify the bisecting angle on the patient. (b) Image of a laser positioning device. The device attaches to the PID to create a red laser crosshair to help identify the bisecting angle on the patient. When acquiring a radiographic image of the left maxillary canine tooth, the sensor is placed within the oral cavity with the tip of the canine tooth contacting the corner of the sensor. The PID should be positioned at a 10–15° angle from the front and side of the tooth with the laser crosshairs centered on the first premolar tooth. Note the red laser crosshairs centered on the first premolar tooth to acquire a diagnostic image of the left maxillary canine tooth. (c) Image of a laser positioning device. The device attaches to the PID to create a red laser crosshair to help identify the bisecting angle on the patient. When acquiring a radiographic image of the mandibular incisors, the sensor should be positioned parallel to the mandibular arcade with the edge of the sensor just in front of the incisors. The PID should be positioned perpendicular to the sensor with a 10–15° angle caudally. The laser crosshairs should be positioned with the center of the beam on midline and the crosshairs centered on the interdental space created by the mandibular canines and the 3rd incisors.

will help to reduce the need for repeated radiographs and decrease radiation exposure to the patient and the radiography technician. The concepts of the bisecting angle can be difficult to understand. Many times, it is more helpful to know what needs to be done to improve or correct an image. Practice is the key. Taking the time to practice on a skull or cadaveric specimen is recommended to reduce the added pressure of having a patient under anesthesia when acquiring images. Do not be afraid to ask for assistance with someone who may have experience in radiographic positioning. While training sessions with individuals who have experience and knowledge in procuring diagnostic images is helpful, it is not a substitute for practicing to attain the images in practice. Remember, radiographic images need to be of diagnostic quality for interpretation, not perfect.

References

1 Altier, B. (2021). Tips for mastering veterinary dental radiography. *DVM360.com*, 18 January. https://www. dvm360.com/view/tips-for-mastering-veterinary-dental-radiography (accessed 19 May 2023).

2 Niemiec, B., Gilbert, A., and Sabatino, D. (2004). Equipment and basic geometry of dental radiography. *J. Vet. Dent.* 21 (1): 48–52.

3 Altier, B. (2019). The ABC's of dental radiology demystified. *DVM360.com* 752–755. https://www.dvm360.com/view/ abc-s-dental-radiology-dental-radiology-demystified-proceedings-pdf.

4 Niemiec, B. and Furman, R. (2004). Canine dental radiography. *J. Vet. Dent.* 21 (3): 186–190.

5 Niemiec, B. and Furman, R. (2004). Feline dental radiography. *J. Vet. Dent.* 21 (3): 252–257.

6 Hardie, E., Spodnick, G., Gilson, S. et al. (1999). Tracheal rupture in cats: 16 cases (1983–1998). *J. Am. Vet. Med. Assoc.* 214: 508–512.

7 Niemiec, B.A. (2007). Foundations digital dental radiography. *J. Vet. Dent.* 24 (3): 192–197.

8 Roy, C.G. (2018). Canine and feline dental radiographic technique. In: *Textbook of Veterinary Diagnostic Radiology*, 7e (ed. D.E. Thrall and W.R. Widmer), 39–57. St. Louis: Elsevier.

9 Charlier, C. (2022). Intraoral Radiographs: Identifying Normal Anatomy. *Today's Veterinary Practice*, April 11,

Issue: May/June 2022. https://todaysveterinarypractice.com/dentistry/intraoral-radiographs-identifying-normal-anatomy.

10 Holmstrom, S.E., Frost, P., and Eisner, E.R. (2004). *Dental Radiology. Veterinary Dental Techniques for the Small Animal Practitioner*, 3e, 131–174. Philadelphia: W.B. Saunders.

11 Niemiec, B. (2019). Oral radiology and imaging. In: *Wigg's Veterinary Dentistry Principles and Practice*, 2e (ed. H.B. Lobrise and B.R. Dodd), 41–62. Hoboken: Wiley.

12 Woodward, T. (2009). Dental radiology. *Top. Companion Anim. Med.* 24 (1): 20–36.

13 Woodward, T. (2005–2023). Simplified positioning for dental radiology. *Animal Dental Care*. https://www.dentalaireproducts.com/simplified-positioning-for-dental-radiology/.

14 Hale, F. (2018). Intraoral radiographic tips and tricks. *Can. Vet. J.* 59 (2): 191–197.

15 Clark, C.A. (1910). A method of ascertaining the relative position of unerupted teeth by means of film radiographs. *Proc. R. Soc. Med.* 3 (Odontol Sect.): 87–90.

3

Interpretation of Normal Radiographic Anatomy

Brenda L. Mulherin

Lloyd Veterinary Medical Center, Iowa State University College of Veterinary Medicine, Ames, IA, USA

CONTENTS

Value of Intraoral Radiographic Imaging

Radiographic imaging of the oral cavity helps the clinician evaluate the structures below the gumline. Canine and feline patients undergoing dental procedures should have dental radiographs taken as part of the accepted standard of care for the patient. The ability to acquire diagnostic radiographs of the dentition and surrounding hard tissue structures allows the clinician to diagnose and potentially treat conditions that they may not have known existed. Dental radiography can reveal pathology that may have been missed if the clinician was basing their treatment plan solely on the clinical oral examination findings [1, 2]. Research has shown that 41.7% of canine patients who did not demonstrate clinical evidence of pathology had incidental radiographic findings consistent with disease [1]. Over 27.8% of dogs without clinical evidence of disease were found to have clinically relevant information observed on intraoral dental radiographs [1]. In canine patients with obvious signs of clinical disease, intraoral radiographs confirmed clinically significant findings in 24.3% of patients [1]. In feline patients without clinical evidence of disease, radiographs yielded clinically important information in 41.7% of patients [2]. Over 53% of feline patients with evidence of disease were found to have clinically relevant information acquired due to the acquisition of dental radiographs [2]. These studies demonstrate the importance of intraoral radiography in the diagnosis of abnormalities within the oral cavity. The ability to acquire diagnostic images and correctly interpret the radiographic findings can provide the clinician the tools they need to create a treatment plan specific for the patient [3]. A clinician needs to use the patient signalment, information collected in the history, and physical examination findings, combined with the acquired diagnostic images and anesthetized oral examination findings to formulate an accurate diagnostic and treatment plan catered to the individual patient's needs [3].

Veterinary Oral Diagnostic Imaging, First Edition. Edited by Brenda L. Mulherin.
© 2024 John Wiley & Sons, Inc. Published 2024 by John Wiley & Sons, Inc.

Quality of Images

Radiographic images of the oral cavity should be well positioned. Positioning depends on what teeth you are attempting to acquire diagnostic images of. (For more information regarding radiographic positioning, see Chapter 2.) Improper positioning can make it difficult for the interpreter to discern pathology from anatomy. The interpretation of radiographic images can also be affected by items used to help position the radiographic film or sensor within the mouth. For effective positioning, the closer the tooth is to the film, the more accurate the image quality. The radiographic beam should be as perpendicular as possible to the bisecting angle for the middle and rostral mandible and for the entire maxilla. For radiographic acquisition of the caudal mandible, the radiographic beam should be as perpendicular as possible to the film and the tooth. The exposure technique of a radiograph can also influence the ability of the interpreter to evaluate for normal and abnormal anatomy and pathology. Radiographic exposure errors can lead to either overinterpretation or under-interpretation of the anatomy or pathology which may be present (see Table 2.4).

Exposure Artifacts

Using appropriate exposure techniques in acquiring radiographic images is extremely important. The image should not be overexposed/too dark or underexposed/too light. If the image appears overexposed or underexposed, the exposure technique needs to be reevaluated so that pathology is not missed, under-interpreted, or so that normal radiographic structures are not overinterpreted as pathology (see Figures 2.42 and 2.43, Table 2.4).

Positioning Techniques

Parallel Technique
For the caudal mandibular premolars and molars, the parallel technique is often utilized. This technique employs the principle of placing the radiographic beam perpendicular to the area of interest and the radiographic film. This radiographic technique is most similar to radiographic image acquisition of any other area of the body, e.g. thorax, abdomen, etc. To avoid distortion of the area of interest, utilization of the parallel technique will yield better image quality (see Figure 2.18a and b, Table 2.2). For more information regarding radiographic positioning, see Chapter 2.

Bisecting Angle Technique
The rest of the oral cavity is imaged most commonly by utilization of the bisecting angle technique. This technique employs placing the radiographic beam perpendicular to the bisecting angle. The bisecting angle is the angle between the long axis of the tooth and the film itself. This angle should always be calculated from inside the patient's mouth. The bisecting angle allows the object to be as accurately represented as possible considering the confines of radiographic imaging (see Figures 2.23–2.26, Table 2.2). For more information regarding radiographic positioning, see Chapter 2.

Positioning Artifacts

When attempting to look at a dental radiograph, it is important to have an organized thought process so that the entire image can be reviewed and both normal and abnormal structures can be identified. The image needs to be well positioned prior to evaluation. This means that the image should have minimal elongation, foreshortening, and cone cutting and have visualization of as much of the apex of the tooth as possible, as positioning artifacts can cause distortion of structures leading to overinterpretation or underinterpretation of a radiographic image.

Elongation
Elongation is where the radiographic beam is not placed perpendicular to the bisecting angle. This causes the area of interest to appear longer than it should be. To correct elongation, the radiographic beam should be placed more on top of the roots or positioned more at a 12 o'clock position (see Figures 2.20, 2.39a, b, 2.40a, and b, Table 2.3). For more information regarding radiographic positioning, see Chapter 2.

Foreshortening
Foreshortening is where the radiographic beam is not placed perpendicular to the bisecting angle. This positioning error causes the area of interest to be smaller than it should be. To correct foreshortening, the radiographic beam should be positioned more lateral to the roots or more toward the horizon (see Figures 2.37a, b, 2.38a, and b, Table 2.3). For more information regarding radiographic positioning, see Chapter 2.

Cone Cutting
Cone cutting is a positioning artifact in which the entire area of the film is not exposed (see Figures 2.39b and 2.41, Table 2.3). It creates a white ring or rim of unexposed film on the radiographic image. There are three main techniques to correct this error: move the film into the radiographic beam, move the radiographic beam over the film, or back the tube head away from the film, so that more scattered radiation exposes the film. For more information regarding radiographic positioning, see Chapter 2.

Missing the Apex

For an ideal radiograph, the interpreter should be able to visualize at least 2 mm of tissue apical to the radiographic apex of the tooth root (see Figures 2.40b and 2.44b, Table 2.3). If at least 2 mm of tissue is not able to be visualized, the interpreter risks the chance of missing pathology present at the apical extent of the tooth. Visualizing at least 2 mm of tissue is thought to be the minimum amount to verify that no evidence of disease is present around the apex of the root. Clear visualization of at least 2 mm of tissue around the apical extent of the root of the tooth is imperative to help diagnose any pathology that may be present which could be an indication of endodontic disease. For more information regarding radiographic positioning, see Chapter 2.

Mounting of Standard Dental Radiographs

In viewing dental radiographs using standard film, there is dimple in the corner of the intraoral film pocket (Figure 3.1). When viewing standard film, all dimples must be placed in the same direction (all dimples are places in a convex position, or all dimples placed in a concave position) when they are mounted for interpretation. The convex surface (raised surface pointing toward viewer) should always be positioned toward the observer.

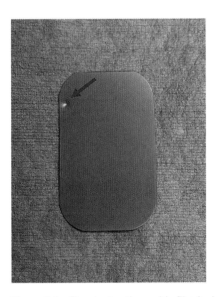

Figure 3.1 Standard radiographic film includes a dimple in the corner of the film. The red arrow identifies the dimple present on the film. The dimple helps the observer in proper placement of the film for interpreting the image. All dimples should be placed in the same direction. Labial mounting of radiographic images is the preferred method of viewing dental radiographs. Bottom line for labial mounting: point your finger to the point of the dimple...POINT TO POINT.

When procuring the radiographic image, the dimple should be positioned toward the radiographic beam. Positioning the raised dimple toward the viewer simulates the viewer in same position as the radiographic generator when it procures the image. This would be the position for labial mounting of the image. If the concave surface (curved surface pointing toward the viewer) is positioned toward the viewer, this would simulate the viewer interpreting the images from inside the patient's mouth. This would be deemed lingual mounting. Labial mounting of radiographic images is the preferred method of viewing dental radiographs.

Types of Mounting

There are two main types of film mounting for dental radiographic images: labial mounting and lingual mounting.

Labial Mounting

If dental radiographic films are placed in a labial mounted format, the films are viewed as if the interpreter is standing outside the patient's mouth looking inward. Therefore, the left side of the patient is on the interpreter's right side and the right side of the patient is on the interpreter's left side. The maxillary arcade would be on top of the mandibular arcade. Labial mounting is the preferred method of viewing the oral cavity (Figure 3.2).

Lingual Mounting

If dental radiographic films are positioned in a lingual mounted format, the films are viewed as if the interpreter is standing inside the patient's mouth looking outward from the mouth. Therefore, the left side of the patient is on the interpreter's left and the right side of the patient is on the interpreter's right. The maxillary arcade would be on top of the mandibular arcade (Figure 3.3).

Labial Mounting of Standard Dental Radiographic Film

On standard radiographic film if the dot or dimple is raised or convex, the interpretation should be performed as if the observer is viewing the images from the outside looking into the patient's mouth, hence labial mounting (Figure 3.4).

Lingual Mounting of Standard Radiographic Film

On standard radiographic film if the raised portion of the dot or dimple is away from the interpreter or in a concave position in relation to the interpreter, the interpretation should be performed as if the observer is inside the mouth of the patient looking out, hence lingual mounting (Figure 3.5).

Labial mounting

Right maxilla   Left maxilla

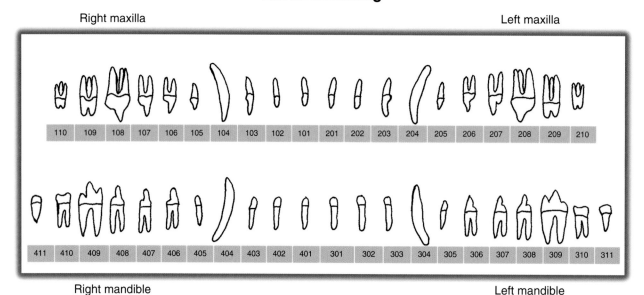

Right mandible   Left mandible

Figure 3.2   Diagram depicts labial mounting of the teeth of a dog. The MAXILLARY teeth should be oriented with the CROWNS of the teeth oriented DOWNWARD, and the CROWNS of the MANDIBULAR teeth oriented UPWARD. The RIGHT MAXILLA and RIGHT MANDIBLE should be viewed on the observers LEFT. The LEFT MAXILLA and LEFT MANDIBLE should be on the observers RIGHT. Labial mounting of the radiographic images depicts the viewer observing the images from OUTSIDE the patient's mouth looking INSIDE.

Lingual mounting

Left maxilla   Right maxilla

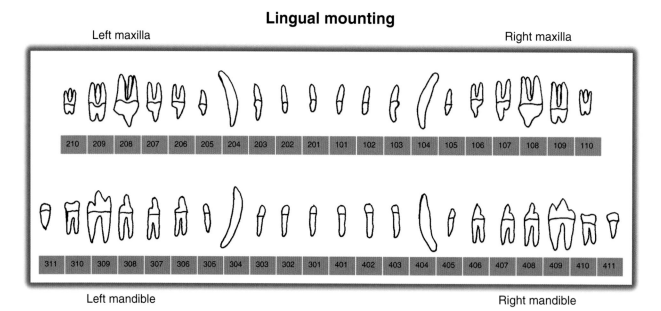

Left mandible   Right mandible

Figure 3.3   Diagram depicts lingual mounting of the teeth of a dog. The MAXILLARY teeth should be oriented with the CROWNS of the teeth oriented DOWNWARD, and the CROWNS of the MANDIBULAR teeth oriented UPWARD. The RIGHT MAXILLA and RIGHT MANDIBLE should be viewed on the observers RIGHT. The LEFT MAXILLA and LEFT MANDIBLE should be on the observers LEFT. Lingual mounting of the radiographic images depicts the viewer observing the images from INSIDE the patient's mouth looking OUTSIDE.

Digital Radiographic Mounting

Computer software created for digital dental radiographic units are designed to appropriately position the image in a standard mounting format. Since labial radiographic mounting is the preferred method of mounting, the rest of the book will focus on the interpretation of radiographic images being viewed and interpreted with standard labial mounting unless specified otherwise.

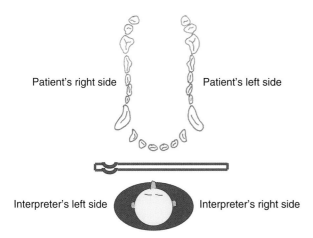

Patient's right side   Patient's left side

Interpreter's left side   Interpreter's right side

Figure 3.4 Diagram depicts labial mounting of the teeth. Note the viewer is OUTSIDE the patient's mouth looking toward the teeth. Also note the dimple of the standard radiographic film is oriented toward the viewer. When labial mounting is utilized the patient's RIGHT side is on the viewer's LEFT side and the patient's LEFT side is on the viewer's RIGHT.

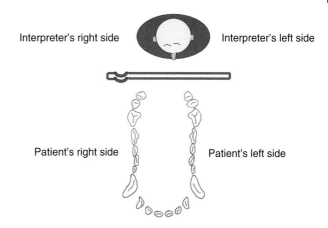

Interpreter's right side   Interpreter's left side

Patient's right side   Patient's left side

Figure 3.5 Diagram depicts lingual mounting of the teeth. Note the viewer is INSIDE the patient's mouth looking toward the teeth. Also note the dimple of the standard radiographic film is oriented away from the viewer. When lingual mounting is utilized the patient's RIGHT side is on the viewer's RIGHT and the patient's LEFT side is on the viewer's LEFT.

Labial Mounting-Positioning of Teeth

For appropriate labial mounting, the maxillary incisors should be positioned with the crowns of the teeth pointing downward and the roots of the maxillary teeth pointing upward. For the mandibular incisors, the crowns of the teeth should be positioned upward, and the roots of the incisor teeth should be pointing downward. Positioning should be as if the patient is looking at the interpreter. For the maxillary canine, premolar and molar teeth, the crowns should be pointing downward, and the roots of these teeth should be pointing upward, just as in the positing of the maxillary incisors. For the mandibular canines, premolars, and molars, the crowns of the teeth should be pointing upward, and the roots of the teeth should be pointing downward, similar to the positioning of the mandibular incisor teeth. The teeth should be viewed as if the patient was looking at the interpreter (Box 3.1) (Figure 3.6).

Determining Maxilla from Mandible

When interpreting images using the labial mounting technique, the interpreter needs to determine the maxilla from the mandible. Maxillary teeth should have evidence of the sinus cavity present. Overall, the maxilla should appear "busier" than the mandible as there are more soft tissue and bony structures present, leading to superimposition of multiple structures in a single area (Figure 3.7a and b). The mandible should have evidence of the mandibular cortex or an increased bony density to the outermost edge of the bone, compared to the airy presence of the nasal concha contained within the maxilla. The mandibular canal which encloses the mandibular artery and vein is visualized

dorsal to the compact bone of the ventral mandible or the mandibular cortex. The mandibular canal is the radiolucent area coursing parallel to the mandibular cortex (Figure 3.8a and b). Again, when interpreting the hard tissues of the mouth, the maxillary teeth should be positioned with crowns down and roots positioned upward, and the mandibular teeth positioned with crowns upward and roots downward as well.

Determining Right from Left
Maxillary and Mandibular Canines, Premolars, and Molars
When viewing a radiographic image of a maxillary or mandibular arcade, it is important to determine whether the left or right side of the patient is being evaluated. For labial mounting and positioning of the radiographic images for interpretation, the right maxillary canine, premolar, and molar teeth that are the most rostral in the mouth should be positioned to the right-hand side of the screen or film, while the caudal most teeth, such as the molars, should be placed more on the left-hand side of the screen or film. When viewing the left arcade, the teeth that are most rostral in the mouth, such as the canines and 1st and 2nd premolar teeth, should be positioned to the left-hand side of the screen or film, while the caudal most teeth should be positioned more on the right-hand side of the screen or film. The mandibular arcade should be positioned similarly (Figure 3.9a and b).

Maxillary and Mandibular Incisors
When viewing the maxillary and mandibular incisor teeth, the first step in discerning the right side from the left side is to confirm the orientation of the radiograph is appropriate.

Box 3.1   Labial mounting

This Box describes the proper way to place radiographic images for appropriate labial mounting. It is recommended that dental radiographic images be mounted in this fashion so that they can be viewed systematically. Traditional dental radiographic images are difficult to label directly on the film due to their size, therefore using consistent labial mounting helps the observer to distinguish the right side from the left side based on the image's positioning.

- Maxillary incisors are positioned with the crowns pointing downward and the roots pointing upward.
- Mandibular incisors are positioned with the crowns pointing upward and the roots pointing downward.
- When viewing the right maxilla or mandible, the teeth closest to the incisors (most rostral teeth) are positioned to the interpreter's right as they are looking at the images.
- When viewing the left maxilla or mandible, the teeth closest to the incisors (most rostral teeth) are positioned to the interpreter's left as they are looking at the images.
- When viewing the maxillary canines, premolars, and molars, the crowns should be pointing downward, and the roots should be pointing upward.
- When viewing the mandibular canines, premolars, and molars, the crowns should be pointing upward, and the roots should be pointing downward.

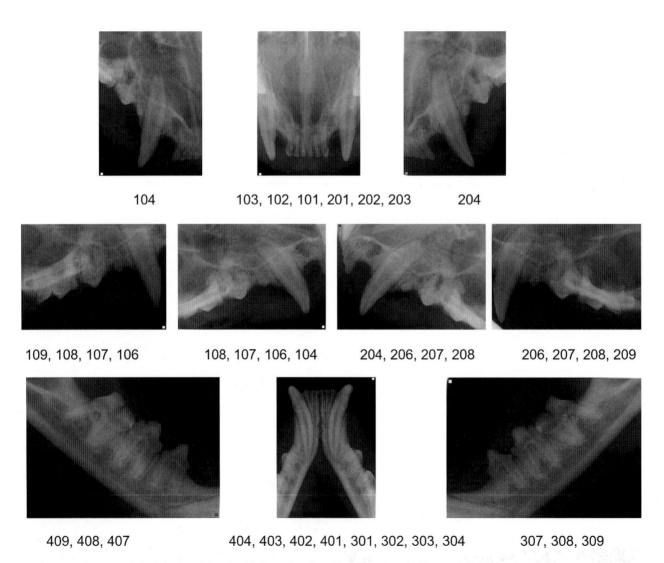

Figure 3.6   Image depicts labial mounting of a full-mouth series of intraoral dental radiographs of a cat. The numbers below the images identify which teeth the radiographs were targeted to acquire.

(a)

(b)

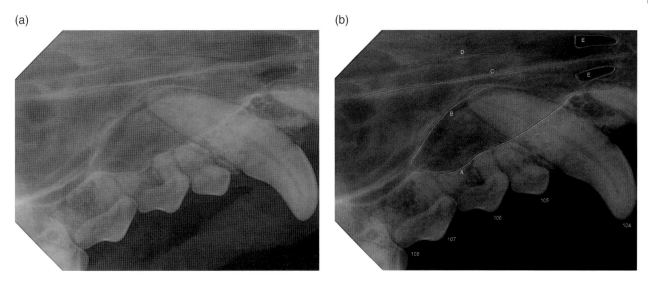

Figure 3.7   (a) Radiographic image of the right maxilla of a dog. Note how the area over the maxillary canine has a "busier" appearance. (b) Radiographic image of the right maxilla of a dog. (Same image as Figure (a).) (A) Nasal surface of the alveolar process of the maxilla, (B) Conchal crest, (C) Vomer, (D) Nasoincisive suture, (E) Palatine fissures.

(a)

(b)

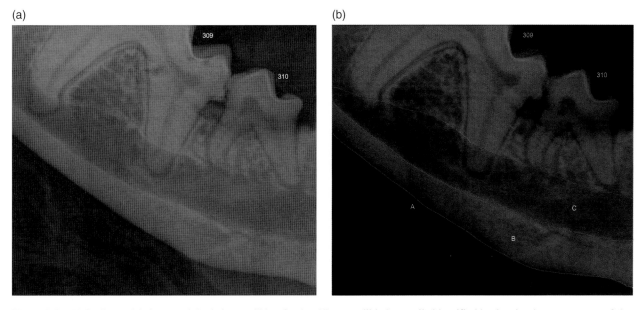

Figure 3.8   (a) Radiographic image of the left mandible of a dog. The mandible is usually identified by the simpler appearance of the image or by visualization of the mandibular cortex. The mandibular canal courses parallel along the length of the body of the mandible and is characterized by a more radiolucent appearing structure that appears close to the ventral cortex. (b) Radiographic image of the left mandible of a dog. (Same image as in Figure (a).) (A) Ventral surface of the mandibular cortex, (B) Compact bone of the ventral mandible, body of the mandibular cortex, (C) Mandibular canal.

For the maxilla, the crowns of the maxillary incisors should be positioned downward, while the roots of these teeth should be positioned upward (Figure 3.10a and b). For the mandibular incisors, the crowns of these teeth should be positioned upward, and the roots should be positioned downward (Figure 3.11a and b). When the images are viewed in this manner, the image can be interpreted as a true radiographic image with the left side of the image described as the patient's right side and the right side of the image described as the patient's left side (Figure 3.12).

(a)

(b)

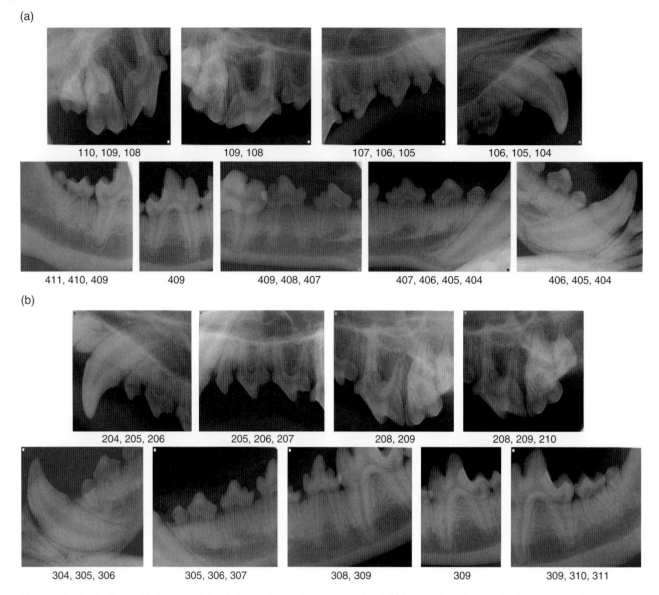

Figure 3.9 (a) Radiographic images of the right maxilla and mandible using labial mounting. The numbering below each radiographic image depicts which tooth or teeth were the target for radiographic procurement. The teeth that are closest to midline should be positioned closer to the arcade being imaged. For example, the right maxillary canine tooth (104) is positioned as far to the right as possible. The right maxillary 2nd molar (110) is the farthest away from the right side for viewing the right side. Similarly, the right mandibular canine tooth (404) is positioned to the right-hand side of the image, while the right mandibular 3rd molar (411) is positioned to the left-hand side of the image. (b) Radiographic images of the left maxilla and mandible using labial mounting. The numbering below each radiographic image depicts which tooth or teeth were the target for radiographic procurement. The teeth that are closest to midline should be positioned closer to the arcade being imaged. For example, the left maxillary canine tooth (204) is positioned as far to the left as possible. The left maxillary 2nd molar (210) is the farthest away from the left side. Similarly, the left mandibular canine tooth (304) is positioned to the left side of the image and the left mandibular 3rd molar tooth (311) is positioned to the right side of the image.

Modified Triadan Numbering System

The modified Triadan numbering system is a systematic method of numbering the teeth within the oral cavity across multiple species. Each tooth within the arcade is given a three-digit number. This number corresponds to whether the tooth is permanent or deciduous, the quadrant in which it resides, and its location within the oral cavity [4]. The first number in the sequence defines which quadrant the tooth is located and whether it is a permanent or deciduous tooth. The numbering system begins with the permanent teeth of the right upper, or maxillary quadrant, being identified as 1,

(a)

(b)

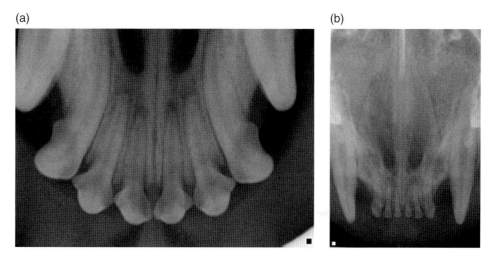

Figure 3.10   (a) Radiographic image of the rostral maxilla of a dog. The radiographic image is diagnostic for the central incisors (right and left maxillary 1st and 2nd incisors) 101, 102, 201, and 202. The image is not diagnostic for the right and left maxillary 3rd incisors as there is less than 2 mm of apex visualized on the image. In an image that utilizes labial mounting, the right maxillary incisors are on the left side of the image and the left maxillary incisors are on the right side of the image. (b) Radiographic image of the rostral maxilla of a cat. The radiographic image is diagnostic for all incisor teeth of the cat (101–103, 201–203). In an image that utilizes labial mounting, the right maxillary incisors are on the left side of the image and the left maxillary incisors are on the right side of the image.

(a)

(b)

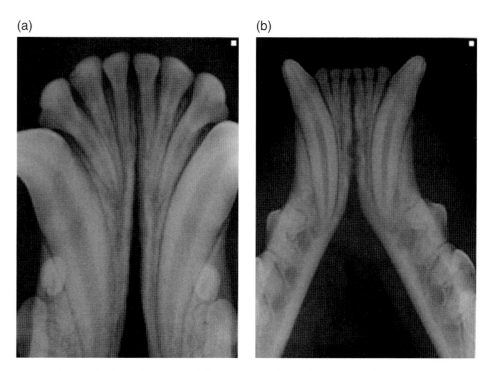

Figure 3.11   (a) Radiographic image of the rostral mandible of a dog. Note the appearance of the mandibular symphysis and the separation between the two mandibles. This is normal as the mandibular symphysis is joined through a fibrocartilaginous union allowing each side of the mandible to move and grow independently. In an image that utilizes labial mounting, the right mandibular incisors are on the left side of the image and the left mandibular incisors are on the right side of the image. This image would be diagnostic for all mandibular incisors. (b) Radiographic image of the rostral mandible of a cat. Note the appearance of the mandibular symphysis and the separation between the two mandibles. This is normal as the mandibular symphysis is joined through a fibrocartilaginous union allowing each side of the mandible to move and grow independently. In an image that utilizes labial mounting, the right mandibular incisors are on the left side of the image and the left mandibular incisors are on the right side of the image. This image would be diagnostic for all mandibular incisor teeth as well as the right and left mandibular canine teeth.

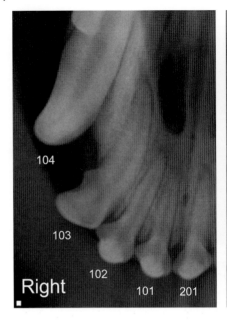
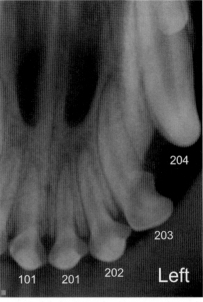

Figure 3.12 Radiographic images of the rostral maxilla of a dog. Two images may be needed to assess all the maxillary incisor teeth depending on the size of the dog. The dog in the images is a beagle. In an image that utilizes labial mounting, the right maxillary incisors are on the left side of the image and the left maxillary incisors are on the right side of the image.

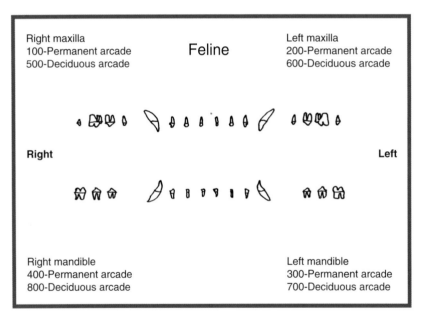

Figure 3.13 Diagram depicts the right and left maxillary and mandibular arcade identification according to the modified Triadan numbering system. In the permanent dentition, arcades are numbered as either 100s, 200s, 300s, or 400s. The deciduous dentition is numbered as 500s, 600s, 700s, or 800s depending on the arcade and side identified.

the permanent dentition of the left maxillary quadrant is identified as 2, left lower or mandibular quadrant as 3, and the right mandibular quadrant as 4. In the deciduous dentition, the numbering begins with the right maxillary quadrant being 5, the left maxillary quadrant 6, the left mandibular quadrant 7, and the right mandibular quadrant 8 [4] (Figure 3.13). The next digits correspond to the location of the tooth within the oral cavity [4]. The numbering of teeth begins just to the right or left of midline. The numbers continue consecutively beginning with 01 and proceed increasing in order distally. This designates their presence in the front of the oral cavity or the caudal aspect of the oral cavity. The next adjacent tooth is 02 followed by 03 and so on. The higher the number, the farther caudal in the mouth the tooth is located (Figure 3.14). The dog and cat do not share the same number of teeth, with the cat having fewer teeth than the dog. The modified Triadan numbering system allows for tooth numbering to be consistent when applied to the different species. Since cats have fewer premolar and molar teeth, the assigned number of the canine tooth and the first molar tooth remain the same between the two species, 04 and 09, respectively [4]. This is considered "The Rule of 4 and 9" [4]. This rule states that all canine teeth end with the digit 04 and all first molars end in

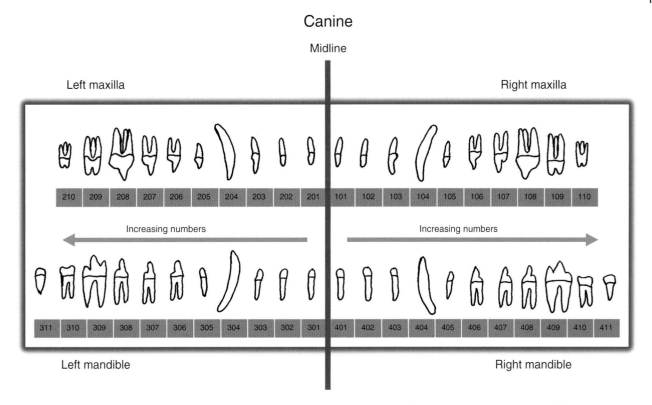

Figure 3.14 Diagram depicts the modified Triadan numbering system for the dog. After designating the arcade and side of the patient, the numbering continues with the individual teeth beginning with the lowest number closest to midline being 01 and the teeth farthest from midline being 10 for the maxilla and 11 for the mandible of the dog.

the digit 09 [4]. Therefore, these numbers remain consistent regardless of the number of teeth present within the oral cavity or the species of the patient [4].

The modified Triadan numbering system numbers the teeth by their association, root structure, and appearance. For species that are anatomically missing teeth, such as the cat, gaps are left in the number sequence where the teeth are normally not present within the oral cavity [4]. Therefore, for the maxillary arcade in the cat, the first tooth behind the canine tooth is deemed the 2nd premolar. This tooth frequently has one to two roots, although they are commonly fused together. This tooth is numbered 06 and is designated as the maxillary 2nd premolar. In the feline mandible, the cat has two premolar teeth between the canine tooth and the first molar tooth. These teeth are designated the 3rd and 4th premolars and are numbered as such with a designation of the third premolar as 07 and the 4th premolar as 08 (Figure 3.15).

Deciduous versus Permanent Teeth

Clinically when evaluating deciduous teeth from permanent teeth, the clinician needs to consider the age of the patient and the clinical and radiographic appearance of the

teeth. Evaluation should include a knowledge of the deciduous and permanent dental formulas accepted as normal for a given species (Tables 3.1–3.4). On clinical evaluation, deciduous teeth in the dog and cat can have similar appearance to the permanent teeth. Especially when evaluating the premolar teeth. In the dog, the deciduous premolar teeth look like the permanent teeth that erupt distally. Therefore, the deciduous maxillary 2nd premolar tooth has the appearance both clinically and radiographically of the permanent 3rd premolar tooth. The deciduous 3rd premolar has the radiographic and clinical appearance of a permanent 4th premolar tooth, and the deciduous 4th premolar tooth has the clinical and radiographic appearance of the first molar tooth. Clinically, the deciduous teeth are generally not as white as the permanent teeth. Deciduous teeth are frequently thinner and wispier looking and have the appearance of being less robust (Figure 3.16a–e).

Eruption Patterns

It is imperative that the interpreter understands the eruption pattern for both the deciduous and the permanent teeth. This allows the clinician to identify what teeth

Feline

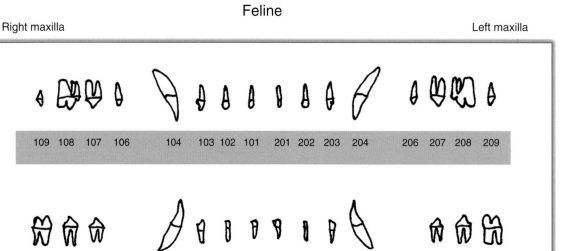

Right maxilla | Left maxilla

| 109 | 108 | 107 | 106 | | 104 | 103 | 102 | 101 | 201 | 202 | 203 | 204 | | 206 | 207 | 208 | 209 |

| 409 | 408 | 407 | | 404 | 403 | 402 | 401 | 301 | 302 | 303 | 304 | | 307 | 308 | 309 |

Right mandible | Left mandible

Figure 3.15 Diagram depicts the modified Triadan numbering system for the cat. After designating the arcade and side of the patient, the numbering continues with the individual teeth beginning with the lowest number closest to midline being 01 and the teeth farthest from midline being 09 for the maxilla and mandible of the cat. Because cats have fewer teeth, the numbering is adjusted to maintain the canine tooth as a 04 and the first molar tooth as a 09. Therefore, for the maxilla of the cat, the first tooth distal to the canine tooth is actually the 2nd premolar, as they do not have a 1st premolar tooth. In the mandible, the first tooth distal to the canine is the 3rd premolar as they do not have a 1st or 2nd premolar tooth.

should be present within the oral cavity based on the reported age of the patient. Deciduous teeth should begin exfoliating from the oral cavity of the cat at approximately three months of age and be finished by approximately six months of age [5]. For the dog, the deciduous teeth begin exfoliating at approximately three months of age, similarly to the cat [5]. All permanent teeth in canine and feline species should show some evidence of eruption of the permanent teeth by seven months of age [5] (Table 3.5). If there is no clinical evidence of eruption occurring, dental radiographs need to be considered to evaluate for the presence of unerupted or impacted teeth, or any additional pathology that may result in delayed eruption or non-eruption of the dentition.

If there are clinically missing teeth in the oral cavity and the dog or cat is over seven months of age, radiographs are warranted to evaluate whether there are unerupted teeth below the gingiva or alveolar bone margin, or whether these missing teeth are truly congenitally missing. Teeth that are found unerupted or impacted are abnormal and may warrant treatment which may include operculectomy, extraction, or orthodontic extrusion into the oral cavity.

Mixed Dentition

Mixed dentition is a condition in which there are both permanent and deciduous teeth present simultaneously within the oral cavity. This condition is undesirable in canine and feline species as it can result in a malocclusion [6]. Appropriate eruption of teeth within dogs and cats occurs with the deciduous teeth exfoliating prior to the eruption of permanent teeth. This allows the permanent teeth to erupt into a more appropriate position. If deciduous teeth persistently remain in the oral cavity, the permanent successors are forced to erupt in the oral cavity in an abnormal position (Figure 3.17a and b). When teeth erupt into the oral cavity, they usually begin with the eruption of the incisors. If there is a mixed dentition present, the permanent incisors erupt lingual or palatal to the deciduous incisor teeth (Figure 3.18a and b). If there are no persistent deciduous teeth present, the permanent teeth erupt through the same eruption pattern as the deciduous teeth that have already exfoliated. Permanent maxillary canine teeth erupt mesial to the deciduous teeth if they are still present (Figures 3.19 and 3.20). Permanent mandibular canine teeth erupt lingual to the deciduous teeth if they are still present (Figures 3.19

Table 3.1 Permanent dental formula of the dog including both maxillary and mandibular teeth and their respective tooth numbers according to the Triadan numbering system.

Dog – permanent maxillary teeth

	Right maxilla										Left maxilla										
Tooth	M2	M1	PM4	PM3	PM2	PM1	C	I3	I2	I1	I1	I2	I3	C	PM1	PM2	PM3	PM4	M1	M2	
Tooth number	110	109	108	107	106	105	104	103	102	101	201	202	203	204	205	206	207	208	209	210	

Dog – permanent mandibular teeth

	Right mandible											Left mandible										
Tooth	M3	M2	M1	PM4	PM3	PM2	PM1	C	I3	I2	I1	I1	I2	I3	C	PM1	PM2	PM3	PM4	M1	M2	M3
Tooth number	411	410	409	408	407	406	405	404	403	402	401	301	302	303	304	305	306	307	308	309	310	311

Table 3.2 Deciduous dental formula of the dog including both maxillary and mandibular teeth and their respective tooth numbers according to the Triadan numbering system.

Dog – deciduous maxillary teeth																
Right maxilla									Left maxilla							
Tooth	pm4	pm3	pm2	pm1	c	i3	i2	i1	i1	i2	i3	c	pm1	pm2	pm3	pm4
Tooth number	508	507	506	*	504	503	502	501	601	602	603	604	*	606	607	608

Dog – deciduous mandibular teeth																
Right mandible									Left mandible							
Tooth	pm4	pm3	pm2	pm1	c	i3	i2	i1	i1	i2	i3	c	pm1	pm2	pm3	pm4
Tooth number	808	807	806	*	804	803	802	801	701	702	703	704	*	706	707	708

The asterisk is placed to identify the normally missing teeth in the dental arcade of the dog.

Table 3.3 Permanent dental formula of the cat including both maxillary and mandibular teeth and their respective tooth numbers according to the Triadan numbering system.

Cat – permanent maxillary teeth																		
Right maxilla										Left maxilla								
Tooth	M1	PM4	PM3	PM2	PM1	C	I3	I2	I1	I1	I2	I3	C	PM1	PM2	PM3	PM4	M1
Tooth number	109	108	107	106	*	104	103	102	101	201	202	203	204	*	206	207	208	209

Cat – permanent mandibular teeth																		
Right mandible										Left mandible								
Tooth	M1	PM4	PM3	PM2	PM1	C	I3	I2	I1	I1	I2	I3	C	PM1	PM2	PM3	PM4	M1
Tooth number	409	408	407	*	*	404	403	402	401	301	302	303	304	*	*	307	308	309

The asterisk is placed to identify the normally missing teeth in the dental arcade of the cat.

Table 3.4 Deciduous dental formula of the cat including both maxillary and mandibular teeth and their respective tooth numbers according to the Triadan numbering system.

Cat – deciduous maxillary teeth																
Right maxilla									Left maxilla							
Tooth	pm4	pm3	pm2	pm1	c	i3	i2	i1	i1	i2	i3	c	pm1	pm2	pm3	pm4
Tooth number	508	507	506	*	504	503	502	501	601	602	603	604	*	606	607	608

Cat – deciduous mandibular teeth																
Right mandible									Left mandible							
Tooth	pm4	pm3	pm2	pm1	c	i3	i2	i1	i1	i2	i3	c	pm1	pm2	pm3	pm4
Tooth number	808	807	*	*	804	803	802	801	701	702	703	704	*	*	707	708

The asterisk is placed to identify the normally missing teeth in the dental arcade of the cat.

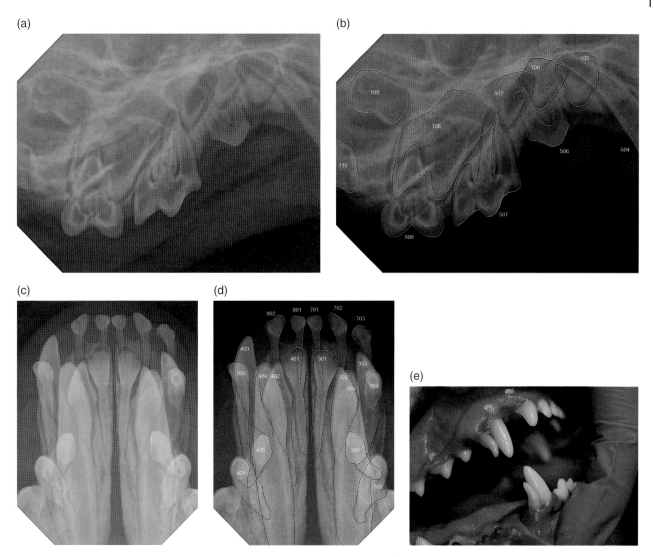

Figure 3.16 (a) Radiographic image of the right maxilla of a dog. The image depicts an erupted deciduous dentition with developing tooth buds of the successor teeth. (b) Radiographic image of the right maxilla of a dog. The image depicts an erupted deciduous dentition. Note how the erupted deciduous teeth have a similar root structure and appearance to the permanent teeth that would erupt behind them. For example, the deciduous maxillary 3rd premolar (507) has the radiographic appearance of a permanent maxillary 4th premolar (108). Also note the appearance of the erupting tooth buds as illustrated by the radiolucent area more apical to the roots of the erupted teeth. Notice the increased radiodensity of the developing crowns of these unerupted successor teeth. (Same image as Figure (a).) (c) Radiographic image of the rostral mandible of a dog. The image depicts an erupted deciduous dentition with developing successor teeth prior to eruption. (d) Radiographic image of the rostral mandible of a dog. The image depicts an erupted deciduous dentition with developing successor teeth prior to eruption. Note the difference in size between the unerupted teeth and the erupted teeth. Also notice the increased radiodensity to the successor teeth. (e) Clinical image of a patient with permanent and persistent deciduous right maxillary and mandibular canine teeth. Note the persistent deciduous canine teeth are not as white as the permanent teeth. They are also smaller, sharper, and pointier than the permanent successor teeth.

and 3.20). Permanent premolar teeth usually erupt beneath or just lingual to the deciduous teeth if they are still present (Figure 3.21a–c). In the author's experience, the most common persistent deciduous teeth observed are the maxillary and mandibular canine teeth as well as the maxillary and mandibular incisors.

If a deciduous tooth is clinically missing in the oral cavity, there is a high likelihood the permanent successor tooth will also be clinically missing. If there is a persistent deciduous tooth that is present with no clinical evidence of a permanent successor, dental radiographs are warranted to evaluate whether a successor exists. It is not uncommon to have a patient with mature permanent teeth present and erupted, and the discovery of a persistent deciduous tooth within the oral cavity without a permanent successor (Figure 3.22a and b). As long as the persistent deciduous

Table 3.5 Expected eruption pattens of the incisors, canines, premolars, and molars of the dog and cat.

Canine and feline eruption patterns	Incisors	Canines	Premolars	Molars
Canine				
Deciduous	3–4 wk	3 wk	2–12 wk	*
Permanent	3–5 mo	4–6 mo	4–6 mo	5–7 mo
Feline				
Deciduous	3–4 wk	3–4 wk	5–6 wk	*
Permanent	3–4 mo	3–5 mo	4–5 mo	5–6 mo

All permanent teeth in the dog and cat should show some evidence of eruption by seven months of age.
The asterisk is placed to identify the normally missing teeth in the dental arcade of the dog and cat.

(a)   (b)

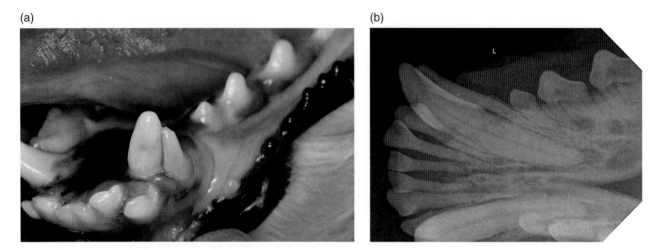

Figure 3.17 (a) Clinical image of a patient with a permanent and persistent deciduous left mandibular canine tooth. For mandibular canine teeth, the permanent successive tooth erupts lingual to the deciduous tooth. If the deciduous tooth persistently remains within the oral cavity as the permanent tooth begins eruption, the permanent tooth is frequently displaced lingually into an abnormal position. (b) Radiographic image of a patient with a permanent and persistent deciduous left mandibular canine tooth. Note how the persistent deciduous tooth root does not demonstrate any evidence of resorption, indicating that it will not likely exfoliate on its own.

tooth is periodontally and endodontically healthy, there may be no need for treatment of the persistent deciduous tooth.

Interpretation of Images

After proper positioning and technique are employed to acquire a diagnostic image, the image needs to be scanned for normal anatomic identifiers as well as confirmation of approximate age of the patient. The age of the patient and the appearance of the teeth should have characteristics of either the deciduous dentition or permanent dentition. Clinically, permanent teeth appear whiter, more robust, and are bigger than deciduous teeth. Clinically, deciduous teeth are thinner, more translucent, and sharper/pointier than permanent teeth. Radiographically,

deciduous teeth appear less mineralized. They usually have a closed root system. An immature permanent tooth radiographically has an open apex until approximately 11 months of age for the canine tooth [7, 8]. If the patient has mixed dentition, the clinical and radiographic appearance of the teeth should correlate with the age of the patient.

Individual teeth have specific anatomic characteristics depending on their appearance (Figure 3.23a and b). Incisor teeth are located in the front of the mouth and have a flat thin edge that is used for cutting food into smaller pieces. They function in tearing and grooming as well as gnawing at the hair or skin. Incisors also function to help hold the tongue in the mouth (Figure 3.24a–f). Canine teeth are the sharp-pointed teeth just distal to the incisor teeth. These teeth are usually the longest teeth and referred to as fangs. Canine teeth function to grab and tear food.

(b)

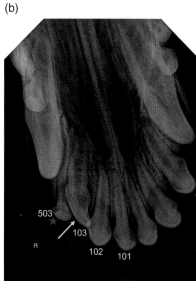

(a)

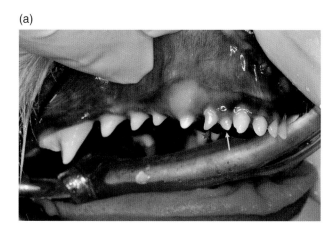

Figure 3.18 (a) Clinical image of the right maxillary arcade of a dog. Note the presence of a persistent deciduous right maxillary 3rd incisor tooth (503) (red star). Also, notice the displacement of the permanent right maxillary 3rd incisor (103) positioned more palatal than normal (yellow arrow). (b) Radiographic image of the rostral maxilla of a dog. Note the presence of a persistent deciduous 3rd incisor (503) (red star). Notice the orientation of the successive permanent incisor (103) (yellow arrow) angled more toward midline. In this patient, the persistent deciduous 503 affected the eruption pattern and position of the successive 3rd incisor (103). Removal of the persistent deciduous tooth may allow the movement of the successive permanent incisor into a more atraumatic position.

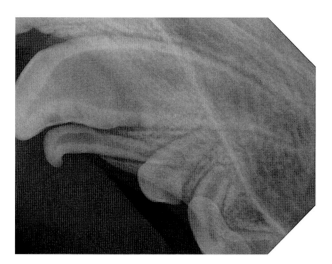

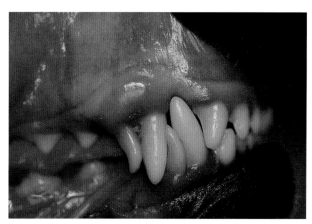

Figure 3.19 Radiographic image of a patient with both a permanent and persistent deciduous left maxillary canine tooth. For maxillary canine teeth, the permanent successive tooth erupts mesial to the deciduous tooth. If the deciduous tooth persistently remains within the oral cavity as the permanent tooth begins eruption, the permanent tooth is displaced mesially into an abnormal position. Note in this patient the large pulp chamber and lack of a formed apex to the permanent successive tooth (204) indicates a juvenile tooth.

Figure 3.20 Clinical image demonstrating the relationship between the permanent and deciduous canine teeth in a dog. The persistent presence of deciduous teeth causes a malocclusion which can result in a traumatic occlusion. Persistent deciduous teeth should be removed as soon as there is evidence of eruption from the permanent successor teeth. This is to allow the permanent teeth to erupt into a more appropriate position. Note the calculus and debris trapped between these two teeth. This can predispose the patient to gingivitis, which can result in loss of attachment as well as eventual loss of both teeth.

They are also used for protection. In working dogs, these teeth function to apprehend individuals or items for the handler (Figure 3.25a–h). Premolar teeth are located on the side of the animal's mouth distal to the canine teeth.

The premolar teeth have a sharper cutting surface and several ridges. Their purpose is to help grind and chew food (Figure 3.26a–i). Molar teeth are located distal to the premolar teeth and round out the caudal aspect of the oral

(a)

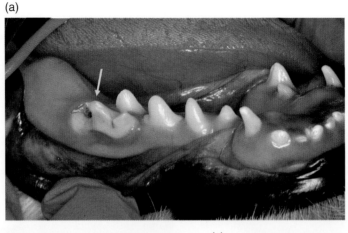

(b)

(c)

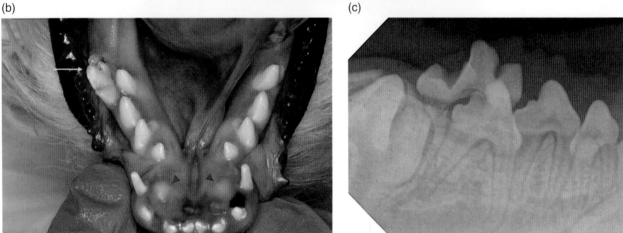

Figure 3.21   (a) Clinical image demonstrating a persistent deciduous right mandibular 4th premolar tooth (808) (yellow arrow). For premolar teeth, persistent deciduous teeth generally erupt more buccally than the permanent successive tooth. Notice how there is a space distal to the persistent deciduous premolar tooth in which there is a raised area of gingiva present. This would be the location of the unerupted right mandibular 1st molar tooth. Note that there is evidence of both right and left deciduous mandibular canine teeth with no obvious evidence of eruption from the permanent mandibular canine teeth. (b) More occlusal clinical image demonstrating a persistent deciduous right mandibular 4th premolar tooth (808) (yellow arrow) which appears more buccally deviated compared to the rest of the teeth in the arcade. For premolar teeth, persistent deciduous premolar teeth generally erupt more buccally than the permanent successor teeth. Note there is evidence of the right and left deciduous mandibular canine teeth. From this view, there is mild blanching (red arrowhead) of the mucosa just lingual to the right and left deciduous canine teeth, which would be suspicious for the start of eruption of the permanent mandibular canine teeth. (c) Radiographic image of the right mandible of a dog. Note the presence of a right mandibular persistent deciduous 4th premolar tooth. Notice how this tooth has the radiographic appearance of a permanent right mandibular 1st molar tooth. There is a more radiolucent halo in the area of the furcation of this tooth and no real recognizable root structure to this tooth. This evidence is consistent with root resorption as expected in a deciduous tooth prior to exfoliation. Also, note in this image the presence of the unerupted right mandibular 1st molar tooth. While there was no obvious clinical evidence of eruption noted with this tooth, it is present and normal eruption is expected.

cavity. The molar teeth are generally the largest teeth. They have a large flat occlusal surface that is used for grinding of food (Figure 3.27a–j).

The maxillary 4th premolar and the mandibular first molar teeth are referred to as carnassial teeth. These teeth function in slicing of meat, shearing meat off the bone as well as slicing through the tough connective tissue of prey that is caught in the wild. These teeth are also referred to as transitional teeth. These transitional teeth have the appearance of being a premolar tooth with a mesial surface that has a point and a ridge and then transition to more of a flat

occlusal surface for grinding as in the molar teeth. These characteristics are significantly more obvious in the mandibular 1st molar tooth in the dog (Figure 3.28a–h).

The interpreting clinician needs to decide whether they are looking at the maxilla or a mandible of the patient when viewing a radiographic image. This is especially important if they are not the ones taking the images. If the interpreter is not present when an assistant is taking the images or if the images are sent from another veterinarian as part of the patient's medical record, the ability to discern maxilla from mandible is imperative.

(a)

(b)

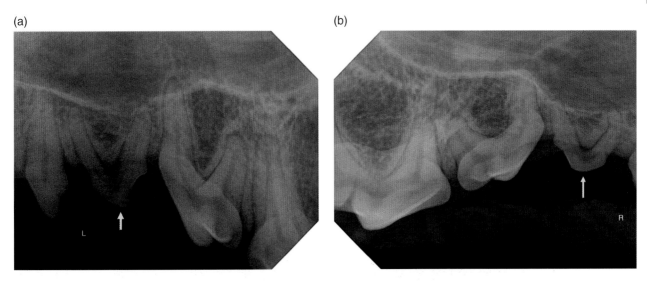

Figure 3.22 (a) Radiographic image of a persistent deciduous left maxillary 2nd premolar tooth (606) (yellow arrow). Note how there is no obvious evidence of an unerupted permanent successor tooth. Notice the appearance of this tooth compared to the surrounding teeth. This tooth is subjectively more radiolucent. The tooth also appears smaller compared to the surrounding teeth. No treatment is necessary for this tooth, provided that there is no clinical or radiographic evidence of disease. (b) Radiographic image of a persistent deciduous right maxillary 2nd premolar tooth (506) (yellow arrow). There is no obvious evidence of an unerupted permanent successor tooth. The tooth is smaller and subjectively more radiolucent than the surrounding teeth. No treatment is necessary for this tooth if there is no clinical or radiographic evidence of disease.

(a)

(b)

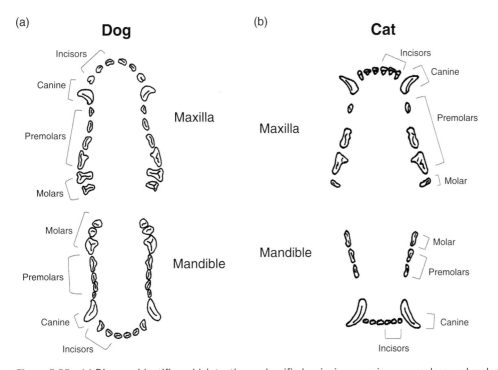

Figure 3.23 (a) Diagram identifies which teeth are classified as incisors, canines, premolars, and molars in the maxilla and mandible of the dog. (b) Diagram identifies which teeth are classified as incisors, canines, premolars, and molars in the maxilla and mandible of the cat.

Radiographs of a patient's maxilla are significantly different from radiographs acquired of the patient's mandible. Maxillary radiographs commonly have evidence of the palatine fissures in the rostral area of the incisors (Figure 3.29a–d). There is also evidence of the nasal cavity and sinuses in the area of the teeth held within the maxilla (Figure 3.30a and b).

Radiographs of the patient's mandible contain evidence of the mandibular symphysis in the rostral area of the oral cavity. At the ventral aspect of the mandible, there is thick

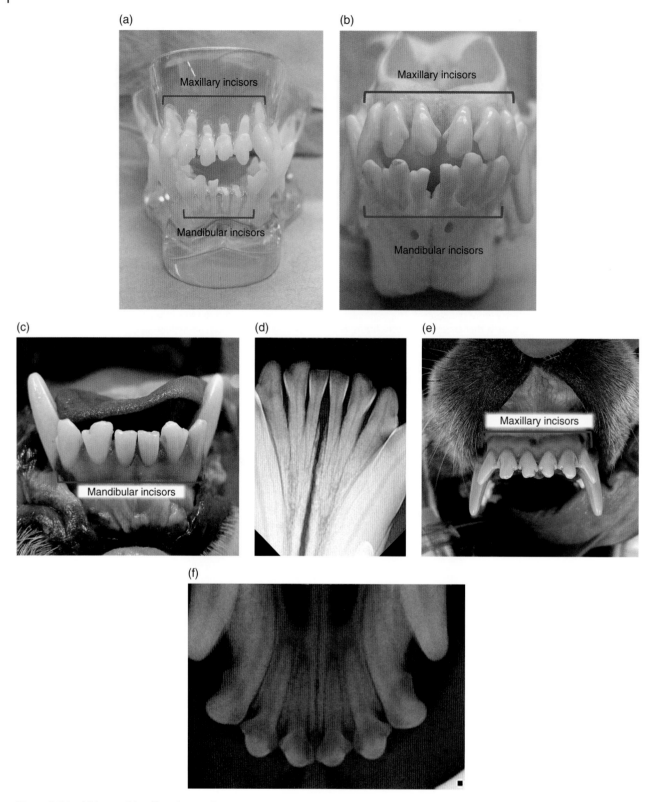

Figure 3.24 (a) Image identifies the maxillary and mandibular incisors on a plastic model of a dog. (b) Image identifies the maxillary and mandibular incisors on a skull of a dog. (c) Clinical image identifies the mandibular incisors of a dog. (d) Radiographic image demonstrates the mandibular incisors of a dog. (e) Clinical image identifies the maxillary incisors of a dog. (f) Radiographic image demonstrates the central maxillary incisors of a dog.

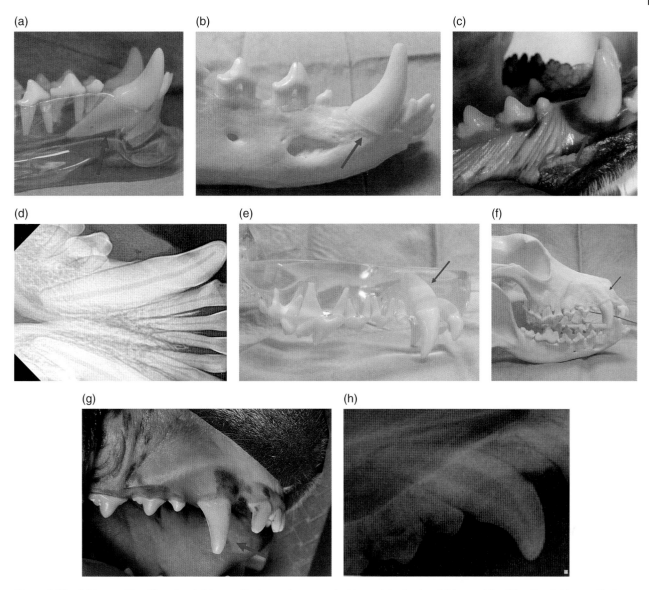

Figure 3.25 (a) Image identifies the right mandibular canine on a plastic model of a dog. (b) Image identifies the right mandibular canine on a skull of a dog. (c) Clinical image identifies the right mandibular canine of a dog. (d) Radiographic image demonstrates the right mandibular canine of a dog. (e) Image identifies the right maxillary canine tooth on a plastic model of a dog. (f) Image identifies the right maxillary canine tooth on a skull of a dog. (g) Clinical image identifies the right maxillary canine tooth of a dog. (h) Radiographic image demonstrates the right maxillary canine tooth of a dog.

cortical bone that comprises the mandibular cortex. In the very caudal aspect of the oral cavity, depending on the size of the patient and the size of the radiographic film, the ramus of the mandible and potentially the angular process of the mandible may be visible (Figure 3.31a and b).

Tooth Root Numbers

Maxillary Teeth

The number of teeth, characteristic size and shape, and individual tooth root numbers vary between the maxilla and mandible. For canine patients, incisor teeth of the maxilla should be single-rooted. The canine teeth should have a single root. The maxillary 1st premolar tooth should have one root. The 2nd and 3rd premolars should have two roots. The 4th premolar and 1st and 2nd molar teeth should all have three roots (Table 3.6). To simplify this, behind the canine tooth, the first tooth has one root, the next two teeth have two roots, and the next three teeth have three roots. While there may be variations of the root structures in which there are fewer or additional roots present, most canine patients maintain this anatomical sequence. When considering the deciduous dentition, the maxillary incisors and canine teeth still

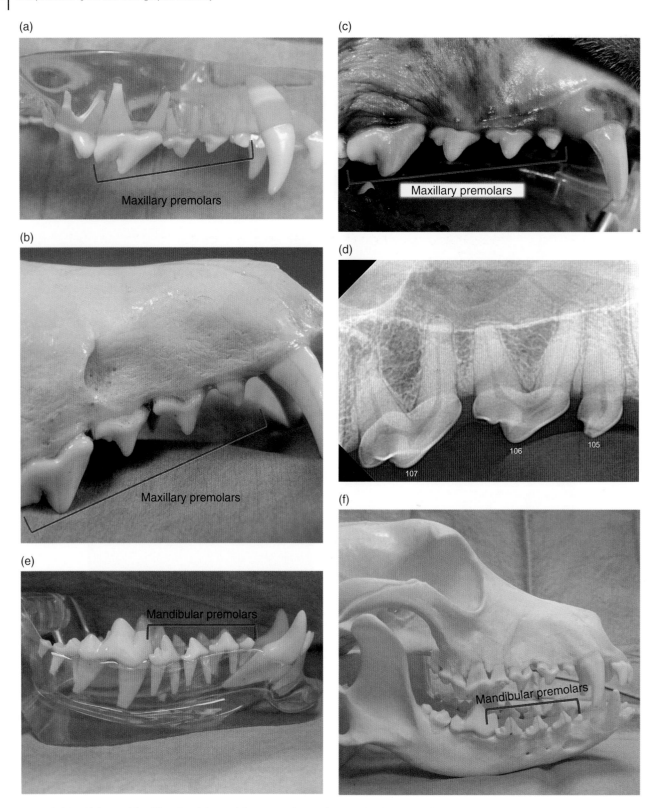

Figure 3.26 (a) Image identifies the right maxillary premolar teeth on a plastic model of a dog. (b) Image identifies the right maxillary premolar teeth on a skull of a dog. (c) Clinical image identifies the right maxillary premolar teeth of a dog. (d) Radiographic image demonstrates the right maxillary 1st, 2nd, and 3rd premolar teeth of a dog. (e) Image identifies the right mandibular premolar teeth on a plastic model of a dog. (f) Image identifies the right mandibular premolar teeth on a skull of a dog. (g) Clinical image identifies the right mandibular premolar teeth of a dog. (h) Radiographic image demonstrates the right mandibular 1st, 2nd, and 3rd premolar teeth of a dog. (i) Radiographic image demonstrates the right mandibular 3rd and 4th premolar teeth of a dog.

(g)

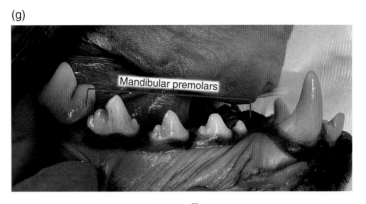

(h)

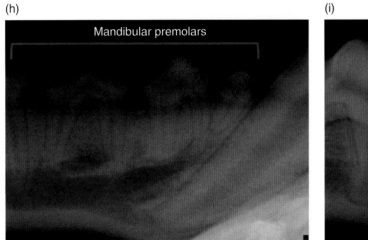

(i)

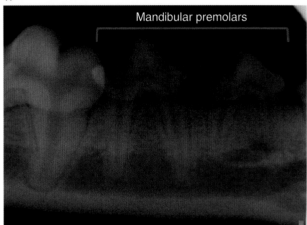

Figure 3.26 (Continued)

maintain one root. There is no deciduous 1st premolar tooth. The first time this tooth makes its appearance within the oral cavity is in the permanent dentition. In observing the deciduous 2nd, 3rd, and 4th premolar teeth, their root structure is similar in appearance to the permanent tooth that erupts *behind* or distal to that deciduous tooth. The deciduous 2nd premolar tooth has two roots, the 3rd premolar has three roots, and the 4th premolar has three roots (Table 3.7). There are no deciduous maxillary 1st or 2nd molar teeth in the dog.

For feline patients, the canines and incisors are single-rooted. The maxillary 2nd premolar has one to two roots. The maxillary 3rd premolar has two roots, while the 4th premolar has three roots. The maxillary 1st molar tooth has one to three roots with much of the time the roots are found fused together to appear as a single root (Table 3.8). The deciduous incisors and canine teeth are single-rooted. The deciduous maxillary 2nd premolar has a single root, the 3rd premolar has two roots, and the 4th premolar has three roots. This is consistent with the permanent dentition (Table 3.9). There are no deciduous maxillary 1st molar teeth in the cat.

Mandibular Teeth

For the permanent dentition of the dog, all mandibular canine and incisor teeth should maintain a single root. The mandibular 1st premolar tooth is single-rooted. The mandibular 2nd, 3rd, and 4th premolars have two roots. The mandibular 1st and 2nd molars also have two roots, while the mandibular 3rd molar is single-rooted (Table 3.10). To simplify this, the first premolar teeth and the 3rd molar teeth are single-rooted, like bookends, while the remaining teeth between these two teeth have two roots. The deciduous mandibular incisors and canine teeth are single-rooted, and the mandibular 2nd, 3rd, and 4th premolars each have two roots. There are no deciduous mandibular 1st premolars or 1st, 2nd, or 3rd molar teeth in the dog (Table 3.11).

For cats, the mandibular canine and incisor teeth maintain a single root in both the permanent and deciduous dentitions. All permanent mandibular premolar and molar teeth have two roots (Table 3.12). The deciduous mandibular premolar teeth also have two roots (Table 3.13). There are no deciduous mandibular 1st molar teeth in the cat.

In addition, as a blanket statement regarding tooth root numbers in the dog and the cat, there should be no three

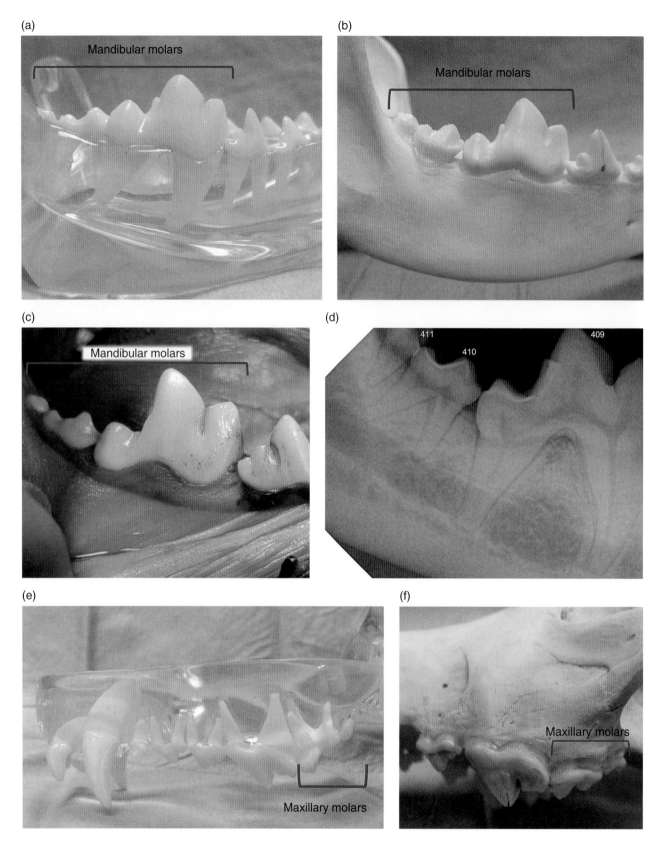

Figure 3.27 (a) Image identifies the right mandibular molar teeth on a plastic model of a dog. (b) Image identifies the right mandibular molar teeth on a skull of a dog. (c) Clinical image identifies the right mandibular molar teeth of a dog. (d) Radiographic image demonstrates the right mandibular 1st, 2nd, and 3rd molar teeth of a dog. (e) Image identifies the left maxillary molar teeth on a plastic model of a dog. (f) Image identifies the left maxillary molar teeth on a skull of a dog. (g) Image identifies the occlusal surface of the left maxillary molar teeth on a skull of a dog. (h) Clinical image of the left maxillary molar teeth of a dog. (i) Clinical image of the occlusal surface of the left maxillary molar teeth of a dog. (j) Radiographic image demonstrates the left maxillary 1st and 2nd molar teeth of a dog. The image would also be diagnostic for the distal root of the left maxillary 4th premolar tooth.

(g)

(h)

(i)

(j)

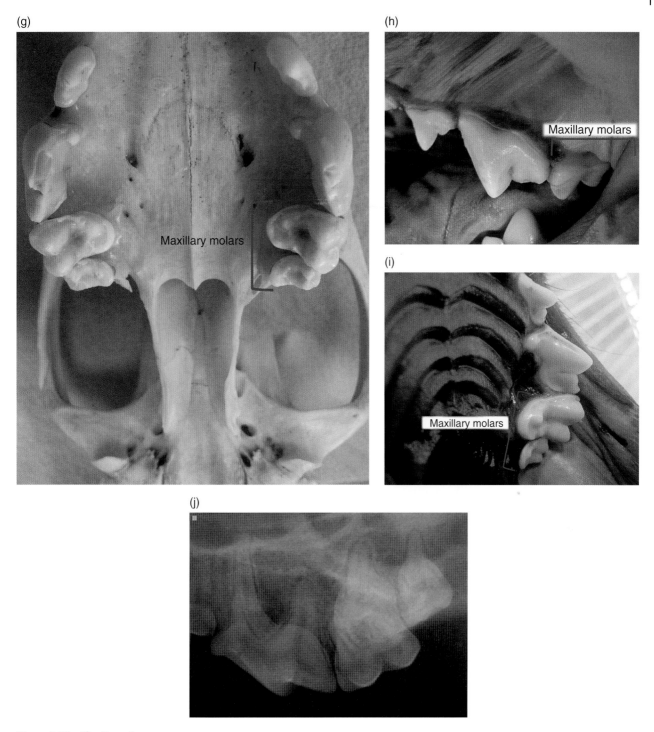

Figure 3.27 (Continued)

rooted teeth in the mandible. If there are three rooted teeth in the mandible, this is an abnormal variation in that specific patient.

Determining whether the right or left side is depicted in a radiographic image depends on whether the image is taken intraorally or extraorally. Most dental radiographic images of canine and feline patients are taken intraorally. If an image is taken extraorally it needs to be marked immediately following image procurement, so the evaluator is aware of the difference in radiographic acquisition. Images of the right side of the patient should be positioned with labial mounting technique with the rostral most teeth

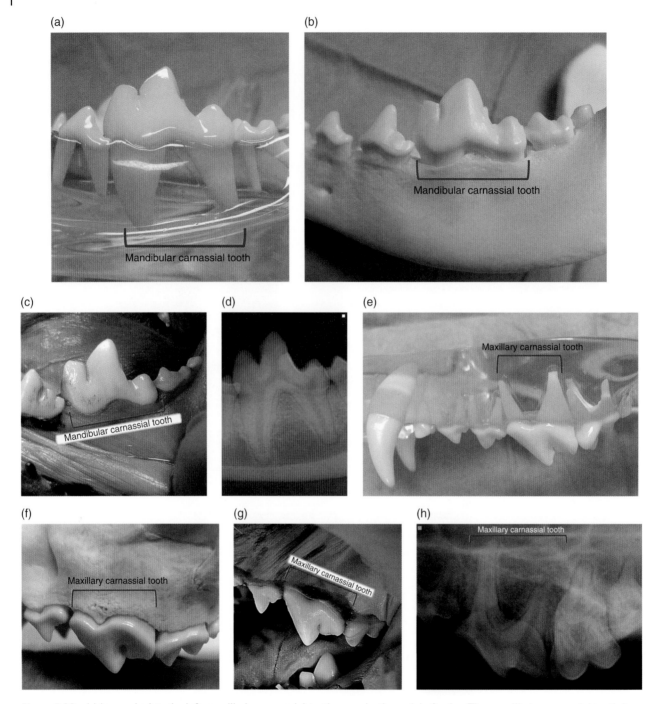

Figure 3.28 (a) Image depicts the left mandibular carnassial tooth on a plastic model of a dog. The mandibular carnassial tooth is identified as the mandibular 1st molar tooth. (b) Image depicts the left mandibular carnassial tooth on the skull of a dog. (c) Clinical image of the left mandibular carnassial tooth of a dog. (d) Radiographic image demonstrates the left mandibular carnassial tooth of a dog. (e) Image depicts the left maxillary carnassial tooth on a plastic model of a dog. The maxillary carnassial tooth is identified as the maxillary 4th premolar tooth. (f) Image depicts the left maxillary carnassial tooth on the skull of a dog. (g) Clinical image of the left maxillary carnassial tooth of a dog. (h) Radiographic image demonstrates the left maxillary carnassial tooth of a dog.

to the viewers right. Images of the patient's left side should be positioned with the rostral most teeth to the viewers left side. The images should also be positioned as if the viewer was looking at the patient with the crowns of the teeth positioned downward for the maxilla and the roots positioned upward. For the mandibular teeth, the crowns should point upward, and the roots should be positioned downward (Figure 3.32a and b).

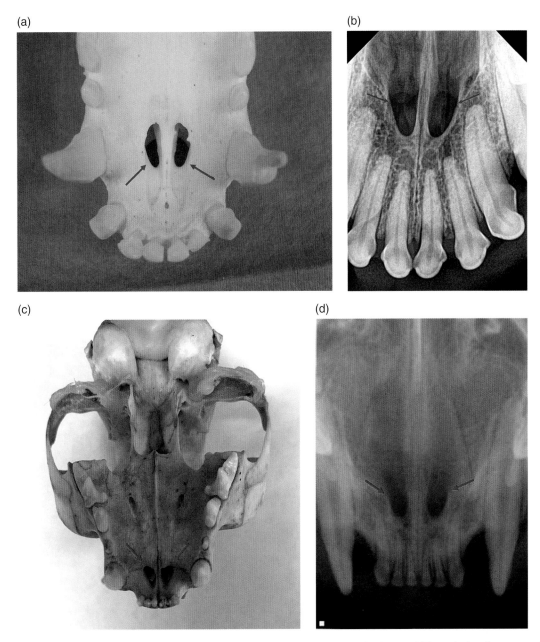

Figure 3.29 (a) Image depicts the palatine fissures on the skull of a dog (red arrows). The palatine fissures are just one way in which the observer can identify the maxilla from the mandible on a radiographic view of the rostral portion of the skull containing the maxillary incisors. (b) Radiographic image of the rostral maxilla of a dog. The positioning is used to procure a diagnostic image of the left maxillary incisors. Note the two symmetrical areas of lucency which lie on either side of midline. The two areas of lucency are the palatine fissures identified by the red arrows. These fissures lie between the premaxilla (ventral surface of the incisive bone) and the maxilla. (c) Image depicts the palatine fissures on the skull of a cat (red arrows). The palatine fissures are positioned on either side of midline within the bone of the premaxilla (ventral surface of the incisive bone) just cranial to the maxillary bone, between the right and left maxillary canine teeth. (d) Radiographic image of the rostral maxilla of a cat. The radiographic positioning is used to procure a diagnostic image of all maxillary incisors of the cat. Note the two symmetrical areas of lucency to the right and left of midline, or the interincisive suture. These lucencies are the palatal fissures of the cat (red arrows).

Once the viewer has identified what teeth they are looking at, they should identify if the normal anatomic characteristics are present. Having the appropriate number of teeth present with the appropriate number of roots will be the first step in interpretation. Patients who are missing multiple teeth can make interpretation of the remaining teeth a bit more difficult. Therefore, using the anatomical markers of the sinuses and superimposition of the bones within the maxilla to identify the sinuses as well as using the mandibular canal and the mandibular symphysis to

(a) (b)

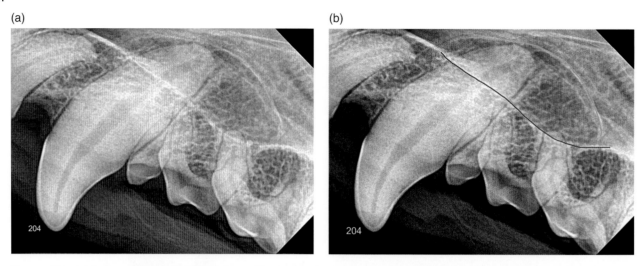

Figure 3.30 (a) Radiographic image of the left maxilla of a dog. The increased radiopaque thin lines depict surfaces of the conchal crest and the nasal surface of the alveolar process. This image shows the much busier appearance of the maxilla as it includes the sinuses. (b) Radiographic image of the left maxilla of a dog. The increased radiopaque thin lines depict surfaces of the conchal crest (yellow line) and the nasal surface of the alveolar process (red line).

(a) (b)

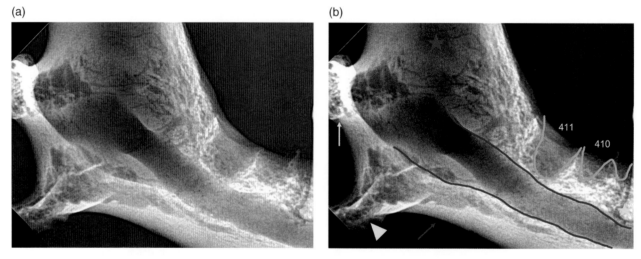

Figure 3.31 (a) Radiographic image of the right caudal mandible of a dog. The radiographic film is placed as far caudal in the oral cavity as possible. This image may not be able to be acquired in all patients due to the size of the patient and the size of the radiographic plate. (b) Radiographic image of the right caudal mandible of a dog. The yellow lines depict the empty alveolus of the missing right mandibular 2nd and 3rd molar teeth (410, 411). The yellow star designates the distal root of the right mandibular 1st molar tooth (409). This image is not diagnostic for this tooth or root. The red lines outline the mandibular canal. The red arrow depicts the ventral surface of the mandibular cortex. The yellow arrowhead demonstrates the angular process of the mandible, and the yellow arrow is the condylar process. The red star is in the location of the ramus of the mandible.

identify the mandible is very important for interpretation (Figure 3.33a–c).

Evaluation of the Structures

All aspects of the teeth should be assessed including any defects or abnormalities in the entire tooth structure. A grasp of what makes up the tooth structure as well as alterations in the normal appearance are helpful to be able to discern normal from abnormal. A tooth is made up of two main portions: the crown and the root. The crown is the visible portion of the tooth that is present above the gingival margin. The root is the portion of the tooth that is most commonly found below the alveolar bone margin (Figure 3.34). The outside covering of the crown of the tooth is comprised of enamel. Enamel is the protective covering of the crown of the tooth. It is highly mineralized and comprised of 96% inorganic material [9]. The root of the

Table 3.6 Permanent tooth root numbers of the maxillary teeth in the dog.

Permanent maxillary tooth root numbers – dog		
Permanent tooth number	**Description of tooth**	**Number of roots**
101–103, 201–203	Maxillary incisors	1
104, 204	Maxillary canine	1
105, 205	Maxillary 1st premolar	1
106, 206	Maxillary 2nd premolar	2
107, 207	Maxillary 3rd premolar	2
108, 208	Maxillary 4th premolar	3
109, 209	Maxillary 1st molar	3
110, 210	Maxillary 2nd molar	3

The table depicts the permanent tooth numbers, the description of the teeth, and the expected number of roots each tooth should have.

Table 3.7 Deciduous tooth root numbers of the maxillary teeth in the dog.

Deciduous maxillary tooth root numbers – dog		
Deciduous tooth number	**Description of tooth**	**Number of roots**
501–503, 601–603	Maxillary incisors	1
504, 604	Maxillary canine	1
*	Maxillary 1st premolar	*
506, 606	Maxillary 2nd premolar	2
507, 607	Maxillary 3rd premolar	3
508, 608	Maxillary 4th premolar	3
*	Maxillary 1st molar	*
*	Maxillary 2nd molar	*

The table depicts the deciduous tooth numbers, the description of the teeth and expected number of roots each tooth should have. The asterisk is placed to identify the normally missing teeth in the dental arcade of the dog.

Table 3.8 Permanent tooth root numbers of the maxillary teeth in the cat.

Permanent maxillary tooth root numbers – cat		
Permanent tooth number	**Description of tooth**	**Number of roots**
101–103, 201–203	Maxillary incisors	1
104, 204	Maxillary canine	1
*	Maxillary 1st premolar	*
106, 206	Maxillary 2nd premolar	1–2 (usually fused)
107, 207	Maxillary 3rd premolar	2
108, 208	Maxillary 4th premolar	3
109, 209	Maxillary 1st molar	1–3 (usually fused)

The table depicts the permanent tooth numbers, the description of the teeth, and the expected number of roots each tooth should have. The asterisk is placed to identify the normally missing teeth in the dental arcade of the cat.

Table 3.9 Deciduous tooth root numbers of the maxillary teeth in the cat.

Deciduous maxillary tooth root numbers – cat		
Deciduous tooth number	**Description of tooth**	**Number of roots**
501–503, 601–603	Maxillary incisors	1
504, 604	Maxillary canine	1
*	Maxillary 1st premolar	*
506, 606	Maxillary 2nd premolar	1
507, 607	Maxillary 3rd premolar	2
508, 608	Maxillary 4th premolar	3
*	Maxillary 1st molar	*

The table depicts the deciduous tooth numbers, the description of the teeth, and expected number of roots each tooth should have. The asterisk is placed to identify the normally missing teeth in the dental arcade of the cat.

tooth is covered with cementum. Cementum is also a mineralized connective tissue structure comprised of approximately 50% inorganic material [9]. Both enamel and cementum cover a structure called dentin. Dentin makes up the bulk of the tooth structure. Dentin is a tubular structure that contains the cells that formed it which are the same cells that help to maintain and repair it throughout the life of the tooth [9]. The cells that form dentin are called odontoblasts. These cells line the outer edge of the pulp of the tooth. Pulp is the soft tissue component within the

tooth which provides nutrients and houses the nerves that give rise to the sensations felt within the tooth. The pulp also provides cells with the ability to repair and produce dentin in response to injury as well as the cells to produce dentin in the initial formation and development of the tooth [9] (Figure 3.35).

Table 3.10 Permanent tooth root numbers of the mandibular teeth in the dog.

Permanent mandibular tooth root numbers – dog		
Permanent tooth number	**Description of tooth**	**Number of roots**
301–303, 401–403	Mandibular incisors	1
304, 404	Mandibular canine	1
305, 405	Mandibular 1st premolar	1
306, 406	Mandibular 2nd premolar	2
307, 407	Mandibular 3rd premolar	2
308, 408	Mandibular 4th premolar	2
309, 409	Mandibular 1st molar	2
310, 410	Mandibular 2nd molar	2
311, 411	Mandibular 3rd molar	1

The table depicts the permanent tooth numbers, the description of the teeth, and the expected number of roots each tooth should have.

Table 3.11 Deciduous tooth root numbers of the mandibular teeth in the dog.

Deciduous mandibular tooth root numbers – dog		
Deciduous tooth number	**Description of tooth**	**Number of roots**
701–703, 801–803	Mandibular incisors	1
704, 804	Mandibular canine	1
*	Mandibular 1st premolar	*
706, 806	Mandibular 2nd premolar	2
707, 807	Mandibular 3rd premolar	2
708, 808	Mandibular 4th premolar	2
*	Mandibular 1st molar	*
*	Mandibular 2nd molar	*

The table depicts the deciduous tooth numbers, the description of the teeth, and expected number of roots each tooth should have. The asterisk is placed to identify the normally missing teeth in the dental arcade of the dog.

Crown

Enamel

Evaluation of the crown of the tooth should consist of identifying the enamel on the tooth surface. The enamel thickness in most feline teeth has been found to be <0.1–0.3 mm [10]. In canine patients, enamel has been found to be <0.1–0.6 mm in thickness [10]. Radiographically, enamel is very thin and can be very difficult to evaluate due to the lack of thickness present in canine and feline patients. Enamel is the most radio-dense tissue associated

Table 3.12 Permanent tooth root numbers of the mandibular teeth in the cat.

Permanent mandibular tooth root numbers – cat		
Permanent tooth number	**Description of tooth**	**Number of roots**
301–303, 401–403	Mandibular incisors	1
304, 404	Mandibular canine	1
*	Mandibular 1st premolar	*
*	Mandibular 2nd premolar	*
307, 407	Mandibular 3rd premolar	2
308, 408	Mandibular 4th premolar	2
309, 409	Mandibular 1st molar	2

The table depicts the permanent tooth numbers, the description of the teeth, and the expected number of roots each tooth should have. The asterisk is placed to identify the normally missing teeth in the dental arcade of the cat.

Table 3.13 Deciduous tooth root numbers of the mandibular teeth in the cat.

Deciduous mandibular tooth root numbers – cat		
Deciduous tooth number	**Description of tooth**	**Number of roots**
701–703, 801–803	Mandibular incisors	1
704, 804	Mandibular canine	1
*	Mandibular 1st premolar	*
*	Mandibular 2nd premolar	*
707, 807	Mandibular 3rd premolar	2
708, 808	Mandibular 4th premolar	2
*	Mandibular 1st molar	*

The table depicts the deciduous tooth numbers, the description of the teeth, and expected number of roots each tooth should have. The asterisk is placed to identify the normally missing teeth in the dental arcade of the cat.

with the tooth structure [11]. If there is loss of enamel associated with a tooth, the tooth should have a corresponding decrease in density related to the affected area (Figures 3.36a–e, 3.37a, and b). Radiographically, enamel can be identified by being the densest area on the crown of the tooth. Due to the extremely thin nature, it is best identified clinically rather than radiographically.

Pulp

When evaluating the internal contents of the tooth, it is important to evaluate the pulp chamber and pulp canal sizes. Dentin is deposited within the tooth throughout the

(a)

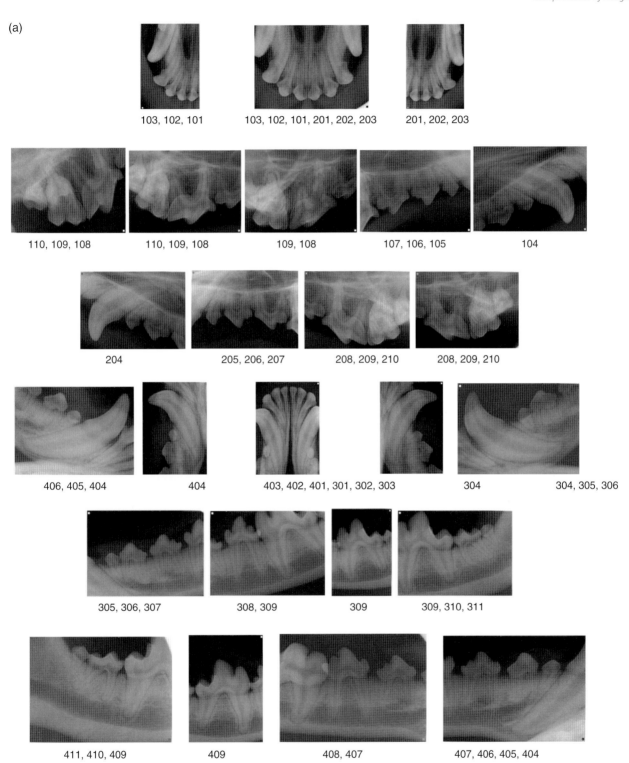

Figure 3.32 (a) Image depicts labial mounting of a complete radiograph set to assess the teeth of a dog. Note that there are numerous images that are necessary to assess all 42 teeth present in the permanent dentition of a dog. Depending on the size of the patient, more or less images may be necessary. The larger the patient, the more images will be needed to assess both the crown and root of the patient. In a smaller patient, more teeth can be captured on one radiographic image. This radiograph set was acquired using a 20-pound beagle dog. (b) Image depicts labial mounting of a complete radiograph set to assess the teeth of a cat. Note how there are two additional images of the maxillary 2nd, 3rd, and 4th premolar and 1st molar teeth that are labeled as extraoral views. These images need to be labeled as extraoral views immediately after acquiring; otherwise, it would be impossible to tell which was the right or left arcade.

(b)

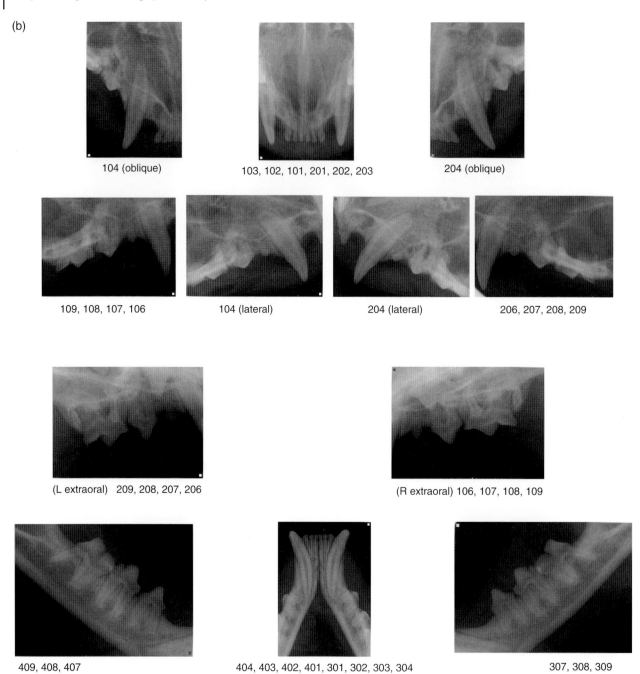

104 (oblique)

103, 102, 101, 201, 202, 203

204 (oblique)

109, 108, 107, 106

104 (lateral)

204 (lateral)

206, 207, 208, 209

(L extraoral)   209, 208, 207, 206

(R extraoral) 106, 107, 108, 109

409, 408, 407

404, 403, 402, 401, 301, 302, 303, 304

307, 308, 309

Figure 3.32   (Continued)

life of the animal or the life of the tooth, whichever comes first. If the pulp chamber or canal is larger than the surrounding pulp chambers or canals, this is an indication that the tooth is no longer vital (Figures 3.38a, b and 3.39a, b).

A pulp chamber or canal that is too small, or smaller than the pulp canals of the surrounding teeth may also be an indication that the tooth is nonvital. In this situation, the pulp was overstimulated to cause increased dentin deposition to the tooth or root, and thus a narrower pulp chamber and canal are observed. While a narrow pulp canal can be an indication that the tooth is no longer vital, an increased pulp canal size compared to the surrounding teeth is significantly more common. Bearing that in mind, a decreased pulp chamber or canal size may still be a radiographic indication the tooth is no longer vital.

In immature teeth, the pulp chamber or canal is very wide prior to tooth eruption. The chambers and canals continue to narrow as teeth mature. The narrowing continues throughout the life of the tooth and the life of the animal (Figure 3.40a–c). All pulp chambers and canals narrow in

(a)

(b)

(c)

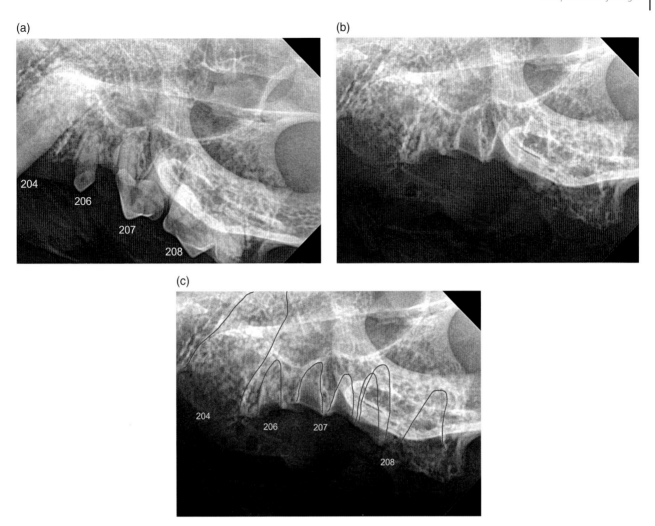

Figure 3.33 (a) Radiographic image of the left maxilla of a cat. The image depicts evidence of the left maxillary canine, 2nd, 3rd, and 4th premolar teeth (204, 206–208). In the radiographic image, there is no obvious evidence of the left maxillary 1st molar tooth (209). (b) Radiographic image of the left maxilla of a cat. The image was taken following a quadrant extraction. Note the empty alveoli from where the teeth had recently been extracted. The radiographic image again depicts the areas of the left maxillary canine, 2nd, 3rd, and 4th premolar and 1st molar teeth (204, 206–209). Notice how it is difficult to appreciate where in the maxilla the image was taken due to the lack of teeth present to use as anatomical markers. (c) Radiographic image of the left maxilla of a cat. This is the same image as seen in Figure (b). The red lines outline the empty alveolus of the left maxillary canine, 2nd, 3rd, and 4th premolar teeth.

size regardless of the specific type of tooth. This is an important point as radiographically when evaluating the pulp sizes of teeth, each tooth should be individually compared to the teeth adjacent to them within the oral cavity or a similar sized tooth on a different arcade. If there is a question or concern of the size of the chamber or canal and the interpreter feels the structure is either too small or too large compared to the adjacent teeth, the contralateral teeth of the same type can be used for comparison as a final assessment.

The pulp chamber or root canal should be uniform in appearance without any irregularities (Figures 3.41 and 3.42a–d). The edges of the canals should be smooth without significant deviation from the canal or chamber

itself. If irregularities are noted within the canal, potential differentials include internal tooth resorption or developmental abnormalities. Further investigation is warranted. The pulp is made of soft tissue; therefore, radiographically this area should be more radiolucent. The entire contents of the pulp canal or chamber should be consistently the same radiographic density.

If there is evidence of increased density to the pulp chamber or canal, or focal areas of radiodensity within the pulp, this could be an indication of the patient having a pulp stone or a denticle (Figure 3.43a and b). Pulp stones and denticles are common incidental radiographic findings. Depending on their location within the chamber or canal, they may cause complications if endodontic therapy is needed as the

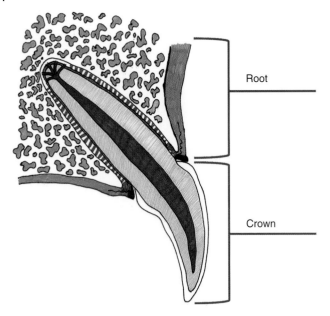

Figure 3.34 The drawing depicts the crown and root of a tooth. The crown of the tooth is identified as the portion of the tooth that is visible above the gumline. The root of the tooth is identified as the portion of the tooth that is encased within the alveolar bone.

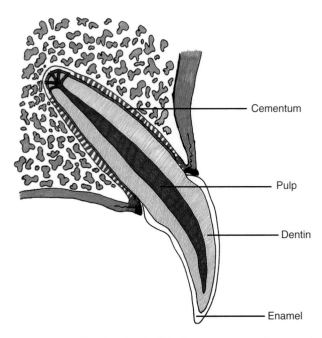

Figure 3.35 The drawing depicts the components of a normal tooth. The outside covering of the crown of the tooth is enamel. The outside covering of the root of the tooth is cementum. The bulk of the tooth is composed of dentin, which is deposited throughout the life of the tooth or the life if the animal. The neurovascular supply is contained within the pulp of the tooth, which is fed by an apical delta at the root apex of the tooth.

specialist would have to navigate around or through the mineralization for completion of their procedure. A pulp stone commonly forms in the coronal portion of the pulp chamber, while a denticle more commonly appears within or near the furcation of a multi-rooted tooth [12].

Irregularities within the pulp canal or pulp chamber can also be indicative of internal tooth resorption. Internal tooth resorption is a pathological process resulting from osteoclastic activity [13]. Internal resorption can be described as surface, inflammatory, or replacement resorption [13]. Internal inflammatory resorption can be observed radiographically as a radiolucent area within the root canal of the tooth [13] (Figures 3.44a, b, 3.45a, and b). In general, internal tooth resorption is a relatively uncommon condition [13].

Dentin

Dentin comprises the bulk of the mature tooth. It supports the enamel and allows it to withstand the forces of mastication and not fracture under pressure [9]. Dentin houses a special cell type called odontoblasts. The odontoblasts are very important for dentin deposition during tooth development. There is a layer of odontoblasts that line the outside of the pulp and continue to form dentin throughout the life of the tooth or the life of the animal whichever ceases first. After the root is formed, secondary dentin is deposited as a continuation of the primary dentin that helped to form the root [14]. If the tooth encounters an injury, tertiary dentin may be deposited within the tooth [14]. The degree of injury determines the amount of tertiary dentin deposited and the rate at which it is produced [14]. Radiographically, there is no difference between the different types of dentin. Clinically, tertiary dentin is commonly deposited on areas where the enamel has been lost and thus has left the tooth with exposed dentin. The odontoblastic processes within the dentinal tubules signal the odontoblasts to protect the pulp and deposit a layer of tertiary or reparative dentin to protect the pulp from additional injury. Radiographically, dentin should have a uniform appearance throughout the tooth. It is mildly less radio-dense than enamel due to the different mineral composition between the two structures. The roots of a mature tooth appear to have a similar radiographic density to the crown of a tooth due to the superimposition of the alveolar bone on the root surface. As a tooth matures, the odontoblasts continue to form secondary dentin until the tooth, or the animal, dies. This is significantly more obvious in a young animal as there is a larger pulp canal present in a young animal (Figure 3.46a and b). Changes in the thickness of the dentin and thus the deposition of dentin are much more radiographically obvious in a young patient compared to a patient with a mature pulp chamber.

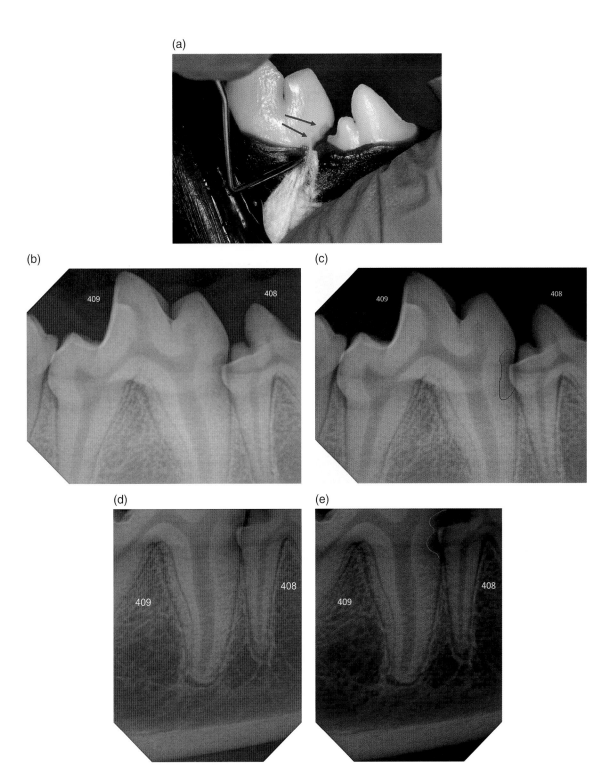

Figure 3.36 (a) Clinical image depicts evidence of two areas of enamel loss on the mesial aspect of the right mandibular 1st molar tooth (409) (red arrows). (b) Radiographic image of the right mandible of a dog. This is the same patient as in Figure (a). The image depicts the crown of the distal aspect of the right mandibular 4th premolar tooth (408) and the mesial aspect of the 1st molar tooth (409). While enamel is the most radiodense portion of the tooth structure, it is not very thick, making it difficult to identify on a radiographic image. When there is loss of enamel on a tooth structure, there is a subtle decrease in density of the tooth associated with the affected area. (c) Radiographic image of the right mandible of a dog. The image depicts the crown of the distal aspect of the right mandibular 4th premolar tooth (408) and the crown of the 1st molar tooth (409). The red line identifies the loss of enamel on the mesial aspect of the crown of the right mandibular 1st molar tooth. This is the same radiographic image as in Figure (b) and the same patient as in Figure (a). (d) Radiographic image of the right mandible of a dog. The image depicts the distal root of the right mandibular 4th premolar tooth (408) and the mesial root of the 1st molar tooth (409). There is a decrease in radiodensity, consistent with an enamel defect present on the mesial root of the right mandibular 1st molar tooth. This is the same patient as in Figure 3.36a–c. (e) Radiographic image of the right mandible of a dog. The image depicts the distal root of the right mandibular 4th premolar tooth (408) and the mesial root of the 1st molar tooth (409). The red line identifies the loss of enamel on the mesial aspect of the crown of the right mandibular 1st molar tooth. This is the same patient as in Figure 3.36a–d.

(a) (b)

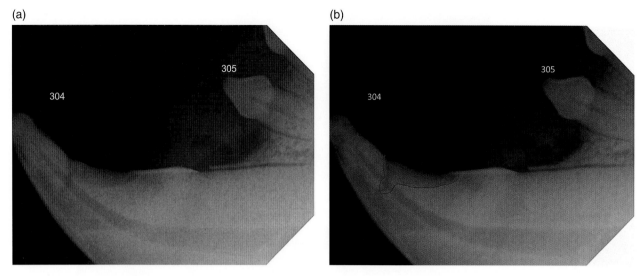

Figure 3.37 (a) Radiographic image of the left mandible of a dog. The image depicts the crown of the distal aspect of the left mandibular canine tooth (304). Notice how there is a decrease in density to the distal aspect of the crown of this tooth.
(b) Radiographic image of the left mandible of a dog. The image depicts the crown of the left mandibular canine tooth. The red line identifies the loss of enamel on the distal aspect of the crown of the left mandibular canine tooth. This is the same image as in Figure (a).

(a) (b)

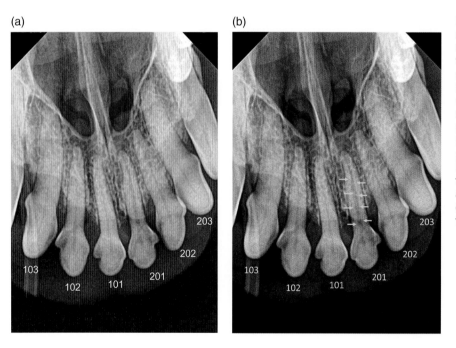

Figure 3.38 (a) Radiographic image of the rostral maxilla of a dog. When evaluating dental radiographs, the viewer needs to appreciate differences in pulp canal size. Note how the pulp canal size in the left maxillary 1st incisor is larger than the surrounding incisor teeth pulp canals. (b) Radiographic image of the rostral maxilla of a dog. Notice the increased pulp canal size associated with the left maxillary 1st incisor compared to the surrounding teeth. The yellow arrows identify the difference in size of the canal associated with this tooth.

Root

Identification of the appropriate number of roots associated with the teeth of the dog or cat is important for proper interpretation of the radiographic images (Tables 3.14–3.17). Root numbers of the various teeth do not vary significantly between the types of teeth within the canine and feline species. Regardless of dog or cat, the maxillary 4th premolar tooth should have three roots. The maxillary 1st molar

also has three roots for both the canine and feline species. The main difference is that within the cat, the maxillary 1st molar demonstrates fusion of one or more of these three roots, giving the appearance of a single-rooted tooth. Occasionally, only two of the roots will be fused together with a separate 3rd root present. The author has never encountered three individual roots in the maxillary 1st molar of a cat. The maxillary 2nd premolar in the dog and

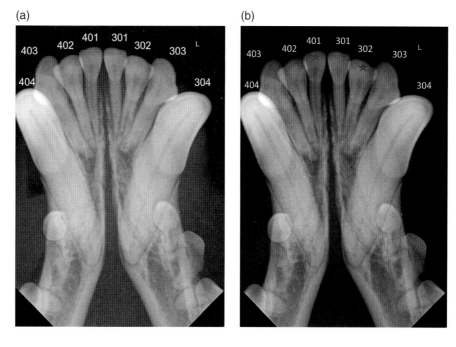

Figure 3.39 (a) Radiographic image of the rostral mandible of a dog. Note there are two mandibular incisor teeth that have increased pulp canal size compared to the surrounding teeth. (b) Radiographic image of the rostral mandible of a dog. This is the same image as in Figure (a). The red stars identify the two incisors which have increased pulp canal size compared to the surrounding incisor teeth. An increased pulp canal size is most commonly associated with teeth that are nonvital.

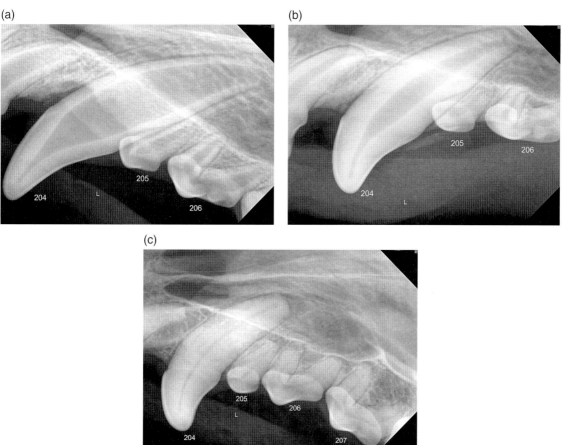

Figure 3.40 (a) Radiographic image of the left maxillary canine tooth of a young dog. Note how the pulp canal is very wide. There is minimal deposition of dentin present. Also note the apex of the tooth does not appear to be fully closed. This would suggest that the patient is less than 11 months of age. (b) Radiographic image of the left maxillary canine tooth of a young adult dog. Note how the pulp canal is significantly smaller than in Figure (a). More dentin is deposited contributing to the decreased size of the pulp canal. Note how the apex of the root appears to be fully formed in this patient. Since the apex of the tooth is formed, it would suggest that the dog is greater than 11 months of age. The size of the pulp canal would suggest that this patient is a young adult between one and three years of age. (c) Radiographic image of a the left maxillary canine tooth of a mature dog. Note the closed apex of the root and the decreased size of the pulp canal. Dentin is deposited by a layer of odontoblasts that line the outside pulp of the tooth. It is deposited throughout the life of the tooth or the life of the animal. As dentin is deposited, the pulp canal decreases in size. The older the patient, the amount of dentin that is deposited is less obvious from year to year. In a young animal such as in Figure (a), the amount of dentin deposited is dramatic compared to Figure (c). The deposition is much less dramatic moving from Figure (b) to (c).

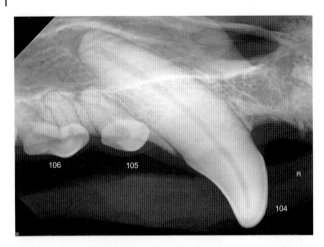

Figure 3.41 Radiographic image of the right maxillary canine tooth of a dog. Note the smooth regular surface of the pulp canal. There does not appear to be any changes in size or irregularities associated with the pulp canal. The patient in this image is a mature adult.

cat has two roots. Again, like the maxillary 1st molar in the cat, the roots are frequently fused together, giving the appearance of a single-rooted tooth in the cat. Simply stated, the radiographic appearance of both the maxillary 2nd premolar tooth and 1st molar tooth in the cat is that of a single-rooted tooth. In the cat, the intimate association of the maxillary 1st molar tooth with the maxillary 4th premolar tooth makes separation of the roots of this tooth radiographically, difficult to acquire. Only if all three roots are not fused together and a root is left behind, there will be the appearance of a retained tooth root on dental radiographs.

Root Formation

As an immature permanent tooth erupts, the root has not yet formed. As the tooth continues to mature, root formation begins. By 11 months of age in canine and feline patients, a definitive root apex should be formed [7, 8]. When a tooth reaches its final length, root formation continues until there is no longer a lucency continuous with the apical root canal contents [8]. Depending on the tooth, formation of the apical extent of each tooth varies slightly, with the maxillary canine tooth being the last tooth to have complete apical closure [7, 8]. A tooth with a closed apex has significantly less vascular supply and therefore an impaired reaction to respond favorably to infection, inflammation, or injury [8] (Figures 3.47a–c and 3.48a–c).

Cementum

The outside covering of the root structure is comprised of cementum (see Figure 3.35). It is the hard structure that covers the dentin which encases the pulp of the tooth [15]. Generally, two forms of cementum are present and need to be considered: cellular and acellular. Depending on the

location of the injury to the tooth depends on the type of cementum encountered. Cellular cementum has the capacity to respond to tooth movement and wear and is usually associated with repair of the periodontal tissues [16]. Acellular cementum is considered more of an attachment structure to the tooth [15, 16]. It has been thought to be a critical structure for the attachment of the tooth to the surrounding periodontal ligament structures that hold the teeth into the alveolar bone [15]. Cellular cementum is generally located in the middle to apical third of the tooth as well as the furcation [16]. Cellular cementum is charged with adaptation and repair. Acellular cementum is located in the coronal third of the tooth but can extend to the apical third [16]. Acellular cementum is charged with attachment and anchorage of the tooth into the alveolar bone and adaptation to the patient's occlusion and chewing habits [15, 16]. Radiographically cellular and acellular cementum cannot be distinguished from each other.

Abnormalities Associated with Cementum When cementum is stimulated, external inflammatory root resorption can occur which will present radiographically as loss of tooth structure with the potential for radiolucencies associated with the periodontal ligament and the bone [17] (Figure 3.49a and b).

Ankylosis is where the cementum or dentin of the root surface directly fuses with the surrounding alveolar bone [18]. This process usually is accompanied by replacement resorption of the root surface [18]. When replacement resorption occurs, the cementum or dentin is usually replaced with bone instead of the original tissue that created it [18]. Clinically, ankylosis results in a lack of mobility to the tooth and root. The difficulty level of extracting these teeth increases dramatically and complete extraction of these teeth can be very frustrating, if not even impossible due to the increased complexity of not being able to identify normal and abnormal tooth structure from the surrounding bone. Replacement resorption and ankylosis have been used interchangeably although they are technically different. Ankylosis should be used as a diagnosis, while replacement resorption should be considered the process by which the tooth is ankylosed to the surrounding bone [18] (Figure 3.50a and b). Radiographically, ankylosis is viewed as a lack of distinction between the lamina dura of the tooth and the root surface [18]. This would be viewed as a lack of a periodontal ligament space radiographically.

Periodontal Ligament

The periodontal ligament is a specialized connective tissue that allows physiologic movement of the tooth within the attached underlying structures, mainly the alveolar bone. One end of the periodontal ligament fibers is

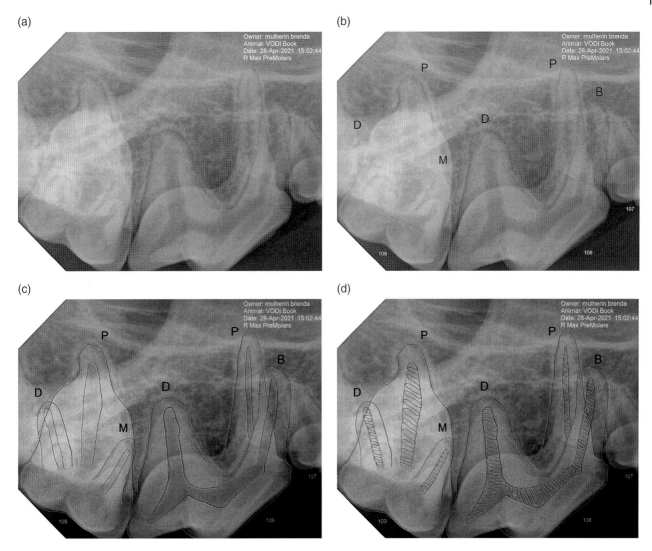

Figure 3.42 (a) Radiographic image of the right maxilla in a dog. The radiograph would be a diagnostic image of the right maxillary 4th premolar and 1st molar teeth (108, 109). Both of these two teeth have three roots. (b) Radiographic image of the right maxilla of a dog. This is the same image as in Figure (a). The black letters on the image identify the three roots associated with each of these teeth. The letter "D" identifies the distal root of each tooth. The letter "M" identifies the mesial root of the maxillary 1st molar tooth. The letter "P" identifies the palatal root of the maxillary 1st molar and the mesiopalatal root of the maxillary 4th premolar. The letter "B" identifies the mesiobuccal root of the maxillary 4th premolar tooth. For identification of the mesiopalatal root and the mesiobuccal root, two images are necessary to identify which root is buccal and which root is palatal. This is when the "SLOB" technique is used to identify these roots from each other. For more information regarding radiographic positioning and the "SLOB" technique, please refer to Chapter 2. (c) Radiographic image of the right maxilla of a dog. This is the same image as in Figure (a) and (b). The red lines outline the root structure of the right maxillary 4th premolar and 1st molar teeth. The letters depict the identification of each individual root. (d) Radiographic image of the right maxilla of a dog. This is the same image as in Figure (a)–(c). The red lines outline the root structure of the right maxillary 4th premolar and 1st molar teeth. The red filling identifies the pulp chamber of the maxillary 4th premolar tooth and the pulp canals of the maxillary 4th premolar and 1st molar teeth. The letters depict the identification of each individual root.

embedded into the cementum of the tooth and the other end is embedded into the alveolar bone [19]. This tissue allows the fibers to stretch and contract in response to forces applied to them [19]. Radiographically, the periodontal ligament is identified as a radiolucent space and not as a soft tissue structure. The periodontal ligament space should be evaluated whether it is present, appropriately sized, larger than normal or the disappearance or absence of the ligament space altogether. If the periodontal ligament space is larger than normal, this could be an indication that there is disease associated with the specific tooth being evaluated. If there is absence of the periodontal ligament space, this could be an indication that ankylosis has occurred and replacement resorption is

(a)

(b)

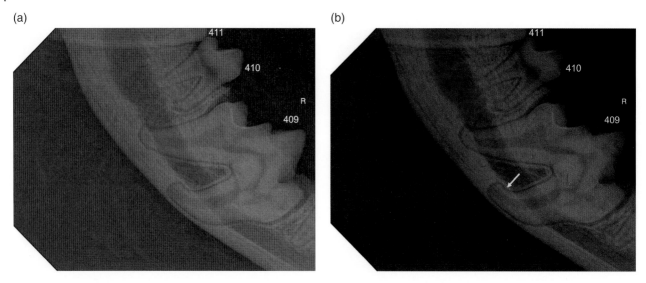

Figure 3.43 (a) Radiographic image of the right mandible of a dog. The radiographic image is diagnostic for the right mandibular 1st and 2nd molar teeth. Note the circular area of radiodensity in the mesial root of the right mandibular first molar tooth. This opacity is a pulp stone. (b) Radiographic image of the right mandible of a dog. The red arrow identifies a pulp stone which is present in the mesial root of the right mandibular 1st molar tooth. The yellow arrow depicts severe dilaceration of the mesial root of the right mandibular 1st molar tooth.

(a)

(b)

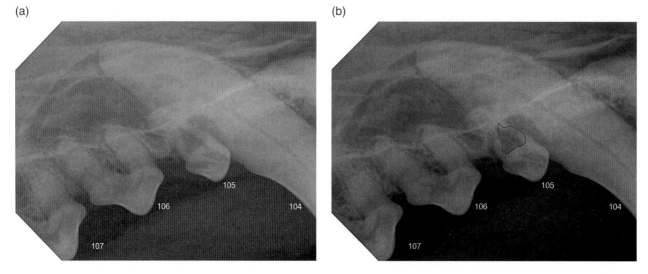

Figure 3.44 (a) Radiographic image of the right maxilla of a dog. The radiograph is diagnostic for the right maxillary canine tooth and the 1st, and 2nd premolar teeth (104–106). Note the triangular shaped lucent space within the right maxillary 1st premolar tooth. This tooth appears to be affected by internal tooth resorption. (b) Radiographic image of the right maxilla of a dog. This is the same image as in Figure (a). An area of internal tooth resorption on the right maxillary 1st premolar tooth is outlined in red.

remodeling the bone and root structure to become one unit (Figure 3.51a–c).

Chevron

A chevron is an inverted V-shape that can be used to describe areas of radiolucency associated with endodontically sound teeth. This radiographic artifact presents as a widening of the apical area in a tooth that is otherwise periodontally and endodontically normal. This chevron lucency is commonly associated with the maxillary and mandibular canine teeth, maxillary incisors, and mandibular molar teeth, although they can be observed in other teeth as well. They generally

(a)

(b)

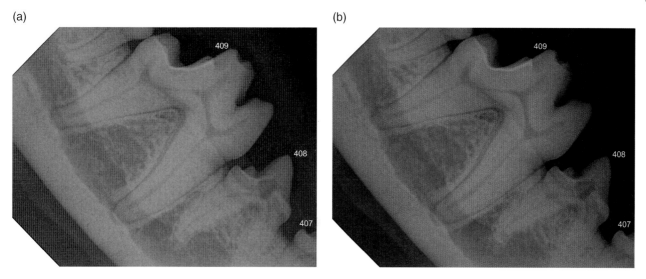

Figure 3.45 (a) Radiographic image of the right mandible of a dog. This image is diagnostic for the right mandibular 1st molar and the distal root of the right mandibular 4th premolar tooth. Note the circular area of lucency observed in the crown, or more specifically the pulp chamber of the right mandibular 4th premolar tooth (408). (b) Radiographic image of the right mandible of a dog. This is the same image as in Figure (a). Note the circular area of radiolucency in the pulp chamber of the crown of the right mandibular 4th premolar tooth (408).

(a)

(b)

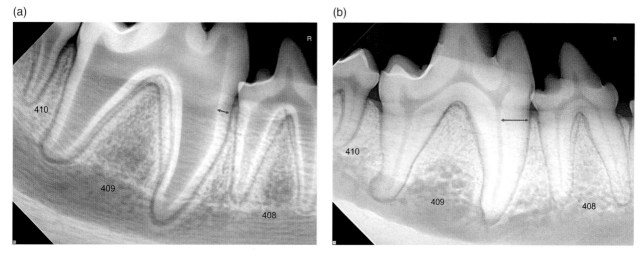

Figure 3.46 (a) Radiographic image of the right mandible of a juvenile dog. Note the thickness of the dentin depicted by the double-headed red arrow. In a juvenile patient, the dentin is very thin. Dentin is deposited by a layer of odontoblasts that line the outside surface of the pulp. As the patient matures, the tooth matures, and more dentin is deposited. The pulp of a juvenile patient is very wide. As the patient matures, the pulp decreases in size and the thickness of dentin deposition increases. (b) Radiographic image of the right mandible of a dog. Note how much thicker the dentin deposition is compared to the same tooth in Figure (a). The thickness is depicted by the double-headed red arrow. This signifies a more mature tooth compared to Figure (a).

have a uniform shape that contours the existing apical shape of the associated root. Due to the close association of the apical extent of a tooth root, chevrons are commonly misdiagnosed as endodontic disease, more specifically a periapical lucency or tooth root abscess.

Endodontic disease results in an irregular shape at the apical extent of the root. While the two radiolucencies are

located in the same region, other factors must be taken into consideration when evaluating a tooth root for either a chevron or periapical lucency (Figure 3.52a–d). A chevron usually has a smooth regular contour that follows the apical third of the root and tapers to a gently rounded point. The periodontal ligament space is generally identified with a very thin lamina dura still intact adjacent to the space

Table 3.14 Deciduous maxillary and mandibular tooth root numbers in the dog using labial mounting.

Dog – deciduous maxillary teeth

Right maxilla

Tooth	m2	m1	pm4	pm3	pm2	pm1	c	i3	i2	i1
Tooth number	*	*	508	507	506	*	504	503	502	501
Number of roots			3	3	2		1	1	1	1

Left maxilla

Tooth	i1	i2	i3	c	pm1	pm2	pm3	pm4	m1	m2
Tooth number	601	602	603	604	*	606	607	608	*	*
Number of roots	1	1	1	1		2	3	3		

Dog – deciduous mandibular teeth

Right mandible

Tooth	m3	m2	m1	pm4	pm3	pm2	pm1	c	i3	i2	i1
Tooth number	*	*	*	808	807	806	*	804	803	802	801
Number of roots				2	2	2		1	1	1	1

Left mandible

Tooth	i1	i2	i3	c	pm1	pm2	pm3	pm4	m1	m2	m3
Tooth number	701	702	703	704	*	706	707	708	*	*	*
Number of roots	1	1	1	1		2	2	2			

The table depicts the description of the tooth, the specific tooth number, and the expected number of roots for each tooth. The asterisk is placed to identify the normally missing teeth within the deciduous dentition of the dog.

Table 3.15 Permanent maxillary and mandibular tooth root numbers in the dog using labial mounting.

Dog – permanent maxillary teeth

Right maxilla

Tooth	M2	M1	PM4	PM3	PM2	PM1	C	I3	I2	I1
Tooth number	110	109	108	107	106	105	104	103	102	101
Number of roots	3	3	3	2	2	1	1	1	1	1

Left maxilla

Tooth	I1	I2	I3	C	PM1	PM2	PM3	PM4	M1	M2
Tooth number	201	202	203	204	205	206	207	208	209	210
Number of roots	1	1	1	1	1	2	2	3	3	3

Dog – permanent mandibular teeth

Right mandible

Tooth	M3	M2	M1	PM4	PM3	PM2	PM1	C	I3	I2	I1
Tooth number	411	410	409	408	407	406	405	404	403	402	401
Number of roots	1	2	2	2	2	2	1	1	1	1	1

Left mandible

Tooth	I1	I2	I3	C	PM1	PM2	PM3	PM4	M1	M2	M3
Tooth number	301	302	303	304	305	306	307	308	309	310	311
Number of roots	1	1	1	1	1	2	2	2	2	2	1

The table depicts the description of the tooth, the specific tooth number, and the expected number of roots for each tooth.

Table 3.16 Deciduous maxillary and mandibular tooth root numbers in the cat using labial mounting.

Cat – deciduous maxillary teeth

	Right maxilla									Left maxilla								
Tooth	m1	pm4	pm3	pm2	pm1	C	i3	i2	i1	i1	i2	i3	c	pm1	pm2	pm3	pm4	m1
Tooth number	*	508	507	506	*	504	503	502	501	601	602	603	604	*	606	607	608	*
Number of roots		3	2	1		1	1	1	1	1	1	1	1		1	2	3	

Cat – deciduous mandibular teeth

	Right mandible									Left mandible								
Tooth	m1	pm4	pm3	pm2	pm1	c	i3	i2	i1	i1	i2	i3	c	pm1	pm2	pm3	pm4	m1
Tooth number	*	808	807	*	*	804	803	802	801	701	702	703	704	*	*	707	708	*
Number of roots		2	2			1	1	1	1	1	1	1	1			2	2	

The table depicts the description of the tooth, the specific tooth number, and the expected number of roots for each tooth. The asterisk is placed to identify the normally missing teeth within the deciduous dentition of the cat.

Table 3.17 Permanent maxillary and mandibular tooth root numbers in the cat using labial mounting.

Cat – permanent maxillary teeth

	Right maxilla									Left maxilla								
Tooth	M1	PM4	PM3	PM2	PM1	C	I3	I2	I1	I1	I2	I3	C	PM1	PM2	PM3	PM4	M1
Tooth number	109	108	107	106	*	104	103	102	101	201	202	203	204	*	206	207	208	209
Number of roots	1–3 (fused)	3	2	1–2 (fused)		1	1	1	1	1	1	1	1		1–2 (fused)	2	3	1–3 (fused)

Cat – permanent mandibular teeth

	Right mandible									Left mandible								
Tooth	M1	PM4	PM3	PM2	PM1	C	I3	I2	I1	I1	I2	I3	C	PM1	PM2	PM3	PM4	M1
Tooth number	409	408	407	*	*	404	403	402	401	301	302	303	304	*	*	307	308	309
Number of roots	2	2	2			1	1	1	1	1	1	1	1			2	2	2

The table depicts the description of the tooth, the specific tooth number, and the expected number of roots for each tooth. The asterisk is placed to identify the normally missing teeth within the permanent dentition of the cat.

(Figure 3.53a and b). A true periapical lucency has a generally broader and unusual or irregular shape. It is difficult to identify a periodontal ligament space, and usually the lamina dura is more indistinct (Figure 3.54a and b). If there is no other clinical or radiographic evidence of disease such as changes in pulp cavity width, periodontal pocketing, or tooth discoloration, a radiographic chevron should be considered.

Missing or Supernumerary Teeth

Visual examination of the oral cavity and documentation of the appropriate number of teeth present within the mouth is important. Knowing the dental formula for the patient being treated is imperative to recognize whether there are an appropriate number of teeth observed, or whether there are too many or too few teeth present (see Tables 3.1–3.4). If there are missing teeth, dental radiography will help discern

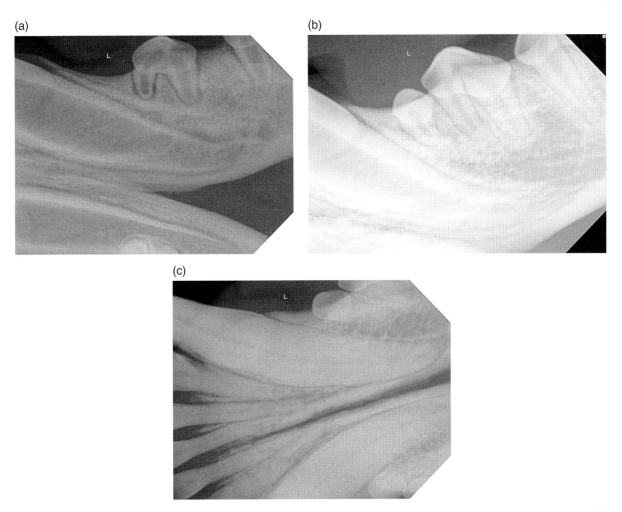

Figure 3.47 (a) Radiographic image of the left mandible of a dog. Note how the apex of the left mandibular canine tooth (304) does not appear to have a closed apex. This would suggest that the patient is less than 11 months of age. Also, notice how the patient in this image is missing a left mandibular 1st premolar tooth and that the first tooth present behind the canine tooth has two roots, suggesting it would be the left mandibular 2nd premolar tooth (306). (b) Radiographic image of the left mandible of a dog. This is an image of a more mature patient than in Figure (a). Note the increased thickness of the dentin and the appearance of a smaller pulp canal. The root of this tooth appears to be fully formed, suggesting the patient is greater than a year of age. (c) Radiographic image of the left mandible of a dog. This is an image of a mature patient. There is significant dentin thickness and a very small pulp canal present radiographically.

whether the missing teeth are impacted or if other reasons exist for their lack of appearance, e.g. tooth resorption, retained tooth roots, previous exfoliation, etc. Dental radiography can also aid in identifying patients that have supernumerary teeth that may be unerupted. Clinically verifying that all teeth are present within the oral cavity may not be enough for definitive treatment of a case. Dental radiography needs to be considered to evaluate for any surprises that may be present within the mouth (Figure 3.55a–e).

Supernumerary Roots

Dental radiography helps to identify if there is an appropriate number of roots associated with the teeth that are present within the oral cavity. Knowing the appropriate tooth root numbers associated with each tooth is crucial to the success of treatment (see Tables 3.6–3.13). While it is important to know the standard number of roots for both canine and feline patients, it is important to recognize that frequently tooth roots have variation in numbers. Dental radiography can help to identify whether there are extra roots associated with the target teeth of interest (Figure 3.56a and b). Knowledge of the root numbers associated with the teeth in a specific patient will help the surgeon identify the proper way to section a tooth, determine if an additional root needs endodontic therapy, or establish if all the roots were removed for definitive treatment of a case.

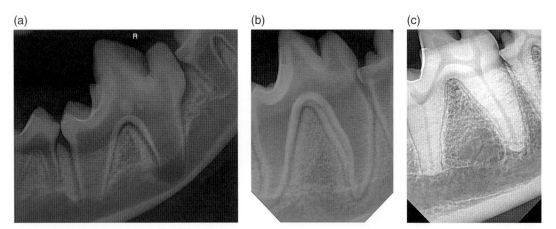

Figure 3.48 (a) Radiographic image of the right mandible of a dog. The tooth in the image is very immature. Note how both apices of the right mandibular first molar tooth and the surrounding roots do not have fully formed apices. This would suggest the patient is much less than 11 months of age. The patient in this image also has evidence that suggests that there are pulp stones within the pulp chamber. Pulp stones are the areas of radiodense material within the pulp chamber. (b) Radiographic image of the right mandible of a dog. The tooth in the image is also very young. Note the significantly large pulp chamber and canal. The apices of both roots appear to be closed, suggesting the tooth has matured to at least 11 months of age. The radiographic image is not diagnostic for the distal root of the mandibular 1st molar tooth as the image does not clearly show at least 2 mm around the entire apex of the tooth root. The dentin is very thin, and the pulp canal and chamber are wide suggesting the tooth would belong to a young adult patient. (c) Radiographic image of the right mandible of a dog. The tooth in the image depicts a tooth with a narrow pulp canal and significant dentin deposition. This would suggest the tooth has matured to a middle-aged to older adult. The tooth also has closed apices.

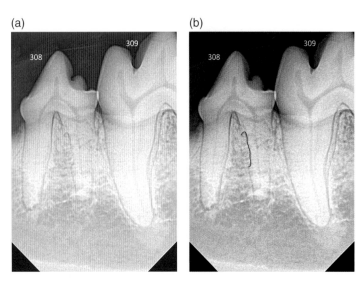

Figure 3.49 (a) Radiographic image of the left mandible of a dog. The left mandibular 4th premolar tooth (308) has evidence of external inflammatory tooth resorption on the mesial surface of the distal root. If the resorption appears to be confined to the root with no clinical evidence of disease, conservative monitoring may be warranted. (b) Radiographic image of the left mandible of a dog. This is the same image as in Figure (a). The area of external inflammatory tooth resorption on the mesial surface of the distal root is outlined in red.

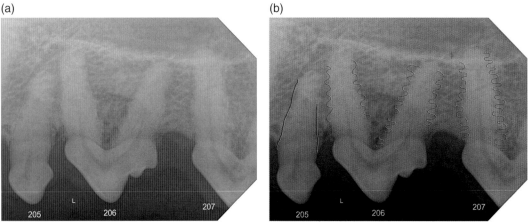

Figure 3.50 (a) Radiographic image of the left maxilla of a dog. This image is diagnostic for the left maxillary 1st and 2nd premolar teeth and the mesial root of the 3rd premolar. Note how the left maxillary 1st premolar has a smooth periodontal ligament space approximately ½–¾ of the length of the root. The left maxillary 2nd premolar tooth and mesial root of the 3rd premolar tooth show evidence of ankylosis of the roots to the surrounding bone. (b) Radiographic image of the left maxilla of a dog. This is the same image as in Figure (a). The periodontal ligament space that is visible on the left maxillary 1st premolar tooth (305), is identified by the red straight lines. The areas of ankylosis that are present in the left maxillary 2nd and 3rd premolars are identified by the red squiggly lines.

(a)

(b)

(c)

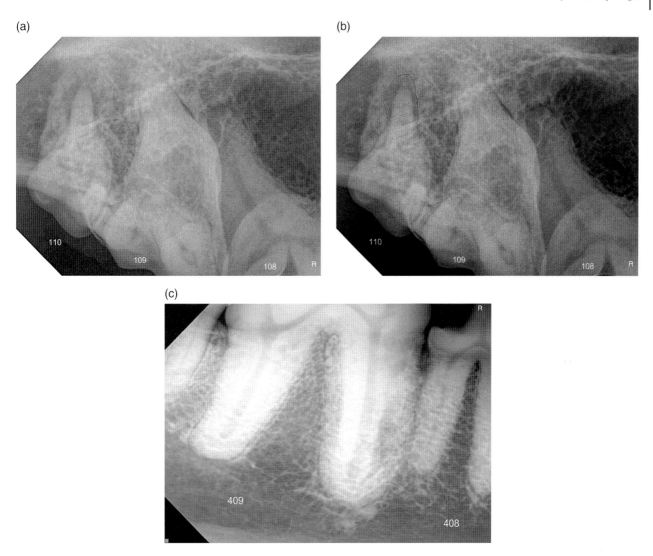

Figure 3.51 (a) Radiographic image of the caudal right maxilla of a dog. This would be a diagnostic image of the right maxillary 1st and 2nd molars. While the distal root of the right maxillary 4th premolar tooth is visible on the image, the entire tooth cannot be visualized. When assessing the image, note the increased area of radiolucency associated with the palatal root of the maxillary 2nd molar. (b) Radiographic image of the caudal right maxilla of a dog. This is the same image as in Figure (a). The red lines outline the periapical lucency associated with the right maxillary 2nd molar tooth (110). Note the smaller "normal" appearing periodontal ligament space of the right maxillary 1st molar tooth (109). (c) Radiographic image of the right mandible of a dog. Note the periodontal ligament space visible on the mesial and distal surfaces of the distal root of the mandibular 1st molar tooth. The periodontal ligament space is also visible on the distal surface of the mesial root. Notice how there is not a distinct periodontal ligament space associated with mesial aspect of the mesial root. This would suggest that there is some ankylosis or replacement resorption of the mesial root.

Reduced Number of Roots and Root Malformations

Clinically, the appearance of the crown of a tooth can give an indication that the roots of a tooth are normal. Unfortunately, what lies beneath the gingival surface may be different. Dental radiography helps to identify root abnormalities which may be of importance when it comes to treatment of a tooth. In humans, malformations of a tooth root frequently arise from developmental disorders of the tooth root itself or an abnormality within the process of radicular development [20]. Root formation is controlled by Hertwigs epithelial root sheath [20]. This structure determines the number, shape, and length of a root. It is also responsible for controlling the formation of cementum on the root [20]. Abnormalities in the shape and number of roots generally are the result of a developmental disorder or a combination of a developmental disorder along with generalized tooth dysplasia [20].

Developmental Root Abnormalities (Fusion, Gemination, and Concrescence) The number of roots can also be

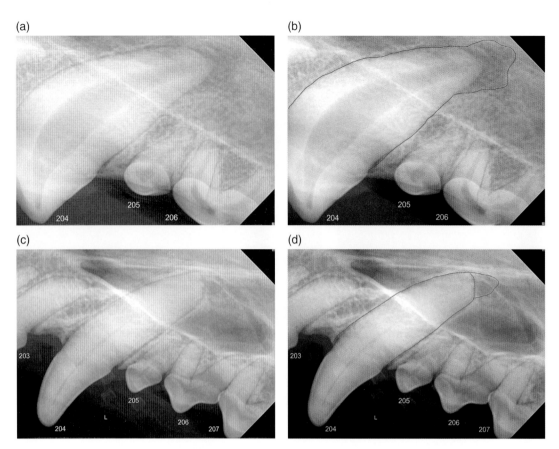

Figure 3.52 (a) Radiographic image of the left maxilla of a dog. This image depicts the left maxillary canine tooth, 1st premolar, and mesial root of the 2nd premolar tooth. Note the periodontal ligament of the maxillary canine tooth is very close to the mesial and distal aspects of the tooth until it reaches the apical 1/3 of the root. At this point, the periodontal ligament space is less distinct, and there is the presence of a periapical lucency associated with the root of this tooth. Also notice the large pulp canal in the left maxillary canine tooth compared to the surrounding teeth. This would suggest that the left maxillary canine tooth is nonvital. Root canal or extraction of this tooth is warranted. (b) Radiographic image of the left maxilla of a dog. This is the same image as in Figure (a). The red line outlines the periodontal ligament space of the mesial and distal surfaces of the left maxillary canine tooth. In the area of the apical 1/3 of the root, the red lines depict the irregular area of radiolucency surrounding the root of the tooth, suggesting a periapical lucency and abscess of the tooth root. (c) Radiographic image of the left maxilla of a dog. This image depicts a more mature left maxillary canine tooth. Note the similar sized pulp canals of this tooth compared to the surrounding teeth. This would suggest the tooth remains vital compared to the pulp chamber discrepancy observed in Figure (a) and (b). Note how the periodontal ligament space is observed all the way around the tooth, including the apical 1/3 of the tooth root and the apex of the tooth. Also notice there is a radiolucent area that is apical to the tooth root with smooth margins. This radiolucent area is consistent with a chevron or radiographic artifact. Note how the margins of the lucency are much smoother compared to the asymmetrical margins of the radiolucency associated with Figure (a) and (b). (d) Radiographic image of the left maxilla of a dog. This is the same image as in Figure (c). The red lines identify the smooth margins of the periodontal ligament space of the left maxillary canine tooth. They also easily demonstrate the periodontal ligament continuing around the apex of the canine tooth and the separate radiolucent area extending from the apex of the canine tooth identified as a radiographic chevron.

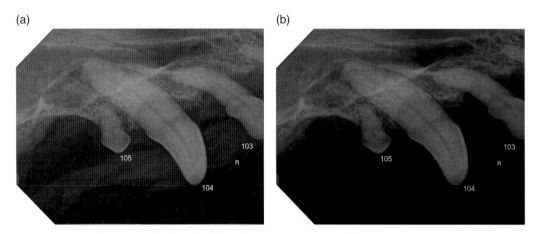

Figure 3.53 (a) Radiographic image of the right maxilla of a dog. This image depicts a mature right maxillary canine tooth. There is the appearance of horizontal bone loss associated with the right maxillary 3rd incisor, canine, and 1st premolar teeth. The right maxillary 2nd premolar tooth appears to be missing. Note the appearance of a chevron associated with the right maxillary canine tooth. (b) Radiographic image of the right maxilla of a dog. This is the same image as in Figure (a). Note the periodontal ligament space is smooth and very closely associated with the right maxillary canine tooth. Also note the connected arrowhead shape of the chevron associated with the apical extent of the canine tooth. The periodontal ligament and the chevron are outlined in red.

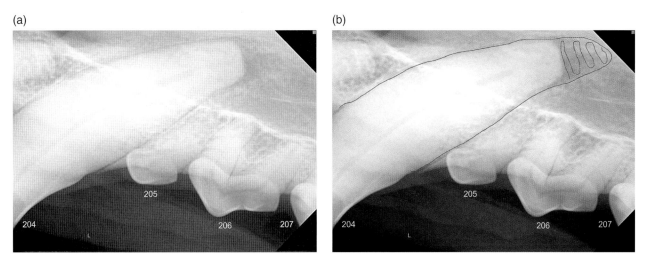

Figure 3.54 (a) Radiographic image of the left maxilla of a dog. The image depicts the left maxillary canine tooth with a loss of the periodontal ligament space beginning at the apical 1/3 of the tooth and extending apically from the tooth. While there are smooth margins of the periodontal ligament space extending apically, there is a loss of the periodontal ligament space directly around the apex of the tooth. The loss of the periodontal ligament space would suggest a periapical lucency or tooth root abscess. (b) Radiographic image of the left maxilla of a dog. This is the same image as in Figure (a). The periodontal ligament space is depicted by the red lines. Note how when the ligament reaches the apical 1/3 of the tooth, there is a loss of the radiolucent space directly around the apex. The radiolucency suggests an apical abscess which is identified by the squiggly lines within the outline of the periodontal ligament space extending apically from the tooth.

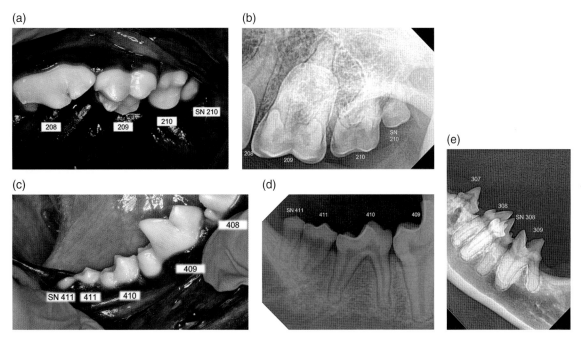

Figure 3.55 (a) Clinical image of the left maxillary 4th premolar, 1st molar, 2nd molar, and a supernumerary (SN) 2nd molar tooth of a dog. A supernumerary tooth may look identical to the tooth it is duplicating. A supernumerary tooth should not be confused with a persistent deciduous tooth. In the case of this patient, it would be unlikely that the extra tooth is a persistent deciduous tooth as there are no deciduous molar teeth present in the deciduous dentition. (b) Radiographic image of the left maxilla of a dog. This is the same patient as in Figure (a). Note how there are three identical teeth on the radiographic image, decreasing in size beginning with the left maxillary 1st molar (209), decreasing in size to the 2nd molar (210) and supernumerary (SN) 2nd molar (SN 210). (c) Clinical image of the right mandibular 1st, 2nd, and 3rd molars and a supernumerary (SN) 3rd molar tooth of a dog. In this patient, it is unlikely that the extra tooth would be classified as a persistent deciduous tooth due to its location in the mouth being in the area of a molar tooth.
(d) Radiographic image of the right mandible of a dog. This is the same patient as in Figure (c). Note the large tooth on the right side of the image. This is the right mandibular 1st molar tooth. The image would be diagnostic for the three teeth seen clearly on the image. These teeth are the caudal molar teeth. The right mandibular 2nd molar tooth clearly has two roots identified. The remaining two teeth are suspected to be 3rd molar teeth. Either of the two teeth could be identified as the supernumerary (SN) tooth. (e) Radiographic image of the left mandible of a cat. There should only be three teeth present caudal to the canine tooth in the cat. In this image, there are four similar sized teeth present. Note tooth 307, while not a diagnostic image for this tooth, shows evidence of tooth resorption, as well as some horizontal bone loss. There are two teeth superimposed on each other. One of these would be designated a supernumerary 4th premolar tooth. All teeth in this image except for the left maxillary 3rd premolar tooth appear to have clear evidence of an intact periodontal ligament space present. There is also evidence of horizontal bone loss associated with all other premolars and molars in the image.

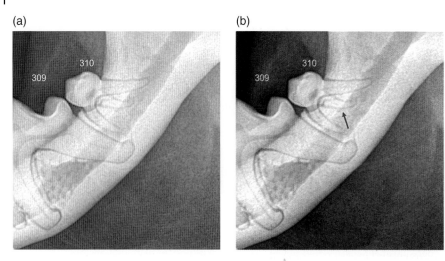

Figure 3.56 (a) Radiographic image of the left mandible of a dog. This image clearly shows the presence of an extra or supernumerary root associated with the left mandibular 2nd molar tooth. This patient is also missing the left mandibular 3rd molar tooth. There should be no three rooted teeth within the mandible. Identifying an extra root prior to extraction will help ensure all roots are removed in their entirety. (b) Radiographic image of the left mandible of a dog. This is the same image as in Figure (a). The red arrow identifies a supernumerary root. Frequently an extra root, if present, will be found in the area of the furcation or "crotch" of a multi-rooted tooth.

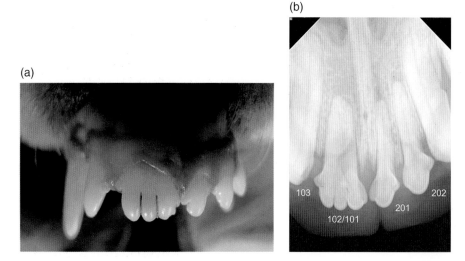

Figure 3.57 (a) Clinical image of the rostral maxilla of a dog. Notice the abnormal appearance of the crown of the right maxillary incisor tooth. The incisor tooth appears to be larger than the surrounding incisor teeth and there is malformation of the crown. (b) Radiographic image of the rostral maxilla of a dog. Note there appears to be a malformed incisor tooth. Without histologic diagnosis, it is difficult to diagnose why the tooth has an abnormal appearance. Differentials for this abnormality would include Fusion, Concrescence, and Gemination. There is a reduced number of incisor teeth present both clinically and radiographically. While there is no obvious separation of two crowns in either the radiograph or the clinical image, the tooth has a singular root, and this would suggest that gemination of the tooth is the most likely diagnosis.

affected by different developmental conditions. These conditions can influence the clinical appearance of the crown and root of the tooth as well as affect the number of roots that would traditionally be associated with a specific tooth. The developmental conditions observed most commonly include fusion, concrescence, and gemination (Figure 3.57a and b).

Fusion Fusion is defined as two adjacent tooth germs merging together to form a singular larger tooth [21, 22]. Histologically, "true fusion" of teeth occurs when there is merging of enamel and dentin. When fusion is observed within teeth, the number of teeth present within the oral cavity is reduced by one, as the two tooth germs fused together to form a singular tooth [22, 23]. Fused teeth usually do not share a common root canal system and maintain their individual root canal components.

Concrescence   Concrescence is similar to fusion in that there is a union of two or more teeth by fusion of the cementum alone [21, 23]. The process of concrescence is identified as a developmental abnormality if the union of the cementum occurs prior to root formation when the roots are in close proximity to each other [23]. Concrescence can also be an acquired condition if it develops following an episode of chronic inflammation, commonly associated with a tooth that was determined to be nonvital. Concrescence can only be diagnosed on a tooth histologically [23]. This means extraction of the tooth would be necessary for the definitive diagnosis of this condition.

Gemination   Gemination is the process by which a single tooth germ fails to divide properly resulting in a tooth with the appearance of two crowns [21, 22]. This "double tooth" anomaly commonly has a single root between the two crowns [22]. Gemination is thought to occur due to the incomplete separation of an individual tooth germ into two separate components due to genetic and/or environmental triggers [22]. The anomaly of gemination commonly gives rise to a singular root with a common root canal system between the bifid crowns. Gemination results in the same number of teeth present within the oral cavity. This is due to an individual tooth germ attempting to divide into two teeth but ultimately fails to complete the process, resulting in the bifid crowned tooth with an individual root canal system [23].

Dilacerated Tooth Roots   Along with having fewer roots due to developmental abnormalities, the roots themselves can be malformed. Root dilaceration is defined by the American Association of Endodontists as displacement of the root of a tooth from its normal alignment with the crown [24] (Figures 3.43b and 3.58a–d). True dilaceration of tooth roots is thought to be a consequence of injury during tooth root development [21]. Additionally, any severe angulation of a tooth root in either a mesial or distal direction is also called dilaceration [24]. Radiographically, identifying teeth with severe dilaceration can help the surgeon formulate the best approach to treatment for the patient and identify potential areas of complication prior to their occurrence.

Bone

The alveolar bone is one of the structures that supports the teeth of mammals within the jaw. The alveolar bone along with the periodontal ligament and cementum provide the needed attachment to help offer teeth the flexibility to withstand the forces of mastication. Specifically, the alveolar bone is the ridge of bone that contains the sockets in which the teeth sit in the bone in both the mandible and the maxilla. Alveolar bone is constantly remodeling and adapting to the forces applied to it by the process of resorption and deposition. There are four layers of alveolar bone: periosteum, compact bone, cancellous bone, and the alveolar process or cribiform plate [24].

The alveolar process is the ridge of compact bone that lies adjacent to the periodontal ligament to provide support to the tooth. It would also be considered the lining of the tooth socket or alveolus. Radiographically this alveolar process is called the lamina dura (Figure 3.59a and b). The lamina dura is the attachment structure by which the periodontal ligament attaches to the cementum. In a periodontally sound tooth, the crest of alveolar bone is normally positioned approximately 1 mm apical to the cementoenamel junction [24]. The vascular and nerve supply penetrate the alveolar bone and alveolar processes to supply nutrients to these areas [24].

Bone Loss

Horizontal Bone Loss   Horizontal bone loss is described as a generalized even degree of bone loss. There is a uniform loss of bone in relation to the height of the tooth. Horizontal bone loss appears across the entire root or tooth or across multiple teeth (Figure 3.60a and b).

Vertical Bone Loss   Vertical bone loss is described as an angular loss of bone. It can result in an uneven reduction of bone in relation to the height of the tooth. Vertical bone loss appears adjacent to an individual tooth or root in a triangular shaped trench (Figure 3.61a and b). This type of bone loss is frequently associated with maxillary canine teeth.

Furcation Bone Loss   The furcation is the area between a multi-rooted tooth in which the roots converge to form a single tooth. Radiographically, a viewer can state that there appears to be loss of bone within the furcation area but cannot make any additional comments to the extent of the loss based on a radiographic evaluation alone. This is because the bone in this area may be less dense due to a disease process, but can be filled with soft tissue or granulation tissue, which is less radiographically dense, maintaining sufficient attachment in the furcation area (Figure 3.62a and b). A clinical evaluation of this area is necessary to correlate the radiographic findings with the clinical findings in these cases.

Interpretation of Radiographic Shadows

When mineralized structures are superimposed on one another, there will be an increase in density to their appearance on the image. For example, when the dental arcade is imaged, the teeth appear to be more radiopaque compared

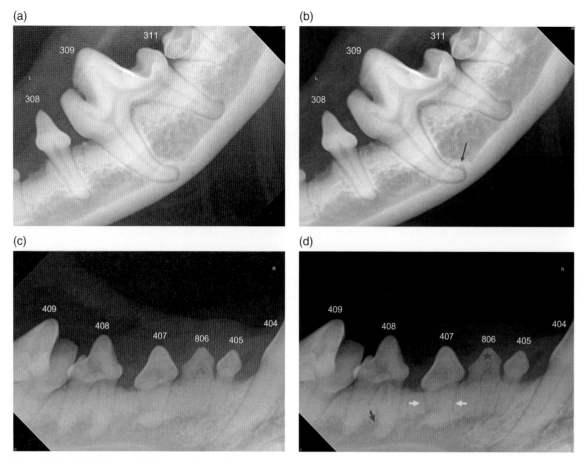

Figure 3.58 (a) Radiographic image of the left mandible of a dog. Note the significant curve to the mesial root of the left mandibular 1st molar tooth. This is an example of dilaceration. Dental radiography helps identify the appearance of the root to help facilitate extraction or treatment of the tooth. Also notice the left mandibular 2nd molar tooth is missing as the tooth caudal to the mandibular 1st molar tooth only has one root present. Also note the mandibular 4th premolar tooth appears to have only one root as well. (b) Radiographic image of the left mandible of a dog. This is the same image as in Figure (a). The red arrow depicts dilaceration of the mesial root of the mandibular 1st molar tooth. The yellow arrows depict the appearance of a single root of the left mandibular 4th premolar tooth. (c) Radiographic image of the right mandible of a dog. Note the dilaceration of the right mandibular 4th premolar tooth. In general, caudal dilaceration of the root occurs more frequently than a cranial or rostral direction. This image also depicts a right mandibular 3rd premolar tooth with fused roots, as there is only one root associated with this tooth. Additionally, there is the appearance of a persistent deciduous right mandibular 2nd premolar tooth and a missing permanent 2nd premolar tooth. (d) Radiographic image of the right mandible of a dog. This is the same image as in Figure (c). The red arrow depicts the caudal dilaceration of the right mandibular 4th premolar tooth. The yellow arrows depict the presence of a fused root associated with the right mandibular 3rd premolar tooth. The star depicts the presence of a persistent deciduous right mandibular 2nd premolar tooth.

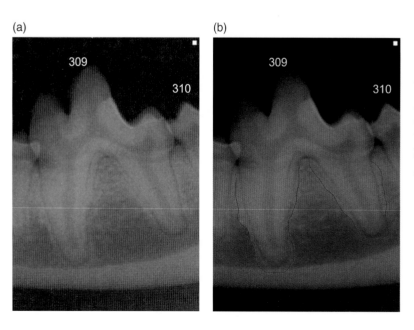

Figure 3.59 (a) Radiographic image of the left mandible of a dog. This is an image of the left mandibular 1st molar tooth (309). The increased radiodensity surrounding the roots and the periodontal ligament is called the lamina dura. This is a normal radiographic appearance of the compact bone that lies adjacent to the periodontal ligament. (b) Radiographic image of the left mandible of a dog. This is the same image as in Figure (a). The red line outlines the area of lamina dura on the left mandibular 1st molar tooth.

Figure 3.60 (a) Radiographic image of the rostral mandible of a dog. This radiographic image of the mandibular incisors demonstrates severe horizontal bone loss associated with these teeth. Horizontal bone loss is a uniform loss of bone in a horizontal plane across either the entire tooth, root, or multiple teeth. (b) Radiographic image of the rostral mandible of a dog. This is the same image as in Figure (a). The white line (A) depicts the expected normal alveolar bone height of the mandibular incisor teeth. The red line (B) depicts the actual alveolar bone margin on this patient, indicating severe horizontal bone loss.

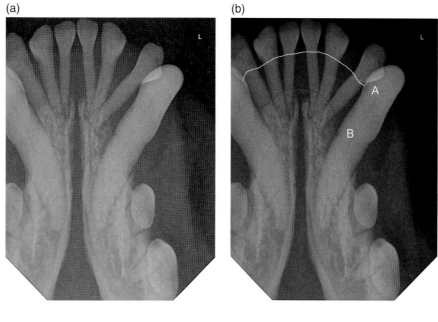

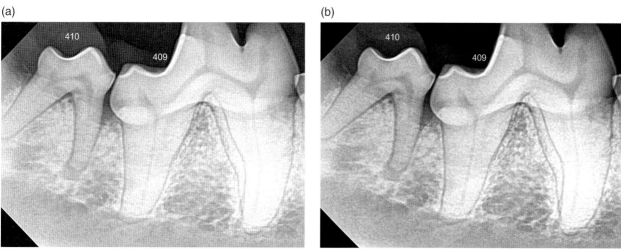

Figure 3.61 (a) Radiographic image of the right caudal mandible of a dog. This radiographic image is diagnostic for the right mandibular 1st molar tooth (409) and the mesial root of the 2nd molar tooth (410). Note the loss of bone between the 1st and 2nd molar teeth. There is a "V" shaped decrease in bone beginning at the distal aspect of the 1st molar extending to the mesial aspect of the 2nd molar tooth. This angular shaped loss of bone is consistent with vertical bone loss. (b) Radiographic image of the right caudal mandible of a dog. This is the same image as in Figure (a). The red line outlines the angular shape of the vertical bone loss associated with the right mandibular 2nd molar tooth.

to the interdental space. This is due to the density of the teeth superimposed on the density of the surrounding alveolar bone Conversely, when air, or air-filled structures are superimposed over the bone, the radiographic area will appear less dense. When fluid, fluid-filled or soft tissue structures are superimposed on mineralized structures, the density of the area appears more radiopaque than air or air-filled structures, but less radiopaque than mineralized structures superimposed over a mineralized area. When pathology is present, more than 30% mineral content may be lost before there is radiographic evidence of disease [25].

Therefore, early lesions may go undetected by the use of radiographs alone depending on the stage of disease and the type of bone that is affected [25].

Nomenclature

Terminology for directions within the oral cavity are different than other areas of the body (Box 3.2, Figures 3.63 and 3.64). The terms cranial and caudal are replaced by the terms mesial and distal respectively, with **mesial** being the

(a) (b)

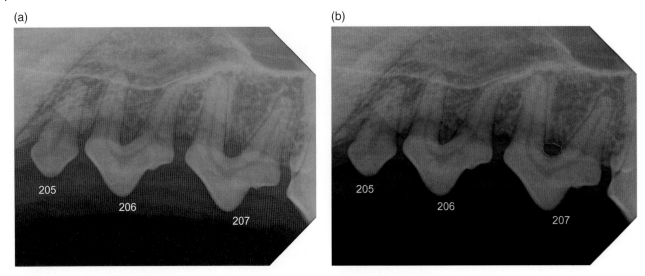

Figure 3.62 (a) Radiographic image of the left maxilla of a dog. This image shows a generalized loss of bone across all teeth on the image, suggesting mild horizontal bone loss. Additionally, there is an increased loss of bone within the furcation of the left maxillary 3rd premolar tooth (207). While true furcation exposure cannot be assessed on radiographic imaging alone, there is a loss of density between the roots of this tooth. (b) Radiographic image of the left maxilla of a dog. This is the same image as in Figure (a). The red outline depicts the suspected loss of bone within the furcation of the left maxillary 3rd premolar tooth (207).

Box 3.2 Nomenclature	
Different terminology is used in the oral cavity compared to other areas of the body. This box describes the common directional terminology used within the oral cavity.	
Vestibular	term used to describe the surface of the teeth facing outward from the inside of the oral cavity
Palatal	term that is used specifically for the maxillary arcade for the surfaces of the incisors, canines, premolars, and molars that face inward toward the hard palate
Facial	term used for the maxillary arcade that holds the canine, premolar, and molar teeth, or the surface that faces the lips or cheeks
Lingual	term that is used for either the maxillary or mandibular arcade for the surfaces if the incisors, canines, premolars, and molars that face inward toward the tongue
Buccal	term used to describe the surface of the teeth that contact or are closest to the cheek surfaces for the premolar and molar region
Labial	term used to describe the surface of the teeth that are closest to the cheek for the incisor region
Coronal	term used to describe the surface toward the clinical crown of a tooth
Apical	term used to describe the area of the root farthest away from the tip of the clinical crown
Mesial	term used to describe the leading edge of the tooth that is closest to midline arching around the arcade. This term can be used to describe a surface or a specific root
Distal	term used to describe surface of the tooth away from midline. This term can be used to describe a surface or a specific root
Occlusal	term used to describe the surface of the tooth used for biting, chewing, and grinding of substances, or the surface that meets the tooth or teeth from the opposite jaw

surface toward midline and **distal** being the surface away from midline. There are also areas of the mouth that can be described using one or more terms, such as the lingual surface. **Lingual** is a term used to describe the inside surface of both the maxillary and mandibular arcades, as both of these arcades contact the tongue, or lingual surface. **Palatal** is a term used to describe only the surfaces of the maxilla that contact the hard palate. The surfaces toward the crown of the tooth are deemed **coronal** and those that are toward the root of the tooth are described as **apical**. **Facial** is used for the surface of the maxillary canine, premolar, and molar teeth that are in contact with the lips and cheek of the patient. The term **buccal** can also be used to describe the surface of the teeth that contact the cheeks. **Vestibular** is reserved for the surfaces of the teeth that face the vestibule or lips or the surfaces that face outward from inside the oral cavity. **Labial** is used to describe the surfaces of the teeth closest to the cheek but in the region of the incisors that is in contact with the lips. The terms labial and buccal can be used to describe areas in the facial or vestibular region of the mouth. **Occlusal** is a term that describes the surface of the tooth that is used for biting, chewing, or grinding, or the surface of a tooth that contacts the tooth or teeth in the opposite jaw.

Where to Begin?

When first beginning to interpret dental radiographic images, the observer needs to understand the basic principles of labial mounting and interpretation (Box 3.3).

Questions that should be pondered should include the following:

1) Is this maxilla or mandible?
2) What teeth are present?
3) Is this the right or left side?
4) Are the teeth deciduous, permanent, or both?
5) Do the teeth have the appropriate number of roots?
6) Do the roots look normal? (i.e. periodontal ligament space too wide or nonexistent)
7) Do the contents of the tooth look normal? (is the pulp chamber too wide or too narrow, does it look irregular)
8) What is the alveolar bone height? (i.e. is there horizontal or vertical bone loss, or is there bone over the tooth)
9) Does what I see radiographically correlate with what I see clinically?

The next several images are unlabeled and labeled radiographic images of anatomic structures associated with the maxillary and mandibular arcades to help familiarize individuals with the normal oral anatomy associated with canine and feline teeth (Figures 3.65a, b, 3.66a–c, 3.67a, b, 3.68a, b, 3.69a, b, 3.70a, b, 3.71a, b, 3.72a, b, 3.73a, b, 3.74a, b, 3.75a, b, 3.76a, b, 3.77a, b, 3.78a, b, 3.79a, b, 3.80a, b, 3.81a, b, 3.82a, b, 3.83a, and b).

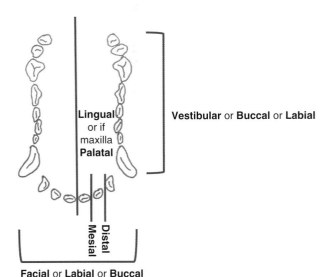

Figure 3.63 Figure identifies the directional terms used within the oral cavity. (A) **Mesial** is the surface toward midline, (B) **Distal** is the surface away from midline, (C) **Lingual** is the inside surface of both maxillary and mandibular arcades facing toward the tongue, (D) **Palatal** is the surface the maxilla that contacts the hard palate, (E) **Facial** is the surface of the maxillary canines, premolar, and molar teeth in contact with the lips and cheek. (Can also use labial and buccal.), (F) **Buccal** is the surface of the teeth in contact with the cheeks, (G) **Labial** is the surface of the teeth in contact with the lips, (H) **Vestibular** is the surface of the teeth that faces outward from inside the oral cavity which are in contact with the vestibule or lips. (Can also use labial and buccal.)

Figure 3.64 Radiographic images used to identify specific areas and surfaces of the tooth and root. (A) **Apical** is used to describe the root portion of the tooth, (B) **Coronal** is used to describe the crown portion of the tooth, (C) **Occlusal** is used to describe the surface of the teeth used for grinding.

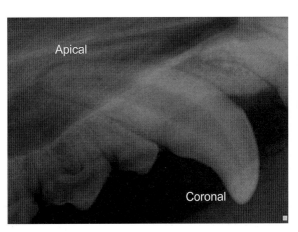
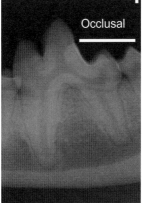

Box 3.3 Steps to reading a dental radiograph

This box describes the approach to reading a dental radiographic image. A logical approach to reading a dental radiograph assists the observer in looking at all portions of the tooth including the crown, root, and alveolar bone. Radiographs need to be well positioned so that the image can demonstrate pathology and not falsely create artifacts that could be interpreted as disease. The observer should be able to identify which arcade they are looking at, whether it is the right or left side, and whether they are looking at the mandible or maxilla. All aspects of the crown, root, and alveolar bone should be evaluated for evidence of disease. As always, the radiographic findings should be correlated with the clinical examination findings, including periodontal probing, to formulate an appropriate treatment plan.

Make sure the image is well positioned	Minimize elongation
	Minimize foreshortening
	Verify at least 2 mm of tissue present apical to tooth root
	Minimize overexposure or underexposure
	Minimize cone cutting
Scan the film for normal anatomic markers	Identify whether maxilla or mandible
	Identify what teeth are present
	Identify whether looking at the right side or left side
	Identify whether the teeth are deciduous or permanent
Evaluate all aspects of the crown	Assess pulp chamber size
	Assess whether there is evidence of resorption
	Assess for presence of pulp stones
Evaluate all aspects of the root	Assess root canal size
	Assess whether there is evidence of resorption
	Assess periodontal ligament space
	Identify appropriate number of roots (supernumerary/fused)
	Assess direction of apical portion of root (dilaceration)
Evaluate all aspects of the alveolar bone	Assess bone height and presence of horizontal bone loss
	Assess for evidence of vertical bone loss
	Assess for mandibular cortical bone loss
	Assess for trabecular bone loss
	Assess for teeth below alveolar bone margin
Correlate radiographic findings with clinical finding on oral examination	Assess periodontal disease score and formulate treatment plan

Conclusion

Having a grasp of the normal radiographic anatomy of the canine and feline oral cavity is imperative for diagnosis and formulation of an appropriate treatment plan. Labial mounting assists with consistent evaluation of the radiographic images. Using appropriate terminology also helps standardize the viewing and interpretation of radiographs. Knowledge of the expected number of teeth within the deciduous and permanent dentition and the anticipated number of roots associated with each tooth is imperative for the assessment and treatment of the patient. Being able to discern normal anatomy and radiographic artifacts from pathology is also essential for formulating an accurate treatment plan for a patient.

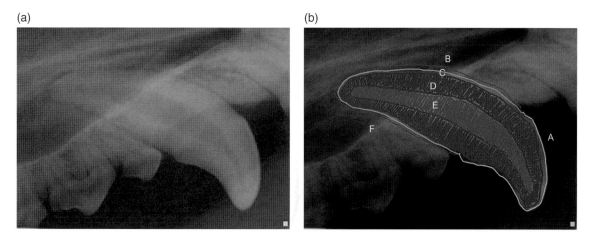

Figure 3.65 (a) Unlabeled radiographic image of the right maxillary canine tooth of a dog. (b) Labeled radiographic image of the right maxillary canine tooth of a dog. (A) Enamel (orange), (B) Periodontal ligament space (pink), (C) Cementum (green), (D) Dentin (blue), (E) Pulp (red), (F) Nasal surface of alveolar process.

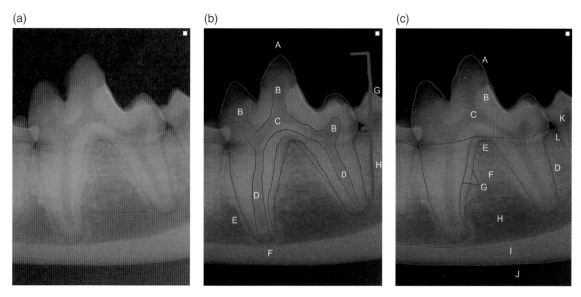

Figure 3.66 (a) Unlabeled radiographic image of the left mandibular 1st molar tooth (309) of a dog. (b) Labeled radiographic image of the left mandibular 1st molar tooth (309) of a dog. (A) Cusp, (B) Pulp horn, (C) Pulp chamber, (D) Pulp canal/root canal, (E) Periodontal ligament space, (F) Apex, (G) Crown, (H) Root. (c) Labeled radiographic image of the left mandibular 1st molar tooth 309 of a dog. (A) Enamel, (B) Dentin, (C) Pulp chamber, (D) Periodontal ligament space, (E) Furcation, (F) Interradicular bone, (G) Radicular groove, (H) Mandibular canal, (I) Compact bone of the ventral mandible, (J) Ventral cortex of the mandible, (K) Alveolar bone margin, (L) Cementoenamel junction.

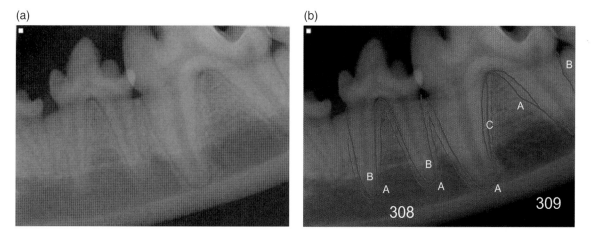

Figure 3.67 (a) Unlabeled radiographic image of the left mandibular 4th premolar and 1st molar teeth of a dog. (b) Labeled image of the left mandibular 4th premolar and 1st molar teeth of a dog. (A) Lamina dura, (B) Periodontal ligament, (C) Radicular groove.

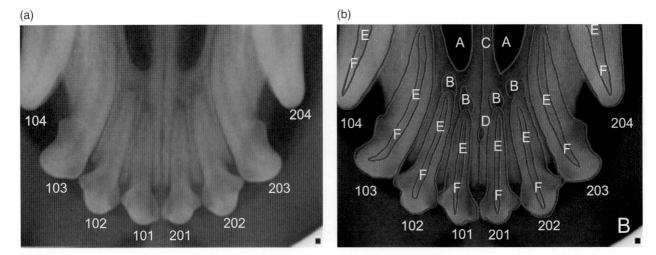

Figure 3.68 (a) Unlabeled image of the maxillary incisors of a dog. (b) Labeled image of the maxillary incisors of a dog. (A) Palatine fissures, (B) "Chevron" lucencies, (C) Interincisive suture, (D) Incisive canal, (E) Pulp canal/root canal, (F) Pulp chamber.

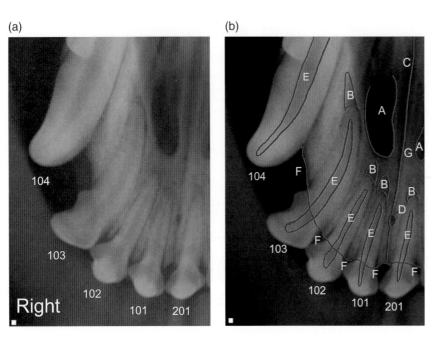

Figure 3.69 (a) Unlabeled image of the right maxillary incisors of a dog. (b) Labeled image of the right maxillary incisors of a dog. (A) Palatine fissures, (B) "Chevron" lucencies, (C) Interincisive suture, (D) Incisive canal, (E) Pulp, (F) Alveolar margin, (G) Vomer bone.

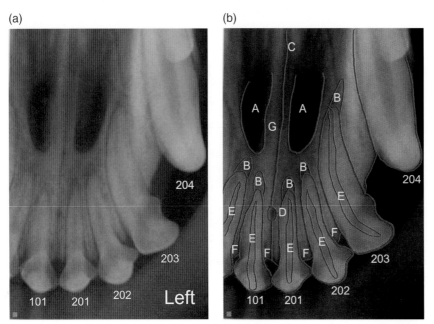

Figure 3.70 (a) Unlabeled image of the left maxillary incisors of a dog. (b) Labeled image of the left maxillary incisors of a dog. (A) Palatine fissures, (B) "Chevron" lucencies, (C) Interincisive suture, (D) Incisive canal, (E) Pulp, (F) Alveolar margin, (G) Vomer bone.

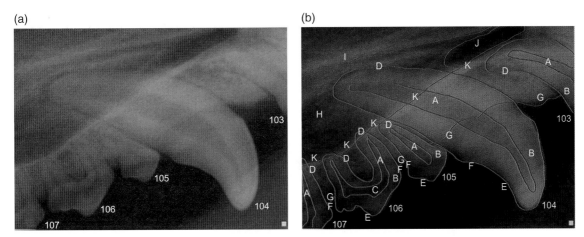

Figure 3.71 (a) Unlabeled image of the right maxillary canine, and 1st and 2nd premolars of a dog. (b) Labeled image of the right maxillary canine, and 1st and 2nd premolar teeth of a dog. (A) Pulp canal, (B) Dentin, (C) Pulp chamber, (D) Periodontal ligament space, (E) Enamel, (F) Cementoenamel junction, (G) Alveolar margin, (H) Nasal cavity, (I) Interincisive suture, (J) Palatine fissure, (K) Nasal surface of the alveolar process.

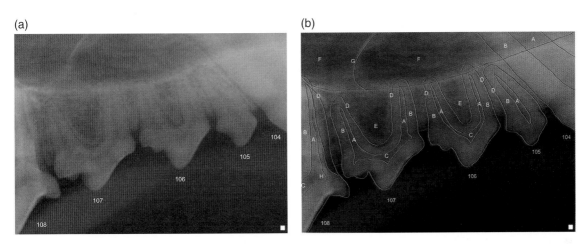

Figure 3.72 (a) Unlabeled image of the right maxillary 1st, 2nd, and 3rd premolar teeth of a dog. (b) Labeled image of the right maxillary 1st, 2nd, and 3rd premolar teeth of a dog. (A) Pulp canal, (B) Dentin, (C) Pulp chamber, (D) Periodontal ligament space, (E) Interradicular bone, (F) Nasal cavity, (G) Conchal crest, (H) Pulp horn.

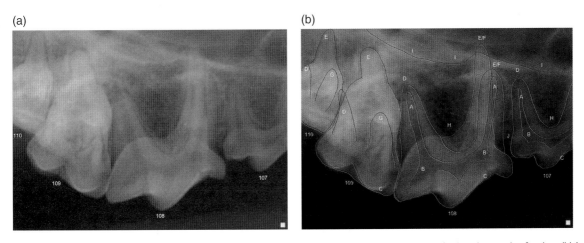

Figure 3.73 (a) Unlabeled image of the right maxillary 3rd and 4th premolars and 1st and 2nd molar teeth of a dog. (b) Labeled image of the right maxillary 3rd and 4th premolars and 1st and 2nd molar teeth of a dog. (A) Pulp canal, (B) Pulp horn, (C) Enamel, (D) Distal or distobuccal roots of the right maxillary 4th premolar, and 1st and 2nd molars, (E) Palatal roots of the right maxillary 1st and 2nd molars, (E/F) Mesiobuccal* or mesiopalatal* roots of the right maxillary 4th premolar tooth. *With a single image it is difficult to appreciate whether the root is the mesiobuccal root or mesiopalatal root of the maxillary 4th premolar tooth as these teeth are superimposed on one another. Two radiographic images are necessary to evaluate the tooth due to the location of their roots, (G) Mesial or mesiobuccal roots of the right maxillary 1st and 2nd molar teeth, (H) Interradicular bone, (I) Nasal surface of the alveolar process, (J) Interproximal bone.

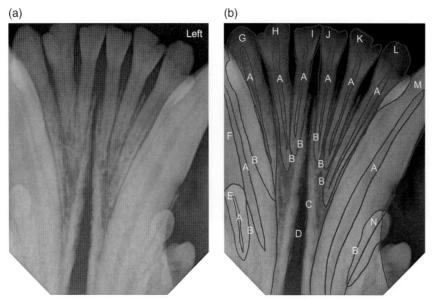

Figure 3.74 (a) Unlabeled image of the mandibular incisors of a dog. (b) Labeled image of the mandibular incisor teeth of a dog. (A) Pulp canal, (B) Periodontal ligament space, (C) Ventral cortex of the left mandible, (D) Ventral cortex of the right mandible, (E) Right mandibular 1st premolar tooth, (F) Right mandibular canine tooth, (G) Right mandibular 3rd incisor tooth, (H) Right mandibular 2nd incisor tooth, (I) Right mandibular 1st incisor tooth, (J) Left mandibular 1st incisor tooth, (K) Left mandibular 2nd incisor tooth, (L) Left mandibular 3rd incisor tooth, (M) Left mandibular canine tooth, (N) Left mandibular 1st premolar tooth.

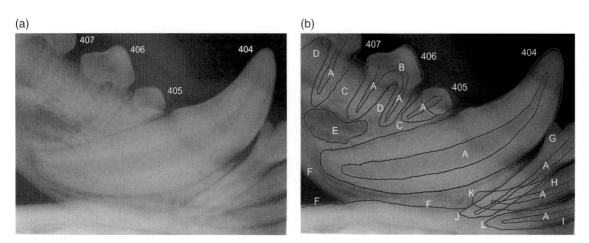

Figure 3.75 (a) Unlabeled image of the rostral right mandible of a dog. (b) Labeled image of the rostral right mandible of a dog. (A) Pulp canal, (B) Pulp chamber, (C) Interproximal bone, (D) Interradicular bone, (E) Middle mental foramen, (F) Ventral cortex of the right and left mandible, (G) Right mandibular 3rd incisor tooth, (H) Right mandibular 2nd incisor tooth, (I) Right mandibular 1st incisor tooth, (J) Apex of the right mandibular 3rd incisor tooth, (K) Apex of the right mandibular 2nd incisor tooth, (L) Apex of the right mandibular 1st incisor tooth.

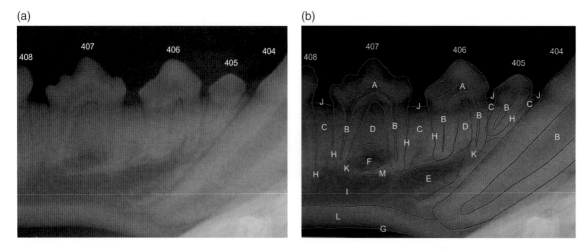

Figure 3.76 (a) Unlabeled image of the right mandible of a dog. (b) Labeled image of the right mandible of a dog. (A) Pulp chamber, (B) Pulp canal, (C) Interproximal bone, (D) Interradicular bone, (E) Middle mental foramen, (F) Caudal mental foramen, (G) Ventral cortex of the mandible, (H) Periodontal ligament space, (I) Mandibular canal, (J) Alveolar bone margin, (K) Dilaceration of a tooth root, (L) Body of the mandible.

Figure 3.77 (a) Unlabeled image of the right mandible of a dog. (b) Labeled image of the right mandible of a dog. (A) Pulp chamber, (B) Pulp canal, (C) Radicular groove, (D) Periodontal ligament space, (E) Mandibular body, (F) Mandibular canal, (G) Interproximal bone, (H) Interradicular bone, (I) Lamina dura (compact alveolar bone), (J) Furcation, (K) Alveolar bone margin, (L) Summation of the enamel (overlap) of the right mandibular 4th premolar and 1st molar teeth.

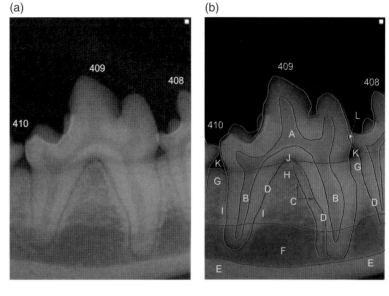

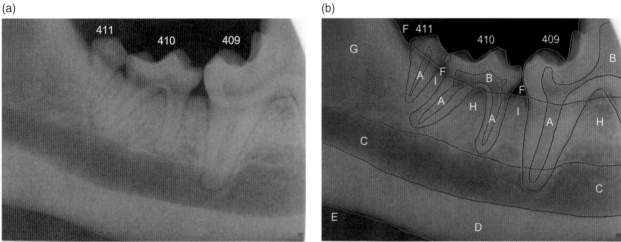

Figure 3.78 (a) Unlabeled image of the caudal right mandible of a dog. (b) Labeled image of the caudal right mandible of a dog. (A) Pulp canal, (B) Pulp chamber, (C) Mandibular canal, (D) Mandibular body, (E) Ventral mandibular cortex, (F) Alveolar bone margin, (G) Ramus of the mandible, (H) Interradicular bone, (I) Interproximal bone.

Figure 3.79 (a) Unlabeled image of the rostral maxilla of a cat. (b) Labeled image of the rostral maxilla of a cat. (A) Pulp canal, (B) Palatine fissures, (C) Interincisive suture, (D) Alveolar bone margin, (E) Incisive canal, (F) Vomer bone, (G) Dentin, (H) Incisive bone (nasal ridge), (I) Trabecular bone, (J) Nasal surface of alveolar process, (K) Nasal bone, (L) Incisive bone (nasal process).

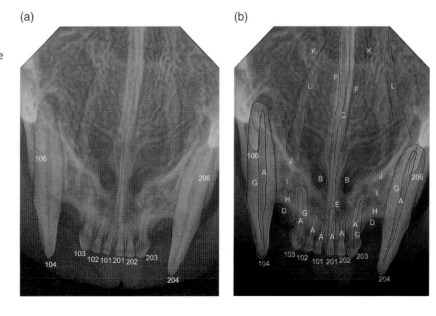

(a)

(b)

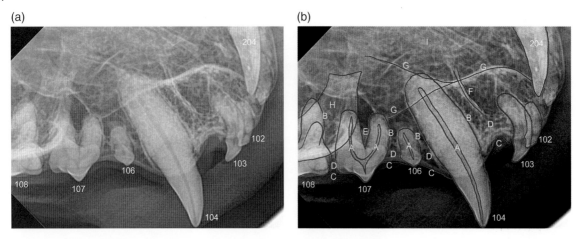

Figure 3.80 (a) Unlabeled image of the right maxilla of a cat. (b) Labeled image of the right maxilla of a cat. (A) Pulp canal, (B) Periodontal ligament space, (C) Alveolar bone margin, (D) Interproximal bone, (E) Interradicular bone, (F) Incisivomaxillary suture, (G) Nasal surface of alveolar process, (H) Zygomatic bone, (I) Nasal cavity.

(a)

(b)

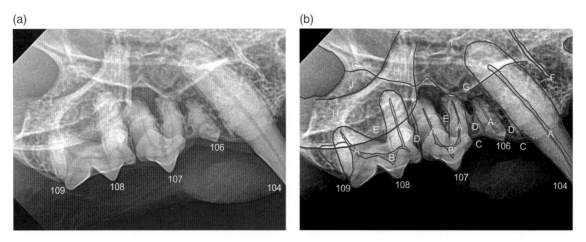

Figure 3.81 (a) Unlabeled image of the right caudal maxilla of a cat. (b) Labeled image of the right caudal maxilla of a cat. (A) Pulp canal, (B) Pulp chamber, (C) Alveolar bone margin, (D) Interproximal bone, (E) Interradicular bone, (F) Incisivomaxillary suture, (G) Nasal surface of alveolar process, (H) Zygomatic bone, (I) Nasal cavity, (J) Maxillary tuberosity.

(a)

(b)

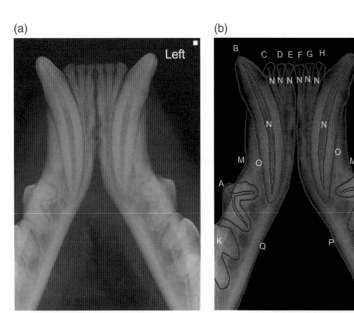

Figure 3.82 (a) Unlabeled image of the rostral mandible of a cat. (b) Labeled image of the rostral mandible of a cat. (A) Right mandibular 3rd premolar tooth, (B) Right mandibular canine tooth, (C) Right mandibular 3rd incisor tooth, (D) Right mandibular 2nd incisor tooth, (E) Right mandibular 1st incisor tooth, (F) Left mandibular 1st incisor tooth, (G) Left mandibular 2nd incisor tooth, (H) Left mandibular 3rd incisor tooth, (I) Left mandibular canine tooth, (J) Left mandibular 3rd premolar tooth, (K) Right mandibular 4th premolar tooth, (L) Left mandibular 4th premolar tooth, (M) Alveolar bone margin, (N) Pulp canal, (O) Periodontal ligament space, (P) Ventral cortex of the left mandible, (Q) Ventral cortex of the right mandible.

(a)

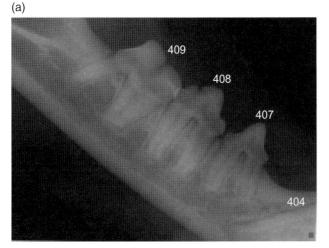

(b)

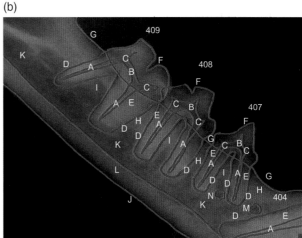

Figure 3.83 (a) Unlabeled image of the right mandible of a cat. (b) Labeled image of the right mandible of a cat. (A) Pulp canal, (B) Pulp chamber, (C) Pulp horns, (D) Periodontal ligament space, (E) Dentin, (F) Enamel, (G) Alveolar bone margin, (H) interproximal bone, (I) Interradicular bone, (J) Ventral mandibular cortex, (K) Mandibular canal, (L) Body of the mandible.

References

1 Verstraete, F.J., Kass, P.H., and Terpak, C.H. (1998). Diagnostic value of full-mouth radiography in dogs. *Am. J. Vet. Res.* 59: 686–691.

2 Verstraete, F.J., Kass, P.H., and Terpak, C.H. (1998). Diagnostic value of full-mouth radiography in cats. *Am. J. Vet. Res.* 59: 692–695.

3 Peralta, S. and Fiani, N. (2017). Interpretation of dental radiographs in dogs and cats. Part 1: principles and normal findings. *Today's Vet. Pract. J.* 2017: 55–66.

4 Floyd, M. (1991). The modified triadan system: nomenclature for veterinary dentistry. *J. Vet. Dent.* 8 (4): 18–19.

5 Wiggs, R.B. and Lobprise, H.B. (ed.) (1997). Oral examination and diagnosis. In: *Veterinary Dentistry Principles & Practice*, 87–103. Philadelphia: Lippencott-Raven.

6 Legendre, L. (1994). Dentistry on deciduous teeth: what, when, and how. *Can. Vet. J.* 35: 793–794.

7 Wilson, G.J. (1998). Atlas of the radiographic closure of the apices of the teeth of the dog. Master'Thesis, The University of Queensland. https://doi.org/10.14264/uqi.2020.268.

8 Wilson, G. (1999). Timing of apical closure of the maxillary canine and mandibular first molar teeth of cats. *J. Vet. Dent.* 16 (1): 19–21.

9 Nanci, A. (ed.) (2008). Structures of the oral tissues. In: *Ten Cate's Oral Histology, Development, Structure and Function*, 1–15. St. Louis: Mosby-Elsevier.

10 Crossley, D.A. (1995). Tooth enamel thickness in the mature dentition of domestic dogs and cats – preliminary study. *J. Vet. Dent.* 12 (3): 111–113.

11 Lacatus, R., Papuc, I., Muste, A. et al. (2010). Dental radiographic examination in dogs. *Cluj Vet. J.* 17 (1): 39–45.

12 Bellows, J. (2017). Image gallery: dental radiology. *Clin. Brief: Dent. Periodontol.* (April): https://www.cliniciansbrief.com/article/image-gallery-dental-radiography (accessed October 2022).

13 Peralta, S., Verstraete, F.J., and Kass, P.H. (2010). Radiographic evaluation of the types of tooth resorption in dogs. *Am. J. Vet. Res.* 71: 784–793.

14 Nanci, A. (2008). Dentin-pulp complex. In: *Ten Cate's Oral Histology, Development, Structure and Function*, 191–238. St. Louis: Mosby-Elsevier.

15 Foster, B.L. (2012). Methods for studying tooth root cementum by light microscopy. *Int. J. Oral Sci.* 4: 119–128.

16 Nanci, A. (2008). Periodontium. In: *Ten Cate's Oral Histology, Development, Structure and Function*, 239–267. St. Louis: Mosby-Elsevier.

17 Abbott, P.V. (2016). Prevention and management of external inflammatory resorption following trauma to teeth. *Aust. Dent. J.* 61: 82–94.

18 Hadi, A., Marius, C., Avi, S. et al. (2018). Ankylosed permanent teeth: incidence, etiology and guidelines for clinical management. *Med. Dent. Res.* 1 (1): 1–11.

19 American Association of Endodontists (2020). *Glossary of Endodontic Terms*, 10e. Chicago: American Association of Endodontists.

20 Luder, H.U. (2015). Malformations of the root in humans. *Front. Physiol.* 6: Article 307.

21 Ahmed, H.M.A. and Dummer, P.M.H. (2018). A new system for classifying tooth, root, and canal anomalies. *Int. Endod. J.* 51: 389–404.

22 Venkatesh, A., Mitthra, S., Prakash, V. et al. (2016). Gemination or fusion?: a case report. *Biomed. Pharmacol. J.* 9 (3): 1225–1228.

23 Sharma, U., Gulati, A., and Gill, N. (2013). Concrescent triplets involving primary anterior teeth. *Contemp. Clin. Dent.* 4 (1): 94–96.

24 Gorrel, C. (ed.) (2013). Anatomy of the teeth and periodontium. In: *Veterinary Dentistry for the General Practitioner*, 2e, 37–41. Edinburgh: Saunders-Elsevier.

25 Bender, I.B. (1982). Factors influencing the radiographic appearance of bony lesions. *J. Endod.* 8 (4): 161–170.

4

Interpretation of Common Oral Pathology in the Canine Patient

Brenda L. Mulherin[1] and Chanda Miles[2]

[1] *Lloyd Veterinary Medical Center, Iowa State University College of Veterinary Medicine, Ames, IA, USA*
[2] *Veterinary Dentistry Specialists, Katy, TX, USA*

CONTENTS

Diagnostic imaging for the interpretation of common oral pathology in the dog is invaluable for formulating a complete and accurate treatment plan. The most common imaging modalities utilized for interpretation of oral pathology in small animals are intraoral dental radiography, cone beam computed tomography (CBCT), and conventional computed tomography (CT). Each of these modalities carries benefits and disadvantages for identifying different types of pathology that can be found in canine and feline patients. Many of the attributes regarding CBCT and conventional CT will be discussed in Chapter 10. Intraoral dental radiography is currently the most readily available imaging modality utilized to diagnose oral pathology in a general practice setting. For this chapter, intraoral dental radiography will be used to demonstrate interpretation of common oral pathology in the canine patient.

Periodontal Disease

Periodontal disease (PD) is without question the most common oral disease diagnosed in companion animals. When disease is present, the periodontium is the most commonly affected tissue. The periodontium is composed of four structures: gingiva (free and attached), periodontal ligament (PDL), cementum, and alveolar bone (Figure 4.1).

Dental radiographs are a crucial diagnostic step when formulating a treatment plan for PD. However, radiographs should not be the sole diagnostic tool used to identify the presence and staging of PD. A comprehensive oral examination with periodontal probing must also be performed on the patient to accompany the dental radiographic findings. Combining the knowledge of the two techniques allows the observer to give an accurate PD stage to create an appropriate treatment plan for each tooth. Additionally,

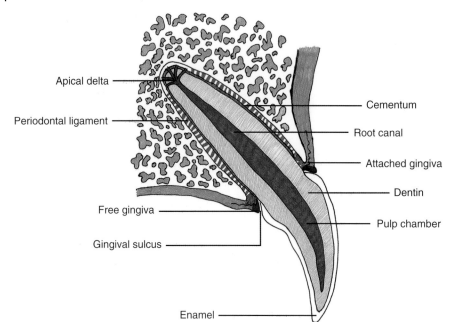

Figure 4.1 Drawing of the periodontium showing the alveolar bone, cementum, gingiva (free and attached), and the periodontal ligament. Enamel is the outside covering of the crown of the tooth. The apical delta is the webbing of neurovascular supply that provides the tooth with nutrients and innervation. The gingival sulcus is the free space around the tooth where the periodontal probe is placed to assess periodontal pocketing. Dentin provides the bulk of the tooth and is produced throughout the life of the tooth. The root canal describes the pulp located within the root of the tooth and the pulp chamber describes the pulp within the crown of the tooth.

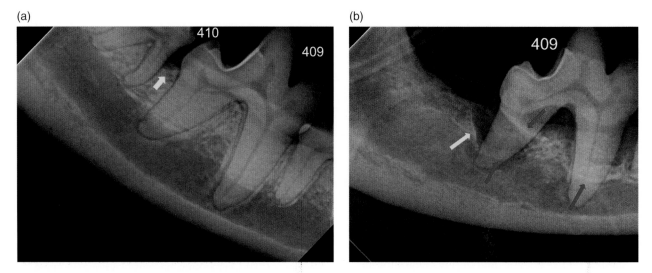

Figure 4.2 (a) Radiograph of the right mandibular 1st molar tooth (409) showing no bone loss present. This image also depicts a portion of the right mandibular 2nd molar tooth (410). Notice slight vertical bone loss on the mesial aspect of tooth 410 (yellow arrow). (b) Radiograph of same patient in Figure (a) showing progressive horizontal (red arrows) and vertical bone (yellow arrow) loss three years later. Also notice the loss of the right mandibular 2nd molar tooth (410) from the image in Figure (a). In this image the right mandibular 3rd molar tooth (411) is also missing.

dental radiography is crucial for monitoring disease progression as well as evaluation of a previously performed periodontal therapy such as bone graft placement for reduction of a periodontal pocket. Utilizing the dental radiographs performed at the initial procedure can provide insight to the success of the therapy provided (Figures 4.2a, b, and 4.3a–c).

Stages of PD

PD is divided into four stages depending on how much inflammation and attachment loss is present both clinically and radiographically (Table 4.1). The first stage of PD is the only reversible stage and will not have any radiographic evidence of disease as there is no bone loss present at this

(a) (b) (c)

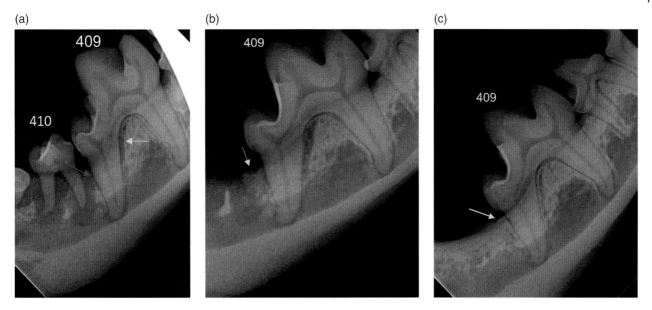

Figure 4.3 (a) Moderate vertical bone loss on the distal aspect of the right mandibular 1st molar tooth (409) (red arrow) secondary to severe bone loss around both the mesial and distal roots of the right mandibular 2nd molar tooth (410). There is also widening of the periodontal ligament space on the mesial aspect of the distal root of 409 (yellow arrow). (b) Radiographic image immediately after extraction of the right mandibular 2nd and 3rd molar teeth (410, 411) and placement of an osteoallograft and bone membrane. The graft and membrane were placed following appropriate cleaning and preparation of the root on the distal aspect of the right mandibular 1st molar tooth (409). The bone graft can be seen as increased mineralization on the distal aspect of tooth 409 (arrow). (c) Radiograph of the right mandibular 1st molar tooth (409) in the same patient as seen in Figure (a) and (b), 10 months following periodontal therapy including bone graft placement. The alveolar bone height and periodontal ligament space have returned to normal.

Table 4.1 Stages of periodontal disease.

Stages of periodontal disease	Description
Stage 1	Gingivitis only. No radiographic evidence of disease
Stage 2	Gingivitis and 25% attachment loss
Stage 3	Gingivitis and 25–50% attachment loss
Stage 4	Gingivitis and >50% attachment loss

The table describes the stages of periodontal disease. Stage 1 periodontal disease is depicted by inflammation of the soft tissues of the gingiva only. At this stage, there is no attachment loss noted either clinically or radiographically, only inflammation of the gingiva is noted. Stage 2 periodontal disease is a progression of Stage 1 in which there is the presence of gingivitis, along with attachment loss. This may consist of loss of the hard tissue structures that attach the teeth into the alveolus including loss of bone, gingival recession, increased periodontal pocketing, or increased mobility. The loss of attachment is <25% of the attachment of the tooth to the alveolus. Stage 3 periodontal disease is gingivitis with 25–50% attachment loss and finally Stage 4 is gingivitis with >50% attachment loss of any of the structures that support the teeth within the alveolus.

stage. The inflammation is strictly confined to the soft tissues of the gingiva. However, the remaining three stages will demonstrate observable radiographic changes. The stage of PD the patient falls into will assist in creating the appropriate immediate and long-term treatment plan for each individual tooth. Truly evaluating a patient for the appropriate PD stage combines the clinical oral evaluation including periodontal probing and assessment of clinical attachment loss with the radiographic assessment of bone loss associated with the teeth.

Attachment loss is defined as the sum of gingival recession and bone loss and is the primary manifestation of PD. Radiographic evidence of attachment loss can simplistically be deemed as bone loss [1]. Normal alveolar bone height can be measured to be just slightly below the cementoenamel junction (CEJ) to the apex of the root (Figure 4.4a–c). A straightforward way to assess the percentage of bone loss would be to visualize normal alveolar bone height from just below the CEJ to the apex of the root as 100% attachment. Next, estimate where the middle of these two points would be to designate the 50% mark. Further, another

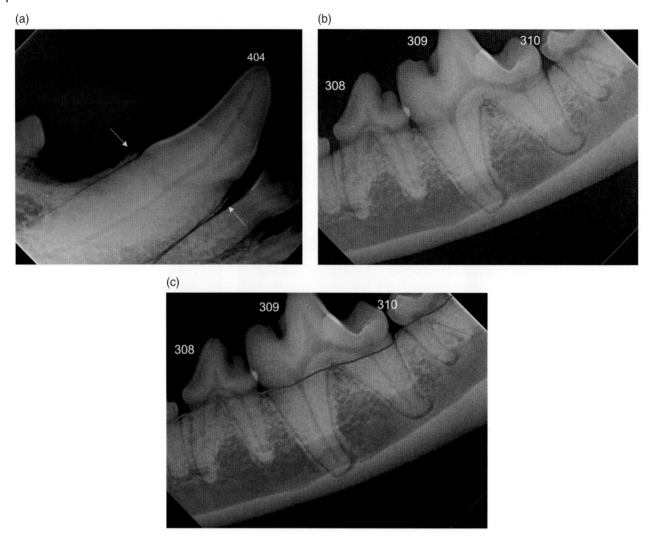

Figure 4.4 (a) Radiograph of the right mandibular canine tooth (404) depicting the alveolar bone that lies just below the cementoenamel junction on both the mesial and distal aspects (yellow arrows). The "knife-edge" appearance of the bone indicates normal, healthy alveolar bone. (b) Normal, healthy alveolar bone in a small breed dog that lies just below the cementoenamel junction of the left mandibular 1st molar tooth (309). (c) Same image as Figure 4.4b with the normal alveolar bone height indicated with the red line.

midline can be established between the alveolar margin and the 50% mark to estimate 25% attachment loss of the bone. This way the root can be imperfectly divided into the different percentages of attachment loss.

The radiographic changes observed in patients exhibiting evidence of periodontitis are horizontal and vertical bone loss, and bone loss within the furcation, but decreased alveolar bone density and widening of the PDL space can also be seen [2]. One tooth or multiple teeth can be affected by bone loss and can be mild, moderate, or severe. The significance of bone loss can be dependent on the individual patient size and the tooth/teeth involved. For example, a mild amount of bone loss on tooth 105 (right maxillary 1st

premolar) in a small breed dog would likely be more significant than the same amount of bone loss with tooth 105 in a large breed dog (Figure 4.5a–d).

When evaluating bone loss, proper radiographic exposure, or even slight under exposure of the radiograph will allow for the best evaluation of the alveolar bone. Overexposure of a radiograph will cause "burn-out" of areas that have less bone density and potentially convey the impression that more advanced pathology (bone loss) is present than what actually is. This is particularly important in the mandibular incisors where the amount of alveolar bone is thinner than in other areas of the mouth.

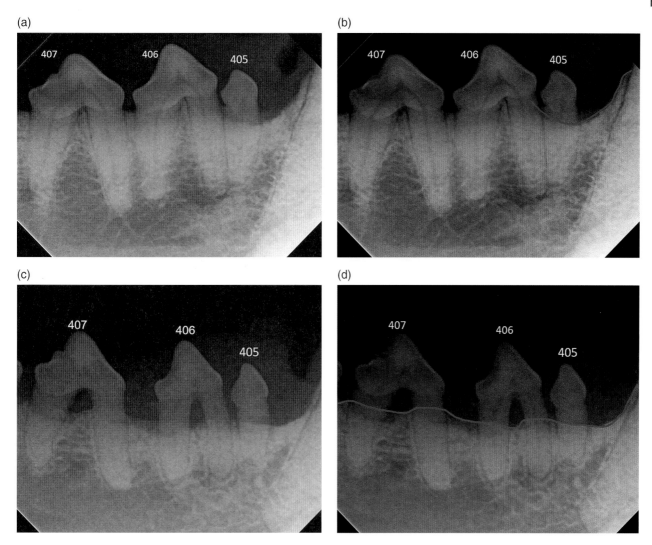

Figure 4.5 (a) Horizontal bone loss of the right mandibular 1st premolar tooth (405) in a large breed dog with a clinically diagnosed 4 mm periodontal pocket depth. (b) Same image as Figure (a), with the horizontal bone loss associated with the right mandibular 1st premolar tooth (405) indicated with the red line. (c) Horizontal bone loss of the right mandibular 1st, 2nd, and 3rd premolar teeth (405–407) in a small breed dog with a clinically diagnosed periodontal pocket depth of 4 mm. Note how the same measurable periodontal pocket depth results in a significant increase in the amount of bone loss observed in the small breed dog (c) compared to the large breed dog (a and b). (d) Same image as in Figure (c), with the horizontal bone loss associated with the right mandibular 1st, 2nd, and 3rd premolar teeth (405–407) indicated with the red line.

Types of Bone Loss

Horizontal Bone Loss

Horizontal bone loss is reduced alveolar bone height across the span of a tooth or teeth, while the bone margin remains perpendicular to the tooth surface [3]. Horizontal bone loss is the most common pattern of bone loss and is due to the bone surrounding the affected tooth/teeth being destroyed at a similar rate [4] (Figures 4.6a–c, 4.7a–d, and 4.8a–d).

Vertical Bone Loss

Vertical bone loss is a boney defect that radiographically carries the shape of a "V" on the mesial or distal aspect of

a tooth (Figure 4.9a–c). The type of defect that is actually present with vertical bone loss can be more complex than what is seen on dental radiographs [3], and therefore probing or even surgical exploration for complete evaluation (to determine how many walls the defect has) is usually warranted.

Vertical bone loss in some areas such as the palatal aspect of a maxillary canine tooth or the mesiobuccal roots of a maxillary 1st molar can be missed or underappreciated due to superimposition of bone and the tooth roots. For example, an oronasal fistula (caused by severe bone loss on the palatal aspect of a maxillary canine tooth) is not pathology

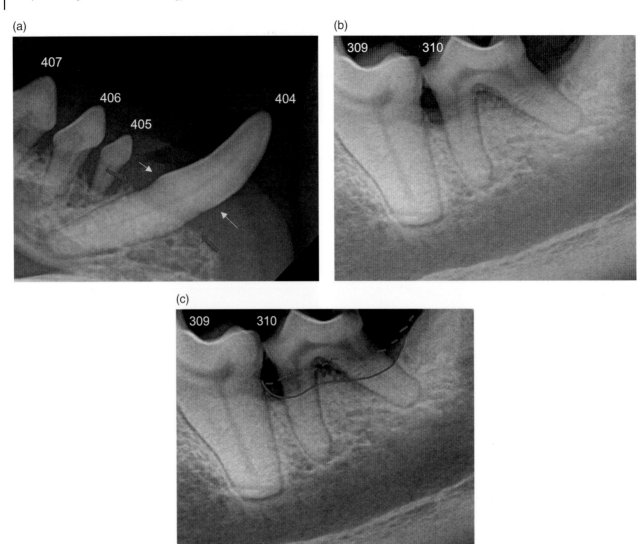

Figure 4.6 (a) Mild horizontal bone loss of the right mandibular canine tooth (404) (red arrow). Notice the alveolar margin is resting approximately 25% below the total distance of the root from the cementoenamel junction (yellow arrow). This amount of bone loss is radiographically consistent with Stage 2 PD. Remember accurate periodontal disease staging needs to be correlated with the clinical findings found with periodontal probing combined with radiographic evidence of disease. This image also depicts severe horizontal bone loss associated with the right mandibular 1st premolar tooth (405). (b) Dental radiographic image of the left caudal mandible of a dog. Mild horizontal bone loss was associated with the left mandibular 2nd molar tooth (310). Also note the left mandibular 3rd molar tooth (311) is missing. (c) Same image as Figure 4.6c with the horizontal bone loss of the left mandibular 2nd molar tooth (310) indicated by the red lines. The solid line indicates the height of the alveolar bone on one side of the tooth and the hashed line indicates the height of the alveolar bone on the opposite side of the tooth, both of which would be associated with <25% attachment loss of the alveolar bone. Again, note that the left mandibular 3rd molar tooth (311) is missing.

that is clearly diagnosed and appreciated with dental radiographs alone and may easily be missed without a comprehensive oral exam and periodontal probing. While not all oronasal fistulas present with obvious radiographic evidence of disease, it is common to see moderate vertical bone loss on the mesial aspect of the maxillary canine tooth when an oronasal fistula is present on the palatal aspect (Figure 4.10).

Furcation Bone Loss

The furcation is the area where a multi-rooted tooth bifurcates. Bone loss in this area is called furcation or furcal bone loss. Identifying the severity of the furcal bone loss helps with treatment planning, e.g. the more severe the furcal bone loss the poorer the long-term prognosis. This is because it is more difficult to clean plaque and debris from a deep furcation particularly if the gingiva is

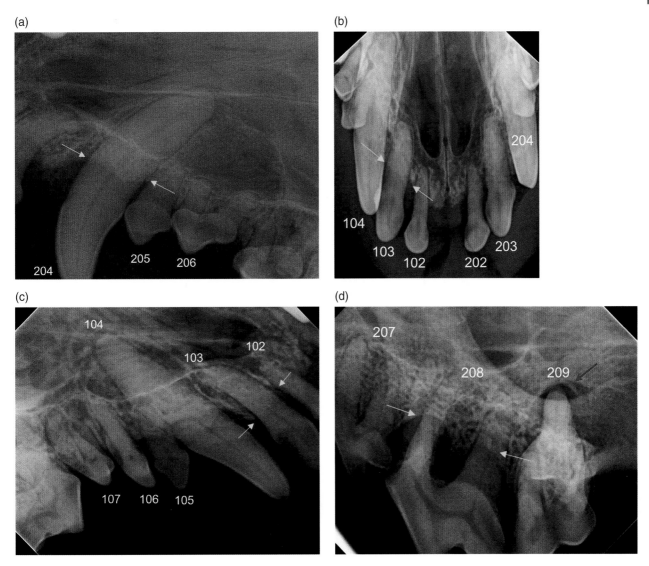

Figure 4.7 (a) Moderate horizontal bone loss of the left maxillary canine tooth (204) (arrows). The alveolar margin rests at >25%, but less than 50% of the total distance of the root. This amount of bone loss is radiographically consistent with Stage 3 PD. *Source:* Courtesy of Debra Nossaman, DVM, DAVDC, FAVD; Dallas Veterinary Dentistry and Oral Surgery. (b) Occlusal view of maxillary incisors showing moderate horizontal bone loss of the right maxillary 3rd incisor tooth (103) (arrows). The amount of bone loss is nearing 50% of the total root and appears more severe than in the view in Figure (c), which is the same patient, but positioned more laterally in Figure (c). Also note the right and left maxillary 1st incisor teeth (101, 201) are missing. There also appears to be >50% bone loss on the right and left maxillary 2nd incisor teeth (102, 202). (c) Lateral view of the right maxillary 3rd incisor tooth (103) in the same patient shown in Figure (b). Two different views (occlusal and lateral respectively) are used to demonstrate moderate horizontal bone loss of tooth 103 (arrows). This amount of bone loss is radiographically consistent with Stage 3 PD. Note the crowding and rotation of the right maxillary 2nd and 3rd premolar teeth (106, 107). (d) Moderate horizontal bone loss of the left maxillary 4th premolar tooth (208) (yellow arrows). The amount is getting very close to affecting nearly 50% of the total root. This amount of bone loss is radiographically consistent with Stage 3 PD. Notice there is also a periapical lucency of the palatal root of the left maxillary 1st molar tooth (209) (red arrow).

covering it. Furcation bone loss is typically more visible on dental radiographs of two rooted teeth rather than three rooted teeth (Figure 4.11a–c). Often additional views of a three rooted tooth are required to detect the furcation bone loss. Slight furcation bone loss may not be detected on dental radiographs due to very little bone missing; hence,

concomitant probing of the furcation area for exposure should be performed in conjunction with radiographs to confirm the diagnosis [5] (Figure 4.12a and b).

PD is a cyclic disease in that there are episodes of active bone and soft tissue destruction and episodes of quiescence [6]. Once there is bone destruction, periodontal

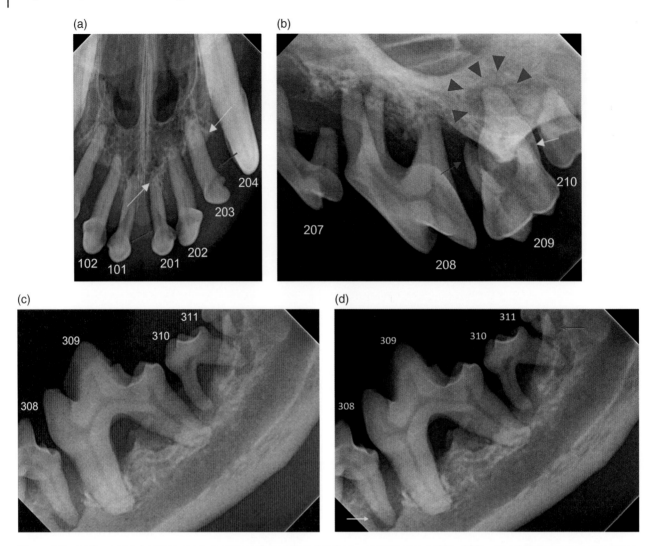

Figure 4.8 (a) Severe horizontal bone loss of the left maxillary 1st, 2nd, and 3rd incisors (201–203) with >50% bone loss associated with these roots (yellow arrows at existing alveolar margin). The red arrows depict the normal alveolar bone height. This amount of bone loss is radiographically consistent with Stage 4 PD. There is also severe horizontal bone loss of the right maxillary 1st and 2nd incisor teeth (101, 102); however, the image is intended to diagnose the left incisors only. (b) Severe horizontal bone loss of the left maxillary 3rd and 4th premolars and 1st molar teeth (207–209) with >50% of the bone missing over all roots of these teeth. There is no bone covering the mesiobuccal (red arrow) or the distobuccal root (yellow arrow) of tooth 209. This amount of bone loss is radiographically consistent with Stage 4 PD. There is no bone covering either root of tooth 207; however, the radiograph is only intended to diagnose 208 and 209. There is also the suspicion of a periapical lucency associated with the palatal root of 209, depicted by the red arrowheads. (c) Severe horizontal bone loss of the left mandibular 1st and 2nd molar teeth (309, 310). The distal root of the left mandibular 4th premolar (308) and 3rd molar tooth (311) (show no bone surrounding these roots). (d) Same image as in Figure (c). The yellow arrow depicts the bone loss surrounding the distal root of the left mandibular 4th premolar tooth (308) and the red arrow depicts the bone loss associated with the root of the left mandibular 3rd molar tooth (311).

pocketing may be present. However, if a tooth has been treated with previous conservative periodontal therapy such as root planing and/or perioceutic placement, healing by formation of long junctional epithelium to the root surface can occur [4, 7]. This in turn reduces the periodontal pocketing, but the surrounding alveolar bone loss is persistent or slightly improved and will present this way on dental radiographs. Therefore, a thorough oral exam with probing is crucial when evaluating a patient's dental

radiographic series to not treat based on radiographic findings alone [8].

Assessment of radiographic bone loss can be challenging in patients with crowded and rotated teeth [9]. Brachycephalic breeds most commonly exhibit tooth crowding and rotation, specifically of the maxillary premolars. The crowding and rotation create a shelter for plaque formation. This abnormal positioning reduces the effectiveness of regular cleansing mechanisms and

(a)

(b)

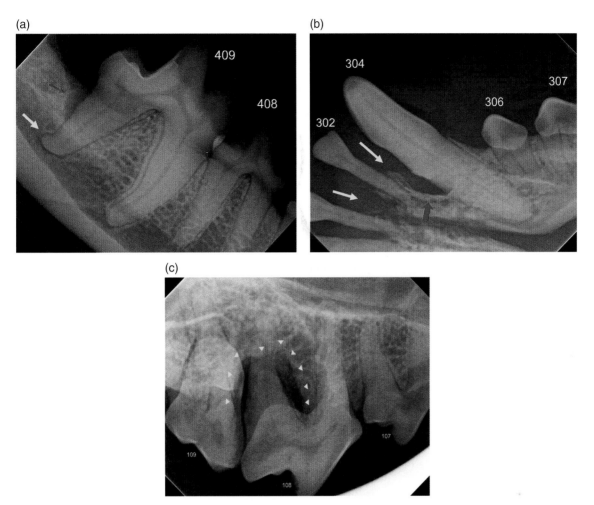

(c)

Figure 4.9 (a) Moderate vertical bone loss on the distal aspect of the right mandibular 1st molar tooth (409) (red arrow). The apical most aspect of this boney defect is nearing 50% of the total root. Also notice the mild dilaceration of the distal root of tooth 409 (yellow arrow). (b) Moderate vertical bone loss on the mesial aspect of the left mandibular canine tooth (304) (red arrow). There is horizontal bone loss of the adjacent mandibular incisors (yellow arrows). (c) Severe vertical bone loss over the distal root of the right maxillary 4th premolar tooth (108) (yellow arrowheads).

Figure 4.10 Radiograph of the left maxillary canine tooth (204) that clinically exhibited a 12-mm periodontal pocket on the palatal aspect and confirmed oronasal fistula. There is moderate vertical bone loss (yellow arrow) on the mesial aspect with moderate horizontal bone loss (red arrow). Although this tooth exhibits evidence of periodontal disease, there is no way to confirm an oronasal fistula on this patient other than with oral exam and associated periodontal probing.

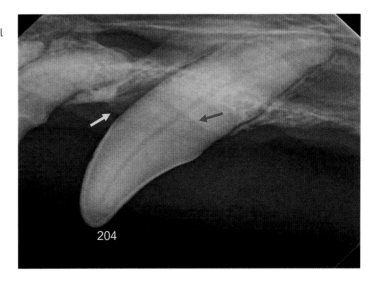

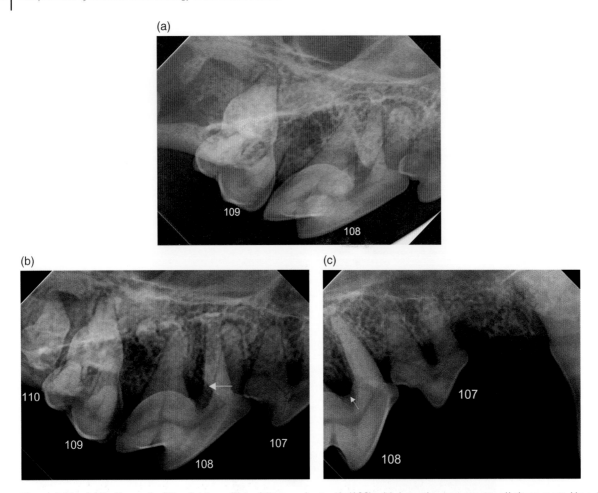

Figure 4.11 (a) Radiograph of the right maxillary 4th premolar tooth (108) with intention to separate all three roots. No evidence of furcation bone loss is present. Note this patient is missing the right maxillary 2nd molar tooth (110). (b) Different angle of the right maxillary 4th premolar tooth (108) with intention to separate all three roots. The furcation bone loss is only slightly visible (arrow). This is a different canine patient from Figure (a). Note this patient does appear to have loss of bone in the furcation area of the right maxillary 3rd premolar tooth (107) (red arrow). (c) Partial lateral radiograph of the right maxillary 4th premolar tooth (108) that shows obvious furcation exposure. There is severe furcation exposure secondary to moderate horizontal bone loss of the right maxillary 3rd premolar tooth (107), which the radiograph was intended to demonstrate (red arrow). This is the same patient as in Figure (b).

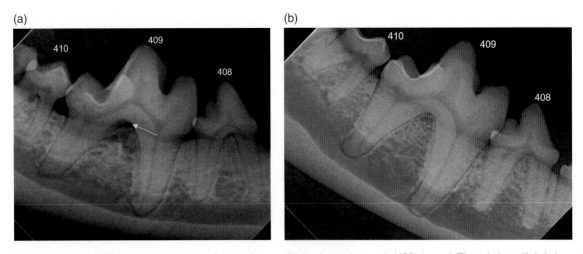

Figure 4.12 (a) Mild furcation bone loss of the right mandibular 1st molar tooth (409) (arrow). There is just slightly less radiodensity at the furcation in comparison to Figure (b). (b) Radiograph of the right mandibular 1st molar tooth (409) with normal bone density at the furcation in a different patient.

(a)

(b)

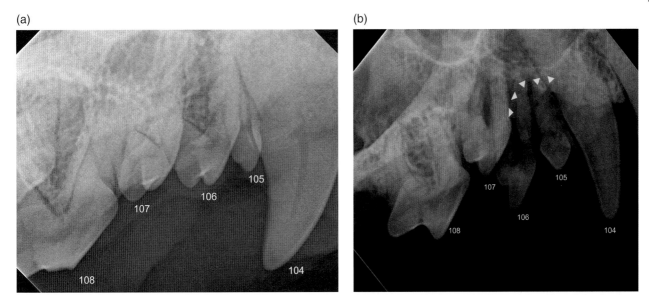

Figure 4.13 (a) Radiograph of the right maxillary premolars in a French Bulldog. There is severe crowding and moderate rotation of the teeth causing superimposition of teeth and difficulty identifying the periodontal structures of each specific tooth. There is no obvious bone loss in this radiograph. (b) Radiograph of the right maxilla in a brachycephalic dog. There is crowding of the premolars and horizontal bone loss of the right maxillary 1st and 2nd premolar teeth (105, 106) (arrowheads), but it is difficult to assess the extent of it radiographically due to the crowding of the teeth.

toothbrushing, propagating accelerated development of PD. Periodontal pocketing and radiographic bone loss can be difficult to diagnose in these patients because a periodontal probe does not fit in the tight, crowded spots easily and superimposition of the teeth radiographically obscures the evidence of radiographic bone loss. Multiple radiographic views may help identify pathology that was not detected on an oral exam (Figure 4.13a and b). A study comparing CBCT to conventional dental radiography to identify dental disorders, including bone loss, showed CBCT was a better imaging modality in diagnosing bone loss in brachycephalic breeds with crowding of teeth [9]. This makes CBCT a valuable diagnostic tool for the diagnosis of PD in brachycephalic breed patients.

Supernumerary Roots and Teeth

All dogs are expected to have 42 teeth, and all of those teeth have an expected number of roots (see Chapter 3). However, supernumerary roots and supernumerary teeth are common incidental findings in veterinary dentistry. If extraction of a tooth is required, knowing the presence of a supernumerary root can lead to successful treatment so all roots of the tooth are properly extracted or treated. The only way to know if a supernumerary root is present, and the condition/orientation/position of the root, is through diagnostic imaging of the tooth. This is commonly accomplished by use of dental radiographs (Figure 4.14).

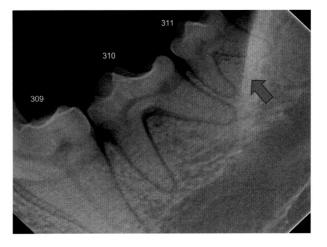

Figure 4.14 Supernumerary root in the left mandibular 3rd molar tooth (311) (blue arrow). This tooth has the same anatomical structure as the left mandibular 2nd molar tooth (310) and therefore could also be considered a supernumerary tooth 310 with tooth 311 missing. No treatment is indicated for this tooth as no radiographic evidence of disease is observed.

One study found supernumerary roots to be present 10.7% of the time in canine patients [10]. Frequently, the maxillary 3rd premolar is found to have a supernumerary root in dogs. If the supernumerary root is large enough, an obvious cusp can be seen clinically on the crown of the tooth located most frequently on the palatal aspect of the tooth (Figure 4.15a and b). Some supernumerary roots will be smaller and exhibit less opacity radiographically than

(b)

(a)

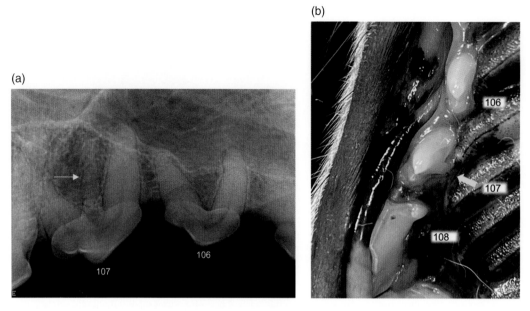

Figure 4.15 (a) Radiograph of the right maxillary 3rd premolar tooth (107) showing a supernumerary root located in the area of the furcation of the tooth (yellow arrow). (b) Clinical image of the tooth in Figure (a) displaying the supernumerary root on the palatal aspect of the right maxillary 3rd premolar tooth (107) (yellow arrow).

(a)

(b)

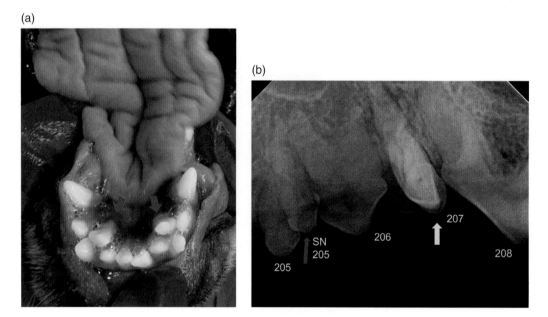

Figure 4.16 (a) Presence of two supernumerary left and right mandibular incisors (red arrow heads) causing significant crowding and rotation in a Labrador mix dog. Extraction of the supernumerary incisors should be considered to reduce risk of periodontal disease and a traumatic malocclusion. (b) Radiograph of the left maxilla in a Boxer showing a supernumerary left maxillary 1st premolar (205) (red arrow) causing crowding. Note the 90° rotation of the left maxillary 3rd premolar tooth (207) (yellow arrow) subsequently allowing more room for the supernumerary 205. This is commonly seen in brachycephalic breeds.

the other predetermined roots. This is important to know prior to extraction as the surgical technique may require a more delicate approach.

Supernumerary permanent teeth and roots are more commonly found in dogs than cats with the Boxer, Bulldog, Greyhound, and Rottweiler breeds being over-represented [11]. Supernumerary teeth can cause crowding which leads to an increased risk of PD, and therefore prophylactic extraction of these teeth can be considered if their existence appears to worsen the presence of PD (Figure 4.16a and b). However, the presence of a supernumerary tooth does not necessarily require

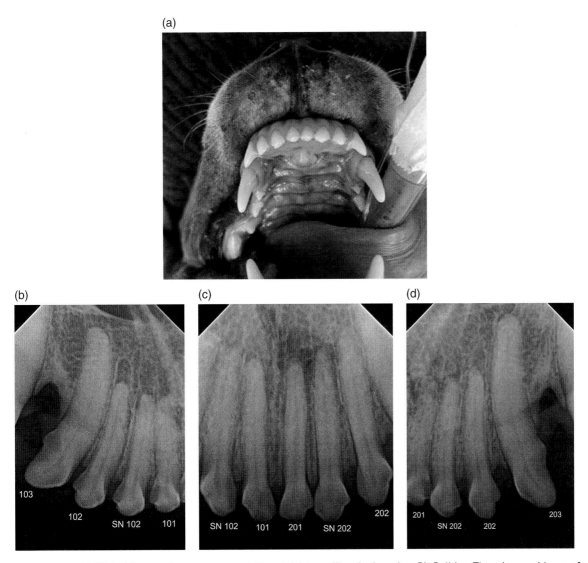

Figure 4.17 (a) Clinical image of supernumerary left and right maxillary incisors in a Pit Bulldog. There is no evidence of crowding or rotation of these teeth, and no obvious malocclusion is present. No treatment is needed. (b) Radiographs of the right maxillary incisors in the patient in Figure (a) indicating the presence of supernumerary teeth but no additional abnormalities and adequate alveolar bone surrounding the teeth. (c) Occlusal radiograph of five of the central maxillary incisors in the patient in Figure (a). Normal and adequate alveolar bone is present. (d) Radiograph of the left maxillary incisors in patient in Figure (a). Normal and adequate alveolar bone is present.

treatment unless it has pathology that indicates disease (Figure 4.17a–d).

Canine Tooth Resorption

Tooth resorption is the process by which the tooth structure is lost by increased osteoclastic activity. Resorption of a tooth can occur from the normal physiologic process seen in young patients exfoliating deciduous teeth (Figure 4.18) but is also seen in mature dogs as a result of increased inflammation (biting forces, orthodontic force, and neoplasia),

infection (apical periodontitis), pressure (cystic or neoplastic lesion), and trauma (concussive injury and luxation). Tooth resorption can typically be diagnosed from radiographic findings but can be diagnosed clinically on oral exam as well [12]. CBCT, if available, would be the modality of choice for diagnosis and assessment of tooth resorption as it can provide a three-dimensional perspective as to the true extent of the lesion [9, 13]. Conventional dental radiography has limitations with two dimensionality which can often mask or cause underappreciation of the extent of disease present, due to superimposition of mineralized structures [9].

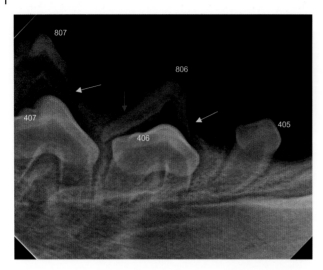

Figure 4.18 Radiograph of the right mandible in a young dog demonstrating normal physiologic resorption. The deciduous 2nd and 3rd premolars (806, 807) are positioned above the permanent counterpart that show evidence of being in an active eruption phase. Resorption of the mesial roots of both teeth can be seen (yellow arrows), while the distal root of 806 is still intact (red arrow).

Types of Tooth Resorption

Tooth resorption can be generally classified as internal or external resorption [14]. External tooth resorption is more commonly seen in dogs and has been further classified into four types. Radiographically, tooth resorption appears as areas of decreased opacity of the crown, root, or both. The four distinct types of external resorption are external inflammatory resorption, external replacement resorption, external surface resorption, and external cervical root surface resorption.

External Tooth Resorption

External Inflammatory Resorption

External inflammatory resorption is typically caused from endodontic or PD with some sort of periapical bone loss (Figure 4.19a and b). Treatment is focused on resolving the underlying endodontic condition and/or PD.

External Replacement Resorption

Radiographically external replacement resorption appears as a loss of PDL space with root tissue blending in with the adjacent alveolar bone (Figure 4.20a and b). It is hypothesized to be both age-related and from increased bite forces as multiple teeth are often affected [12]. These bite force injuries are thought to lead to necrosis of the PDL fibers resulting in the replacement resorption seen radiographically and histologically. A study showed that 53% of dogs who exhibited tooth resorption of any kind, most commonly showed evidence of external replacement and external inflammatory resorption [12].

External Surface Resorption

External surface resorption radiographically appears as a shallow depression in the cementum and into dentin on the lateral margin of the root. There is still obvious PDL and lamina dura present as these structures are not affected (Figure 4.21). The external surface resorption is thought to be an early lesion of the external replacement resorption [12].

(a)   (b)

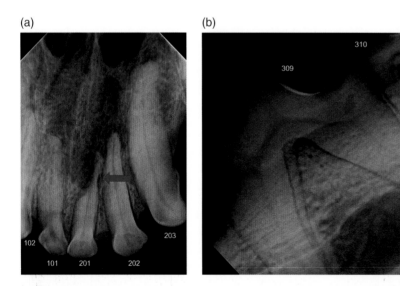

Figure 4.19 (a) External inflammatory resorption of the root of the left maxillary 1st incisor tooth (201) with endodontic disease from a complicated crown fracture. There is significant loss of the apical tooth structure (red arrow). Note the periapical bone loss around this root consistent with endodontic disease. (b) External inflammatory resorption of the mesial root of the left mandibular 2nd molar tooth (310) with a periapical lucency (red arrow).

(a)

(b)

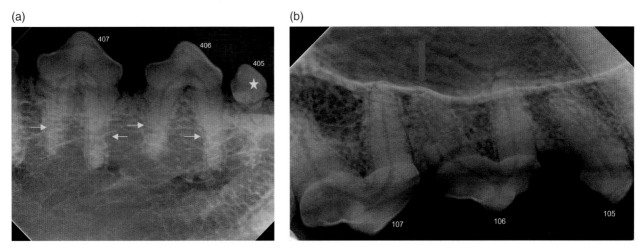

Figure 4.20 (a) Near complete root replacement resorption of the right mandibular 1st premolar tooth (405) (yellow star). The roots of the right mandibular 2nd and 3rd premolar teeth (406, 407) are also showing evidence of root replacement resorption (yellow arrows). (b) The distal root of the right maxillary 2nd premolar tooth (106) is showing root replacement resorption of the entire root (red arrow). Notice the lack of periodontal ligament space and less radiopacity of this root in comparison to the mesial root.

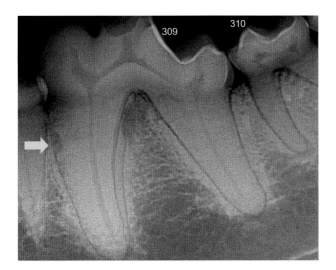

Figure 4.21 External surface resorption on the coronal mesial aspect of the left mandibular 1st premolar tooth (309) (arrow). Notice that the periodontal ligament space is intact.
Source: Courtesy of Debra Nossaman, DVM, DAVDC, FAVD; Dallas Veterinary Dentistry and Oral Surgery.

External Cervical Root Surface Resorption

External cervical root surface resorption starts at the cervical area of the tooth and is progressive and aggressive. This type of resorption results in a massive loss of tooth structure (Figure 4.22). The cause is unknown [12]; however, in humans, it is suspected to be prompted by an insult such as periodontal treatment, trauma, or orthodontic treatment; all of which can be performed in companion animals in facilities that provide advanced dentistry procedures [13]. Treatment in humans is aimed at aggressive removal of the osteoclastic cells within the lesion followed

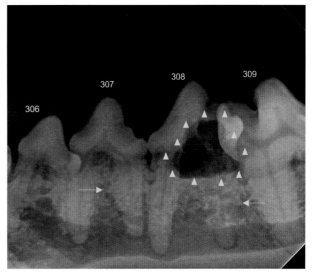

Figure 4.22 External cervical inflammatory resorption of the left mandibular 4th premolar tooth (308) (yellow arrowheads). Notice the large ovoid radiolucency at the cervical region. There is significant tooth structure missing. There is some overlap of the left mandibular 1st molar tooth (309) obscuring the entire lesion on the distal aspect. There is also external root resorption of both mesial and distal roots of the left mandibular 4th premolar tooth (308) and beginning of the distal root of the left mandibular 3rd premolar tooth (307) (yellow arrows).

by restoration of the defect [13]. This carries a guarded long-term prognosis. Debridement and restorative therapy of these lesions by a veterinary dentist can be considered; however, extraction is likely to be recommended given the challenges with treatment availability and the follow-up care required in companion animals.

(a)

(b)

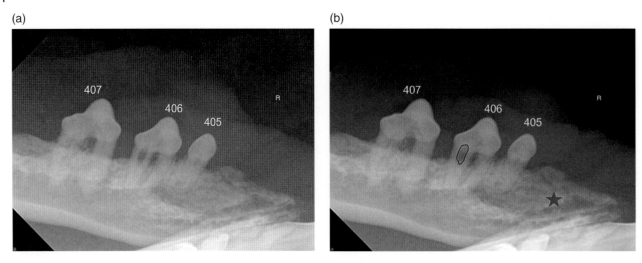

Figure 4.23 (a) Internal tooth resorption is seen radiographically directly adjacent to the pulp chamber of the distal root of the right mandibular 2nd premolar tooth (406). (b) Same image as Figure (a). The red line identifies the area of internal tooth resorption associated with the distal root of the right mandibular 2nd premolar tooth (406). The red star depicts the area of the canine tooth which appears to be radiographically missing.

Internal Tooth Resorption

Three types of internal resorption have been described: internal surface resorption, internal replacement resorption, and internal inflammatory resorption [12]. Radiographically, the first two present as small ovoid structures that follow the path of the pulp canal [12]. Internal surface resorption is typically seen in the apical portion of the root canal, while the internal replacement resorption is seen in the coronal portion of the canal [12]. Both types of internal resorption are self-limiting. Internal inflammatory resorption is radiographically seen as an ovoid lucency within or directly adjacent to the pulp chamber and the cervical area of the tooth. This type of resorption is associated with endodontic disease [12] (Figure 4.23a and b).

Treatment of Tooth Resorption

Tooth resorption in dogs is a disease process that is not well understood. It is known, however, that there are several types of resorption and that the process is progressive with limited treatment options to stop the progression of disease. The decision of how to treat an affected tooth should be based on what area of the tooth is affected and the severity of destruction to the tooth. General criteria for formulating a treatment plan would include extraction of any teeth with overt clinical lesions of the crown eroding into deeper tooth tissues and lesions that show radiographic or clinical evidence of periapical periodontitis (Figure 4.24). Minor lesions suspected to be from endodontic disease could be treated with endodontic therapy with a guarded prognosis, as the condition is thought to be progressive. A study showed that root canal therapy as a treatment for

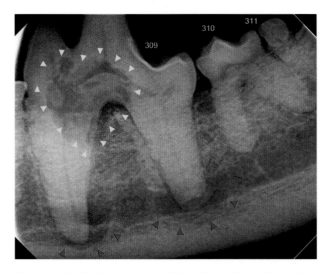

Figure 4.24 Tooth resorption of the left mandibular 1st molar tooth (309) with extensive tooth structure missing (yellow arrowheads) and periapical periodontitis of both roots (red arrowheads). The resorptive lesion is affecting both the crown and root and has caused pulp exposure leading to endodontic disease indicated by the periapical lucencies of both mesial and distal roots. Extraction would be the best treatment for this tooth.

teeth with endodontic disease and root resorption was successful in only 50% of the teeth [15]. Progressive root resorption was radiographically present at follow-up radiographic assessments, and therefore endodontic therapy was deemed unsuccessful [15]. The effect of minor lesions (both internal and external) of the roots in canine and feline patients and how to treat them is not well established in veterinary dentistry. Continued radiographic monitoring of small external lesions is reasonable if there is owner compliance to return for at least annual radiographic evaluation and the lesions are not clinically appreciated on the crown of the tooth. Progressive resorption is expected, and repeated radiographic monitoring is necessary. It is noteworthy to mention that extraction of teeth with advanced tooth resorption can be particularly challenging as the tooth structure is frequently compromised, and clinically it is difficult to distinguish the difference between tooth root structure and the surrounding alveolar bone.

Odontogenic Cysts

An odontogenic cyst is a cavity (typically fluid filled) that is lined by odontogenic (arising from a tooth) epithelium [16]. Odontogenic cysts can be classified as either developmental or inflammatory [16]. The two most common odontogenic cysts in dogs are the dentigerous cyst and the radicular or periapical cyst. Odontogenic cysts arise from stimulated epithelial cells that are otherwise quiet either at the crown of an embedded tooth (dentigerous cyst) or the apex (periapical cyst) of the tooth. Radiographic imaging of a cystic structure is an important diagnostic tool to aid in the diagnosis of the type of cyst present (dentigerous or radicular). This is by identifying the relationship between the cyst and the surrounding region of the tooth. It is important to discern whether the cyst appears to originate from the crown or root of the tooth. Odontogenic cysts have general radiographic features of an ovoid shape and a central lucency and are generally associated with a tooth (Figure 4.25). However, some odontogenic cysts can have more of a scalloped appearance of the periphery of the cyst (multi-loculated) [16] due to cavitation (Figure 4.26). More advanced odontogenic cysts often alter one's ability to determine what tooth the cyst originated from because the cyst may span over several teeth (Figure 4.27a and b). Larger cysts cause significant adjacent bone resorption and remodeling, thereby compromising the bone which raises concern for pathologic fractures (primarily of the mandible) [16]. Resorption of tooth roots within the cyst may also be seen (Figure 4.28a and b). More information regarding radiographic evidence of cystic structures can be found in Chapter 6.

Dentigerous Cysts

Dentigerous cysts are odontogenic cysts which are classified as developmental [16]. They are caused by an unerupted or impacted tooth whereby the epithelial cells of the follicular sac that envelop the crown of the tooth begin to produce fluid [16]. Dentigerous cysts are most commonly associated with the mandibular 1st premolar

tooth in dogs, although they have also been observed with the maxillary and mandibular canine teeth [10, 16, 17]. Brachycephalic breeds are the most common skull type that exhibit the presence of dentigerous cysts [10, 16, 18].

The distinct radiographic feature of a dentigerous cyst is the presence of an unerupted tooth, commonly in an abnormal (horizontal) orientation [17], either within the cyst or immediately adjacent to the crown of the tooth

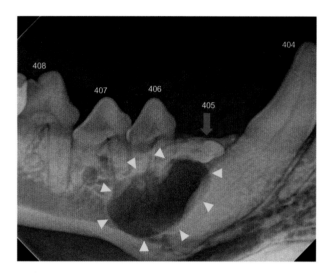

Figure 4.25 Dentigerous cyst likely associated with the unerupted right mandibular 1st premolar tooth (405) (red arrow). The appearance of the cyst has a typical ovoid shape with a central lucency (yellow arrowheads). The cyst does not appear to be directly associated with a particular tooth; however, the horizontal orientation of tooth 405 is an indication that tooth 405 is likely the cause of the dentigerous cyst.

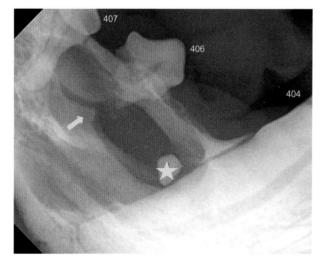

Figure 4.26 Dentigerous cyst from an unerupted right mandibular 1st premolar tooth (405) (yellow star) that is seen within the center of the radiolucency. There are scalloped edges of this cyst (yellow arrow). Note the resorption of the roots of both 405 and 406.

(a)

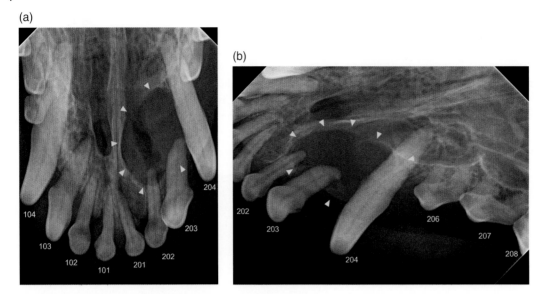

Figure 4.27 (a) Occlusal radiographic image of a large cystic structure associated with the left rostral maxilla. There is a large radiolucency (yellow arrowheads) overlying the apices of both the left maxillary 2nd and 3rd incisor teeth (202, 203). This lesion is likely a periapical cyst as there is not an unerupted tooth associated with the lucency. It is difficult to discern which tooth (202 or 203) the cyst is originating from. (b) Lateral radiographic image of the same large cystic structure of the left rostral maxilla from Figure (a) with a radiolucency (yellow arrowheads) overlying the apices of both the left maxillary 2nd and 3rd incisor teeth (202, 203).

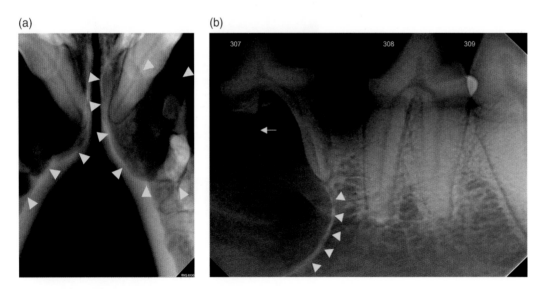

Figure 4.28 (a) Occlusal radiograph of the rostral mandible in a Pug dog with bilateral dentigerous cysts that have caused resorption of alveolar bone (yellow arrowheads) that could result in bilateral pathologic mandibular fractures. *Source:* Courtesy of Christopher J. Snyder, DVM, DAVDC, Founding Fellow, AVDC Oral and Maxillofacial Surgery, University of Wisconsin-Madison, School of Veterinary Medicine. (b) The caudal aspect of a large dentigerous cyst in a large breed dog. There is clear root resorption of the mesial root of the left mandibular 3rd premolar tooth (307) (yellow arrow). The distinct cyst border between the radiolucent filled cyst and alveolar bone can be easily detected (yellow arrowheads).

depending on the size of the cyst (Figure 4.29a and b). Clinically, with more developed dentigerous cysts, a swelling over the missing tooth may be present and some may have a blue hue to the clinical appearance of the gingiva (Figure 4.30).

While not all unerupted teeth will form dentigerous cysts, it is essential to radiograph all areas where there are clinically missing teeth to rule out the presence of either an unerupted tooth, or the presence of an unerupted tooth with cystic formation (Figure 4.31). Importantly, some patients may have

(a)

(b)

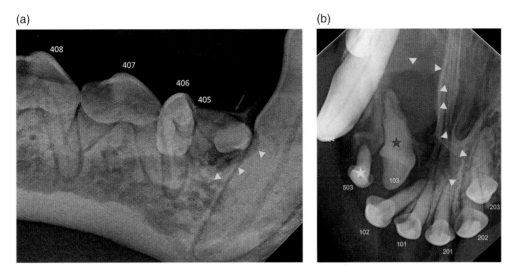

Figure 4.29 (a) A small radiolucency can be seen surrounding the crown of the right mandibular 1st premolar tooth (405) (yellow arrowheads) with a slight amount of alveolar bone on the dorsal aspect of the tooth (red arrow). These radiographic findings are consistent with a small dentigerous cyst. (b) Occlusal radiograph of the rostral mandible in a dog with an unerupted right maxillary 3rd incisor tooth (103) (red star) and persistent deciduous right maxillary 3rd incisor tooth (503) (yellow star). There is a large indistinct radiolucency surrounding tooth 103 (yellow arrowheads), consistent with a dentigerous cyst. There is obvious root resorption of tooth 103.

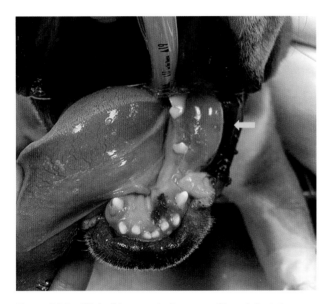

Figure 4.30 Clinical image of a large swelling of the left mandible secondary to a dentigerous cyst (yellow arrow). Note the bluish-tinged color to the area of soft tissue.

supernumerary teeth that can form dentigerous cysts, and therefore routinely acquiring full-mouth radiographs is recommended so as not to miss this potential pathology [16].

Periapical Cysts

As the name implies, periapical cysts (also called radicular cysts) are cysts associated with the apex of a tooth. Periapical cysts form when the dormant epithelial cells at

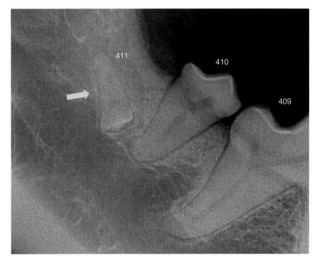

Figure 4.31 Image depicts an unerupted tooth in the right caudal mandible. The right mandibular 3rd molar (411) appears to be completely embedded in bone with no evidence of cyst development. Note that the larger tooth in the image appears to be the right mandibular 1st molar tooth (409). The tooth distal to 409 has only a single root. This would indicate that either the unerupted tooth is an unerupted supernumerary 3rd molar tooth, or the right mandibular 2nd molar (410) is malformed, with only a single root, instead of two roots as is normally seen. *Source:* Courtesy of Debra Nossaman, DVM, DAVDC, FAVD; Dallas Veterinary Dentistry and Oral Surgery.

the apex of the root that are present from initial tooth development are stimulated by chronic inflammation (pulpitis/pulp necrosis) followed by subsequent fluid accumulation.

Radiographically, periapical cysts are similar in appearance to dentigerous cysts as they are lucent structures at the apex of the tooth. As with dentigerous cysts, they can be very destructive to the surrounding bone and involve multiple teeth (Figure 4.27a and b). A widened pulp chamber may also be seen with a tooth affected by a radicular cyst, indicating the tooth is nonvital, with the nonvitality caused by pulpitis/pulp necrosis.

Treatment for Odontogenic Cysts

Treatment for odontogenic cysts is removal of the embedded tooth (dentigerous cyst) or causal tooth (periapical) and complete enucleation of the cyst lining. It is also recommended that the cystic lining and affected tooth/teeth be submitted for a histopathologic diagnosis. For advanced cystic structures extraction of teeth that no longer have sufficient alveolar bone surrounding the roots or teeth that show evidence of root resorption is recommended (Figure 4.32a and b). Annual radiographic monitoring of the affected area is also recommended to monitor for cyst recurrence, regardless of the type of cyst present.

Tooth Fractures

Next to PD, tooth fractures are one of the more common pathoses seen in canine patients. The American Veterinary Dental College (AVDC) describes fractures based on the extent of the fracture and location on the tooth (Figure 4.33a–g):

- Enamel infraction
- Enamel fracture
- Uncomplicated crown fracture
- Uncomplicated crown-root fracture
- Complicated crown fracture
- Complicated crown-root fracture
- Root fractures

Regardless of the specific type of fracture, there is an indication that the tooth sustained trauma and therefore is at risk of developing pathology. Any fractured tooth can develop pulpitis from a concussive injury (enamel infraction, enamel fracture, or uncomplicated crown fracture) or bacterial invasion into the pulp either through exposed dentin (uncomplicated crown fracture) or direct pulp exposure (complicated crown fracture). While teeth affected with enamel infractions or small enamel fractures are at less risk of developing pulpitis or periodontitis, any trauma to a tooth can result in discomfort or pathology which may or may not show radiographic evidence of disease.

Fractures with direct pulp exposure must be treated either with endodontic therapy, if the tooth is a candidate, or extraction. Pulp exposure allows for direct invasion of bacteria into the endodontic system (Figure 4.34a and b). These teeth should not be conservatively monitored, as the risk for developing periapical periodontitis is extremely high. Teeth that have complicated crown-root fractures (slab fracture) have both the endodontic system and the

(a)

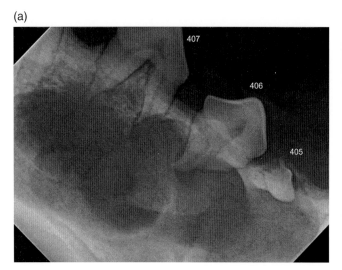

(b)

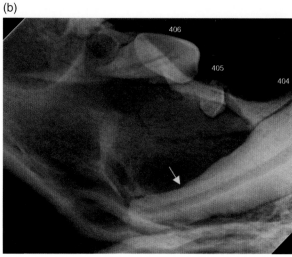

Figure 4.32 (a) Radiograph of the right mandible in a large breed dog with a large dentigerous cyst. There is severe resorption of the alveolar bone and of the tooth roots of the right mandibular 1st, 2nd, and 3rd premolar teeth (405–407). Tooth 405 is likely the causal tooth as it is in a horizontal orientation indicating it never erupted into occlusion. (b) This radiograph is from the same patient in Figure (a) with a more rostral positioning to capture the severe bone loss and root resorption of the root of the right mandibular canine tooth (404) (yellow arrow). Extraction of this tooth may be warranted.

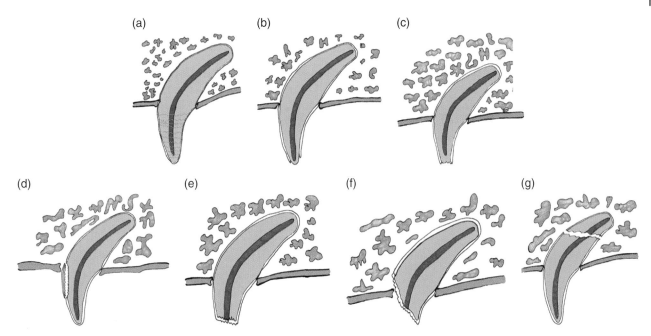

Figure 4.33 (a) Enamel infraction: an enamel infraction is seen as a microcrack in the tooth surface that is limited to the enamel. There is no actual enamel loss or loss of tooth structure in this condition. (b) Enamel fracture: an enamel fracture is trauma to the tooth that causes loss of the tooth structure that is limited to the enamel only. The dentin is still intact although it is exposed to the external environment. (c) Uncomplicated crown fracture: an uncomplicated crown fracture is trauma to the tooth resulting in enamel loss extending into the dentin. This type of fracture does not penetrate into the pulp of the tooth. (d) Uncomplicated crown-root fracture: an uncomplicated crown-root fracture is trauma to the tooth resulting in enamel loss extending into the dentin of both the crown and root surface. This type of fracture extends below the free gingival margin. The loss of tooth structure does not extent into the pulp. (e) Complicated crown fracture: a complicated crown fracture is trauma to the tooth resulting in loss of tooth structure through the enamel and dentin which extends into the pulp exposing the neurovascular supply (pulp) to the tooth. (f) Complicated crown-root: a complicated crown-root fracture is trauma to the tooth resulting in loss of tooth structure through the enamel and dentin which extends into the pulp exposing the neurovascular supply (pulp) to the tooth both above and below the free gingival margin of the tooth. (g) Root fracture: a root fracture is trauma to the tooth resulting in trauma to the cementum, dentin, and potentially the neurovascular supply (pulp) of the tooth. Trauma of this type is confined to the root surface and is predominately only observed radiographically.

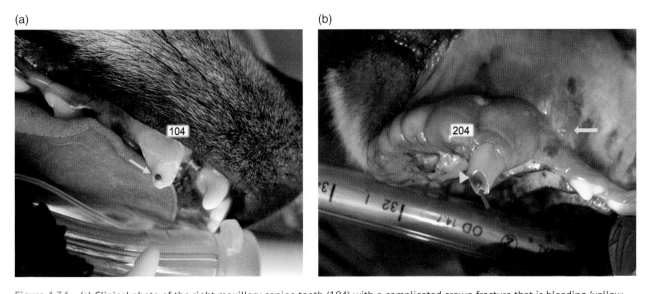

Figure 4.34 (a) Clinical photo of the right maxillary canine tooth (104) with a complicated crown fracture that is bleeding (yellow arrow) from the pulp canal indicating a recent fracture. This tooth was treated with root canal therapy. (b) Chronic complicated crown fracture of the left maxillary canine tooth (204) that has calculus within the pulp canal (red arrow) and discoloration of the exposed dentin (yellow arrowhead). There is also a parulis (draining wound) present apical to the mucogingival line (yellow arrow). This tooth was extracted due to the extent of periapical bone loss present.

periodontium affected and although treatment for this type of fracture can be accomplished with both endodontic therapy and periodontal surgery, careful selection of this treatment is warranted due to a guarded long-term prognosis (Figure 4.35a–d).

Complicated crown fractures that occur in young animals (<18 months) are candidates to receive an endodontic treatment, called vital pulp therapy. This therapy attempts to preserve the vitality of the pulp of the tooth and allows the tooth the opportunity to continue to mature (Figure 4.36a–e). Unfortunately, this type of therapy is

time-sensitive and should be performed within 48 hours of the injury, if possible, to provide the best outcome [19].

Uncomplicated crown fractures are at risk of developing pathology, while the dentinal tubules are exposed. This process occurs when bacteria traverse through the exposed dentinal tubules and invade into the pulp canal space causing infection and resulting apical periodontitis (Figure 4.37a and b). Fortunately, the tooth does have a reparative process whereby tertiary dentin develops within the dentinal tubules to seal the tubules from the external environment. The development of tertiary dentin requires the tooth to

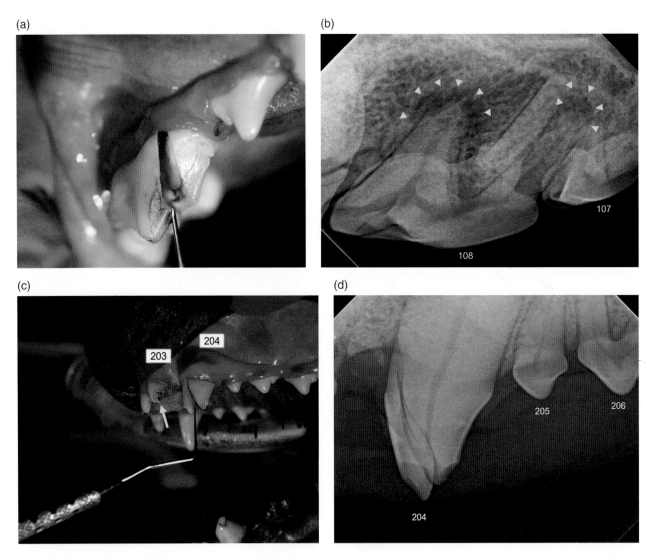

Figure 4.35 (a) Clinical photo of a complicated crown-root fracture (slab fracture) of the right maxillary 4th premolar tooth (108) showing complete separation of a buccal portion of the tooth that is still attached to the gingiva. Both the endodontic system and periodontium of this tooth are affected and carry a guarded prognosis for treatment. (b) Radiographic image of the patient in Figure (a) showing the tooth has significant endodontic disease as evidenced by the periapical lucency of the distal and mesiobuccal roots (yellow arrowheads). The slab fracture seen in the clinical picture is not obvious in the radiographic image. (c) Complicated crown-root fracture (slab fracture) of the left maxillary canine tooth (204). Note there is also an additional complicated crown fracture of the left maxillary 3rd incisor tooth (203) (yellow arrow). (d) Radiograph of the crown of the left maxillary canine tooth (204) in the patient in Figure (c) showing the subgingival fracture extending to the alveolar bone margin and has multiple fragments.

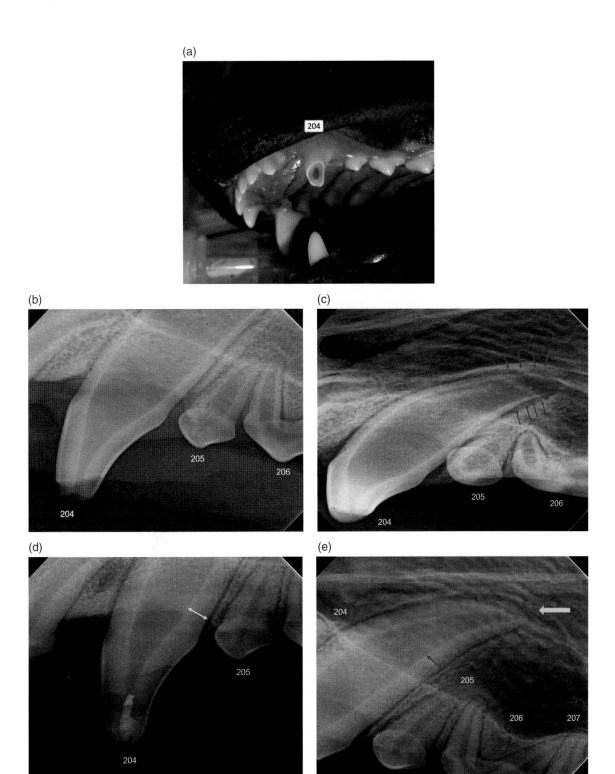

Figure 4.36 (a) Clinical image of a complicated crown fracture of the left maxillary canine tooth (204) in a five-month-old patient. Notice the very large size of the exposed pulp due to immaturity of the patient and the tooth. (b) Radiograph of the crown of the left maxillary canine tooth (204) of the patient in Figure (a) showing the complicated crown fracture. (c) Radiographic image of the apical portion of the left maxillary canine tooth (204) as seen in Figure (a) and (b). Note the presence of an open apex indicating immaturity of the tooth. The red arrows depict the extent of dentin deposition and root development/formation. As stated previously, this patient is approximately five months old. (d) Radiographic image of left mandibular canine tooth 204 of the patient in Figure (a)–(c) six months following treatment with vital pulp therapy. Vital pulp therapy was performed in attempt to save the tooth following a complicated crown fracture. Observe how there is more dentin deposition to the tooth structure (yellow double arrow). Evidence of dentin deposition and continued tooth maturation is an indication that the tooth still remains vital following the trauma and endodontic treatment. (e) Radiographic image of the left mandibular canine tooth 204 in the patient in Figure (a)–(d) six months following treatment with vital pulp therapy. (Same visit as Figure (c and d.) Note how the apex of the root is closed (yellow arrow) and the continued deposition of dentin (thickness) of the tooth (red double arrow). This observed evidence of apical tooth root closure and continued dentin deposition are indications the tooth remains vital and is continuing to mature.

(a)   (b)

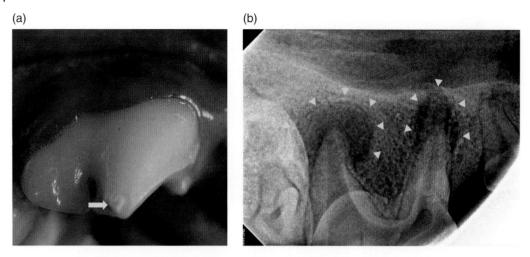

Figure 4.37   (a) Clinical photo of the right maxillary 4th premolar tooth (108) with an uncomplicated crown fracture that does not have obvious evidence of pulp exposure. There is clinical evidence of dentin exposure (yellow arrow). (b) Radiographic image of the right maxillary 4th premolar tooth (108) in the patient in Figure (a) showing severe periapical lucencies of all roots indicating periapical periodontitis (yellow arrowheads) is present. It is important to note that the absence of pulp exposure can still result in periapical periodontitis. *Source:* Courtesy of Christopher J. Snyder, DVM, DAVDC, Founding Fellow, AVDC Oral and Maxillofacial Surgery, University of Wisconsin-Madison, School of Veterinary Medicine.

remain vital and the insult to the tooth to be somewhat minor. The deposition of tertiary dentin and tooth vitality are positive signs of repair; however, radiographs of these teeth are still warranted. These teeth sustained trauma and other pathology may be present or develop in the future, which warrants continued radiographic monitoring. Clinically, tertiary dentin typically appears as darker colored dentin, or hard tissue at the center of the tooth where the pulp of the tooth would normally be located (Figure 4.38a–c). Continued radiographic monitoring of these teeth is warranted at least one year post-fracture or injury diagnosis to ensure that pathology does not develop given that frequently it is unknown when the trauma occurred.

Root Fractures

Root fractures are solely fractures of the root alone, involving the cementum, dentin, and pulp and are classified according to their location (apical, middle, and cervical) [20] (Figure 4.39a–c). Root fractures are typically incidental findings and are commonly seen in the incisor region. The mobility of the root fracture depends on the location of the fracture; cervical root fractures will exhibit more mobility of the crown than apical root fractures. Radiographically, these fractures appear as a lucent line through the root of the tooth. These types of fractures can be easily missed radiographically if the angulation of the radiographic beam is not positioned to reveal the fracture. Therefore, if a root fracture is suspected, multiple radiographic views may be necessary for confirmation, combined with clinical evidence and suspicion of pathology [20] (Figure 4.40a–c).

Prognosis for a root fracture is dependent on the location of the fracture within the root. The recommended treatment for root fractures is splinting of the teeth to the adjacent teeth to drastically reduce their mobility [20]. This is ideally performed within 48 hours of the injury [20]. Treatment for root fractures can be challenging as these fractures go undetected for extended periods of time, thereby making extraction of the affected teeth more common. Cervical root fractures have more clinical mobility and therefore cause stretching of the pulp leading to subsequent pulp necrosis [20]. Prognosis is much more guarded with cervical root fractures [20]. Middle and apical root fractures can heal with fibrous tissue or hard tissue with splinting, but pulp vitality must be present. This can be difficult to assess based on radiographic and clinical evaluation of the affected tooth upon presentation [20]. If treatment is initiated, radiographic monitoring of root fractures is recommended every three to six months for at least one year to assess for subsequent endodontic disease [20].

Retained Tooth Roots

Cervical root fractures or severe complicated crown-root fractures that cause the crown of the tooth to be completely fractured and displaced from the root leave behind retained tooth roots. Depending on when the fracture occurred and

(a)

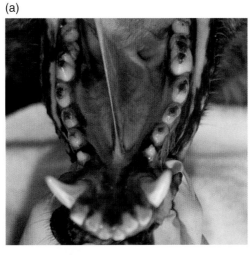

(b)   (c)

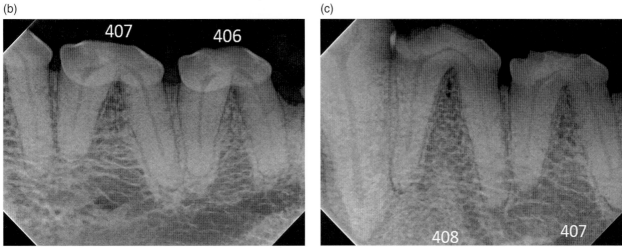

Figure 4.38 (a) Clinical image of the mandible of a dog with multiple uncomplicated crown fractures. It is important to note that trauma to the teeth without pulp exposure will not definitively develop into periapical disease. The clinical photo shows uncomplicated crown fractures with tertiary dentin present on multiple mandibular premolar and molar teeth in a dog. (b) Radiographic images of the right mandibular 2nd and 3rd premolar teeth 406, 407 of the patient depicted in Figure (a). The radiograph does not indicate any evidence of endodontic disease. The loss of crown structure of the cusp tips of the premolar teeth is observed in the radiographs. (c) Radiographic images of right mandibular 3rd and 4th premolar teeth 407, 408 in the patient depicted in Figure (a and b). The radiograph indicates no radiographic evidence of endodontic disease. Note the wear of the cusp tip of the crowns can also be appreciated in the radiographs.

to what severity, clinical presentation can range from a visible tooth root protruding through the gingiva, to a small area of erythema in the gingiva, to a draining tract in the gingiva, to an area of a clinically missing tooth completely covered by healthy gingiva. Radiographically, these tooth roots can have a variety of pathology present. This may depend on how long the retained tooth root(s) has been present and the extent of the injury which caused it (Figure 4.41a and b). Some tooth roots can be difficult to see radiographically and may require multiple images from different angles to visualize the retained tooth roots clearly. If other external pathology is present and a tooth root is not appreciated initially, this would warrant multiple radiographic views

(Figure 4.42a–d). All retained tooth roots have pulp exposure regardless of what pathology is observed. Frequently, retained tooth roots require extraction as they have the potential to develop endodontic disease.

Endodontic Disease

Etiology

Endodontic disease is inflammation or necrosis of the pulp within a tooth. There are multiple factors that can contribute to the development of endodontic disease including

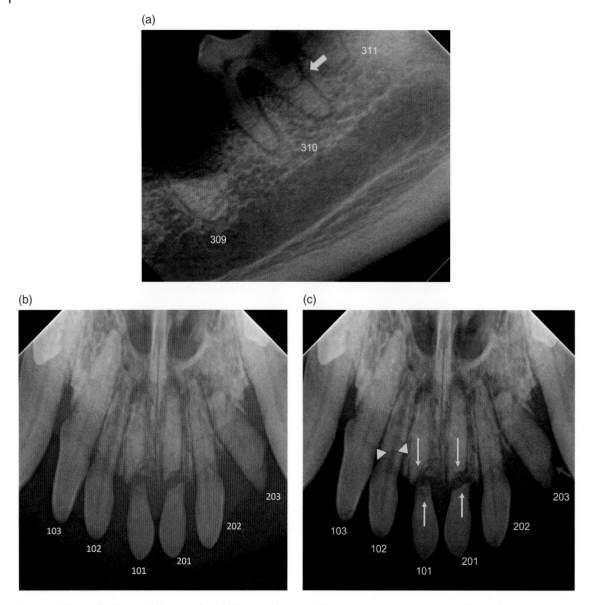

Figure 4.39 (a) Radiographic image of a middle root fracture of the distal root of the left mandibular 2nd molar tooth (310) (yellow arrow) with no evidence of periapical changes. There is also a retained tooth root of the distal root of the left mandibular 1st molar tooth (309) (red arrow). (b) Cervical root fractures of the right and left central, or 1st incisors (101, 201). These teeth were very mobile on oral examination. (c) Same image as in Figure 4.39b. Cervical root fractures of the right and left 1st incisors (101, 201) (yellow arrows). Note the retained tooth root of the left maxillary 3rd incisor, 203 (red arrow), and the wide pulp chamber on the right maxillary 2nd incisor tooth, 102 (yellow arrowheads).

tooth fractures with and without pulp exposure, PD, concussive traumas, carious lesions, anachoresis, and tooth resorption. Early inflammation of the pulp (pulpitis) can be quite difficult to discern in patients both clinically and radiographically. Typical pulp testing that is performed in humans to gain more information on what tooth is affected and the extent of discomfort that is experienced cannot be performed in animals and therefore presents a huge limitation in the diagnosis of early pulpitis in veterinary patients. Additionally, animals are inherently stoic and frequently will not show signs of oral discomfort. However, clinical signs such as ptyalism, jaw chattering, reluctance or slow to chew hard kibble or chew on toys can be signs of both acute and chronic pulpitis.

The limitations in detecting clinical signs of endodontic disease compels veterinarians to rely on dental radiographs or CBCT for diagnosis of the condition. Proper technique and positioning for acquiring diagnostic images is essential for the detection of endodontic disease, particularly if the radiographic and clinical findings are subtle. Angulation

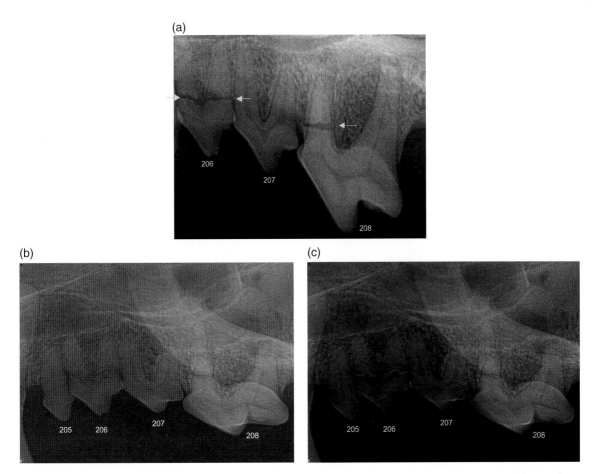

Figure 4.40 Dental radiographic images of the left maxillary premolar teeth in a dog. This is the same patient in all three images. Note how varying the radiographic positioning affects the ability to visualize the extent of the root fractures. (a) Lateral radiograph of the left maxilla showing cervical root fractures of the mesial and distal roots of the left maxillary 2nd premolar (206) and a mesial root of the left maxillary 4th premolar (208) (yellow arrows). (b) Radiograph of the left maxillary 1st, 2nd, 3rd, and 4th premolar teeth (205–208) with slight foreshortening of the images from the patient in Figure (a) causing the root fractures to be much less visible. *Source:* Courtesy of Debra Nossaman, DVM, DAVDC, FAVD; Dallas Veterinary Dentistry and Oral Surgery. (c) Radiograph of the left maxillary 1st, 2nd, 3rd, and 4th premolar teeth (205–208) with slight foreshortening of the patient in Figure (a) causing the fractures to be much less visible. This is the same image as in Figure (b). Note the red lines depicting the fracture lines of the mesial and distal roots of 206 and one of the mesial roots of 208.

Figure 4.41 (a) Clinical image of the rostral mandible of a dog with a clinically missing right mandibular 2nd incisor tooth (402). The gingiva is smooth with no evidence of inflammation. (b) Radiographic image of the patient in Figure (a) displaying a retained tooth root of the right mandibular 2nd incisor tooth (402) that is fractured into multiple pieces (red arrow). No endodontic disease is observed. *Source:* Courtesy of Debra Nossaman, DVM, DAVDC, FAVD; Dallas Veterinary Dentistry and Oral Surgery.

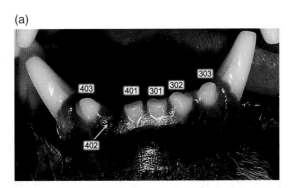

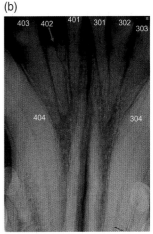

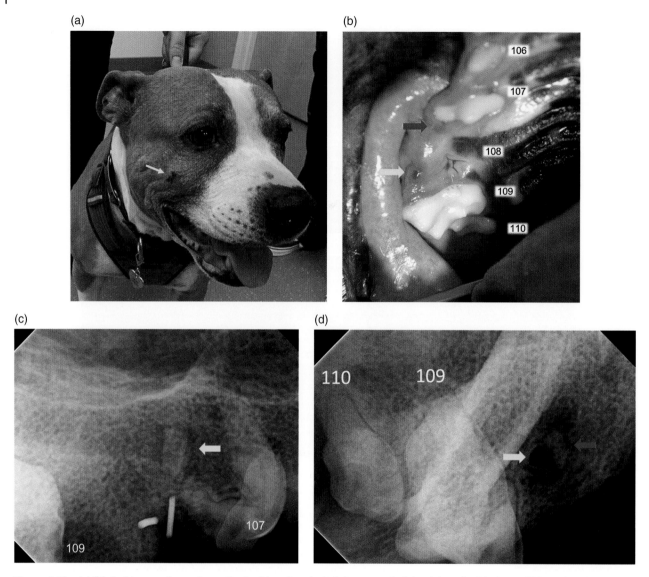

Figure 4.42 (a) Clinical image of a canine patient with a chronic draining wound of the right suborbital area. This patient had a history of having the right maxillary 4th premolar tooth (108) extracted. (b) Clinical intraoral image in the area of the missing right maxillary 4th premolar tooth (108) in the patient in Figure (a). There is inflammation at the location of the distal root of 108 (yellow arrow) with a very small focal area of inflammation where the mesiobuccal root should be located (red arrow). (c) Radiograph of the area of the right maxillary 4th premolar tooth (108) locating one of the retained mesial roots (yellow arrow). The radio-opaque structures are pieces of gutta percha used as markers to identify the location of the root. (d) Radiograph of the retained distal root of the right maxillary 4th premolar tooth (108). Multiple views were acquired to try to isolate this tooth root. This view shows a radiolucent area in the bone (yellow arrow) adjacent to the tooth root (red arrow).

and superimposition of bone or tooth structures can obscure the presence of endodontic disease [21]. Appropriate exposure parameters and interactive manipulation of the brightness and contrast of an image with or without filters is strongly recommended when assessing dental radiographs for endodontic disease.

Having knowledge of the normal oral anatomy of a patient, in particular the different foramina of the skull, will help determine normal anatomy from true pathology.

For example, a foramen present within the alveolar bone will move away from the apex of a tooth with different radiographic positioning angles, whereas a periapical lucency will always follow the apex of the tooth regardless of the radiographic angle (Figure 4.43a–d). For more information on normal radiographic anatomy, see Chapter 3.

Early endodontic disease, however, is often not detected radiographically. This is because not enough time has passed to allow for bone loss at the apex to occur thereby

(a)

(b)

(c)

(d)

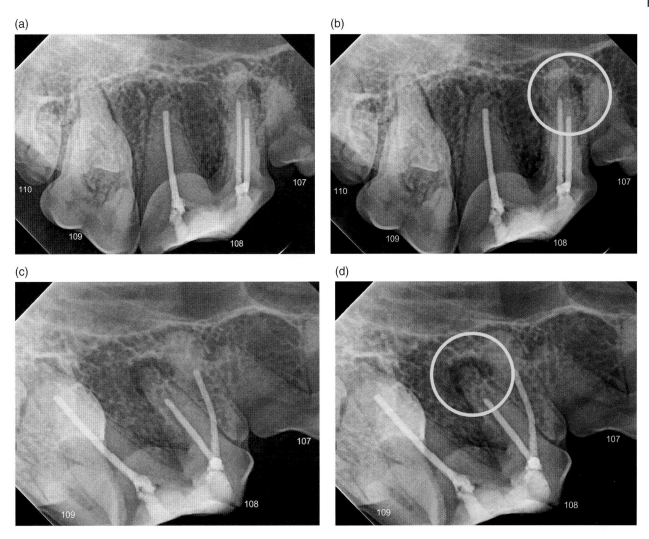

Figure 4.43 (a) Lateral radiograph of the right maxillary 4th premolar tooth (108) that has received root canal therapy. A subtle decrease in alveolar bone can be detected over the superimposed mesial roots. (b) Lateral radiograph of the right maxillary 4th premolar tooth (108) that has received root canal therapy. A subtle decrease in alveolar bone can be detected over the superimposed mesial roots (circle). This is the same image as in Figure (a). (c) Radiograph taken with the bisecting angle technique splitting the mesial roots of the right maxillary 4th premolar tooth (108). A very clear radiolucency can be appreciated over the mesiobuccal root demonstrating that multiple radiographs with different angulation and correct positioning can help identify pathology. (d) Radiograph taken with the bisecting angle technique splitting the mesial roots of the right maxillary 4th premolar tooth (108). A very clear radiolucency can be appreciated over the mesiobuccal root (circle) demonstrating that multiple radiographs with different angulation and correct positioning can help identify pathology. This is the same radiographic image as in Figure (c).

allowing for radiographic changes to be observed, thus making dental radiographs unreliable at times for accurate diagnosis of disease. About 30–40% of the mineral content in bone must be lost before pathology can be identified radiographically [2, 22]. CBCT is currently the favored imaging modality in human dentistry for the detection of early endodontic disease [9]. This imaging modality is becoming more widely used among board certified veterinary dentists for the assessment of disease [9] (see Chapter 10, for more information).

Endodontic disease affects both the pulp and the surrounding periodontal structures. When interpreting diagnostic images, the PDL and surrounding alveolar bone are the structures that are specifically being evaluated radiographically. Lesions of endodontic origin (LEO) occur because of the infected pulp tissue [23]. The bacterial toxins emerge through the apical delta or lateral canals of the tooth into the periradicular tissues which then initiate an inflammatory response. This results in an osteoclastic response of the bone and subsequent resorption of alveolar bone, appearing radiographically as a periapical lucency [23].

Radiographic Signs of Endodontic Disease

There are several radiographic signs to indicate that endodontic disease is present (Table 4.2).

Widened PDL Space

A widened PDL space is the first radiographic sign that a LEO is present [24, 25]. One of the more difficult diagnoses to make is when a tooth has a widened PDL space, but little to no pathology to support this radiographic finding is observed. If there is obvious pathology such as a fracture (complicated or uncomplicated), significant periodontal pocketing, discoloration of the tooth (indicating non-vitality), or a carious lesion, then one can feel more comfortable with the diagnosis correlating with the radiographic image (Figure 4.44).

Table 4.2 The table describes the common radiographic signs of endodontic disease.

Radiographic signs of endodontic disease
Widened periodontal ligament space
Loss of lamina dura around the apex
Periapical lucency
External and internal root resorption
Widened pulp canal
Pulp canal calcification

Loss of Lamina Dura

The lack of lamina dura is another radiographic sign indicating the presence of the beginning stages of a LEO [23, 24, 26] which are frequently more consistent with acute apical periodontitis (Figure 4.45).

Periapical Lucency

A periapical lucency can take on many different appearances based on how long the LEO has been present. An early lesion, from acute apical periodontitis for example, will likely have indistinct borders (Figure 4.46). While a more chronic lesion, like what would be consistent with

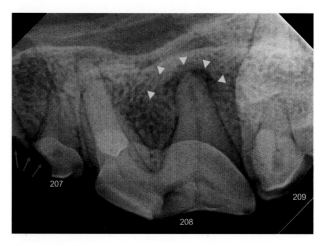

Figure 4.45 Loss of the lamina dura (yellow arrowheads) of the distal root of the left maxillary 4th premolar tooth (208). Also note the loss of crown structure associated with the left maxillary 3rd premolar tooth 207 (red arrows).

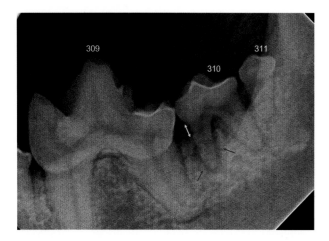

Figure 4.44 The periodontal ligament surrounding mesial root of the left mandibular 2nd molar tooth (310) is wider than the distal root (red arrows). There is also mild–moderate horizontal bone loss of this tooth (yellow double arrow). This is one of the first indications that endodontic disease is present and may be seen at the apex only as well.

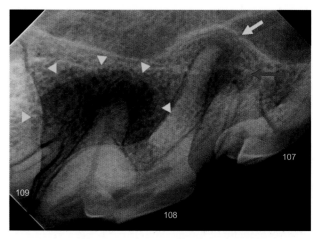

Figure 4.46 Periapical lucencies of all roots of the right maxillary 4th premolar tooth (108) can be seen. They have indistinct borders with the distal root (yellow arrowheads) exhibiting a more prominent radiolucency than the mesiobuccal (red arrow) and palatal (yellow arrow) roots.

(a) (b)

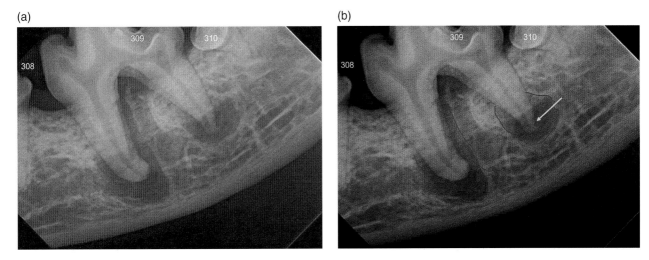

Figure 4.47   (a) Periapical lucencies of the mesial and distal roots of the left mandibular 1st molar tooth (309) with indistinct borders. There is also external root resorption present on the distal root. (b) Periapical lucencies of the mesial and distal roots of the left mandibular 1st molar tooth (309) with indistinct borders (red outline). There is also external root resorption present of the distal root (yellow arrow).

chronic apical periodontitis, will have distinct, discernable borders (Figure 4.47a and b). Sclerosing or condensing osteitis surrounding a periapical lucency can also be observed as a radiographic feature that is present in more chronic lesions (Figure 4.48). A periapical lucency cannot be distinguished from a cyst, granuloma, or abscess as these diagnoses are made histologically [23, 26]. They all have a similar appearance radiographically, which can be described as a diffuse or circumscribed radiolucent lesion [23]. Abscesses form from the presence of bacteria and the toxins produced by them. A cyst or granuloma forms from stimulation of the epithelial cell rests of Malassez that reside at the apex of a tooth [23]. These epithelial cells form and are stimulated secondary to chronic inflammation [26].

A chevron is a lucency observed at the apex of maxillary canine teeth. Occasionally, maxillary incisors can also have a chevron lucency resulting from decreased bone density and radiographic angulation. Chevron lucencies are not present in all patients and can vary in size. They have a distinct shape of a chevron or arrowhead at the apex and are frequently mistaken for a periapical lucency (Figure 4.49a and b). Periapical lucencies have more of a rounded appearance, compared to the angular appearance of a chevron. To aid in distinguishing between the two, a radiograph of the contralateral tooth should be taken as the contralateral tooth will likely have a chevron sign as well. Lack of a cause for a periapical lucency can also influence the interpretation of a tooth having a chevron rather than a periapical lucency.

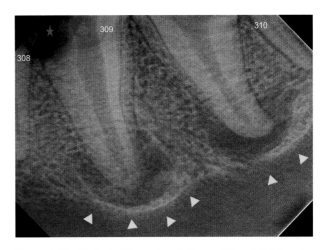

Figure 4.48   Periapical lucencies of the mesial and distal roots of the left mandibular 1st molar tooth (309) with condensing osteitis (yellow arrowheads). Note the loss of crown structure on the mesial surface of the crown (red star).

External and Internal Root Resorption

External root resorption is another radiographic sign indicative that a chronic LEO is present. This radiographic finding is often paired with the presence of a periapical lucency (Figure 4.47a and b). These lesions can be difficult to detect radiographically if they are present on the buccal, palatal, or lingual surfaces of the tooth as the superimposition of the mineralized structures can mask an early lesion. For these lesions, the use of CBCT to allow a three-dimensional view of the tooth is preferred [27].

(a)　　　　　　　　　　　　　　　　　　　　　　(b)

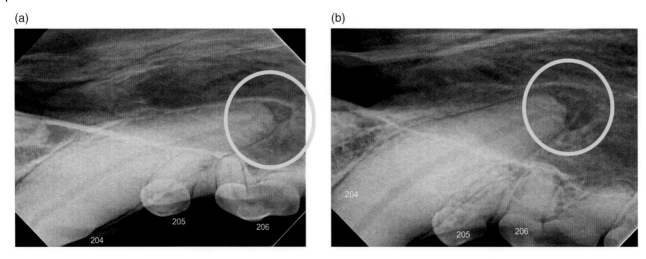

Figure 4.49 (a) Dental radiographic images of the left maxillary canine tooth (204) in two different patients demonstrating the difference between the "chevron lucency" and a true periapical lucency. The left maxillary canine tooth (204) demonstrates a chevron lucency (yellow circle). Notice the unique chevron shape, which follows "the waist" of the apex. A chevron has a more "V"- shaped or arrowhead appearance. (b) The left maxillary canine tooth (204) with a periapical lucency exhibiting a more rounded appearance (yellow circle) when compared to Figure (a). Note how the lucency is more irregular in appearance and extends further onto the body of the tooth root than the more organized chevron appearance in Figure (a).

Internal root resorption as the name implies occurs within the root canal system and progresses outward. They appear as round or ovoid radiolucent enlargements with defined margins in the root canal system [27] (Figure 4.23a and b).

Prognosis is guarded with teeth affected with either internal or external root resorption as the process is typically progressive. Performing root canal therapy has the potential to stop the progress, but this treatment can be unpredictable [15]. Therefore, extraction of teeth affected with tooth resorption is commonly elected over endodontic therapy.

Widened Pulp Canal

A widened pulp canal is an indication of a nonvital tooth. As teeth mature, the odontoblasts that reside on the outer layer of the pulp–dentin complex continue to perform dentinogenesis, causing the pulp canal to continually decrease in diameter with age [28, 29] (Figure 4.50a–c). The process of dentinogenesis continues throughout either the life of the tooth or the life of the animal, whichever comes first. Thus, when a pulp canal appears more widened than another tooth, this demonstrates the tooth has ceased to mature due to pulp death. When a widened pulp canal is suspected radiographically, comparison of this tooth to the pulp width of the contralateral tooth or a tooth of comparable size can help aid in the diagnosis (Figure 4.51a–d). Subtle widening of the pulp chamber can be easily missed with improper angulation; thus, multiple views may be necessary for a definitive diagnosis.

The cause of the death of a tooth is not always obvious, particularly when the tooth structure appears to be intact. Close observation of the tooth may show discoloration of the tooth or only part of a tooth ranging from an obvious pink, purple, gray, or brown color to a more subtle darker yellow or overall dull color (Figure 4.52a–c). The discoloration frequently occurs from a concussive injury to the tooth without causing a fracture or loss of any tooth structure. The concussive injury leads to hemorrhage of the pulp which then permeates into the dentinal tubules. The hemorrhage trapped within the dentinal tubules can be visibly seen through the thin enamel. As the blood products break down within the tooth, the color may change as well (like bruised skin). While the blood products may change color, they remain trapped within the dentinal tubules as there is no direct blood supply to remove the necrotic cells from the root canal or chamber of the tooth. The pulp is usually unable to recover from the trauma, and therefore irreversible pulpitis and death of the pulp and tooth occurs. Although these nonvital teeth have no direct bacterial contamination immediately, they can succumb to eventual contamination and therefore endodontic treatment, or extraction is the recommendation for these teeth.

Pulp Canal Calcification

Pulp canal calcification is another radiographic sign of endodontic disease; however, this should be distinguished from the normal aging process that causes narrowing of a pulp canal over time. Radiographically pulp calcification

(a)

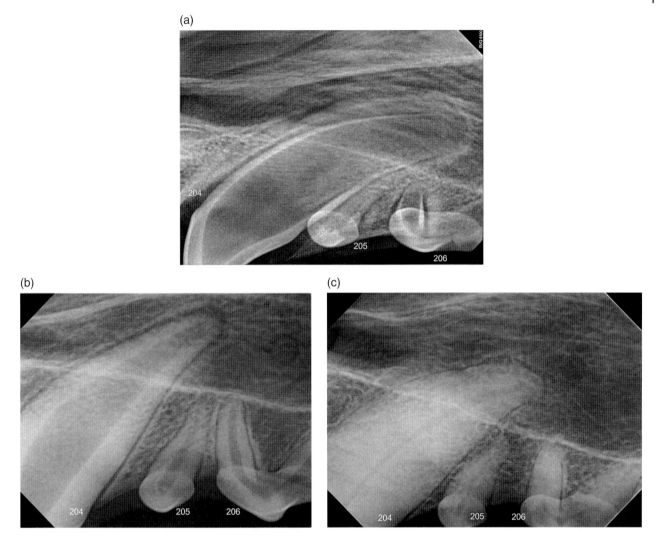

(b)

(c)

Figure 4.50 (a) Dental radiographic image of a left maxillary canine tooth in progressive stages of development and formation of an apex. This depicts the left maxillary canine tooth (204) in a young patient (six months). The apex is open with very little dentin present and a very wide pulp canal. (b) Radiograph of the left maxillary canine tooth (204) in an adolescent patient (18 months). The apex is now closed with more dentin development in comparison to Figure (a). (c) Radiograph of the left maxillary canine tooth (204) in a mature patient (eight years) showing significant narrowing of the pulp canal as a result of dentin development in comparison to Figure (a, b).

is complete disappearance of the normally radiolucent pulp canal (Figure 4.53a–c). Discerning the difference between pulp calcification and narrowing due to age is simply by the observation of the patient's teeth radiographically. If the narrowing observed is due to an aging process, it will be present in all or most of the patient's teeth. Pulp calcification would have the appearance of narrowing only in the specific teeth affected by the pulpal irritation causing increased dentinogenesis in response to an inflammatory stimulus. Pulp calcifications should also be distinguished from pulp stones, which are intrapulpal mineralized structures not associated with disease [1] (see Figures 3.43a, 3.48a, 4.43b).

Apical Periodontitis

Acute Apical Abscess

When inflammation is present at the apex of the tooth, it is referred to as apical periodontitis [30]. This is because the surrounding periodontium of the tooth is also affected [30].

Apical periodontitis can progress to an acute apical abscess or a chronic apical abscess. With an acute apical abscess, the patient has an acute onset of clinical signs and can present with obvious external facial swelling in the region of the affected tooth (Figure 4.54a and b). The most commonly affected teeth that frequently display this type of presentation are the maxillary 4th premolars and the

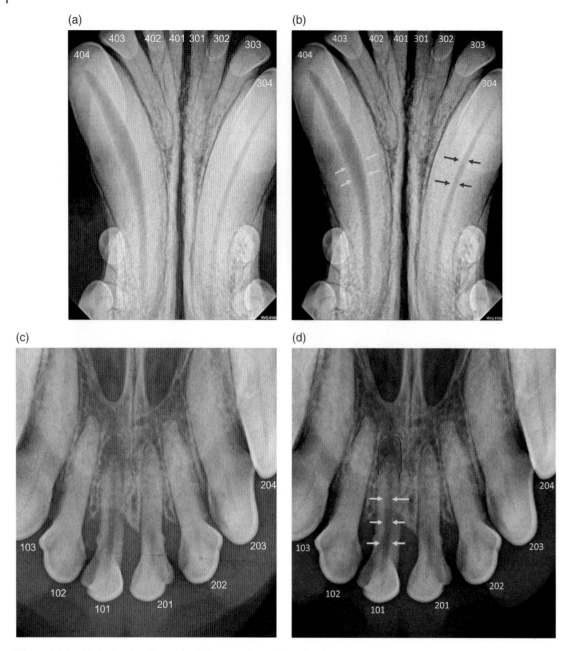

Figure 4.51 (a) Occlusal radiograph of the rostral mandible showing widened pulp canal of the right mandibular canine tooth (404) in comparison to the left mandibular canine tooth (304). (b) Occlusal radiograph of the rostral mandible showing widened pulp canal of the right mandibular canine tooth (404) (yellow arrows) in comparison to the left mandibular canine tooth (304) (red arrows). This is the same image as in Figure (a). *Source:* Courtesy of Christopher J. Snyder, DVM, DAVDC, Founding Fellow, AVDC Oral and Maxillofacial Surgery, University of Wisconsin-Madison, School of Veterinary Medicine. (c) Widened pulp canal of the right maxillary 1st incisor tooth (101) with evidence of a periapical lucency. (d) Widened pulp canal (yellow arrows) of the right maxillary 1st incisor tooth (101) with a periapical lucency (red outline). This is the same image as seen in Figure (c).

maxillary 1st and 2nd molars. This type of facial swelling can be misdiagnosed as a hypersensitivity reaction because overt dental pathology may not be seen intraorally. Radiographically, the appearance of an acute apical abscess can range from a widened PDL space to an overt periapical lucency.

Chronic Apical Abscess

A chronic apical abscess has a more gradual onset and does not typically cause any obvious swelling, but visualization of purulent material coming from a draining tract intraorally, called a parulis, may be present [30]. A parulis originating from a maxillary tooth with endodontic disease will be

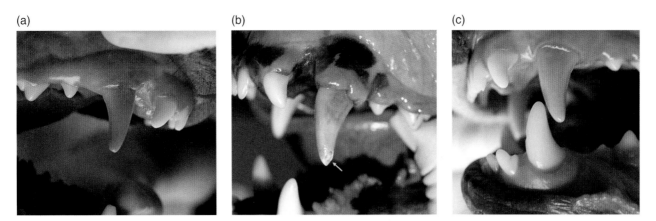

Figure 4.52 (a) Clinical images of different observable changes in the color of canine teeth affected with intrinsic staining. Images a–c were taken from three different patients. Intrinsically stained right maxillary canine tooth (104) with a pink/purple hue indicating a more recent concussive injury. (b) The left maxillary canine tooth (204) has a brown hue to it. Note the suspected uncomplicated crown fracture to the cusp tip of this tooth (yellow arrow). (c) The left maxillary canine tooth (204) has just a slight darker discoloration to it in comparison to the opposing left mandibular canine tooth (304) indicating a chronically nonvital tooth. In this case, the tooth has a duller appearance, rather than an obvious color change.

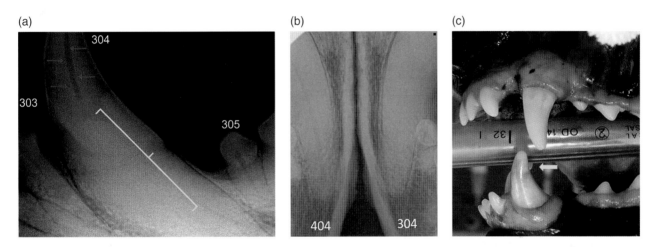

Figure 4.53 (a) A lateral radiograph of the left mandibular canine tooth (304) showing calcification of the pulp canal starting in the crown and extending into the apex (yellow bracket). There is an obvious pulp canal in the coronal one half (red arrows). This tooth had intrinsic staining of one half of the crown (Figure c) where the tooth was discolored. (b) Occlusal radiograph of the same patient in Figure (a) showing calcification of the root of the left mandibular canine tooth (304) in comparison to the contralateral right mandibular canine tooth (404). (c) Clinical image of intrinsic staining of the left mandibular canine tooth (304) (yellow arrow) of the patient in Figure (a) and (b). *Source:* Courtesy of Debra Nossaman, DVM, DAVDC, FAVD; Dallas Veterinary Dentistry and Oral Surgery.

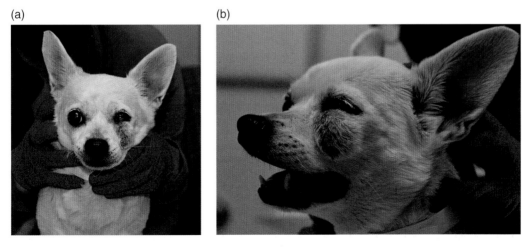

Figure 4.54 (a) Clinical image of a patient with significant left-sided facial swelling secondary to acute periapical periodontitis (acute apical abscess). The swelling is causing the lower eyelid to obstruct a portion of the eye. (b) Clinical image of the left side of the same patient as in Figure (a) with severe left sided facial swelling. This view demonstrates how large and demarcated the swelling is.

(a)　　　　　　　　　　　　　　　　　　　(b)

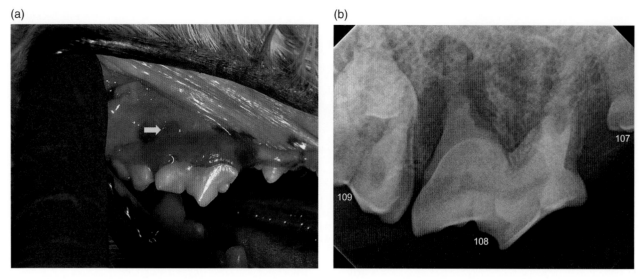

Figure 4.55 (a) Clinical image of a parulis from apical periodontitis of the right maxillary 4th premolar tooth (108) (arrow) that is present apical to the mucogingival line. (b) Radiograph of the left maxillary 4th premolar tooth (208) in Figure (a) showing periradicular bone loss and external root resorption in multiple places of all roots.

present apical to the mucogingival line (toward the apex of the tooth root) (Figure 4.55a and b). The suppurative material from a maxillary chronic apical abscess will penetrate through the bone and take the path of least resistance, which is above, or apical to the mucogingival line. The gingival tissue at the area of the mucogingival line is firmly adhered and will not allow the purulent material to penetrate, thus directing the necrotic fluid to infiltrate through the less rigid mucosa. A parulis may not always be located adjacent to the affected tooth. Therefore, dental radiographs are crucial for identifying specifically which tooth has been affected by pathology observed on the clinical exam and which tooth or teeth should receive appropriate treatment (Figure 4.56a–d). A draining tract or fistula of a mandibular tooth with endodontic disease will generally either drain in the vestibule or externally to the skin through the ventral mandible but can also present as a parulis (Figure 4.57a–c).

An external draining facial wound at the suborbital area can also be present secondary to a chronic apical abscess associated with a tooth. Often these draining wounds will improve with antibiotic +/− lavage therapy, but soon return if the causal tooth is not treated. These wounds can be misdiagnosed as a primary skin condition. Radiographically, a chronic apical abscess will exhibit a periapical lucency +/− distinct border around the lucency associated with the diseased tooth (Figure 4.58a–c).

Endodontic Therapy

Root Canal Therapy
Endodontic therapy includes both root canal therapy and vital pulp therapy and implies that some form of pulp treatment has been performed. Root canal therapy is the

process of complete removal of the entire pulp, cleaning/disinfecting and shaping of the root canal system, obturation (placement of materials to fill the pulp canal), and restoration. Once the pulp canal is disinfected and filled, the pathway of constant bacterial infiltration from the mouth to the pulp canal is eliminated. The immune system is then responsible for the eradication of the periapical infection (if present) followed by regeneration of the periradicular tissues of the affected tooth or teeth.

Radiographs are essential for determining if a tooth is a suitable candidate for endodontic therapy as well as determination of the success or failure of the procedure. The clinical and radiographic presence of endodontic disease is an indication that root canal therapy or extraction is warranted. Some signs of endodontic disease have a poorer prognosis than others; for example, a tooth with a large, apical radiolucency will have a more guarded prognosis than a tooth with a widened PDL space and no periapical lucency appreciated.

Root canal therapy can bring many procedural complications such as inadequate cleaning, shaping or obturation of the canal, instrumentation mishaps such as ledging, instrument breakage within the canal, and extrusion of materials through lateral or apical canals. The overall prognosis following treatment can change when these types of complications occur (Figure 4.59a–d). If failure of endodontic therapy is suspected following treatment, the presence of any of these complications can be suspected, therefore aiding in consideration for endodontic retreatment or extraction.

Continued radiographic monitoring is imperative to appropriately assess for success or failure of root canal therapy. Typically, follow-up radiographs are recommended at least

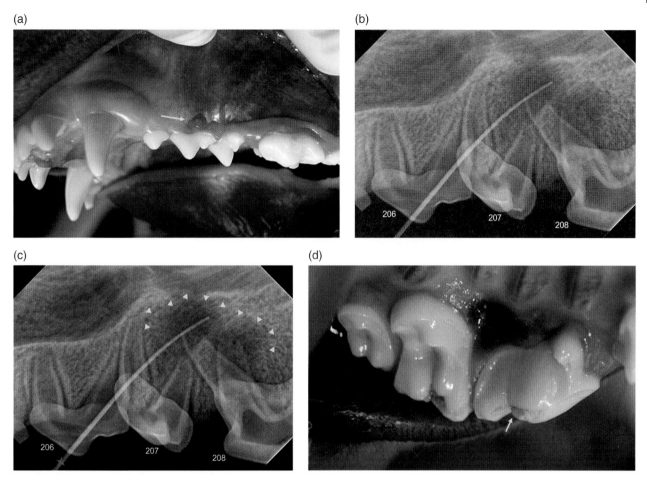

Figure 4.56   (a) Clinical and radiographic images of a dog with a draining tract associated with the left maxillary 2nd premolar tooth, which originated from a developmental abnormality associated with the left maxillary 4th premolar tooth. Photograph of a parulis present at the furcation of the left maxillary 2nd premolar tooth (206) (yellow arrow). (b) Radiograph of the patient in Figure (a) showing a radio-opaque gutta percha cone inserted into the draining tract that traverses directly to a periapical lucency of one of the mesial roots of the left maxillary 4th premolar tooth (208). There is also a periapical lucency of the other mesial root. (c) Radiograph of patient in Figure (a) showing a radio-opaque gutta percha cone (red star) that was inserted into the draining tract that traverses directly to a periapical lucency of one of the mesial roots of the left maxillary 4th premolar tooth (208) (yellow arrowheads). There is also a periapical lucency of the other mesial root (yellow arrowheads). This is the same image as in Figure (b). (d) Clinical image of the left maxillary 4th premolar tooth (208) showing a developmental abnormality of the crown (yellow arrow) that was likely the impetus for the endodontic disease demonstrated both clinically and radiographically in Figure (a)–(c).

at one year, two years, then four years post-procedure, although this can vary among veterinary dentists. Radiographic follow-up has also been recommended once every six months for the first two years following therapy and then annually indefinitely. Root canal therapy has been deemed successful if the PDL space appears radiographically normal apically (indicating periapical lucency is completely resolved), if there was radiographic evidence of a periapical lucency or loss of lamina dura, prior to the endodontic treatment [15] (Figure 4.60a and b). Root canal therapy is deemed to have no evidence of failure if the periapical lucency noted prior to presentation was stable or subjectively smaller (no larger than at the time of treatment) with cessation of root resorption (if present) [15] (Figure 4.61a–d). If the radiographs post-treatment noted a

smaller radiolucency on interpretation of the image, it would be an indication that root canal therapy was likely successful. Root canal therapy would be considered unsuccessful if a periapical lesion increased in size, appeared when one was not previously present, or root resorption progressed (if previously present) or was observed if not previously present [15] (Figure 4.62a and b).

A study assessing success of root canal therapy found that failure of root canal treatment could be determined relatively quickly following the procedure; however, long-term follow-up is recommended for evaluating a definitive outcome [15]. This is because a periapical lucency can take several years to fully remodel and repair the apical tissues of the root and surrounding bone [15]. Timely follow-up of patients receiving endodontic therapy is recommended

(a)

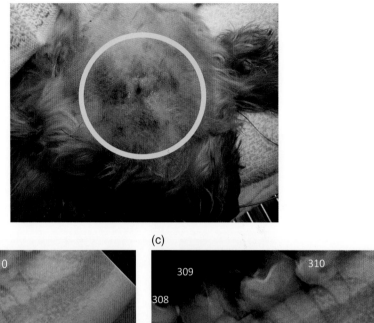

(b) (c)

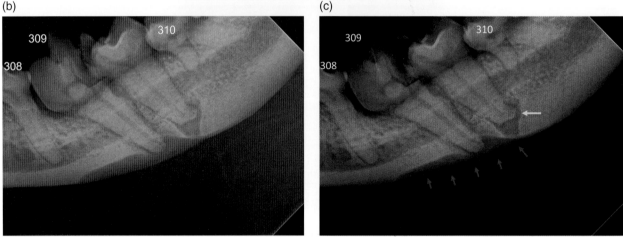

Figure 4.57 (a) Chronic draining wound of the ventral mandible (yellow circle) from a chronic LEO (lesion of endodontic origin) of the left mandibular 1st molar tooth (309) because of a condition called dens in dente. The patient is in dorsal recumbency, and the area has been clipped and cleaned. (b) Radiograph of the left mandibular 1st molar tooth (309) of the patient in Figure (a) showing a significant periapical lucency of the distal root and complete periapical bone loss of the ventral cortical bone surrounding the mesial root. The crown is severely deformed due to the developmental abnormality. (c) Radiograph of the left mandibular 1st molar tooth (309) of the patient in Figure (a) and (b) showing a significant periapical lucency of the distal root (yellow arrow) and complete periapical bone loss of the ventral cortical bone surrounding the mesial root (red arrows). The crown is severely deformed due to the developmental abnormality.

due to the patient's inability to communicate discomfort, potentially indicating a need for retreatment. Following endodontic treatment, if the patient becomes symptomatic or has radiographic evidence which could be interpreted as having evidence of failure, retreatment would be recommended.

CBCT has become the preferred imaging modality for the evaluation of both the presence of endodontic disease and the response to treatment following endodontic therapy. CBCT aids in identifying lesions earlier than intraoral dental radiographs. It has recently become standard of care for human endodontists [27] and is also becoming more commonly used by veterinary dentists.

Vital Pulp Therapy

Vital pulp therapy is an endodontic treatment option for recently complicated crown fractures in young animals. This procedure is usually recommended for patients who have fractured a tooth and are presented for treatment within 24–48 hours of the injury. Presentation and treatment of the patient within 48 hours has been shown to have an 88% success rate for this procedure. The prognosis drops to 41% if they present for treatment within one week and 23% success if the procedure is performed within three weeks of pulp exposure [31]. Vital pulp therapy consists of removing 2–4 mm of the exposed pulp and placement of a series of materials within the pulp canal.

(a)

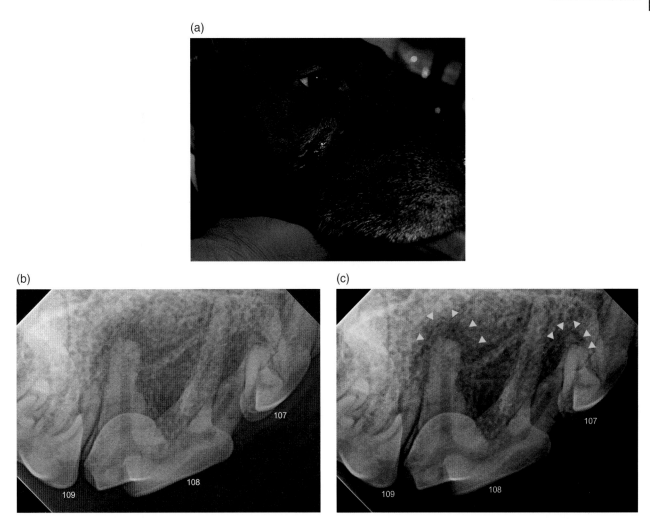

(b)

(c)

Figure 4.58 (a) Clinical and radiographic images of a dog presenting with a draining tract associated with a lesion of endodontic origin (LEO). Note the draining facial wound in the right suborbital region from a chronic LEO of the right maxillary 4th premolar tooth (108). (b) Radiograph of the right maxillary 4th premolar tooth (108) causing a draining wound in the patient in Figure (a) showing periapical lucencies of the distal root and a mesial root. These lucencies do not have a distinct border despite the chronic nature of the lesion. Note the radiographic evidence of resorption of the mesial surface of the distal root of tooth 108. (c) Radiograph of the right maxillary 4th premolar tooth (108) causing a draining wound in the patient in Figure (a) showing periapical lucencies of the distal root and a mesial root (yellow arrowheads). These lucencies do not have a distinct border despite the chronic nature of the lesion. Note the radiographic evidence of resorption of the mesial surface of the distal root of tooth 108 (red arrow). This is the same image as in Figure (b).

Mineral trioxide aggregate (MTA) is placed directly on the pulp followed by two different restorative materials (frequently glass ionomer and composite) (Figure 4.63). This type of endodontic therapy, as the name implies, allows the tooth to remain vital for continued maturation. Continued radiographic monitoring at 6 and 12 months post-procedure is recommended to assess for progressive narrowing of the pulp chamber and canal +/− dentinal bridge development under the MTA layer (Figure 4.64). While dentinal bridge formation can be a sign of vital pulp therapy success, the lack of dentinal bridge formation does not indicate vital pulp therapy failure as the bridge does not always form.

Attrition and Abrasion

Attrition is tooth wear caused by tooth-on-tooth contact, while abrasion is wear of a tooth caused by tooth contact with an inanimate object. The wear can range from mild to severe and may carry no significant ramification to the tooth if the process occurs slowly. As previously mentioned, the tooth has a reparative mechanism by which it produces tertiary dentin in response to an inflammatory response. The wear must be slow enough for the body to have a reciprocal response that generates tertiary dentin at the same rate in which the tooth structure wear occurs (Figure 4.65a and b). If the wear occurs faster than the

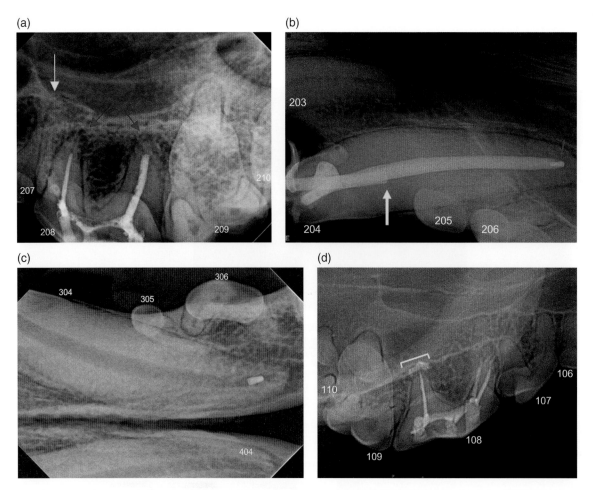

Figure 4.59 (a) Various radiographic images of different patients documenting complications of root canal therapy in Figure (a)–(d). Dental radiographic image of incomplete obturation of the palatal root of the left maxillary 4th premolar tooth (208) (yellow arrow) as there is no radio-opaque obturation material within the canal. There is also a widened periodontal ligament space of the mesiobuccal and distal roots (red arrows) indicating failure of this endodontic treatment. (b) Intraoperative radiograph after partial filling of sealant material of the left maxillary canine tooth (204) showing a ledge in the canal (yellow arrow). An instrument tip is also present at the apex that appears as a metal opacity (red arrow). *Source:* Courtesy of Debra Nossaman, DVM, DAVDC, FAVD; Dallas Veterinary Dentistry and Oral Surgery. (c) Instrument separation at the apex of the left mandibular canine tooth (304) during the instrumentation phase of root canal therapy. (d) Extrusion of sealant of the distal root of the right maxillary 4th premolar tooth (108) during the obturation phase of root canal therapy (yellow bracket). *Source:* Courtesy of Debra Nossaman, DVM, DAVDC, FAVD; Dallas Veterinary Dentistry and Oral Surgery.

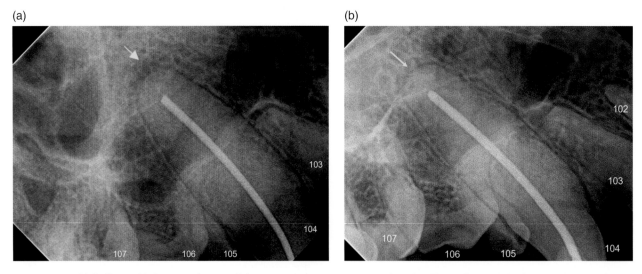

Figure 4.60 (a) Radiographic images of successful root canal therapy treatment in a dog. The radiograph depicts the right maxillary canine tooth (104) immediately following root canal therapy with evidence of endodontic disease (loss of lamina dura) at the apex of the root (yellow arrow). (b) Radiograph of patient in Figure (a) at one year follow-up. There is a normal periodontal ligament space and mineralization of the bone at the apex indicating successful endodontic therapy.

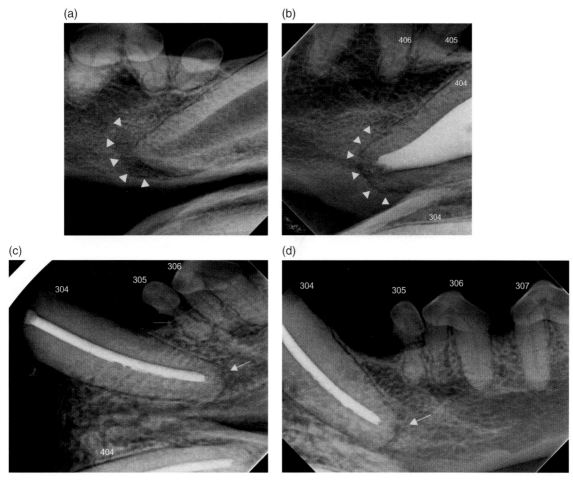

Figure 4.61 (a) Dental radiographic images of a dog who received staged root canal therapy of the right mandibular canine tooth. Preoperative radiograph of the right mandibular canine tooth (404) prior to staged root canal therapy with a periapical lucency present (yellow arrowheads). (b) Radiograph of patient in Figure (a) one year following root canal therapy. There is a normal periodontal ligament space (yellow arrowheads) and complete resolution of the periapical lucency indicating root canal therapy success. (c) Radiograph of the left mandibular canine tooth (304) in a canine patient immediately after root canal therapy. There is very slight evidence of root resorption at the apex (yellow arrow). Note there appears to be tooth resorption associated with the left mandibular 1st premolar tooth (red arrow). (d) Dental radiograph of the left mandibular canine tooth (304) in Figure (c) two years following root canal therapy. There appears to be no progression of the resorption indicating successful root canal therapy. Note there continues to be evidence of root resorption associated with the roots of the left mandibular 1st premolar tooth and the mesial root of the 2nd premolar tooth (305, 306).

body can respond, subsequent pulpitis or pulp exposure can occur (Figure 4.66a–c). Radiographic evaluation of teeth with clinical wear is recommended to ensure that endodontic disease is not present radiographically.

Eruption Abnormalities

Persistent Deciduous Teeth

A persistent deciduous tooth is identified when there is delayed exfoliation of a deciduous tooth a few days beyond the initial eruption of the permanent tooth through the gingiva [11]. Persistent deciduous teeth are commonly observed in small breed dogs, with the maxillary and mandibular canine teeth being most commonly affected (Figure 4.67). A persistent deciduous tooth may not have a permanent counterpart and therefore continue to remain as a functional tooth within the oral cavity throughout the life of the animal (Figure 4.68). In either case, radiographic monitoring of a persistent deciduous tooth is necessary to assess how much or how little of the tooth root is resorbed or if a permanent successor tooth exists (Figure 4.18). If a deciduous tooth and its permanent successor are both present, extraction of the deciduous tooth is recommended as there is likely unnecessary crowding of the teeth. This crowding creates an increased

(a)

(b)

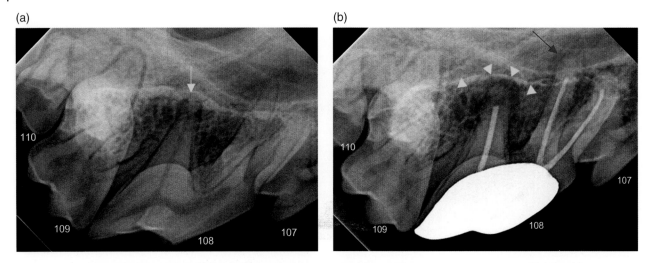

Figure 4.62 (a) Dental radiographic images of root canal therapy failure in a right maxillary 4th premolar tooth of a dog. Preoperative radiograph of the right maxillary 4th premolar tooth (108) prior to root canal therapy to treat a complicated crown fracture. There is a loss of the lamina dura of the distal root (yellow arrow). (b) Two year follow up for the patient in Figure (a) showing a periapical lucency with an indistinct border (yellow arrowheads) of the distal root and possible widening of the periodontal ligament space of the one of the mesial roots (red arrow) indicating root canal therapy failure. The metal opacity is a full metal crown.

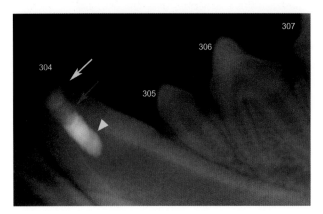

Figure 4.63 Radiograph of the left mandibular canine tooth (304) immediately after vital pulp therapy treatment showing the different opacities of the three materials used. MTA (yellow arrowhead) is placed directly on the pulp, glass ionomer is placed on the MTA (red arrow), and the final restorative material is composite (yellow arrow).

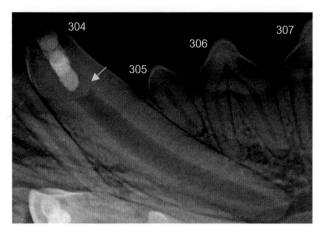

Figure 4.64 The left mandibular canine tooth (304) at a post-procedure recheck at least six months following vital pulp therapy exhibiting a dentinal bridge (arrow). Presence of the dentinal bridge is usually a sign of a successful vital pulp therapy treatment.

risk of PD. Surgical planning for extraction of a deciduous tooth requires radiographic evaluation to determine how much of the tooth root, if any, has evidence of resorption. Persistent deciduous premolars have a distinct clinical appearance, typically being smaller and having a wider base of the roots (Figure 4.68). Deciduous teeth radiographically are frequently less radiopaque than the permanent successor teeth. Deciduous teeth which persistently remain in the oral cavity have the same anatomical structure as the successive permanent teeth. Caudal to the deciduous canine tooth, deciduous tooth roots have the clinical and radiographic appearance of the permanent tooth that erupts behind it. More clearly, the deciduous 2nd premolar has the clinical and radiographic appearance of the permanent 3rd premolar, the deciduous 3rd premolar has the clinical and radiographic appearance of the permanent 4th premolar, and the deciduous 4th premolar has the clinical and radiographic appearance of the permanent 1st molar tooth. This can be confusing as the clinical appearance needs to be correlated with the age of the patient as to whether the teeth present within the oral cavity are permanent or deciduous.

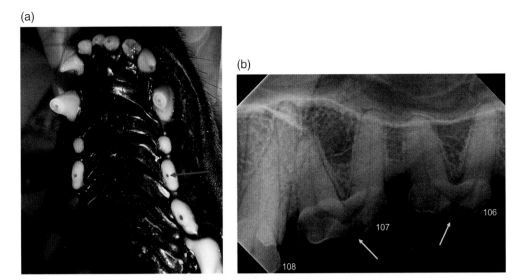

Figure 4.65   (a) Clinical image of patient with severe abrasion on multiple teeth from a tennis ball resting on the premolars and canine teeth. The brown central discoloration (red arrow) is tertiary dentin. No pulp exposure is present on the worn teeth. (b) Dental radiographic image of the right maxillary 2nd and 3rd premolar teeth (106, 107) of the patient in Figure (a). There is no evidence of endodontic disease of either tooth. The wear can be appreciated on the crown of these teeth radiographically as well (yellow arrows).

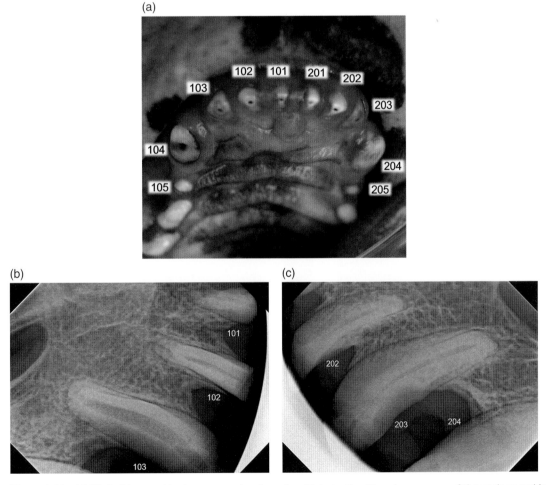

Figure 4.66   (a) Clinical image showing severe abrasion of multiple teeth with pulp exposure of the canines and incisors from rapid wear against an inanimate object. (b) Dental radiographic image of the right maxillary 3rd incisor tooth (103) with a wide pulp canal in comparison to the right maxillary 2nd incisor tooth (102) in the same image. When comparing tooth 103 to the left maxillary 3rd incisor tooth (203) in Figure (c), notice the significant difference in pulp canal size between the two teeth indicating tooth 103, with the larger pulp canal to have endodontic disease and tooth nonvitality. (c) Radiograph of the left maxillary 3rd incisor tooth (203) with a narrower pulp canal compared to the right maxillary 3rd incisor tooth (103) in Figure (b). Although both 103 and 203 are pulp exposed only tooth 103 has radiographic evidence of endodontic disease. *Source:* Courtesy of Christopher J. Snyder, DVM, DAVDC, Founding Fellow, AVDC Oral and Maxillofacial Surgery, University of Wisconsin-Madison, School of Veterinary Medicine.

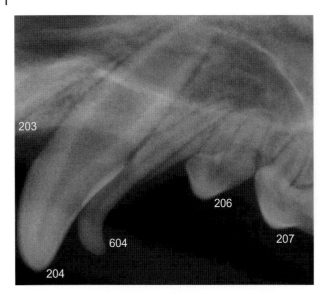

Figure 4.67 Radiograph of a persistent deciduous left maxillary canine tooth (604) alongside the permanent left maxillary canine tooth (204). There is crowding of the two canine teeth with no evidence of root resorption of tooth 604. Note there is no radiographic evidence of the left maxillary 1st premolar tooth (205) within the maxilla. The tooth that has erupted distal to the deciduous 604 has radiographic evidence of two roots which would be consistent with the left maxillary 2nd premolar tooth.

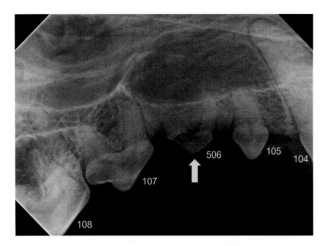

Figure 4.68 The deciduous right maxillary 2nd premolar tooth (506) is present and serving as a functional tooth without a permanent counterpart (yellow arrow). The smaller size and wider deviation of the root is characteristic of a deciduous tooth.

An additional common misconception when extracting a deciduous tooth is that if the deciduous root is fractured during the extraction procedure, the remaining root tip will continue to resorb. This may likely not happen, and all attempts to extract the entire tooth root are recommended regardless of it being identified as a persistent deciduous tooth (Figure 4.69). If there is no permanent successive tooth present, and there is no radiographic or clinical

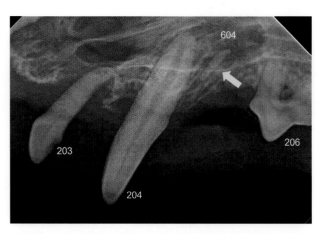

Figure 4.69 Retained tooth root of the deciduous left maxillary canine tooth (604) (yellow arrow). It is difficult to discern if there is bone loss surrounding it as this patient has decreased mineralization of the bone in that area normally. Note the patient is also missing the left maxillary 1st premolar (205) and has significant alveolar bone loss associated with the remaining maxillary 3rd incisor (203). The patient also has mild horizontal bone loss associated with the maxillary canine tooth, as well as a wide pulp chamber indicating likely endodontic disease of this tooth and non-vitality.

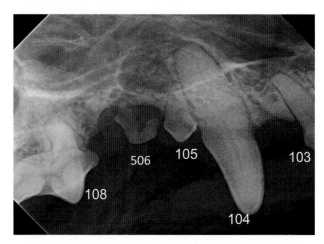

Figure 4.70 Root resorption and horizontal bone loss over the persistent right maxillary 2nd premolar tooth (506) with no permanent counterpart in a six-year-old dog. Note this patient is radiographically and clinically missing the permanent right maxillary 3rd premolar tooth (107).

evidence of disease associated with the persistent deciduous tooth, conservative monitoring of the persistent deciduous tooth is acceptable. Persistent deciduous teeth frequently exhibit resorption and bone loss as the patient ages, so continued radiographic monitoring annually is recommended (Figure 4.70).

Unerupted Teeth

Impacted (aka embedded or unerupted) teeth are defined as teeth that have not properly erupted due to a physical barrier such as bone or soft tissue [11] or teeth that lack

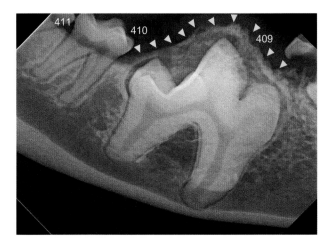

Figure 4.71 Radiograph of the right mandibular 1st molar tooth (409) with alveolar bone over the crown impeding eruption of this tooth (yellow arrowheads).

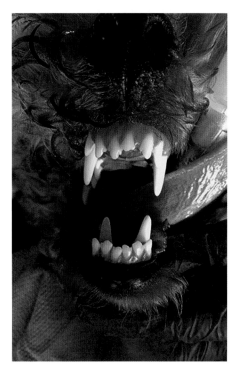

Figure 4.72 Clinical image of a patient with severe linguoversion of the mandibular canines causing hard palatal trauma.

sufficient eruption forces [17]. Frequently unerupted teeth are in an abnormal orientation, commonly positioned in a horizontal orientation [17]. In brachycephalic breeds, the most commonly observed unerupted teeth are 305 and 405 (the left and right mandibular 1st premolar teeth) [9, 17]. Radiography is crucial to visualizing the cause of impaction (bone or soft tissue), the orientation, as well as aid in appropriate treatment planning for the patient.

If the physical barrier can be removed while the tooth is still developing and in the eruption period, the tooth may likely still erupt in the proper position but be delayed (Figure 4.71). If the tooth is more mature and past the eruption process, extraction or orthodontic extrusion could be considered as unerupted teeth are prone to develop dentigerous cysts [17] (Figures 4.25, 4.26, 4.29a, b, 4.32a, and b). Orthodontic extrusion would only be considered in very select patients and specific teeth as this is a very technique sensitive and difficult procedure.

Abnormal Eruption

Eruption abnormalities in companion animals are usually derived from a genetic abnormality or from trauma sustained as a young animal during the development/eruption process. Abnormal eruption from a genetic component can cause a variety of malocclusions in a variety of breeds. Abnormal eruption and orientation of teeth can lead to other pathology such as inappropriate and traumatic contact of a tooth with apposing soft tissues. An example of this would be linguoversion of the mandibular canine teeth, which is commonly seen in dolichocephalic breeds (Figure 4.72). This type of abnormal contact can cause pain and ulceration of the adjacent tissues, frequently including the hard palate.

Brachycephalic breeds often exhibit infraeruption (incomplete or under eruption) of the mandibular canines (Figure 4.73) as well as severe crowding of the maxillary premolars allowing for the patient to succumb to PD more readily (Figure 4.13b). Other breeds may exhibit mesioversion of the maxillary canine teeth causing the diastema to be narrowed. This frequently results in a reciprocal positioning of the opposing mandibular canine teeth in an abnormal position which may cause soft tissue damage or inappropriate attrition (Figure 4.74). Any abnormally positioned tooth should be radiographed to provide as much information as possible prior to treatment. If orthodontic movement is performed to correct a malocclusion, follow-up radiography of those teeth is recommended at 6 and 12 months following treatment. This is to ensure that root resorption has not occurred secondary to moving the tooth too rapidly (Figure 4.75a–d).

Maxillofacial trauma early in life can also lead to abnormal eruption and development of the tooth/teeth in the area of insult. The eruption can range anywhere from complete cessation of tooth development or eruption to partial or delayed development or eruption. Radiographic imaging is key in these instances to assess both tooth vitality and whether the tooth is deformed or malformed. A tooth that sustains trauma in the stages of development can result in malformation of the tooth.

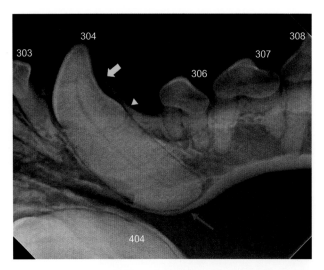

Figure 4.73 Severe infraeruption (incomplete eruption) of the left mandibular canine tooth (304) in a Shih Tzu. The alveolar bone can be seen well above the cementoenamel junction (CEJ) (yellow arrow). The alveolar bone is supposed to be positioned just below the CEJ (yellow arrowhead). The infraeruption causes the canine tooth to occupy a majority of the mandible and therefore there is very little cortical bone below the apex (red arrow). Note this patient is radiographically missing the left mandibular 1st premolar tooth (305).

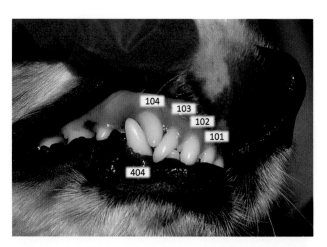

Figure 4.74 Clinical image of a Class 1 malocclusion in which mesioversion of the right maxillary canine tooth (104) has closed the diastema between the right maxillary canine tooth and 3rd incisor (104, 103) which led to buccoversion of the right mandibular canine tooth (404).

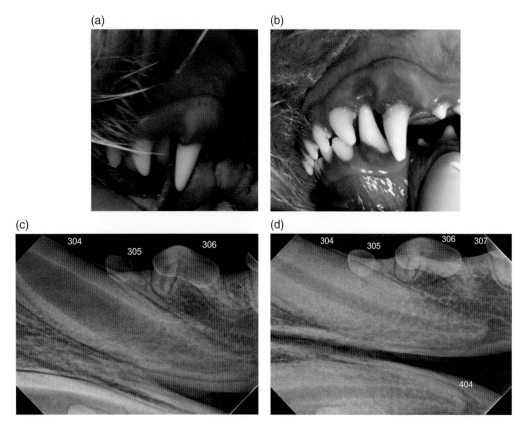

Figure 4.75 (a) Clinical image of a 10-month-old canine patient with a linguoverted left mandibular canine tooth. The patient was treated with an orthodontic appliance. The radiographic images demonstrate continued maturation of the tooth following treatment. Clinical image of a linguoverted left mandibular canine tooth (304) striking the hard palate mucosa causing palatal trauma. An orthodontic appliance (inclined plane) was used to begin lateral orthodontic movement of the tooth. (b) Same patient in Figure (a); clinical image after removal of the inclined plane and prior to placement of an additional orthodontic appliance (crown extension). The first appliance allowed significant lateral movement of the tooth. A crown extension was applied for completion of the orthodontic movement into an atraumatic position and retention of the tooth into the natural diastema between the maxillary canine tooth and third incisor. (c) Radiograph of the left mandibular canine tooth (304) in the patient depicted in Figure (a) and (b) at the time of inclined plane placement. There is a wide pulp chamber associated with the tooth, consistent with the patient's young age. (d) Radiograph of the left mandibular canine tooth (304) in the patient depicted in Figure (a)–(c) two years following orthodontic treatment. The pulp canal is narrower demonstrating maturation of the tooth and no evidence of root resorption observed indicating a healthy normal tooth.

(a)

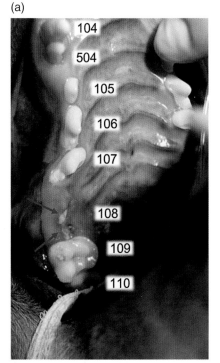

(b)

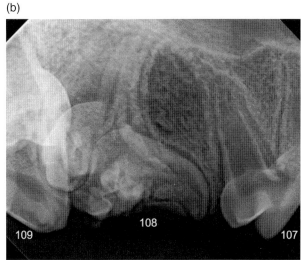

Figure 4.76 (a) Clinical image of a patient with a malformed right maxillary 4th premolar tooth (108) exhibiting incomplete eruption. Only a small portion of the tooth is visible (red arrows). Note this patient also has clinical evidence of a persistent deciduous right maxillary canine tooth (504). (b) Radiograph of the right maxillary 4th premolar tooth (108) in patient in Figure (a) showing severe deformity of the tooth.

This malformation has the potential to compromise the integrity of the tooth making it susceptible to infection in the future (Figure 4.76a and b). Depending on when and what stage of development these teeth are radiographed will determine how often they should be monitored for the development of endodontic disease if extraction is not elected. An immature tooth, which is considered to be such in dogs <11 months old, should be radiographed every three to six months for at least one year following the injury, then annually thereafter. If endodontic disease is observed during the monitoring process, treatment is considered on a case-by-case basis. A compromised tooth, however, is often not a viable candidate for root canal therapy and extraction is often elected.

Conclusion

Radiographic evaluation of all dental pathology identified on the oral examination is imperative for developing an appropriate treatment plan particularly for PD, tooth resorption, and endodontic disease diagnosed in canine patients. Full-mouth radiographs are recommended to ensure that all pathology is identified which may not have been recognized on oral examination alone. Comparison radiographs of the contralateral tooth (when possible) is also recommended to help gain a definitive diagnosis. Even if treatment is not indicated at the time of diagnosis, radiographic monitoring is important for continued assessment of disease in the canine patient.

References

1 Reiter, A. (2018). Commonly encountered dental and oral pathologies. In: *BSAVA Manual of Canine and Feline Dentistry and Oral Surgery*, 4e (ed. A. Reiter and M. Gracis), 89–118. Gloucester: British Small Animal Veterinary Association.

2 DuPont, G. and DeBowes, L. (2009). Periodontal disease. In: *Atlas of Dental Radiography in Dogs and Cats*, 1e, 32–33. St. Louis: Elsevier-Saunders.

3 Camargo, P., Takei, H., and Carranza, F. (2019). Bone loss and patterns of bone destruction. In: *Newman and Carranza's Clinical Periodontology*, 13e (ed. M. Newman, H. Takei, P. Klokkevold, and F. Carranza), 316–327. Philadelphia: Elsevier.

4 Stepaniuk, K. (2019). Periodontology. In: *Wigg's Veterinary Dentistry Principles and Practice*, 2e (ed. H. Lobprise and B. Dodd), 81–108. Hoboken: Wiley.

5 Tetradis, S., Mallya, S., and Takei, H. (2019). Radiographic aids in the diagnosis of periodontal disease. In: *Newman and Carranza's Clinical Periodontology*, 13e (ed. M. Newman, H. Takei, P. Klokkevold, and F. Carranza), 397–409. Philadelphia: Elsevier.

6 Takei, H. (2019). Phase II periodontal therapy. In: *Newman and Carranza's Clinical Periodontology*, 13e (ed. M. Newman, H. Takei, P. Klokkevold, and F. Carranza), 585–589. Philadelphia: Elsevier.

7 Takei, H. (2019). Phase I periodontal therapy. In: *Newman and Carranza's Clinical Periodontology*, 13e (ed. M. Newman, H. Takei, P. Klokkevold, and F. Carranza), 505–510. Philadelphia: Elsevier.

8 Wolf, H., Rateitschak, E., Rateitschak, K. et al. (2005). *Color Atlas of Dental Medicine*, 3e, 278–279. New York: Thieme Stuttgart.

9 Doring, S., Arzi, B., Kass, P.H., and Verstraete, F.J. (2018). Evaluation of the diagnostic yield of dental radiography and cone-beam computed tomography for the identification of dental disorders in small to medium sized brachycephalic dogs. *Am. J. Vet. Res.* 79: 62–72.

10 Verstraete, F.J., Kass, P.H., and Terpak, C.H. (1998). Diagnostic value of full mouth radiography in dogs. *Am. J. Vet. Res.* 59: 686–691.

11 Shope, B.H., Mitchell, P.Q., and Carle, D. (2019). Developmental pathology and pedodontology. In: *Wigg's Veterinary Dentistry Principles and Practice*, 2e (ed. H. Lobprise and B. Dodd), 81–108. Hoboken: Wiley.

12 Peralta, S., Verstraete, F., and Kass, P. (2010). Radiographic evaluation of the types of tooth resorption in dogs. *Am. J. Vet. Res.* 71: 784–793.

13 Rotondi, O., Waldon, P., and Kim, S. (2020). The disease process, diagnosis and treatment of invasive cervical resorption: a review. *Dent. J. (Basel)* 8 (64): 1–12.

14 Lobprise, H. (2019). General oral pathology. In: *Wigg's Veterinary Dentistry Principles and Practice*, 2e (ed. H. Lobprise and B. Dodd), 155–176. Hoboken: Wiley.

15 Kuntsi-Vaattovaara, H., Verstraete, F., and Kass, P. (2002). Results of root canal treatment in dogs: 127 cases (1995–2000). *J. Am. Vet. Med. Assoc.* 220 (6): 775–780.

16 Murphy, B., Bell, C., and Soukup, J. (2020). Odontogenic cysts. In: *Veterinary Oral and Maxillofacial Pathology*, 207–216. Hoboken: Wiley.

17 Bellei, E., Ferro, S., Zini, E. et al. (2019). A clinical, radiographic and histological study of unerupted teeth in dogs and cats: 73 cases (2001–2018). *Front. Vet. Sci.* 8: 6.

18 Babbitt, S., Krakowski Volker, M., and Luskin, I. (2016). Incidence of radiographic cystic lesions associated with unerupted teeth in dogs. *J. Vet. Dent.* 33 (4): 226–233.

19 Niemiec, B. (2001). Assessment of vital pulp therapy for nine complicated crown fractures and fifty-four crown reductions in dogs and cats. *J. Vet. Dent.* 18 (3): 122–125.

20 Soukup, J. (2019). Traumatic dentoalveolar injures. In: *Wigg's Veterinary Dentistry Principles and Practice*, 2e (ed. H. Lobprise and B. Dodd), 109–130. Hoboken: Wiley.

21 Campbell, R.D., Peralta, S., Fiani, N. et al. (2016). Comparing intraoral radiography and computed tomography for detecting radiographic signs of periodontitis and endodontic disease in dogs: an agreement study. *Front. Vet. Sci.* 31: 3.

22 Fiorellini, J., Kim, D., and Chang, Y. (2019). Anatomy, structure, and function of the periodontium. In: *Newman and Carranza's Clinical Periodontology*, 13e (ed. M. Newman, H. Takei, P. Klokkevold, and F. Carranza), 19–49. Philadelphia: Elsevier.

23 Boyd, R. (2019). Basic endodontic therapy. In: *Wigg's Veterinary Dentistry Principles and Practice*, 2e (ed. H. Lobprise and B. Dodd), 311–334. Hoboken: Wiley.

24 DuPont, G. and DeBowes, L. (2009). Endodontic disease. In: *Atlas of Dental Radiography in Dogs and Cats*, 1e, 34–40. St. Louis: Elsevier-Saunders.

25 Niemiec, B. (2019). Oral radiology and imaging. In: *Wigg's Veterinary Dentistry Principles and Practice*, 2e (ed. H. Lobprise and B. Dodd), 41–62. Hoboken: Wiley.

26 Roda, R. and Gettleman, B. (2016). Nonsurgical retreatment. In: *Cohen's Pathways of the Pulp*, 11e (ed. K. Hargreaves, L. Berman, and I. Rotstein), 324–386. St. Louis: Elsevier.

27 Nair, M., Levin, M., and Nair, U. (2016). Radiographic interpretation. In: *Cohen's Pathways of the Pulp*, 11e (ed. K. Hargreaves, L. Berman, and I. Rotstein), 33–70. St. Louis: Elsevier.

28 Lemmons, M. (2019). Oral anatomy and physiology. In: *Wigg's Veterinary Dentistry Principles and Practice*, 2e (ed. H. Lobprise and B. Dodd), 1–24. Hoboken: Wiley.

29 Fouad, A. and Levin, L. (2016). Pulpal reactions to caries and dental procedures. In: *Cohen's Pathways of the Pulp*, 11e (ed. K. Hargreaves, L. Berman, and I. Rotstein), 573–598. St. Louis: Elsevier.

30 Berman, L. and Rotstein, I. (2016). Diagnosis. In: *Cohen's Pathways of the Pulp*, 11e (ed. K. Hargreaves, L. Berman, and I. Rotstein), 2–32. St. Louis: Elsevier.

31 Clark, D. (2001). Vital pulp therapy for complicated crown fracture of permanent canine teeth in dogs: a three-year retrospective study. *J. Vet. Dent.* 18 (3): 117–121.

5

Interpretation of Common Pathology in the Feline Patient

Brenda L. Mulherin[1] and Chanda Miles[2]

[1] Lloyd Veterinary Medical Center, Iowa State University College of Veterinary Medicine, Ames, IA, USA
[2] Veterinary Dentistry Specialists, Katy, TX, USA

CONTENTS

Feline patients seen in general practice have conditions that affect their oral cavities on a regular basis. Many of these disorders are similar to those that are also observed in canine patients as discussed in depth in Chapter 4. In general, for feline patients, full-mouth radiographs are recommended when performing dental procedures to assist in identifying pathology that may not be seen with oral examination alone. This chapter focuses on common abnormalities seen in feline patients along with the characteristic radiographic findings observed to appropriately diagnose and treat the conditions.

Periodontal Disease

The specific details and stages of periodontal disease in canine patients are discussed in Chapter 4 and apply to feline patients as well. The reader is directed to Chapter 4 for general information on periodontal disease and a more detailed discussion of horizontal, vertical, and furcation bone loss.

Radiographically, periodontal disease in cats presents very similarly to periodontal disease in dogs. The periodontium including the gingiva, alveolar bone, cementum, and periodontal ligament is affected (see Figure 4.1). The stages of disease are the same as described in the dog. Stage 1 is defined as gingivitis with no attachment loss. Stage 2 is described as gingivitis with less than 25% attachment loss. Stage 3 is defined as gingivitis with 25–50% attachment loss. Finally, Stage 4 is described as gingivitis with greater than 50% attachment loss. Horizontal, vertical, and furcation bone loss are the types of bone loss observed in feline patients, as is seen in dogs. The same principles of dental radiography in dogs such as proper exposure, technique, and positioning apply to feline patients as well. For more information on radiographic technique and diagnostic image acquisition in cats, please refer to Chapter 2.

Feline skulls tend be more consistent in size and therefore the individual tooth size typically remains uniform among most cats. Skull shape can vary with different breeds, but this does not tend to influence the size of the teeth. Consequently, probing depths and the amount of

---

gingival recession observed indicate a similar amount of disease comparing one cat to another. This differs from periodontal disease observed in the dog, where the same measurement of periodontal pocketing depth and attachment loss in a chihuahua would not equal the same amount of attachment loss seen in a Great Dane. This is because larger dogs can tolerate increased attachment loss better than smaller dogs due to the size of the teeth and the amount of surrounding bone associated with the teeth. In dogs, the periodontal probing depth that is accepted is 1–3 mm. For cats, the periodontal probing depth is 0.5–1 mm, or in general, less than 1 mm. The smaller range accepted for feline species supports less variation between feline patients compared to canine patients.

Types of Bone Loss

Horizontal, vertical, and furcation bone loss in feline patients have a similar radiographic presentation to canine patients. Horizontal and vertical bone loss is classified as mild, moderate, and severe, which corresponds with the stages of periodontal disease and how much attachment loss is appreciated (see Table 4.1). Stage 1 will not demonstrate any radiographic or clinical evidence of bone loss as only gingivitis is present at this stage. Stage 1 periodontal disease is the only reversible stage as this stage is comprised of inflammation of the soft tissues with no evidence of attachment loss. Reducing the inflammation to the soft tissues with a professional, anesthetized dental cleaning, followed by providing homecare to the affected patient, should help to resolve or stabilize the level of periodontal disease before attachment loss occurs.

Horizontal bone loss presents as a reduced alveolar bone height across the span of a tooth or teeth, while the alveolar bone margin remains parallel to the occlusal tooth surface. Horizontal bone loss can be over one root of a multirooted tooth (Figure 5.1a–d), the entire tooth (one rooted or multi-rooted) (Figure 5.1e–g), or across multiple teeth (Figure 5.1h–k). Horizontal bone loss is the most common type of bone loss observed in cats [1].

Vertical bone loss is a boney defect that radiographically carries the shape of a "V" on the mesial or distal aspect of a tooth (Figure 5.2a and b). It has also been described as an angular-shaped defect associated with a specific tooth.

Furcation bone loss is loss of bone where a multirooted tooth bifurcates. The furcation area can also be considered the "crotch" of the tooth (Figure 5.3a–d).

Vertical and furcation bone loss is not as commonly observed in cats as horizontal bone loss. When furcation bone loss is observed, it is frequently combined with horizontal bone loss and can be associated with multiple teeth (see Figures 5.1h, i, 5.3c, and d).

It is important to note that all types of bone loss, particularly when minor, can be difficult to appreciate radiographically on teeth of the maxilla due to superimposition of the zygomatic arch. Radiographically altering the bisecting angle of an image (elongating or foreshortening) can be helpful in moving the zygomatic arch out of the field of view from being superimposed on the target teeth (Figure 5.4a–c).

Buccal Alveolar Expansile Osteitis (BAEO)

BAEO is a descriptive term used for clinically enlarged periodontal tissues, primarily of the gingiva and alveolar bone, that is commonly observed in cats. There are many other terms for this condition in the literature such as buccal or alveolar bone expansion, peripheral buttressing, and alveolar osteitis [2, 3]. Studies have shown BAEO to be prevalent in 35% to >50% of cats [1, 3, 4]. This condition most commonly affects the maxillary canine teeth but occasionally affects the mandibular canine teeth as well. The primary cause for BAEO is unknown; however, periodontitis is suspected to be the principal inciting factor [2, 3]. Additionally, osteomyelitis and a traumatic malocclusion have also been reported as potential etiologies [2, 3].

Clinically, BAEO appears as bulbous buccal alveolar bone with or without periodontal pocketing. Extrusion (supraeruption) of the tooth may also be observed (Figure 5.5a and b). Patients usually present with concurrent gingivitis, but this can vary. Radiographically, BAEO appears as thickened and rounded alveolar bone, with varying amounts of associated horizontal and vertical bone loss [1, 3]. Additionally, evidence of tooth resorption of the affected tooth/teeth is commonly appreciated [1, 3] (Figure 5.6). The bone tends to have a slightly decreased radiographic density compared to normal bone (Figures 5.6 and 5.7a–d). This is because it is composed of areas of loose fibrous stroma [5]. Buccal alveolar bone width of greater than 1 mm is considered abnormal and therefore deemed BAEO [1, 3].

If mild BAEO is the only clinical and radiographic finding, continued monitoring without surgical intervention can be considered. Concurrent periodontal disease and/or tooth resorption along with BAEO usually indicates that extraction of the tooth should be considered (Figure 5.8a–d).

Tooth Resorption

Tooth resorption (TR) in cats is a process by which odontoclasts are signaled to destroy hard dental tissue. The etiology is unknown despite multiple studies attempting to

(a)　　　　　　　　　　　　　(b)

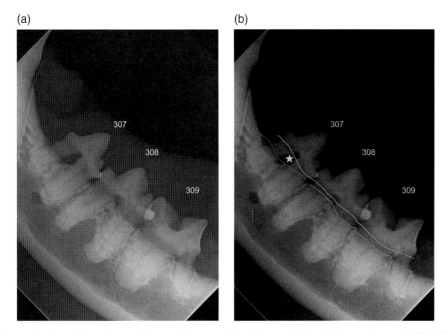

Figure 5.1 (a) Moderate horizontal bone loss of the mesial root of the left mandibular 3rd premolar tooth (307). The amount of bone loss observed would be consistent with Stage 3 periodontal disease as there appears to be almost 50% bone loss of the root. There is also furcation bone loss of tooth 307. The mild horizontal bone loss associated with the left mandibular 4th premolar and 1st molar teeth (308, 309) would be consistent with Stage 2 periodontal disease. If giving an overall stage of periodontal disease, it should be based on the worst tooth in the mouth. Based on this radiographic image, the cat would be diagnosed with Stage 3 periodontal disease. (b) Moderate horizontal bone loss of the mesial root of the left mandibular 3rd premolar tooth (307) (red line). The amount of bone loss would be consistent with Stage 3 periodontal disease as there appears to be almost 50% bone loss of the root. There is also furcation bone loss of tooth 307 (yellow star). The yellow line depicts the presumed alveolar bone margin height in a normal patient. There is also mild horizontal bone loss associated with the left mandibular 4th premolar and 1st molar teeth (308, 309) (green line) which would be consistent with Stage 2 periodontal disease. The red arrow identifies the middle mental foramen. (c) Severe horizontal bone loss on the distal root of the right mandibular 1st molar (409) with >50% attachment loss. Bone loss on the distal roots of the mandibular 1st molar is a common finding with periodontal disease in feline patients. (d) Severe horizontal bone loss on the distal root of the right mandibular 1st molar (409) with >50% attachment loss on both the buccal and lingual surfaces of bone (red and yellow lines). Bone loss on the distal roots of the mandibular 1st molar is a common finding with periodontal disease in feline patients. Additionally, there appears to be bone loss within the furcation area of 409 (yellow star). While it cannot be confirmed with a radiograph that there is complete furcation exposure, the radiograph demonstrates bone loss within the area of the furcation. (e) Moderate horizontal bone loss consistent with Stage 3 periodontal disease affecting the entire right mandibular 3rd premolar tooth (407). Note the mesial root is more affected than the distal root. (f) Moderate horizontal bone loss consistent with Stage 3 periodontal disease affecting the entire right mandibular 3rd premolar tooth (407) (red line). Note the mesial root is more affected than the distal root (yellow arrow). (g) Mild horizontal bone loss of the right mandibular canine tooth (404) indicated by the alveolar bone margin (red arrow) just slightly below the cementoenamel junction (blue arrow). This amount of bone loss is consistent with Stage 2 periodontal disease. Also note in this image the severe horizontal bone loss associated with the right mandibular 4th premolar tooth (408) (red lines) and bone loss within the furcation of this tooth (yellow star). Additionally, there is a retained tooth root associated with the right mandibular 3rd premolar tooth (407) (yellow arrow). (h) Moderate horizontal bone loss of the right mandibular 3rd and 4th premolars and 1st molar teeth (407–409). This amount of bone loss is consistent with Stage 3 periodontal disease (25–50% attachment loss). Note there is tooth resorption of the distal root of 409. (i) Moderate horizontal bone loss (red line) of the right mandibular 3rd and 4th premolars and 1st molar teeth (407–409). This amount of bone loss is consistent with Stage 3 periodontal disease (25–50% attachment loss). The anticipated alveolar bone margin is indicated with the yellow line. Note there is tooth resorption (red arrow) of the mesial surface of the distal root of 409. The caudal mental foramen is identified with the yellow arrow. (j) Severe horizontal bone loss consistent with Stage 4 periodontal disease across the maxillary incisors. There is also tooth resorption affecting all incisor teeth. Additionally, there is a fractured right maxillary 1st incisor tooth (101) with the crown of the tooth displaced from the root. (k) Severe horizontal bone loss consistent with Stage 4 periodontal disease across the maxillary incisors (red line). There is tooth resorption affecting all incisor teeth (yellow arrows). Additionally, there is a fractured right maxillary 1st incisor tooth (101) with the crown of the tooth displaced from the root (red arrow).

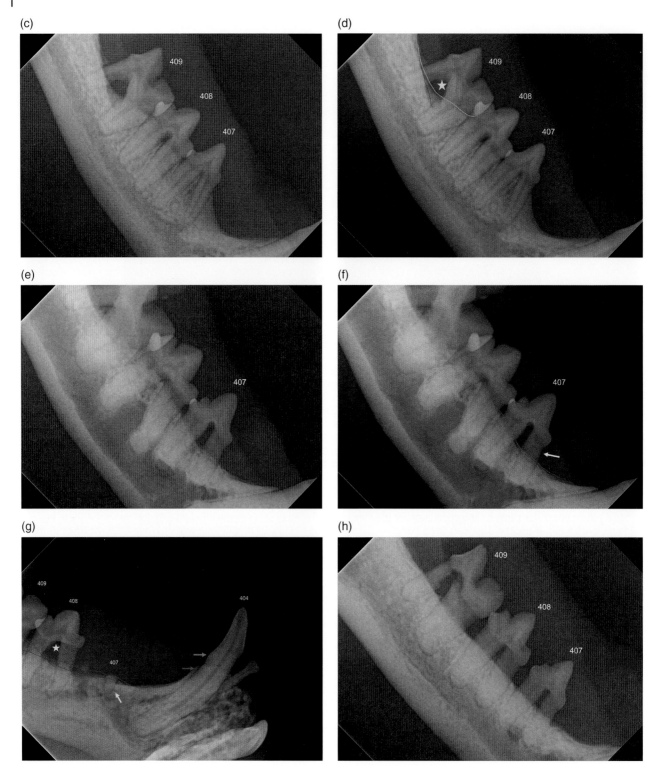

Figure 5.1 (Continued)

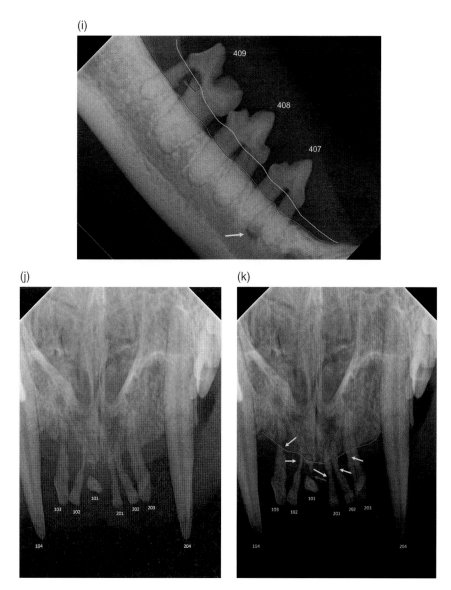

Figure 5.1 (Continued)

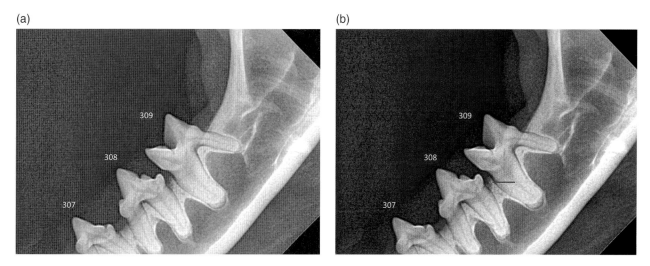

Figure 5.2 (a) Vertical bone loss observed on the distal aspect of the left mandibular 4th premolar tooth (308). (b) Vertical bone loss observed on the distal aspect of the left mandibular 4th premolar tooth (308). Note the angular-shaped defect that is present between the mandibular 4th premolar (308) and first molar tooth (309) (red arrow).

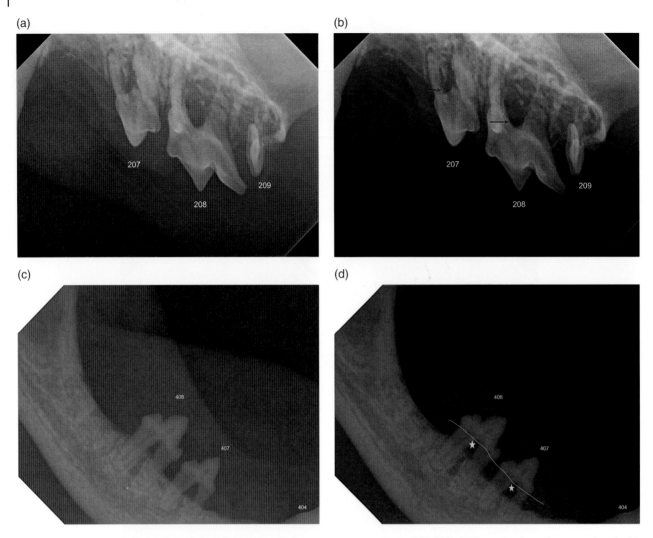

Figure 5.3 (a) Furcation bone loss of the left maxillary 3rd and 4th premolar teeth (207, 208). (b) Furcation bone loss associated with the left maxillary 3rd and 4th premolar teeth (207, 208) (red arrows). (c) Furcation bone loss associated with the right mandible of a cat. There is loss of bone within the furcation of the right mandibular 3rd and 4th premolar teeth (407, 408) as well as moderate horizontal bone loss. (d) Furcation bone loss associated with the right mandible of a cat. There is horizontal bone loss indicated by the red line. The yellow line depicts the presumed normal alveolar bone height. The yellow stars indicate the bone loss within the furcation. Additionally, the distal surface of the mesial root of the right mandibular 3rd premolar tooth (407) has evidence of root resorption. This patient is also missing the right mandibular 1st molar tooth.

correlate it with other disease processes such as periodontal disease [6]. Tooth resorption affects 25–75% of cats making it one of the most common diseases impacting the teeth of feline patients. This wide range is dependent on the population of cats being investigated and what methods of diagnosis were employed to identify the disease [6–8]. Tooth resorption is rarely seen in cats less than two years of age, and the prevalence of disease has been shown to increase with age [6, 7].

Tooth resorption is progressive with no identified treatment to stop it. It can be painful for the patient and therefore extraction is the recommended treatment for teeth that demonstrate clinical evidence of resorption. Careful evaluation of how and where each tooth is affected is necessary before treatment is considered. Any tooth can be affected with TR. Research has determined the left and right mandibular third premolars (307, 407) are the teeth most frequently affected by tooth resorption [6, 9]. Dental radiography is essential for diagnosis and treatment because TR can affect either the crown only, the root only, or both the crown and the root of the tooth simultaneously.

Clinically, early lesions can appear as small focal areas of gingivitis at the gingival margin (frequently adjacent to the

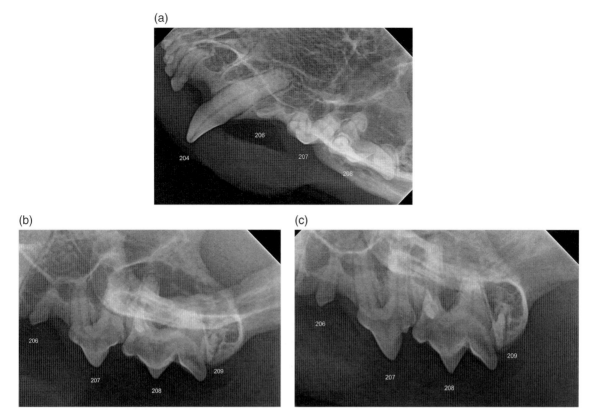

Figure 5.4   (a) Intraoral dental radiograph of the left maxilla of a cat demonstrating how positioning of an image by intentionally using foreshortening or elongation can reveal certain aspects of the tooth and its roots. In this image, severe foreshortening of the left maxillary premolar teeth is observed. Note the zygomatic arch is superimposed over the premolars. Although all premolars are in this radiograph, the angle is intended to show the left maxillary canine tooth (204). (b) Intraoral dental radiograph of the left maxillary premolar and molar teeth (206–209) of the same cat as shown in (a) with proper angulation. Note the zygomatic arch lies over these teeth causing some superimposition of bone on the distal root of the left maxillary 3rd premolar (207) and all roots of the left maxillary 4th premolar (208). This feline patient does not appear to have any bone loss. (c) Intraoral dental radiograph of the left maxilla using an elongated view of the left maxillary premolar and molar teeth (206–209) of the same cat as seen in Figure (a) and (b). Note the elongation of the image allows better visibility of the periodontal ligament space of the distal root of the left maxillary 3rd premolar (207) and all roots of the left maxillary 4th premolar (208) because there is less superimposition of the zygomatic bone over these roots.

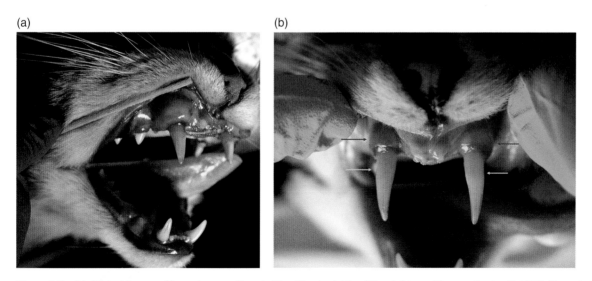

Figure 5.5   (a) Clinical image of buccal expansile osteitis with gingivitis of the right maxillary canine tooth (104). No periodontal pocketing was present. Note there is supraeruption of the tooth as you can see root structure below the cementoenamel junction (yellow arrow). A more bulbous appearance of the maxillary canine tooth is observed in the image. (b) Clinical photograph of a cat with buccal alveolar expansile osteitis of the right (104) and left (204) maxillary canine teeth (red arrows). The cat in this image also demonstrates supraeruption of both maxillary canine teeth. The yellow arrows depict the cementoenamel junction of the canine teeth. Note the extensive supraeruption of the canine teeth from the maxilla. The patient in this image has a normal periodontal pocketing depth.

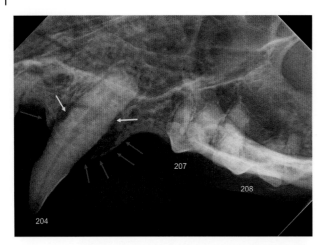

Figure 5.6   Intraoral dental radiograph of the left maxilla of a cat. There is evidence of buccal alveolar expansile osteitis associated with the left maxillary canine tooth (204). Notice the rounded edges and moth-eaten appearance of the alveolar bone which is due to the loose fibrous tissue that is within the bone (red arrows). The patient in this image is missing the left maxillary 2nd premolar tooth. There is also suspicion of tooth resorption associated with the left maxillary canine tooth (204) (yellow arrows). Appreciate how there is a loss of a crisp border to the edges of the canine tooth.

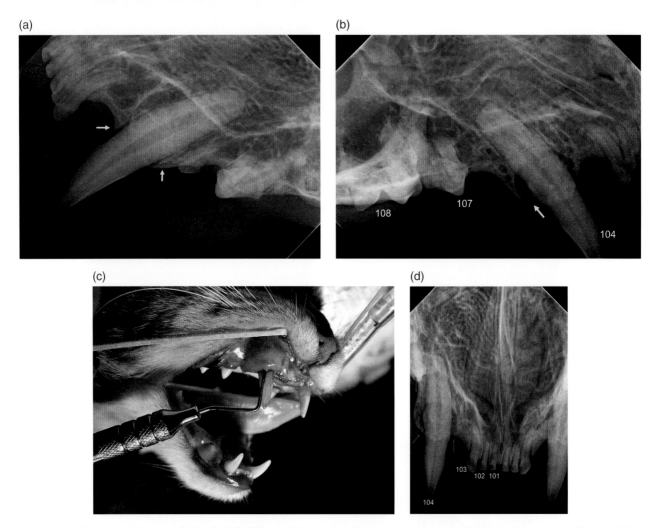

Figure 5.7   (a) Intraoral dental radiograph of the left maxilla of a cat with normal appearance of alveolar bone surrounding the left maxillary canine tooth (204). Note the sharp edges of the mesial and distal bone (yellow arrows) at the alveolar margin. (b) Intraoral dental radiograph of the right maxilla of a cat. The radiograph demonstrates moderate expansile osteitis and vertical bone loss on the distal aspect of the right maxillary canine tooth (104) (yellow arrow) with associated periodontal pocketing. The patient in this image is missing the right maxillary 2nd premolar tooth. (c) Clinical image of the right maxillary canine tooth (104) in same patient depicted in Figure (b) demonstrating the depth of the periodontal pocket. The periodontal probing depth of this patient is 9 mm. The normal probing depth accepted in the cat is 0.5–1 mm. Note the more bulbous appearance of the alveolar bone surrounding the canine tooth indicative of buccal alveolar expansile osteitis. (d) Intraoral dental radiograph utilizing the occlusal view of the same cat as seen in Figure (b) and (c) with moderate expansile osteitis (red arrows). Note the vertical bone loss is not as obvious in this occlusal view as it was utilizing the bisecting angle technique in Figure (b).

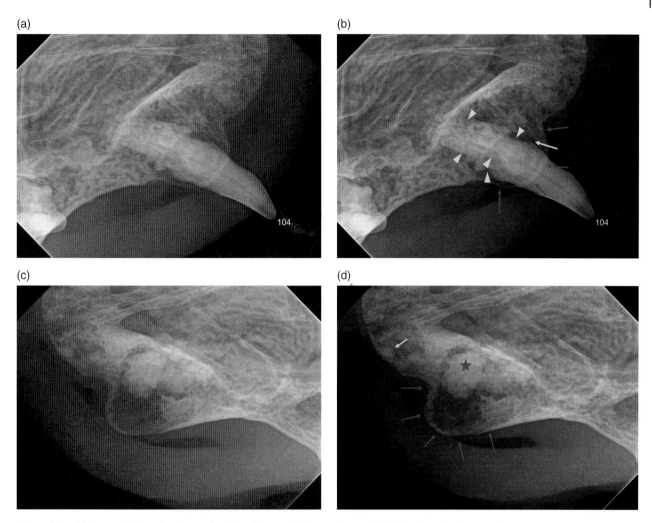

Figure 5.8 (a) Intraoral dental radiograph of the right maxillary canine tooth (104) affected with buccal alveolar expansile osteitis, tooth resorption, and vertical bone loss. The patient is missing multiple teeth. (b) Intraoral dental radiograph of the right maxillary canine tooth (104) affected with buccal alveolar expansile osteitis (red arrows), tooth resorption (yellow arrowheads), and vertical bone loss on the mesial aspect of the tooth (yellow arrow). (c) Intraoral dental radiograph of the left maxillary canine tooth (204) of the same patient as seen in Figure (a) and (b) showing significant buccal alveolar expansile osteitis. There is root structure remaining of tooth 204. This tooth is severely affected by tooth resorption with only evidence of the root remaining. (d) Intraoral dental radiographic image of the left maxillary canine tooth (204) of the same patient as seen in Figure (a)–(c) showing evidence of buccal alveolar expansile osteitis (red arrows) and root resorption with a remaining root tip (red star). The patient is missing multiple teeth. Additionally, there is evidence of a retained tooth root associated with one of the maxillary incisors (yellow arrow).

cementoenamel junction) or areas of gingiva that are covering more of the tooth structure than normal (Figure 5.9a–c). When these areas are probed, the resorptive lesion will appear as a defect in the tooth (missing tooth structure), with gingiva or granulation tissue present within the void of missing structure (Figure 5.10). The granulation tissue will bleed easily when probed. Secondary inflammation of the periodontal tissues can often be seen as well. As TR progresses, more of the crown is missing and in more advanced lesions, almost the entire crown can be missing with only a small remnant of tooth structure seen protruding through the gingiva (Figure 5.11a and b).

When a root or roots of a tooth are affected with TR, they may undergo a process of slowly being replaced with bone. The periodontal ligament space may no longer be present and as the process advances, the root may eventually be resorbed and no longer identifiable radiographically compared to the surrounding bone (Figure 5.12a–c). Root replacement resorption is only seen radiographically. This is the most important reason dental radiographs are so imperative when diagnosing and treating TR (Figure 5.13). Dental radiographs can be utilized to provide additional information and guide the practitioner in the most appropriate treatment options for the patient (Figure 5.14a and b).

(a)

(b)

(c)

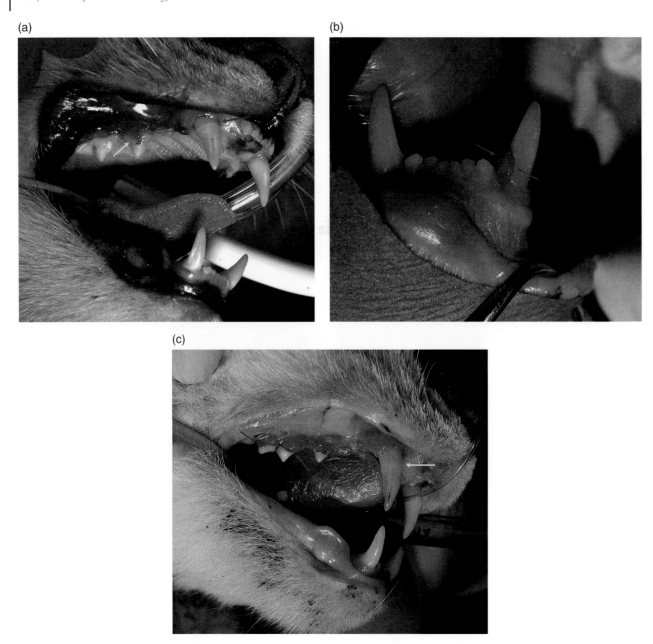

Figure 5.9 (a) Clinical image of the right maxillary 3rd premolar tooth (107) affected with tooth resorption. The missing tooth structure is filled with granulation tissue giving the appearance of a focal area of gingivitis (yellow arrow). Generalized gingivitis is present on the right maxillary 3rd and 4th premolar teeth (107, 108) as well. Supraeruption of the right maxillary canine tooth (104) is also observed (red arrow). (b) Clinical image of tooth resorption affecting the lingual aspect of the left mandibular canine tooth (304). There is missing tooth structure that has filled in with granulation tissue (red arrows). (c) Clinical image of the right maxillary 3rd and 4th premolar teeth (107, 108) affected with tooth resorption. The gingiva is inflamed and covers a large portion of the crowns of these teeth (red arrows). Beneath the inflamed gingiva, there is loss of crown structure that can be appreciated only on the anesthetized oral examination. Additionally, there is supraeruption of the right maxillary canine tooth (104) (yellow arrow).

Radiographically, TR lesions that affect the crown will be seen as focal or multifocal radiolucent areas observed primarily in the crown of an affected tooth (Figure 5.15a–d).

Although tooth resorption commonly progresses and eventually causes pulp exposure and endodontic compromise, radiographic evidence of a periapical lucency does not occur as frequently in cats as it does in dogs (see Figure 4.24).

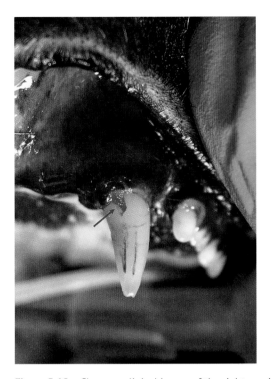

Figure 5.10 Close-up clinical image of the right maxillary canine tooth (104) showing a tooth resorptive lesion just below the cementoenamel junction that is filled with granulation tissue (red arrow). The missing tooth structure can be appreciated in this image.

Stages and Types of Feline Tooth Resorption

When TR is diagnosed, understanding the stages and types of resorption present and to what extent the resorption is affecting the tooth can be crucial for treatment. The American Veterinary Dental College has classified feline tooth resorption based on the severity (stages) and location (types) of the TR, both of which affect the radiographic appearance of the tooth.

There are five stages and three types of TR in cats as described in Boxes 5.1 and 5.2.

Stages of Tooth Resorption

Stage 1: Mild loss of tooth structure limited to cementum or cementum and/or enamel of a tooth. These lesions typically occur subgingivally and are difficult to identify. The lesions are not seen radiographically (Figure 5.16).

Stage 2: Moderate loss of tooth structure that extends into dentin, but not the pulp cavity (cementum or cementum and enamel with loss of dentin that does not extend to the pulp cavity) (Figure 5.17a and b).

Stage 3: Loss of tooth structure that extends into the dentin and into the pulp cavity; most of the tooth maintains its integrity and structure (Figure 5.18a–c).

(a)

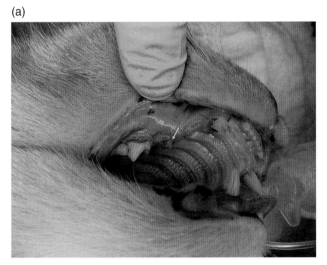

(b)

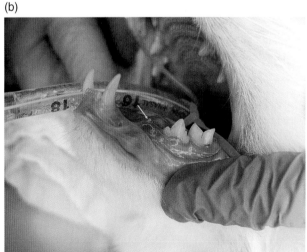

Figure 5.11 (a) Clinical image of the right maxilla of a cat. The cat has been diagnosed with tooth resorption. Note how there is significant granulation tissue present in the area of the right maxillary 3rd premolar tooth (107), with only a small amount of crown remaining, protruding from the free gingival margin. Additionally, there is suspicion of tooth resorption associated with the right maxillary canine tooth which should be explored both clinically and radiographically for a definitive diagnosis (red arrow). (b) Clinical image of the left mandible of a cat. There is significant inflammation in the area of the left mandibular 3rd premolar tooth (307), with only a small amount of the crown remaining visible (yellow arrow). The right and left mandibular 3rd premolar teeth are the teeth most commonly affected by tooth resorption.

(a)

(b)

(c)

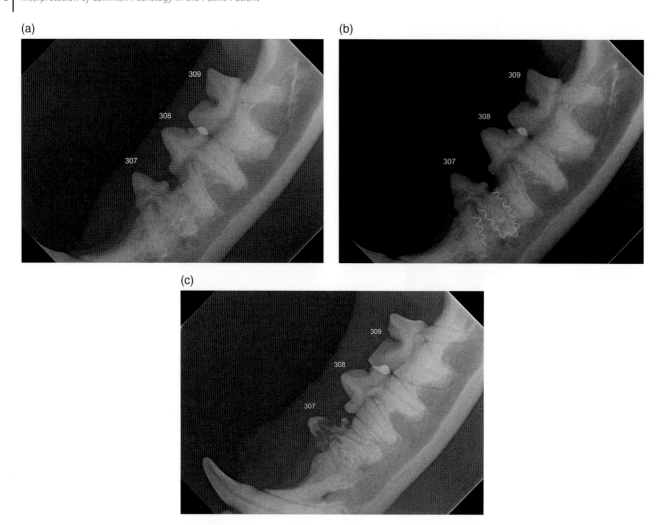

Figure 5.12 (a) Intraoral dental radiograph of the left mandibular 3rd premolar tooth (307) showing beginning stages of root replacement resorption. Notice the periodontal ligament space of the roots has disappeared and there is less distinction between the tooth roots and the surrounding bone. Additionally, there is a subtle radiolucency within the crown of this tooth. (b) Intraoral dental radiograph of the left mandibular 3rd premolar tooth (307) demonstrating beginning stages of root replacement resorption. The periodontal ligament space has disappeared (yellow lines), and there is less distinction between the tooth roots and the surrounding bone. Additionally, there is a radiolucency consistent with a resorptive process present within the crown of this tooth (red star). (c) Intraoral dental radiograph of the left mandibular 3rd premolar tooth (307) showing severe root replacement resorption of both roots. Note how there is no radiolucent distinction of the periodontal ligament space when comparing this tooth to the surrounding teeth. Adjacent teeth maintain a clearly visible radiolucent periodontal ligament space. Additionally, note the loss of crown structure and difficulty identifying the presence of an entire 3rd premolar tooth on the radiographic image.

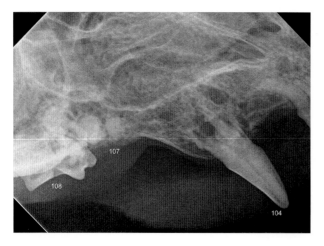

Figure 5.13 Type 2 tooth resorption of tooth 104. There is near complete root replacement resorption of the root while the crown is still intact. This pathology would only be seen radiographically as there was no clinical evidence the crown was affected with a tooth resorption lesion. Also note there is evidence of retained tooth roots associated with the right maxillary 3rd premolar tooth (107). The right maxillary 2nd premolar tooth is missing.

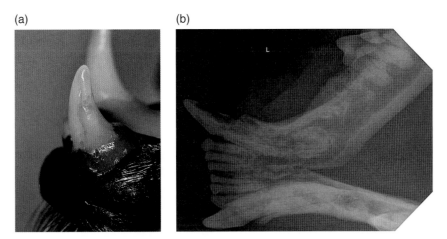

Figure 5.14 (a) Clinical image of the left mandibular canine tooth of a cat that is affected with tooth resorption. Note the granulation tissue present over the distal and buccal surface of the tooth. Additionally, note how the affected area appears to originate from below the free gingival margin of the tooth. (b) Intraoral radiographic image of the same left mandibular canine tooth affected with tooth resorption as seen clinically in Figure (a). There is significant loss of the architecture of the tooth. There is no identifiable pulp canal present nor is there an obvious periodontal ligament space present. The distinction between the root and the surrounding alveolar bone is lost. While the crown of this tooth has clinical evidence of being affected with tooth resorption, the radiographic evidence of resorption is much more dramatic.

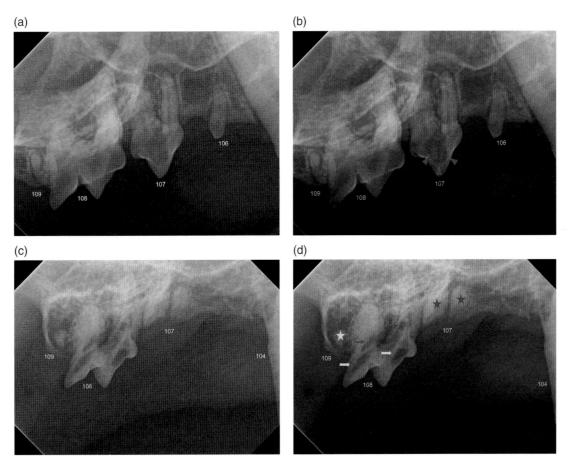

Figure 5.15 (a) Intraoral dental radiograph of the right maxillary 3rd premolar tooth (107) that is affected with tooth resorption. Note the focal irregular lucency present within the center of the crown from the missing tooth structure. (b) Intraoral dental radiograph of the right maxillary 3rd premolar tooth (107) that is affected with tooth resorption. There is a focal irregular radiolucency that is present within the center of the crown of the affected tooth, identified by the red arrowheads. This would be diagnosed as a Type 1 tooth resorption lesion due to an obvious periodontal ligament space around each tooth root. (c) Intraoral dental radiograph of the right maxilla of a cat diagnosed with tooth resorption. There are multiple, multifocal lucent areas within the crown of the right maxillary 4th premolar tooth (108). Additionally, there is evidence of retained tooth roots associated with the right maxillary 3rd premolar (107) and 1st molar teeth (109). (d) Intraoral dental radiograph of the right maxillary 4th premolar tooth (108) showing multiple, multifocal lucent areas of tooth resorption within the crown of the tooth (yellow arrows). Some lucent areas extend into the distal and mesial roots (red arrows). Note the presence of retained tooth roots associated with the right maxillary 3rd premolar (107) (red stars) and the 1st molar (109) teeth (yellow star). Additionally, this cat is radiographically missing the right maxillary 2nd premolar tooth (106).

Box 5.1   The stages of tooth resorption

Stages of tooth resorption. The five stages of tooth resorption are described.

Stage 1	Loss of tooth structure limited to cementum and/or enamel of a tooth
Stage 2	Loss of tooth structure extending into the dentin
Stage 3	Loss of tooth structure extending into the pulp, tooth maintains its integrity and structure
Stage 4	Loss of tooth structure extending into pulp, loss of integrity to the tooth structure
	4a: Crown and root are equally affected
	4b: Crown is more affected than the root
	4c: Root is more affected than the crown
Stage 5	Loss of clinical evidence of the tooth structure, irregular radiopacities that resemble tooth structure observed radiographically

Box 5.2   Types of tooth resorption

Types of tooth resorption. The three types of tooth resorption are described.

Type 1	Roots maintain radiographic evidence of a periodontal ligament space
Type 2	Roots do not maintain clear evidence of a periodontal ligament space
Type 3	Components of both a Type 1 lesion and a Type 2 lesion in a multirooted tooth. Presence of an intact periodontal ligament space in one root and absence of a periodontal ligament space in another root

Stage 4: Extensive loss of tooth structure. Resorption of dentin and the pulp cavity; most of the tooth has been resorbed. This stage has three subcategories based on what portion of the tooth has been affected.

TR4a: The crown and root are equally affected (Figure 5.19a–c).

TR4b: The crown is more affected than the root (Figure 5.19d–f).

TR4c: The root is more affected than the crown (Figure 5.19g–i).

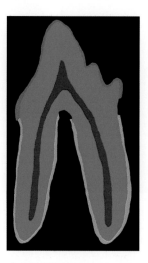

Figure 5.16   Diagram of Stage 1 tooth resorption. This stage of tooth resorption is not readily identified radiographically. Stage 1 tooth resorption is confined to the cementum and/or enamel of a tooth. Frequently, it is associated with the cementoenamel junction. Diagnosis of this stage of tooth resorption is more of a clinical diagnosis found on oral examination if it is associated with the enamel of an affected tooth.

Stage 5: All the tooth structure is missing and covered by gingiva. There are only irregular radiopacities present radiographically that resemble root structure within the underlying alveolar bone (Figure 5.20a–c).

Types of Tooth Resorption

Type 1: Only the crown of the tooth is affected with a focal or multifocal radiolucency, while the roots maintain normal radiopacity and periodontal ligament space (Figure 5.21a–c). These teeth can typically be extracted with a normal surgical extraction technique.

Type 2: There is missing periodontal ligament space of all or parts of the roots with radiolucency of part or most of the crown (Figure 5.22a–c). Teeth affected with Type 2 tooth resorption may be treated with either extraction or crown amputation. Specific patient criteria needs to be met in order to perform a crown amputation (Box 5.3).

Type 3: Components of both Types 1 and 2 are present in the same tooth (Figure 5.23a–c). Teeth affected with Type 3 tooth resorption are generally treated with extraction of the root with the Type 1 lesion and treated with either extraction or crown amputation of the root affected with the Type 2 lesion, provided the criteria for performing a crown amputation has been met.

Criteria for Performing Crown Amputation/Intentional Root Retention

Treatment for patients affected with tooth resorption presents multiple challenges. The treatment of choice for teeth that are affected with tooth resorption is

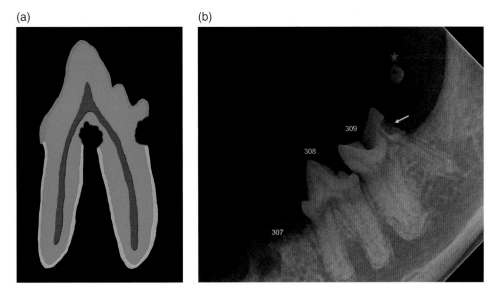

Figure 5.17 (a) Diagram of Stage 2 tooth resorption. This stage of resorption affects the cementum and/or enamel and extends into the dentin. This is the first stage of tooth resorption that demonstrates radiographic evidence of disease. (b) Stage 2 tooth resorption on the distal aspect of the crown of the left mandibular 1st molar tooth (309) (yellow arrow). The lesion is affecting the enamel and dentin only. There is also a mineral opacity of unknown origin (red star). This could be a portion of the affected tooth, a piece of calculus, or other mineralized structure. Although this radiograph is not positioned to assess the rostral mandible, there appears to be resorption of the left mandibular 3rd premolar tooth (307) as well. The type of tooth resorption affecting this tooth is difficult to discern. There are areas in which a periodontal ligament space is clearly visualized, and other areas in which the periodontal ligament space is difficult to appreciate. If there is a question as to the Type of tooth resorption present, all attempts should be made to remove the roots in their entirety. Annual clinical and radiographic monitoring of the site to observe for evidence of abnormalities associated with the remaining tooth roots is recommended.

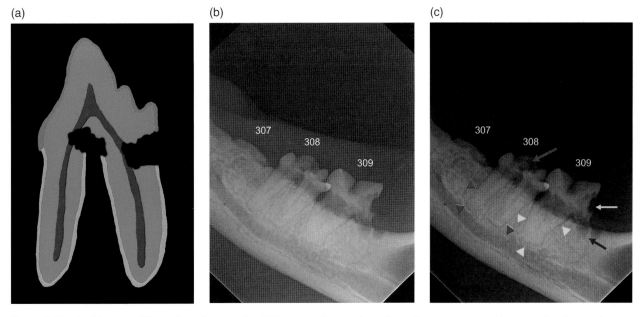

Figure 5.18 (a) Diagram of Stage 3 tooth resorption. This stage of resorption affects the cementum and/or enamel and extends through the dentin into the pulp of a tooth. At this stage, there is mild structural damage of the tooth. (b) Stage 3 tooth resorption of the left mandibular 4th premolar tooth (308) and 1st molar tooth (309). (c) Stage 3 tooth resorption of the left mandibular 4th premolar tooth (308). The lesion extends into the pulp within the crown of the tooth, but most of the tooth structure is still present (red arrow). Tooth 308 is also categorized as a Type 1 lesion because the roots have a clear periodontal ligament space visualized (red arrowheads). Tooth 309 also appears to be affected with Stage 3 tooth resorption as the resorptive process appears to extend into the pulp of the tooth (yellow arrow). This tooth differs from the left mandibular 4th premolar tooth (308) because it would be categorized as a Type 3 lesion. Note there is complete root replacement resorption of the distal root (purple arrow) and missing tissue of the crown as well. The mesial root appears to have a clearly visible intact periodontal ligament space (yellow arrowheads). Additionally, appreciate the left mandibular 3rd premolar tooth (307) is likely at end stage tooth resorption (Stage 5; see Figure 5.20a–c). Recommended treatment for tooth 308 would be complete extraction of the tooth and associated roots. Recommended treatment for tooth 309 would be extraction of the mesial root and either extraction or crown amputation of the distal root if the patient meets the criteria for performing a crown amputation.

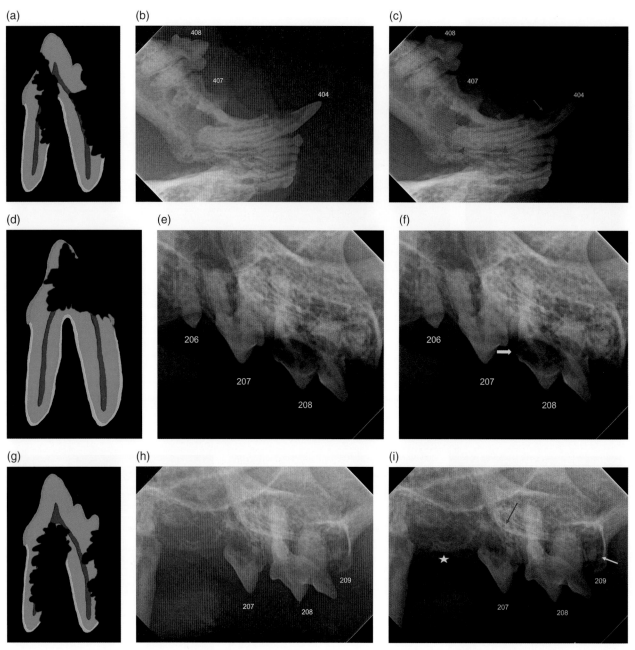

Figure 5.19 (a) Diagram of Stage 4a tooth resorption. Stage 4 tooth resorption is when the resorptive lesion has entered through the cementum and/or enamel, through the dentin and into the pulp similarly to Stage 3 tooth resorption. In Stage 4 tooth resorption, there is significant structural damage of the tooth. Additionally, the stage is divided into what portion of the tooth is more affected. Stage 4a tooth resorption is described as the crown and the root being equally affected. (b) Stage 4a tooth resorption of tooth 404. There is significant loss of tooth structure in which the crown and the root are equally affected. Tooth 407 is also missing. (c) Stage 4a tooth resorption of the right mandibular canine tooth. There is loss of the crown structure of this tooth (red arrow) as well as a loss of distinction between the root of this tooth and the surrounding alveolar bone (red arrowheads). This tooth would be classified as a Type 2 lesion as there is no clear radiolucent periodontal ligament space observed. The right mandibular 3rd premolar tooth (407) appears to be clinically missing. There is a hint of retained tooth roots of this tooth. (d) Diagram of Stage 4b tooth resorption. This stage is described as an extension of the resorption into the pulp of the tooth, with the crown of the tooth being more affected than the root of the tooth. (e) Stage 4b tooth resorption of the left maxillary 4th premolar tooth (208). Invasion into the pulp has occurred, and the crown is more affected than the root. (f) Stage 4b tooth resorption of the left maxillary 4th premolar tooth. There is a large lucency within the crown indicating loss of a large amount of tooth structure (yellow arrow). The loss of structure also supports invasion of the lesion into the pulp of the tooth. The roots of the tooth are visible as well as the periodontal ligament space, classifying this tooth as a Type 1 lesion. (g) Diagram of Stage 4c tooth resorption. This stage is described as an extension of resorption into the pulp of the tooth, with the root of the tooth being more affected than the crown of the tooth. (h) Stage 4c tooth resorption of the left maxillary 3rd premolar tooth (207). The roots, which are nearly completely resorbed, are more severely affected than the crown. (i) Stage 4c tooth resorption of the left maxillary 3rd premolar tooth (207). There appears to be minimal radiographic evidence of a root structure present in the affected tooth (red arrows). There is evidence of a retained tooth root associated with the left maxillary 1st molar tooth (209) (yellow arrow). The left maxillary 2nd premolar also appears to be missing (yellow star). This tooth would be classified as Type 2 tooth resorption as there is no evidence of a periodontal ligament space present.

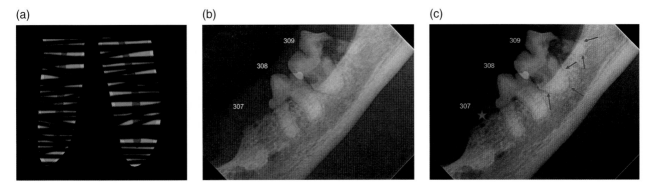

Figure 5.20 (a) Diagram of Stage 5 tooth resorption. This stage is also described as end-stage tooth resorption. Clinically, there is usually no obvious tooth structure present. Radiographically, there may be no recognizable tooth structure present or potentially a radiographic hint of the location of tooth roots when they were previously present. This has been described as "ghost roots." (b) Stage 5 tooth resorption of the left mandibular 3rd premolar tooth (307). Stage 4c and Type 1 tooth resorption are affecting the left mandibular 1st molar tooth (309) as well. (c) Stage 5 tooth resorption of the left mandibular 3rd premolar tooth (307). There is no recognizable tooth structure (crown or roots) visible in the radiographic image (red star). Assuming there is gingiva covering the missing tooth, no treatment is necessary. The left mandibular 1st molar tooth (309) appears to have a Type 1 lesion in which the periodontal ligament space is visible in both the mesial and distal roots (red arrows). The roots of this tooth appear to be more affected than the crown of this tooth staging this tooth as a Stage 4c. Treatment of this tooth would be extraction of both roots.

extraction of the entire tooth and associated root or roots [10]. This can be complicated by the weakened tooth structure as well as the ankylosis of the tooth root to the surrounding bone that is commonly seen in these patients.

Crown amputation or intentional root retention has been demonstrated as a possible treatment option for teeth affected with tooth resorption [10]. This procedure is described as amputating the crown of an affected tooth to the level of the alveolar crest, or just below the level of the alveolar crest [10]. The sharp edges of the remaining alveolar bone are then smoothed, and the gingiva is closed over the amputation site [10].

Unfortunately, crown amputations are not recommended in all teeth that are diagnosed with tooth resorption. There are several criteria that need to be met prior to considering crown amputation as a potential treatment option for an affected tooth.

1) The affected tooth should be radiographically classified as a Type 2 lesion (there should be no radiographic evidence of a periodontal ligament space present associated with the affected tooth).

2) The patient should not exhibit any clinical evidence of gingivostomatitis [also known as FCGS (feline chronic gingivostomatitis), caudal faucitis, CGS (chronic gingivostomatitis), etc.].

3) The patient should not demonstrate clinical or radiographic evidence of endodontic disease associated with the affected tooth/teeth.

4) The patient should not display clinical or radiographic evidence of periodontal disease associated with the affected tooth/teeth.

5) The patient should have a negative viral status [FELV (feline leukemia) and FIV (feline immunodeficiency virus) negative].

Even if all these criteria are met, all efforts should be taken to remove as much tooth structure as possible without jeopardizing the surrounding hard and soft tissues associated with the affected tooth. Radiographic diagnosis of a Type 2 resorptive lesion is necessary for a crown amputation to be performed. Therefore, if there is no radiographic capability of verifying that a Type 2 resorptive lesion is present, crown amputations should not be performed.

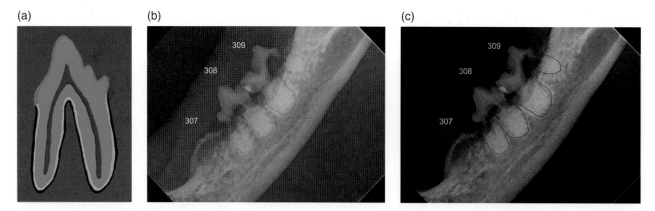

Figure 5.21 (a) Diagram of Type 1 tooth resorption. Type 1 tooth resorption is described as the affected tooth having evidence of an intact periodontal ligament space present radiographically around both roots. (b) Type 1 tooth resorption of the left mandibular 4th premolar and 1st molar teeth (308, 309). The crowns of these teeth have lucent areas where the tooth structure is missing while having an intact periodontal ligament space all the way around each root. (c) Type 1 tooth resorption of the left mandibular 4th premolar and 1st molar teeth (308, 309). There is an intact periodontal ligament space around both the mesial and distal roots of each tooth, classifying these teeth as Type 1 lesions (red lines). Note the end stage tooth resorption of tooth 307 indicated by the missing crown of the tooth with irregular radiopacities above the alveolar margin consistent with tooth resorption of the underlying tooth and roots.

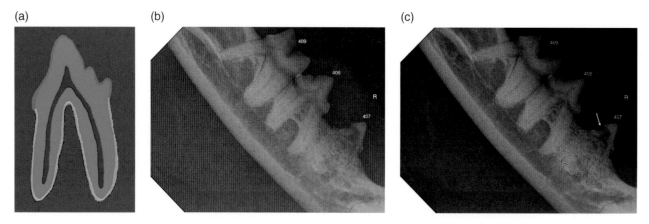

Figure 5.22 (a) Diagram of Type 2 tooth resorption. Type 2 tooth resorption is described as a tooth affected by tooth resorption in which there is no radiographic evidence of a periodontal ligament space. There is an inability to distinguish the remaining tooth root structure from the surrounding alveolar bone. (b) Type 2 tooth resorption of the right mandibular 3rd premolar tooth (407). (c) Type 2 tooth resorption of the right mandibular 3rd premolar tooth (407). There is no visible periodontal ligament space visible (red lines). Additionally, there is minimal crown structure remaining (yellow arrow). Crown amputation may be indicated as treatment of this tooth.

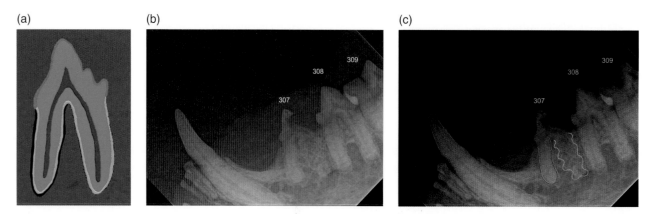

Figure 5.23 (a) Diagram of Type 3 tooth resorption. Type 3 tooth resorption is described as a multirooted tooth that has the radiographic appearance of both Type 1 and 2 lesions. This would be demonstrated as one root having clear evidence of a periodontal ligament space radiographically visible and one root in which there is no obvious periodontal ligament space radiographically appreciable. (b) Type 3 tooth resorption of the left mandibular 3rd premolar tooth (307). There is near complete root replacement resorption of the distal root, while the mesial root still has a visible periodontal ligament space. (c) Type 3 tooth resorption of the left mandibular 3rd premolar tooth (307). There is a clear periodontal ligament space present on the mesial root of this tooth (red lines). A lack of distinction between the distal root of this tooth and the periodontal ligament space and the surrounding bone is observed (yellow lines).

Supraeruption/Extrusion

Supraeruption or abnormal extrusion of the canine teeth in cats is a relatively common abnormality observed in middle-aged and geriatric cats [8]. Research has demonstrated that supraeruption of the canine teeth becomes clinically apparent when the distance between the alveolar margin and the cementoenamel junction on clinical examination is found to be greater than or equal to 2.5 mm [8]. Additionally, no evidence of horizontal and vertical bone loss is appreciated when supraeruption occurs [8]. Similarly to cats diagnosed with BAEO, tooth resorption is frequently appreciated in patients that are diagnosed with supraeruption. It has been demonstrated that up to 63% of cats that were diagnosed with tooth resorption of the maxillary canine teeth also demonstrated evidence of supraeruption of the affected teeth [8] (Figure 5.24). Supraeruption alone does not require treatment unless there is clinical and/or radiographic evidence of disease (Figure 5.25a and b).

Osteomyelitis and Osteitis

Osteomyelitis and osteitis are inflammation of the bone usually secondary to infection [2, 11]. Osteomyelitis varies from osteitis by involvement of the bone marrow and medullary cavity [12]. Osteitis is defined as a more superficial inflammation of the bone, more specifically of the cortex of the bone, while osteomyelitis affects the bone marrow and medullary cavity [12]. Frequently, infections of both the medullary cavity and the cortex are observed due to the intimate association of the haversian canals and the periosteum [12]. Osteomyelitis in the cat is observed less frequently than the other pathological conditions discussed in this chapter but is still worth mentioning. There are several routes in which bacteria can be introduced into the bone to cause osteomyelitis. Exposure of bone to the oral cavity environment either by trauma or surgical site contamination, periodontal and endodontic infection, or

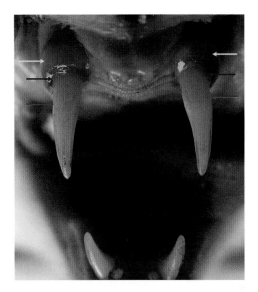

Figure 5.24 Clinical image of supraeruption of the maxillary canine teeth of a cat. The cementoenamel junction (red arrows) should be encased within the bone of a normal tooth. The cementoenamel junction of a tooth depicts the transition from the crown to the root of the tooth. The amount of exposed root can vary between patients when supraeruption occurs. The purple arrows indicate the free gingival margin and alveolar bone margin of these teeth. This patient does not have any periodontal pocketing associated with the supraeruption. The cat also demonstrates bilateral buccal alveolar expansile osteitis (yellow arrows).

hematogenously (carried by the blood) are the most frequent routes of infection [2, 11]. Hematogenous spread is the least common route of introduction of infection into the bone [2, 11].

Clinically osteomyelitis can be seen as a firm swelling of the jawbone (maxilla or mandible) that can be painful [11] (Figure 5.26). The patient may also exhibit ptyalism (excessive drooling) because of the pain (Figure 5.27). The two most common differentials for a maxillary or mandibular swelling are osteomyelitis or neoplasia. Osteomyelitis can occur secondary to neoplasia; therefore, both can be present concurrently.

(a)   (b)

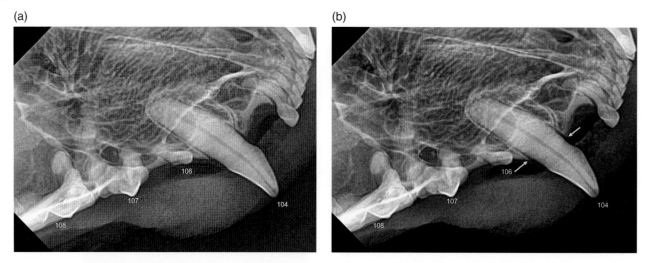

Figure 5.25 (a) Intraoral dental radiograph of the right maxillary canine tooth (104) that exhibits radiographic evidence of supraeruption. (b) Intraoral dental radiograph of the right maxillary canine tooth (104) that exhibits radiographic evidence of supraeruption. Note how there is a sharp demarcation where the alveolar crest of bone contacts the root surface (yellow arrows). There is no radiographic evidence of vertical bone loss, a periapical lucency, buccal alveolar expansile osteitis, or tooth resorption associated with this tooth. Note the subtle bulge of the crown of the tooth as it tapers to demarcate the transition to the root of the tooth (red arrows). Between the red and yellow arrows denote the amount of supraeruption associated with this tooth. Assuming there is no other clinical evidence of disease associated with the patient, no treatment is indicated.

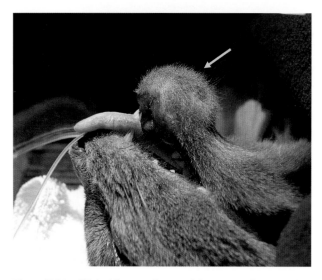

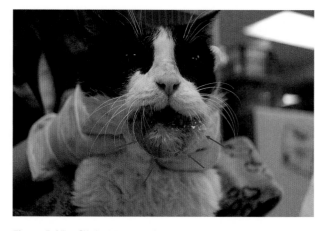

Figure 5.27 Clinical image of a cat with a severe, firm swelling of the rostral mandible (red arrows). The patient was exhibiting significant ptyalism as a result of discomfort from his mouth.

Figure 5.26 Clinical image of a cat with a severe, firm swelling of the rostral mandible (yellow arrow). The patient presented with complicated crown fractures (pulp exposed) of the left and right mandibular canine teeth (304, 404). Endodontic disease with secondary osteomyelitis was suspected to be the cause of the firm swelling. The patient is in dorsal recumbency.

Radiographically, osteomyelitis appears as a proliferation of bone that can have a moth-eaten or less commonly a star-burst appearance. This can be very similar to the appearance of a neoplastic lesion (Figures 5.28a–d, 5.29a, and b). There may also be the appearance of a periosteal bone reaction, which is demonstrated by a thickened and/or irregular cortical bone margin (Figure 5.30a and b). Grossly distinguishing between osteomyelitis and neoplasia can be difficult. If there is evidence of tooth pathology within or surrounding the lesion, it may indicate that osteomyelitis is the cause of the bony abnormality, rather than neoplasia (Figure 5.31a–d). Additionally, a neoplastic process can cause secondary changes such as lysis, alveolar bone loss, and tooth resorption; therefore, biopsy of the bone is imperative to give a definitive diagnosis (Figure 5.32a–e).

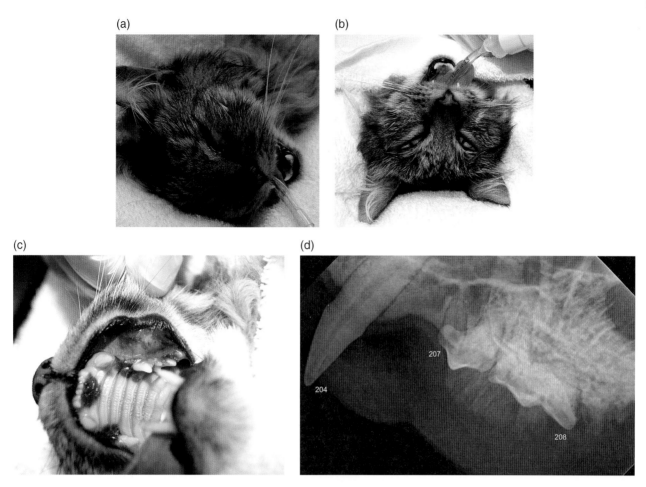

Figure 5.28 (a) Left maxillary swelling of a cat with confirmed osteomyelitis of the maxilla. (b) Left maxillary swelling of a cat diagnosed with osteomyelitis. This is the same cat as seen in Figure (a) positioned in dorsal recumbency. The left maxilla has a firm swelling and is causing the lower (ventral) eyelid to protrude slightly. (c) Left maxillary swelling of a cat diagnosed with osteomyelitis as seen in Figure (a) and (b). This is an intraoral view of the swelling. (d) Intraoral dental radiograph of the left maxilla of the cat seen in Figure (a)–(c). There is significant proliferation of bone. The bone also has a starburst appearance which can be consistent with osteomyelitis. There is no obvious tooth pathology that would indicate the etiology of the swelling to be osteomyelitis. Diagnosis was confirmed with a bone biopsy. Additionally, the left maxillary 2nd premolar tooth (206) is missing. It is also difficult to appreciate the presence of the left maxillary 1st molar tooth (209).

Retained Tooth Roots

Retained tooth roots are discussed in Chapter 4, and the reader is directed to this section for a more complete review of this common finding.

Radiographic evidence of retained tooth roots is frequently observed in the cat. The two most common causes of retained tooth roots include root fractures and tooth resorption (Figure 5.33a and b). When tooth resorption is the inciting cause, the root may be in any state of resorption at the time of discovery. This can range from the crown recently exfoliating from the root with the entire periodontal ligament space observed around the residual intact root to end-stage root replacement resorption with minimal recognizable tooth structure remaining (Figure 5.34a

and b). An additional cause for retained tooth roots is incomplete surgical extraction. As mentioned in Chapter 4, multiple radiographic views may be required to appropriately visualize and locate a retained tooth root (Figure 5.35a–c). When possible, extraction of (an intact) retained tooth root is recommended. A retained tooth root left unaddressed within the bone can be an inciting factor for endodontic disease.

Endodontic Disease

Endodontic disease is discussed more in depth in Chapter 4, and the reader is directed to this chapter for a general review. The most common causes of endodontic disease in

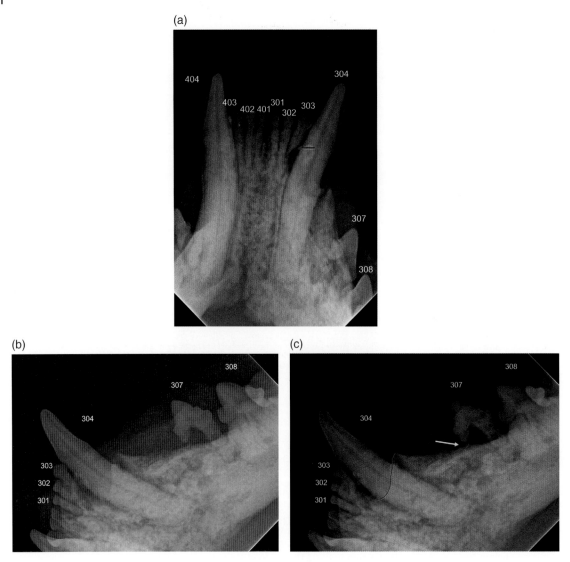

Figure 5.29 (a) Intraoral dental radiograph using the occlusal view of the rostral mandible of a cat diagnosed with osteomyelitis. Note the significant proliferation of bone associated with the left mandible. The bone has a somewhat moth-eaten appearance from the symphysis to the left mandibular 3rd premolar tooth (307). There is also root resorption of the left mandibular 3rd incisor tooth 303 (red arrow). (b) Lateral radiograph of the rostral left mandible of the cat in Figure (a). The mandibular bone has an abnormal appearance surrounding the left mandibular incisors, canine, and 3rd premolar teeth. The bone begins to look normal again at the left mandibular 4th premolar tooth (308). There is horizontal bone loss of the left mandibular canine (304) and tooth resorption of the left mandibular 3rd premolar tooth (307). (c) Intraoral dental radiograph of the left rostral mandible of the cat in Figure (a) and (b). There is the appearance of abnormal bone present extending from the incisors to the left mandibular 3rd premolar tooth (307). Additionally, there is horizontal bone loss associated with the left mandibular canine tooth (304) (red line) and tooth resorption associated with the left mandibular 3rd premolar tooth (307) (yellow arrow).

the cat are tooth fractures, tooth resorption, and periodontal disease. The canine teeth are most frequently affected with complicated and uncomplicated crown fractures. There are, however, some differences in endodontic disease presentation when comparing the cat to the dog. The etiology of endodontic disease is similar in both species, but some radiographic features and clinical signs that exist in the dog are not as commonly observed in the cat. In cats, small fractures of the cusp tip of the canine tooth frequently lead to pulp exposure. This is because the pulp canal terminates only millimeters away from the cusp tip.

There is not nearly as much enamel present in cat teeth as compared to dog teeth [13]. Research has demonstrated that there is <0.1–0.3 mm of enamel thickness present in cat teeth compared to <0.1–0.6 mm of enamel thickness in teeth of the dog [13]. Clinical signs of endodontic disease that are frequently observed in the dog but not as commonly seen in the cat include facial swelling, external facial draining wound, or a parulis (intraoral draining tract associated with the mucogingival line) (Figure 5.36). The typical suborbital swelling from endodontic disease commonly seen in dogs is rarely appreciated in cats. In cats,

(a)　　　　　　　　　　　　　　　　　(b)

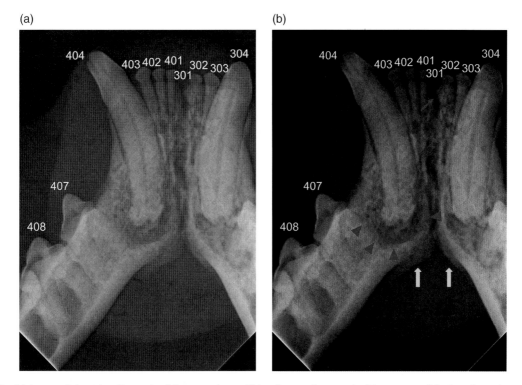

Figure 5.30 (a) Intraoral dental radiograph of the rostral mandible of a cat diagnosed with osteomyelitis. A periosteal reaction secondary to osteomyelitis can be appreciated which is associated with the right and left mandibular canine teeth. There is a periapical lucency associated with the right mandibular canine tooth (404). Additionally, there is a suspected retained tooth root associated with the left mandibular 1st incisor. (b) Intraoral dental radiograph of the rostral mandible showing a periosteal reaction (yellow arrows) secondary to osteomyelitis from endodontic disease of the left and right mandibular canine teeth (304, 404). The right side is more visualized than the left side which may be due to angulation of the radiograph. A periapical lucency is present associated with the right mandibular canine tooth (404) (red arrowheads). There also appears to be a retained tooth root associated with the left mandibular 1st incisor (301) (red arrow).

osteomyelitis with alveolar bone expansion of the maxillary canine teeth is a much more common presentation when endodontic disease is present (Figures 5.37a–e, 5.38, 5.39a, and b).

As mentioned earlier, tooth resorption is frequently observed in cats and can be secondary to pathology such as periodontal disease. Development of root resorption secondary to endodontic disease in cats is no exception. Radiographically, endodontic disease of a tooth will most commonly present as external resorption of the root (Figure 5.40a and b). Periapical lucency of a tooth that is affected with endodontic disease is rare in cats but can be observed (Figures 5.41a–c, 5.42a, and b). As with dogs, radiographs of the contralateral tooth for comparison as well as multiple views of a tooth with suspected endodontic disease should be taken in attempt to reveal if a periapical lucency is present.

When multiple different pathological processes of a tooth are seen in a cat, determining the initial cause and thus the treatment can be challenging. Ultimately, when deciding what treatment to initiate, it is important to note if tooth resorption is radiographically or clinically present. Extraction of the affected tooth may be the best option as this condition is a progressive process. Predicting the outcome of root canal therapy on a canine tooth that has evidence of tooth resorption at the apex is difficult. While theoretically the root canal will remove the bulk of the infection by disinfecting and sealing the canal, there still may be periapical periodontitis present that can continue to stimulate the progression of root resorption. This can eventually lead to destruction of the remaining tooth structure leaving behind root canal material within the bone which can cause additional inflammation of the surrounding tissues. However, root canal therapy in a tooth that does not show evidence of tooth resorption is an excellent treatment for a tooth with evidence of endodontic disease (pulp exposed fracture, widened pulp canal) (Figure 5.43a and b). Root canal therapy in cats is customarily only performed on canine teeth as it can be very challenging and near impossible in other teeth due to the size of the teeth and associated pulp canals.

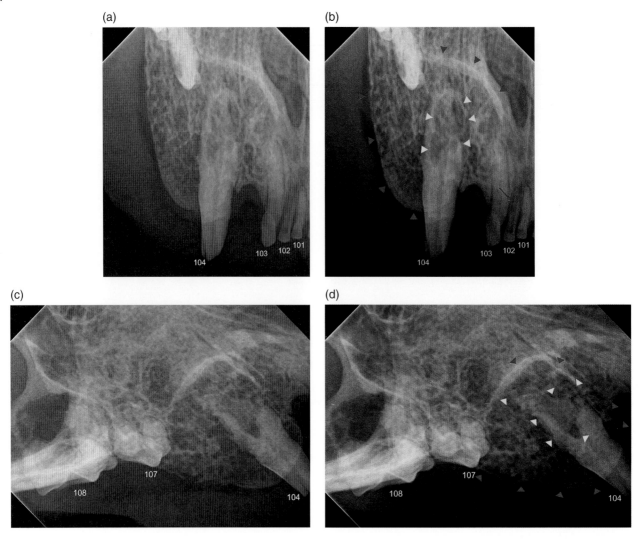

Figure 5.31 (a) Intraoral dental radiograph taken with an occlusal view of the right maxillary canine tooth (104) demonstrating osteomyelitis of the alveolar bone. (b) Intraoral dental radiograph utilizing an occlusal view of the right maxillary canine tooth (104) demonstrating the presence of osteomyelitis. Note the proliferation and moth-eaten appearance of the bone (red arrowheads). There is also severe root resorption of the right maxillary canine tooth (104) (yellow arrowheads). The right maxillary canine tooth (104) had a complicated crown fracture with endodontic disease, which was the cause of the osteomyelitis. There is also suspicion of tooth resorption associated with the right maxillary 2nd incisor (102) (red arrow). (c) Intraoral lateral radiograph of the right maxillary canine tooth (104) of the same cat as seen in Figure (a) and (b). Significant proliferation of the alveolar bone and root resorption can be appreciated. This presentation is similar to expansile osteitis; however, given the pulp exposure and severe root resorption, osteomyelitis was the diagnosis. (d) Intraoral lateral radiograph of the right maxillary canine tooth (104) of the same cat as seen in Figure (a)–(c) diagnosed with osteomyelitis. There is significant proliferation of the alveolar bone (red arrowheads) and tooth resorption of the right maxillary canine tooth (yellow arrowheads). The right maxillary 2nd premolar appears to be missing in this patient.

Conclusion

While the clinical and radiographic appearance of periodontal disease and endodontic disease in dogs and cats is similar, they do have their individual differences. The appearance of horizontal, vertical, and furcation bone loss and the staging of periodontal disease is identical between the species. In feline patients, dental radiography is crucial for the identification and subsequent treatment of tooth resorption lesions in cats. Full-mouth radiographs are recommended to ensure that pathology not detected on oral examination is identified radiographically and addressed, as necessary. Expansile bone lesions in cats will usually have an underlying etiology, such as endodontic disease or osteomyelitis. These primary conditions typically require treatment such as

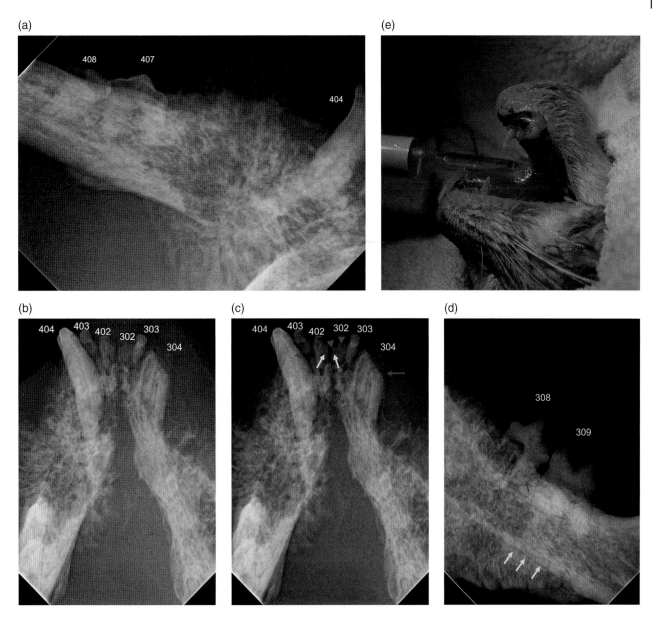

Figure 5.32 (a) Intraoral dental radiograph of the right mandible of a cat diagnosed with fungal osteomyelitis. Notice there is proliferation of the bone with a star-burst appearance. There is also root resorption of the right mandibular canine tooth (404). (b) Intraoral occlusal radiograph of the rostral mandible of a cat diagnosed with fungal osteomyelitis. This is the same cat as seen in Figure (a). Note the majority of the rostral mandible of both the right and left side appears to be affected. The left and right mandibular cortices show significant boney changes. The crown of the left mandibular canine tooth (304) is no longer present and severe root resorption of both mandibular canine teeth (304, 404) is observed. Additionally, the patient appears to be missing several mandibular incisor teeth. (c) Intraoral occlusal radiograph of the rostral mandible of a cat diagnosed with fungal osteomyelitis. This is the same cat as seen in Figure (a) and (b). Note the star-burst appearance of the bone. The crown of the left mandibular canine tooth (304) appears to be missing (red arrow). There are multiple missing incisor teeth (yellow arrows). There is also evidence of tooth resorption associated with the incisor teeth (red arrowheads). (d) Intraoral dental radiograph of the left mandible of the cat seen in Figure (a)–(c) demonstrating significant proliferation and moth-eaten appearance of the mandibular bone. The ventral cortical bone is severely affected and almost not visible (yellow arrows). There is root resorption of the mesial and distal roots of the left mandibular 4th premolar tooth (308) (red arrows). (e) Clinical image of the patient in Figure (a)–(d) diagnosed with fungal osteomyelitis demonstrating severe swelling of the rostral mandible. The patient is in dorsal recumbency.

(a)

(b)

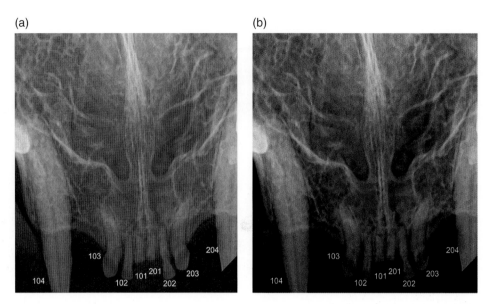

Figure 5.33 (a) Intraoral dental radiographic image of the rostral maxilla. There are retained tooth roots of the right and left maxillary 1st incisor teeth (101, 201) with no apparent pathology associated with them. (b) Intraoral dental radiograph of the rostral maxilla of a cat with retained tooth roots associated with the right and left maxillary 1st incisor teeth (101, 201) (red arrows). There does not appear to be any pathology associated with the roots of these teeth.

(a)

(b)

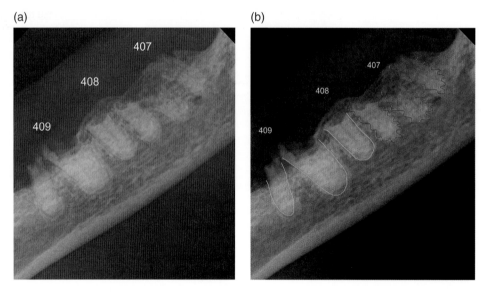

Figure 5.34 (a) Intraoral dental radiograph of the right mandible of a cat with retained tooth roots of the right mandibular 3rd and 4th premolar and 1st molar teeth (407–409). Several different types of root replacement resorption are observed in this image. (b) Intraoral dental radiograph of the right mandible of a cat demonstrating all three types of tooth resorption with associated retained tooth roots. The right mandibular 3rd premolar tooth (407) is near end stage tooth resorption and has very little root structure remaining with no periodontal ligament space observed. This tooth would be classified as a Type 2 resorptive lesion (red lines mesial and distal roots of 407). The right mandibular 4th premolar tooth (408) has more apparent tooth structure present with the periodontal ligament space seemingly absent on the mesial root (red lines mesial root 408) and areas of the periodontal ligament space being observed on the distal root (yellow lines distal root of 408), classifying this tooth as a Type 3 resorptive lesion. The right mandibular 1st molar tooth (409) shows retained tooth roots with the periodontal ligament space being observed on both the mesial and distal roots, classifying this tooth as a Type 1 resorptive lesion (yellow lines).

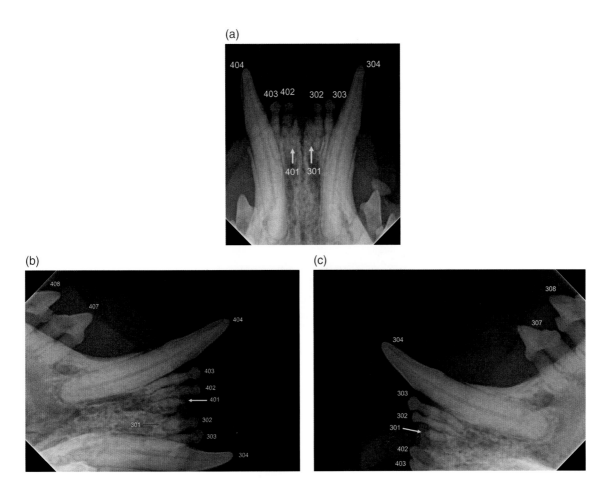

Figure 5.35 (a) Intraoral dental radiograph of the rostral mandible of a cat with retained tooth roots. Retained tooth roots of the left and right mandibular 1st incisors (301, 401) are present (yellow arrows) but very difficult to visualize. (b) Intraoral dental radiograph of the right rostral mandible of a cat with retained tooth roots. This is a lateral view of the rostral mandible of the patient seen in Figure (a). This lateral radiograph shows a retained tooth root of the right mandibular 1st incisor tooth (401) more clearly (yellow arrow). The retained tooth of the left mandibular 1st incisor (301) is superimposed over the root of the left mandibular 2nd incisor tooth (302) (red arrow). (c) Intraoral dental radiograph of the left rostral mandible of the patient seen in Figure (a) and (b) demonstrating a retained tooth root of the left mandibular 1st incisor tooth (301) more clearly (yellow arrow). Multiple radiographic views may be necessary to identify retained tooth roots and other radiographic pathology.

Figure 5.36 Clinical image of a cat who was diagnosed with a parulis, or intraoral draining tract associated with the mucogingival line. Frequently a parulis is associated with an endodontic infection.

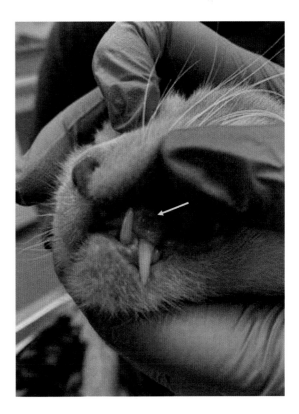

(a)

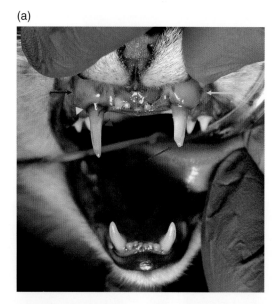

(b)   (c)

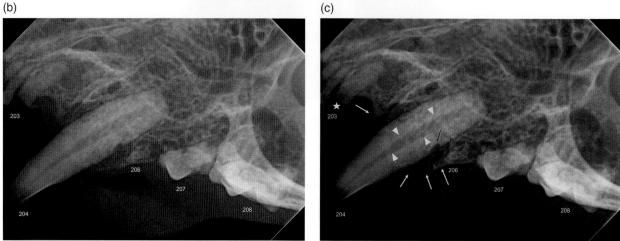

Figure 5.37 (a) Clinical image of a patient with a complicated crown fracture of the left maxillary canine tooth (204) (red arrow) with secondary expansile osteitis (yellow arrow) and mild supraeruption. There is a mild expansile osteitis (purple arrow) and supraeruption (red and yellow arrowheads) of the right maxillary canine tooth (104) with gingivitis only. (b) Intraoral dental radiograph of the left maxillary canine tooth (204) in the patient seen in Figure (a). A widened pulp chamber is consistent with a nonvital tooth secondary to a complicated crown fracture. Note there is expansile osteitis present as well. There is evidence of root resorption associated with the distal surface of the root, thus making this tooth a poor candidate for root canal therapy. Considering the changes appreciated within the surrounding alveolar bone as well as the suspicion for root resorption associated with this tooth, root canal therapy would have a guarded prognosis. It is difficult to determine if the expansile osteitis of 204 was present before or after the fracture occurred making treatment planning more challenging. (c) Intraoral dental radiograph of a nonvital canine tooth secondary to a complicated crown fracture. This is the same patient as seen in Figure (a) and (b). Note the widened pulp chamber of the left maxillary canine tooth (yellow arrowheads). Also appreciate expansile osteitis associated with the left maxillary canine tooth (204) (yellow arrows). The left maxillary 3rd incisor (203) appears to be missing the crown of the tooth (yellow star). The left maxillary 2nd premolar tooth (206) appears to have evidence of a retained tooth root (red star). Additionally, there appears to be vertical bone loss associated with distal aspect of the root of 204 (red arrowheads). The suspicion of root resorption on the left maxillary canine tooth is identified by the red arrow. (d) Intraoral dental radiograph of the right maxillary canine tooth (104) of the same patient as seen in Figure (a)–(c) showing slight expansile osteitis and vertical bone loss of the distal aspect of the root. Note the pulp chamber is narrower in the right maxillary canine tooth (104) than is observed in the left maxillary canine tooth (204) as seen in Figure (b) and (c). (e) Intraoral dental radiograph of the right maxillary canine tooth (104) of the same patient as seen in Figure (a)–(d). The image demonstrates a smaller pulp chamber of the right maxillary canine tooth (104) indicated by the yellow arrowheads. There is evidence of mild expansile osteitis (yellow arrows). There is vertical bone loss associated with the distal aspect of the right maxillary canine tooth (red arrowheads). There appears to be retained tooth roots associated with the right and left maxillary 1st incisors (101, 201) (yellow stars).

(d)

(e)

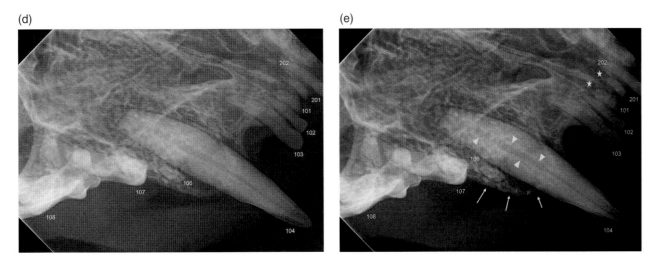

Figure 5.37   (Continued)

Figure 5.38   Clinical photo of a patient with a complicated crown fracture of the right maxillary canine tooth (104) (yellow star) with expansile osteitis (red arrow) that is likely secondary to endodontic disease related to the fractured tooth.

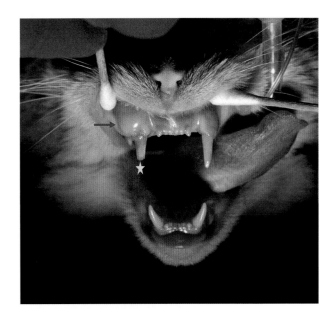

(a)

(b)

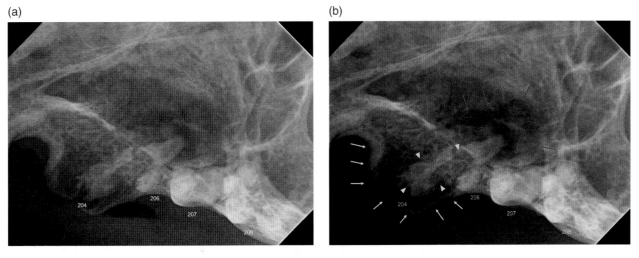

Figure 5.39   (a) Intraoral dental radiograph of a retained tooth root of the left maxillary canine tooth (204) with severe periapical bone loss (endodontic disease). There is severe tooth resorption and buccal alveolar expansile osteitis of this tooth. (b) Intraoral dental radiograph of a retained tooth root of the left maxillary canine tooth (204) with severe periapical bone loss (red arrows). There is severe tooth resorption (yellow arrowheads) and buccal alveolar expansile osteitis of this tooth (yellow arrows).

(a)

(b)

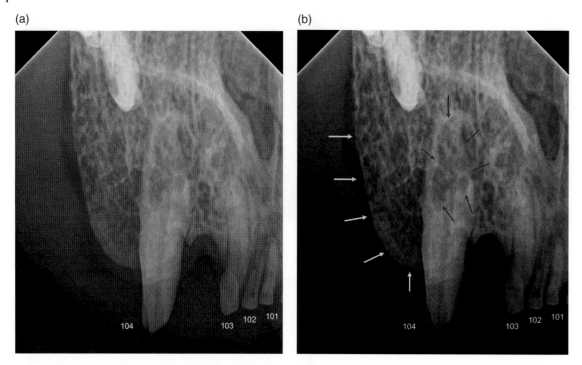

Figure 5.40 (a) Intraoral dental radiograph of a patient demonstrating severe root resorption of the right maxillary canine tooth (104) and significant expansile osteitis secondary to the periapical periodontitis. This tooth is not a candidate for root canal therapy because of the root resorption and secondary bone inflammation. (b) Intraoral dental radiograph of a patient demonstrating severe root resorption of the right maxillary canine tooth (104) (red arrows). There is also significant expansile osteitis noted associated with the tooth (yellow arrows).

(a)

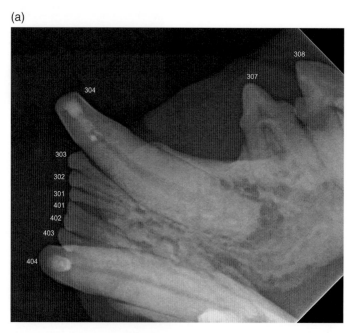

Figure 5.41 (a) Intraoral dental radiograph of the left mandibular canine tooth (304) with a periapical lucency from a failed crown reduction and vital pulp therapy procedure. (b) Intraoral dental radiograph of the left mandibular canine tooth (304) with a periapical lucency (red arrows) from a crown reduction and vital pulp therapy procedure that failed. There appears to be some root resorption at the apex of the canine tooth (yellow arrowheads) as there is a slight irregularity of the apex when compared to the contralateral tooth seen in Figure (c). (c) Intraoral dental radiograph of tooth 404 in the same patient as seen in Figure (a) and (b) showing no evidence of endodontic disease. Note the apex is round and a periodontal ligament space can be seen around the entire apex indicating a healthy, vital tooth.

(b) (c)

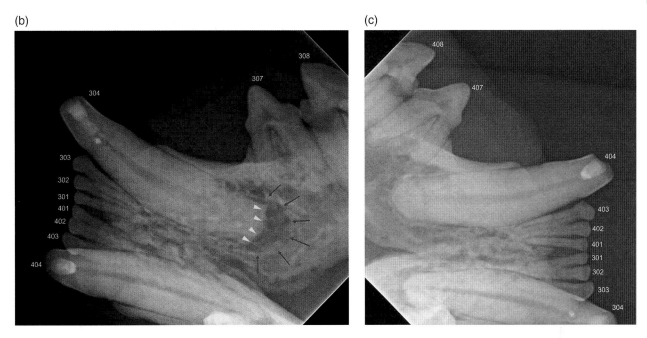

Figure 5.41 (Continued)

(a) (b)

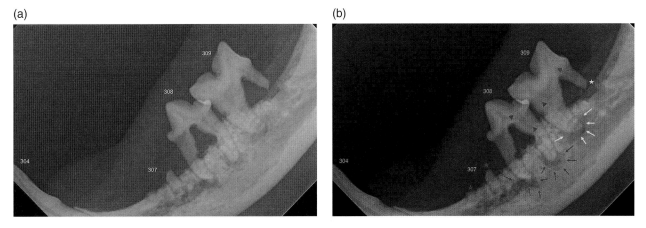

Figure 5.42 (a) Intraoral dental radiograph of the left mandibular 3rd and 4th premolars and 1st molar teeth (307–309) with periapical lucencies of the mesial and distal roots of 308 and the mesial root of 309. These teeth are affected with severe horizontal bone loss and tooth resorption. This radiograph is an example of multiple radiographic pathologies present in the same image. Note there are also retained tooth roots of 307. (b) Intraoral dental radiograph of the left mandible of a cat affected with multiple radiographic pathologies. There are periapical lucencies associated with the mesial and distal roots of the left mandibular 4th premolar (308) (red arrows) and the mesial root of the 1st molar (309) (yellow arrows). There appears that there is root resorption associated with the distal root of the 1st molar tooth (309) (yellow star). There are also retained tooth roots associated with the mesial and distal roots of the left mandibular 3rd premolar tooth (307) (red stars). Note the root resorption of both the 4th premolar and 1st molar teeth (red arrowheads).

extraction of the diseased tooth. Additionally, definitive diagnosis of an expansile lesion may require a bone biopsy. The radiographic and clinical presentation of endodontic disease in cats makes it difficult to differentiate it from other oral manifestations of disease. Frequently multiple abnormalities are observed within the affected teeth including tooth resorption and expansion of the buccal alveolar bone associated with the tooth. While treatment of the affected teeth may be similar, identification of the underlying cause may provide a better overall prognosis for the patient to help manage client expectations and patient comfort.

(a)

(b)

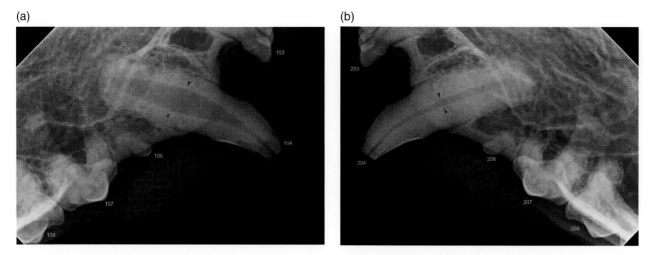

Figure 5.43 (a) Intraoral dental radiograph of the right maxillary canine tooth (104) with a complicated crown fracture and endodontic disease, causing nonvitality of the tooth as indicated by a widened pulp chamber (red arrowheads). Note there is no evidence of root resorption or periapical lucency observed. This tooth would be a reasonable candidate for root canal therapy. (b) Intraoral dental radiograph of the left maxillary canine tooth (204) in the same patient as seen in Figure (a), demonstrating a much narrower pulp canal (red arrowheads) in comparison to the contralateral tooth.

References

1 Lommer, M. and Verstratete, F. (2001). Radiographic patterns of periodontitis in cats: 147 cases (1998–1999). *J. Am. Vet. Med. Assoc.* 218 (2): 230–234.

2 Bell, C. and Soukup, J. (2015). Histologic, clinical, and radiologic findings of alveolar bone expansion and osteomyelitis of the jaws of cats. *Vet. Pathol.* 52 (5): 910–918.

3 Peralta, S., Fiani, N., and Scrivani, P. (2020). Prevalence, radiographic, and demographic features of buccal bone expansion in cats: a cross-sectional study at a referral institution. *J. Vet. Dent.* 37 (2): 66–70.

4 Farcas, N., Lommer, M., Kass, P., and Verstraete, F. (2014). Dental radiographic findings in its with chronic gingivostomatitis (2002–2012). *J. Am. Vet. Med. Assoc.* 244 (3): 339–345.

5 Murphy, B., Bell, C., and Soukup, J. (2020). Inflammatory lesions of the oral mucosa and jaws. In: *Veterinary Oral and Maxillofacial Pathology*, 49–77. Hoboken: Wiley.

6 Reiter, A., Johnston, N., Anderson, J. et al. (2019). Domestic feline oral and dental diseases. In: *Wigg's Veterinary Dentistry Principles and Practice*, 2e (ed. H. Lobprise and B. Dodd), 439–461. Hoboken: Wiley.

7 Gorrel, C. (2015). Tooth resorption in cats: pathophysiology and treatment options. *J. Feline Med. Surg.* 17 (1): 37–43.

8 Lewis, J., Okuda, A., Shofer, F. et al. (2008). Significant association between tooth extrusion and tooth resorption in domestic cats. *J. Vet. Dent.* 25 (2): 86–95.

9 Ingham, K., Gorrel, C., Blackburn, J. et al. (2001). Prevalence of odontoclastic resorptive lesions in a population of clinically healthy cats. *J. Small Anim. Pract.* 42: 439–443.

10 DuPont, G. (1995). Crown amputation with intentional root retention for advanced feline resorptive lesions: a clinical study. *J. Vet. Dent.* 12 (1): 9–13.

11 Lobprise, H. (2019). General oral pathology. In: *Wigg's Veterinary Dentistry Principles and Practice*, 2e (ed. H. Lobprise and B. Dodd), 155–176. Hoboken: Wiley.

12 Krakowiak, P.A. (2011). Alveolar osteitis and osteomyelitis of the jaws. *Oral Maxillofac. Surg. Clin. North Am.* 23 (3): 401–413.

13 Crossley, D.A. (1995). Tooth enamel thickness in the mature dentition of domestic dogs and cats-preliminary study. *J. Vet. Dent.* 12 (3): 111–113.

6

Oral Surgery: Neoplasia and Cystic Conditions
Megan Mickelson

University of Missouri Veterinary Health Center, Columbia, MO, USA

CONTENTS

Radiographic Indications of Neoplasia (Benign and Malignant)

Imaging is an important component of a complete clinical evaluation for oral abnormalities found on physical examination or identified at the time of a routine prophylactic dental treatment. Presentation varies from no knowledge of a mass to owners visualizing an oral mass, to external facial deformity created from the presence of a mass. Clinical signs for oral tumors vary and can be absent or subtle early in the stage of disease. Clinical signs may progress to include ptyalism, blood-tinged saliva, epistaxis, halitosis, dysphagia, decreased appetite, and/or weight loss [1, 2]. Mobile teeth in an otherwise normal animal with minimal periodontal disease could be an indication of an underlying oral tumor [3]. Certain differential diagnoses should be considered based on the external appearance of the lesion, patient clinical history, anatomic location and/or signalment of the patient, and potentially clinical behavior of the lesion. Diagnostic imaging will help determine the extent of the lesion to aid in surgical planning and can also be used for staging of the disease. In the case of malignant oral tumors, diagnostic imaging is used to

evaluate for evidence of underlying metastasis with advanced imaging modalities, such as computed tomography (CT). This chapter will outline certain underlying features of the most common oral masses – and cystic lesions in the canine and feline patient.

A definitive diagnosis is confirmed by obtaining an incisional biopsy and submission of the sample to a histopathologist. Diagnostic imaging is utilized to aid in surgical margin planning. With certain benign oral lesions, such as odontogenic cysts, the origin of the lesion directs the surgeon to the most appropriate treatment. Depending on the origin of the mass, an intracapsular excision with tooth extraction and/or enucleation of the cystic lining with curettage can be utilized and is considered effective [4]. Marginal, en bloc excisions can be pursued for benign odontogenic tumors [4]. With oral malignant neoplasms, the general rule followed by oncologic surgeons is a minimum of 1 cm margin of normal bone needs to be removed based upon gross tumor and bone infiltration on imaging [5–8]. If possible, following historical recommendations of removing 2–3 cm of normal appearing bone from the gross tumor, especially for highly infiltrative tumors, such as oral fibrosarcoma (FSA), is still

---

Veterinary Oral Diagnostic Imaging, First Edition. Edited by Brenda L. Mulherin.

recommended [1, 9, 10]. Oral surgeons generally consider the tooth roots when planning their surgical margins. This means some margins will fall greater than the recommendation by the nature of planning alveolar bone cuts around surrounding tooth roots. Following surgical excision, it is important to evaluate the specimen for evidence of transected tooth roots and remove any remaining tooth roots within the surgical field. Dental radiography should be utilized to confirm tooth roots have not been left behind, as these retained roots could lead to future problems with oral pain and abscessation [11].

Benign Oral Tumors

Odontogenic tumors, including canine acanthomatous ameloblastoma (CAA) and peripheral odontogenic fibromas (POFs), are common in dogs, encompassing up to 34% of oral pathologic lesions found in this species [12]. These tumors are considered rare in cats, making up only 3% of all reported oral pathology cases [12].

Canine Acanthomatous Ameloblastoma (CAA)

CAA was previously referred to as either acanthomatous epulis or epithelial mass in literature [13]. This oral lesion commonly presents as a raised, irregular gingival mass [14] (Figure 6.1a–c). There is a predilection for the rostral mandible in up to 51% of cases [15], but lesions also occur in other locations. The mean age for patients is 7–10 years [16, 17], and it is most common in medium- and large-breed

dogs [18, 19], especially Sheepdogs [16, 18] and Golden retrievers [15, 18].

While considered benign, CAA behaves aggressively, locally, with significant underlying cortical bone infiltration and surrounding bone destruction, commonly displacing teeth without causing tooth resorption [14]. Radiographically, the lesion varies with either a unilocular or multilocular, honeycomb or *soap-bubble* appearance reported [20, 21]. There are no reported metastatic lesions associated with CAA [1, 3]. Using CT, both intraosseous and extraosseous locations are reported, with all lesions having alveolar bone lysis of varying severity. Frequently, CAA are found to cause tooth displacement, bone expansion, periosteal bone reaction, and thinning of the cortical bone. In 93–100% of cases, the lesions are contrast-enhancing [22, 23], usually involving multiple teeth [23]. Specific lysis of the apical border is considered a characteristic feature of CAA on CT [19] (Figures 6.2a1, a2, b, and 6.3a–d).

Wide excision with 1 cm margins is recommended due to the incidence of local recurrence [16]; however, despite dirty margins in 33% of cases, no local recurrence was noted on follow-up [15], and the prognosis is considered excellent with surgery [15, 16].

Peripheral Odontogenic Fibroma (POF)

POFs were previously referred to as fibromatous epulis or ossifying epulis [13] and are considered a benign mesenchymal tumor consisting of a proliferation of fibrous

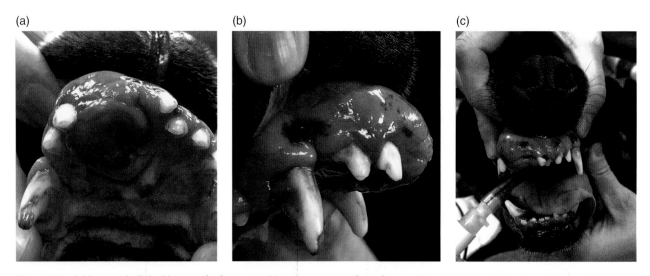

(a)   (b)   (c)

Figure 6.1 (a) Intraoral clinical image of a four-year old male castrated Cane Corso with a right-sided rostral maxillary canine acanthomatous ameloblastoma. (b) Right lateral clinical image of the rostral maxilla of a dog with a canine acanthomatous ameloblastoma. (c) Clinical image of the rostral maxilla of a dog with a canine acanthomatous ameloblastoma. Note the clinically missing right maxillary 2nd incisor, and mesial displacement of the right maxillary 1st incisor. *Source:* Courtesy of Richard Meadows, DVM, DABVP, University of Missouri, College of Veterinary Medicine.

(a1) (a2) (b)

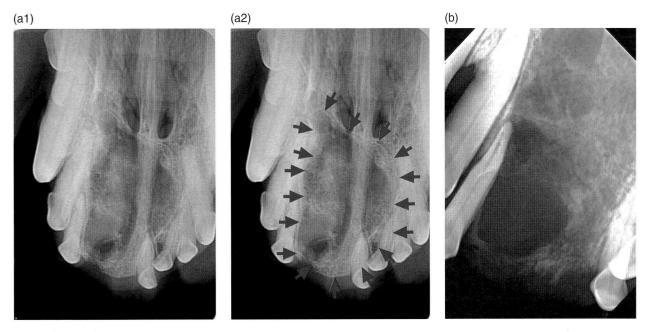

Figure 6.2 (a1) Intraoral dental radiographic images from the dog pictured in Figure 6.1a–c diagnosed with a canine acanthomatous ameloblastoma. (a2) Note the red arrows surrounding the radiolucent lesion of affected tissue, diagnosed as a canine acanthomatous ameloblastoma. (b) (post-biopsy) Note the absence of the right maxillary 1st incisor following incisional biopsy of the mass for definitive diagnosis of a canine acanthomatous ameloblastoma. *Source:* Courtesy of Richard Meadows, DVM, DABVP, University of Missouri, College of Veterinary Medicine.

tissue [14]. Clinically, lesions appear as raised, smooth, gingival masses along the dental arcade, arising from the periodontal ligament [18]. They are most commonly found in older (eight- to nine-year-old), castrated male dogs [18] and are rare in young cats [24]. The gross appearance consists of intact epithelium with a predilection for the rostral maxilla to the level of the third premolar [17, 18] (Figures 6.4a–c and 6.5). Due to the osteoid content, lesions can be difficult to biopsy because of their firm nature [18].

Regarding the diagnostic imaging of these lesions, there are no underlying lytic boney changes or changes to dentition. Depending upon the degree and variation of the mineral component [21], there is either a smooth proliferative change of bone or a simple gingival and/or soft tissue proliferation of the affected area [14] (Figures 6.6a1, a2, b1, b2, and 6.7a–c).

Feline Inductive Odontogenic Tumor (FIOT)

Feline inductive odontogenic tumors (FIOT) were previously called fibroameloblastomas because of the mixed mesenchymal and epithelial content found on histopathology [25]. These lesions are most commonly found in young cats (8–18 months) within the rostral maxilla [25, 26]. Grossly, they appear as raised gingival proliferations [26] (Figure 6.8a and b).

Radiographically, the lesions consist of an expansile, circumscribed lytic region with deformity of teeth and/or absence of teeth, as well as distortion and invasion of the underlying alveolar bone [1, 14, 21] (Figure 6.9a–d).

Malignant Oral Tumors

Malignant oral tumors comprise up to 37% of all reported oral lesions in dogs [12] and 47% of those in cats [12].

Nontonsillar Squamous Cell Carcinoma (SCC)

Nontonsillar squamous cell carcinoma (SCC) is the most common malignant oral tumor found in cats [27, 28], encompassing up to 37% of all oral pathology [12] and 60–75% of reported oral neoplasms [29, 30]. It is typically diagnosed in older cats [3], most commonly in the sublingual region (Figures 6.10, 6.11a, and b). Nontonsillar SCC is typically considered the second most common malignant oral neoplasm in dogs [5], encompassing up to 26% of all reported oral tumors [30], but it has also been reported to be the most common oral tumor found in the canine species [12]. These lesions are most common in older (eight- to nine-year-old) dogs [31]. A predilection for the rostral mandible has been reported [32, 33]. Gross lesions

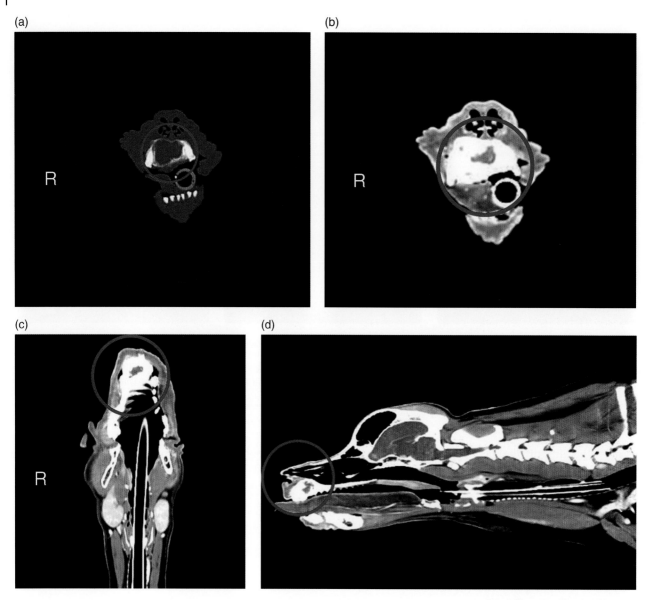

Figure 6.3 (a) Computed tomography scan from the dog pictured in Figurs 6.1(a–c) and 6.2a1–a2 and b diagnosed with a canine acanthomatous ameloblastoma. Axial/transverse bone window image of a dog diagnosed with a canine acanthomatous ameloblastoma. Note the expansile appearance of the cortical bone and lytic area of the affected tissues of the right maxilla. (b) Axial/transverse soft tissue window post-contrast image of a dog diagnosed with a canine acanthomatous ameloblastoma. Note the contrast enhancement of the affected tissue in the right maxilla. (c) Coronal/dorsal reconstruction soft tissue window post-contrast administration image of a dog diagnosed with a canine acanthomatous ameloblastoma. Note the contrast enhancement of the affected tissue in the right maxilla appearing to extend across midline of the patient. (d) Sagittal reconstruction, soft tissue window post-contrast administration image of a dog diagnosed with a canine acanthomatous ameloblastoma. Note the expansile nature of the affected tissue with a smooth dorsal border. Note the contrast enhancement of the affected tissue. Also note the lytic lesion (marked with a red circle) in the right rostral maxilla on all views (Figure a–d). There is extraosseous bone formation and contrast enhancement of the affected tissues.

are typically red, raised masses which are occasionally associated with a historical tooth extraction at the site of tumor occurrence [34]. Lesions oftentimes consist of mucosal ulceration and inflammation [29, 35] (Figure 6.12).

Radiographically, lesions are classified as expansile with extensive boney invasion [1, 3, 36]. Osteolysis, tooth resorption, and periosteal proliferation are commonly observed with SCC [32, 34, 36, 37] (Figure 6.13a–c). Concerning advanced diagnostic imaging, such as CT, lesions are heterogenous with soft tissue contrast enhancement, osteolysis, and osteoproliferation [32, 35] with poor margination and cortical destruction [38]. They have been

(a)   (b)   (c)

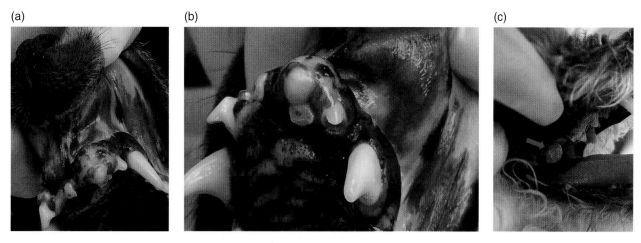

Figure 6.4 (a) Clinical image of the rostral maxilla of an eight-year-old, male castrated mixed breed dog diagnosed with a peripheral odontogenic fibroma. Note the soft tissue proliferation appears to be associated with the left maxillary 2nd incisor. The left maxillary 1st incisor appears to be displaced mesially. The right maxillary 1st and 2nd incisors appear to be clinically missing. (b) Intraoral view of the left rostral maxilla of the same dog in Figure (a). Note there appears to be palatal displacement of the left maxillary second incisor. *Source:* Courtesy of Richard Meadows, DVM, DABVP, University of Missouri, College of Veterinary Medicine. (c) Clinical image of a 12-year-old female spayed Terrier mix with a peripheral odontogenic fibroma, ossifying type. Clinically, a pedunculated, mucogingival lesion is noted in the diastema of the right maxillary 3rd and 4th premolar teeth which appear to be clinically missing.

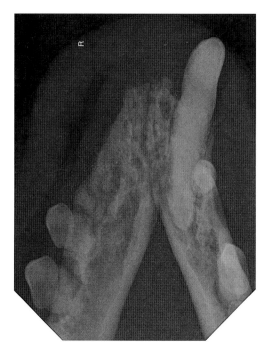

Figure 6.5 Radiographic image of the rostral mandible of a dog with a peripheral odontogenic fibroma. There was gross evidence of a soft tissue swelling located over the right mandibular canine tooth (404) extraction site. The mandibular canine tooth was previously extracted due to a complicated crown fracture two years prior to presentation. There is no radiographic evidence of boney changes, as is consistent with this lesion. The radiographic image also depicts that the left mandibular 1st, 2nd, and 3rd incisors (301–303) and right mandibular 1st, 2nd, and 3rd incisors (401–403) were also missing.

described as having an "amorphous/pumice stone-like periosteal reaction" in maxillary lesions and mixed solid/lamellar appearance versus irregular/pumice-like changes in mandibular lesions [38] (Figure 6.14a–d). Maxillary mass extension into the orbit is common, as well as invasion into the sinonasal cavity [35, 38] (Figure 6.15a–d). With the biologic behavior of these tumors, it is important to evaluate the extent of disease along with evaluation for cervical lymphadenopathy and locoregional metastasis.

Papillary Squamous Cell Carcinoma (PSCC)

Oral papillary squamous cell carcinomas (PSCCs) are a distinct histopathologic subset of oral nontonsillar SCC. Historically, they have been reported primarily in young dogs (<five months old) [39–41], but they have also been reported in adult dogs (>six years old) [41]. The mean age is four years old, and they are found in primarily large-breed dogs [42]. Although originally thought to be associated with papillomavirus, no virus has been confirmed using histopathologic studies [40, 43]. The tumor arises from the gingiva surrounding the dentition, with the majority of tumors being located rostrally, especially within the rostral maxilla [41, 42]. Grossly, the lesions vary from papillomatous to ulcerative and proliferative in nature and can cause loss or displacement of surrounding teeth [41]. It is imperative to differentiate oral PSCC from oral SCC due to the potentially better outcomes and decreased risk of metastasis associated with PSCC [42, 43].

(a1) (a2)

(b1) (b2)

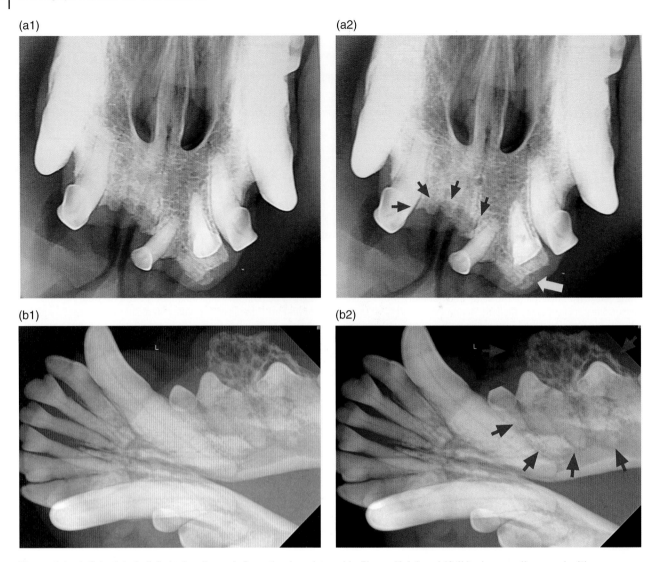

Figure 6.6 (a1) (unlabeled) Dental radiograph from the dog pictured in Figure (6.4a) and (6.4b) who was diagnosed with a peripheral odontogenic fibroma of the rostral maxilla. (a2) (labeled) The right maxillary 1st and 2nd incisors are absent (101, 102), and the left maxillary 1st first incisor (201) is displaced mesially. Note the maxillary bone defect with focal radiolucency (red arrows) that is not associated with the peripheral odontogenic fibroma, but more likely associated with previously diagnosed periodontal disease necessitating the extraction of the right maxillary 1st and 2nd incisor teeth. The yellow arrow depicts the location of the ossifying-type peripheral odontogenic fibroma due to the radiographic appearance of mineralization within the lesion with no bony destruction noted. *Source:* Courtesy of Richard Meadows, DVM, DABVP, University of Missouri, College of Veterinary Medicine. (b1) (unlabeled) Radiographic image of the left mandible of a dog with an ossifying-type peripheral odontogenic fibroma of the left mandible centered around the left mandibular 2nd and 3rd premolar teeth (306, 307). (b2) (labeled) Radiographic image of a dog with an ossifying-type peripheral odontogenic fibroma. Note the honeycomb appearance of the periosteal proliferation (red arrows) within the surrounding soft tissue opacity that appears to be affecting the left mandible. The swelling is focused between the 2nd and 3rd premolar teeth of the left mandible. *Source:* Courtesy of Brenda Mulherin, DVM, DAVDC, Iowa State University, College of Veterinary Medicine.

Radiographically, PSCCs are observed to be locally aggressive, soft tissue opacity masses, associated with significant amounts of underlying bone lysis [40, 44]. No metastatic lesions have been reported in PSCC lesions [44], in contrast to nontonsillar SCC lesions. On CT evaluation, contrast-enhancing, infiltrative, and expansile masses are observed, oftentimes with cavitation, similar to cysts. PSCC lesions are found to be observed with osteolysis, with or without boney proliferation [41, 42] (Figure 6.16a–e).

Oral Malignant Melanoma (MM)

Oral melanoma is considered the most common malignant oral tumor in dogs [5, 30]. Interestingly it is a tumor

(a)

(c)

(b)

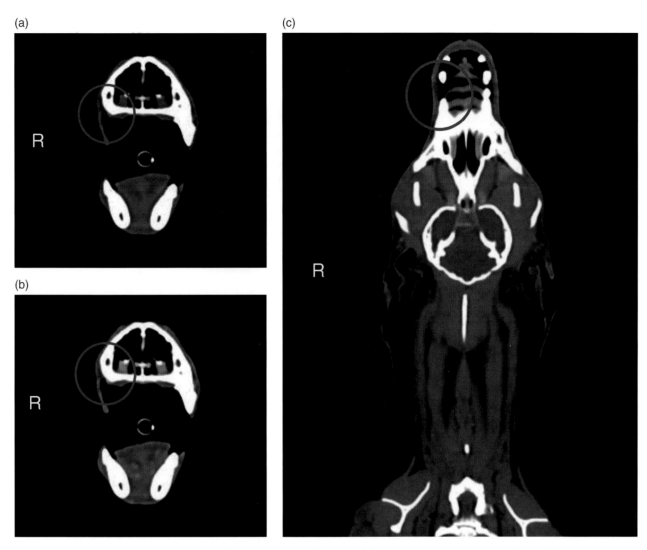

Figure 6.7 (a) Computed tomography scan of the dog pictured in Figure 6.4c demonstrating no evidence of underlying bone involvement nor contrast -enhancement of the soft tissue mass in the region of the pedunculated peripheral odontogenic fibroma pictured in the right caudal maxilla (red circle in region of interest). The CT is largely unremarkable. Axial/transverse soft tissue window image of the dog pictured in Figure 6.4c demonstrating no evidence of disease, which is consistent with a peripheral odontogenic fibroma. (b) Axial/transverse soft tissue window post-contrast image of the dog pictured in Figure 6.4c demonstrating no radiographic evidence of disease, consistent with a peripheral odontogenic fibroma. (c) Coronal/dorsal reconstruction bone window image of the dog pictured in Figure 6.4c demonstrating no radiographic evidence of disease, consistent with a peripheral odontogenic fibroma. The gross lesion is noted in the diastema of the right maxillary 3rd and 4th premolar teeth which are noted to be missing on the CT.

that is very rarely reported in cats [12, 29]. It has frequently been associated with a higher incidence in small body-weight dogs, especially Cocker spaniels [34, 45], miniature Poodles, Pekingese, Poodles, and Chow Chows [45]. The mean age of diagnosis is in older dogs (11 years) [45] and older cats (12–13 years) when reported [46–48]. In dogs, the labial mucosa and gingiva of the mandible are the most common sites to be affected [45] (Figure 6.17a–c). Grossly, two-thirds of the masses are pigmented black or

brown and are frequently accompanied by ulceration and hemorrhage [3, 44].

When using imaging alone, it can be difficult to differentiate malignant melanoma (MM) from other tumors. MM lesions have a tendency towards exhibiting less underlying boney changes compared to other oral neoplasms; however, bone invasion is more frequently reported in melanomas found in the maxillary region of cats [48] (Figure 6.18a–c). There is a very high metastatic rate to locoregional

(a) (b)

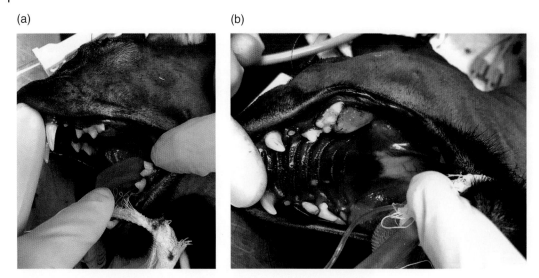

Figure 6.8   (a) Clinical images of a two-year old castrated male domestic longhair with a feline inductive odontogenic tumor (FIOT) of the left caudal maxilla. Clinical image of the lateral view of a feline inductive odontogenic tumor (FIOT), distal to the left maxillary 4th premolar tooth. (b) Clinical image of the intraoral view of the feline inductive odontogenic tumor (FIOT), distal to the left maxillary 4th premolar tooth. Note the clinical absence of the left maxillary 1st molar tooth (209).

lymph nodes associated with MM, so advanced imaging using a CT +/− utilization of indirect CT lymphangiography (ICTL) is recommended to fully stage patients [1, 3]. Many surgeons advocate for complete cervical lymph node removal in MM patients at the time of oral surgery.

Fibrosarcoma (FSA)

Oral FSA is considered the second most common malignant oral tumor in cats [5, 29, 30], and the third most common malignant oral tumor in dogs [31]. In dogs, the gingiva of the maxilla and hard palate are the most commonly reported locations affected [31]. Given the frequent caudal and palatal presentation of these masses, they are oftentimes discovered late in the course of disease [49]. The clinical presentation may begin with facial deformity from the mass growing externally from the maxilla, potentially causing displacement of teeth [50]. The lesions are commonly reported in large-breed dogs, such as Golden retrievers and Labrador retrievers [1, 31, 50, 51] at a median age of eight years old [3, 31, 51]. Cats are typically young-to-middle age at diagnosis (8–10 years) [29, 52] with no breed predilection observed.

Grossly, lesions appear as a firm, erythematous swelling or mass, frequently with ulceration and facial deformity that is noted to have a quick clinical progression [3, 49, 50]. FSA lesions are classically characterized by a rapid clinical growth with significant boney invasion and osteolysis [31] noted on both dental radiography and CT imaging [50, 53] (Figure 6.19a–d).

A unique subset of FSA tumors present as histologically low-grade, biologically high-grade (high-low) tumors in dogs and are found mainly within the maxilla at the level of the canine tooth to the level of the carnassial teeth [50]. These have aggressive boney involvement on diagnostic imaging [50]. Because of the high risk for local recurrence, aggressive, wide surgical resection with or without adjuvant radiation therapy postoperatively is indicated to treat these tumors in dogs [50].

Osteosarcoma (OSA)

Oral osteosarcoma (OSA) is considered the fourth most common malignant oral tumor in dogs [3]. This malignant oral tumor is considered to be rare in cats [30, 52, 54]. OSAs are very aggressive tumors that affect both the appendicular and axial skeleton. The appendicular skeletal regions commonly affected are the long bones of the limbs, while in the axial skeleton, the skull, ribs, vertebra, and pelvis are the most common locations. In dogs, tumors have been reported on the skull, mandible, and maxilla [55] in middle-to-older age, medium- and large-breed dogs [55] (Figure 6.20).

Radiographically, lesions in the axial skeleton have been described to be more osteoblastic in nature compared to appendicular locations, with granular areas of calcification and well-defined borders [32]. In cats, they have been characterized by periosteal new bone formation along with bone lysis [56]. On CT scan, contrast-enhancing soft tissue masses often surround the underlying boney lesion [57] (Figure 6.21a–d).

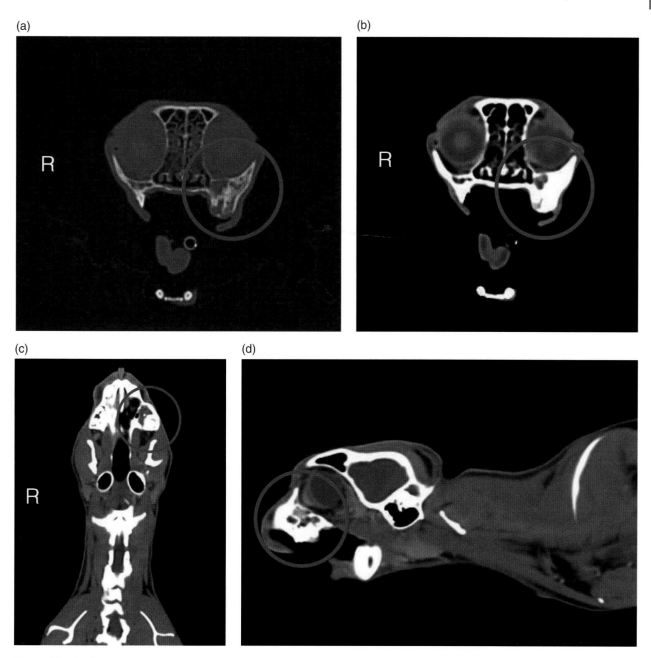

Figure 6.9 (a) Computed tomographic imaging of a two-year old castrated male domestic long hair with a feline inductive odontogenic tumor (FIOT) of the left maxilla (affected area circled). This is the same patient as described in Figure 6.8a–b. Axial/ transverse bone window image of a feline inductive odontogenic tumor (FIOT). Note the expansile bone lysis of the left caudal maxilla and displacement of surrounding teeth. (b) Axial/transverse soft tissue window post-contrast image of the feline inductive odontogenic tumor (FIOT) associated with the patient in Figure 6.8. Note the expansile bone lysis of the left caudal maxilla and mild intralesional contrast enhancement. (c) Coronal/dorsal soft tissue window, post-contrast image of the feline inductive odontogenic tumor (FIOT) associated with the patient in Figure 6.8. Note the expansile bone lysis of the left caudal maxilla, mild intralesional contrast enhancement, and displacement of surrounding teeth. (d) Sagittal soft tissue window, post-contrast image of the same patient as in Figure 6.8 diagnosed with a feline inductive odontogenic tumor (FIOT). Note the expansile bone lysis of the left caudal maxilla, mild intralesional contrast enhancement, and displacement of surrounding teeth along with absence of the left maxillary 1st molar tooth.

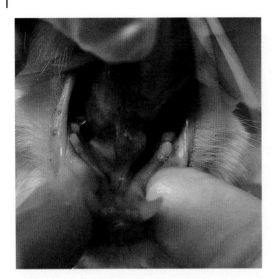

Figure 6.10 Clinical image of a 13-year-old castrated male domestic shorthair with a classic sublingual oral squamous cell carcinoma.

Multilobular Osteochondrosarcoma (MLO)

Multilobular osteochondrosarcoma (MLO), historically referred to as multilobular tumor of bone, OSA, chondroma rodens, or multilobular osteoma [58], is an uncommon tumor in dogs, and an even rarer tumor in cats. This tumor is reported to occur in the flat bones of the skull, including the maxilla and mandible [44, 59]. These tumors are reported in older age, large-breed dogs [59]. Patients commonly present with a firm, palpable swelling, occasionally accompanied by exophthalmos, ocular signs, pain, and/or

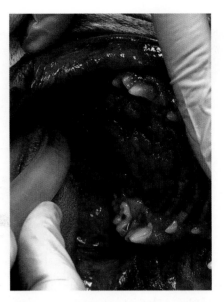

Figure 6.12 Clinical image of an eight-year-old, male castrated American Staffordshire Terrier with a large oral squamous cell carcinoma of the caudal maxilla with involvement of the hard and soft palate. Intraoral clinical image demonstrating both a grossly proliferative and ulcerated appearance of the squamous cell carcinoma. There is no absence of dentition. Significant ulceration is a common clinical presenting appearance of squamous cell carcinoma.

neurological signs, especially if the tumor involves the caudal maxilla, zygomatic arch, and/or calvarium [59, 60].

On radiographs, MLO tumors are classically well-defined bone lesions with coarse and stippled areas of granular calcification and mineralized proliferation with minimal

(a) (b)

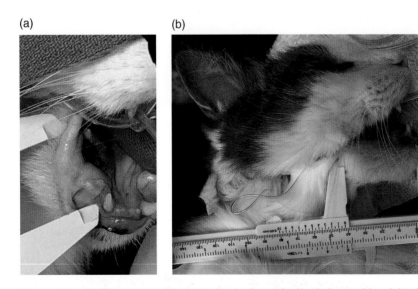

Figure 6.11 (a) Fifteen-year-old castrated male domestic shorthair cat with a right-sided mandibular squamous cell carcinoma demonstrating significant ulceration and loss of dentition. Intraoral clinical image of a squamous cell carcinoma of the right mandible of a cat. (b) Extraoral image of the extent of the intraoral mass shown with calipers. The squamous cell carcinoma extended along the length of the ventral mandible. This is the same patient as imaged in Figure (a).

(a)　　　　　　　　　　(b)　　　　　　　　　　(c)

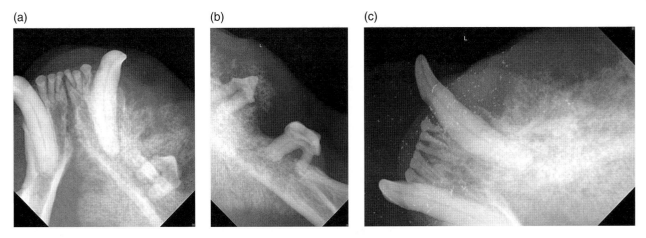

Figure 6.13　(a) Intraoral dental radiographs of an oral squamous cell carcinoma in a twenty-one-year-old castrated male domestic long-hair cat showing extensive periosteal proliferation and underlying alveolar bone lysis. Intraoral dental radiographic image of the rostral mandible of a domestic long-hair cat diagnosed with an oral squamous cell carcinoma. Note how the affected area appears to involve the left mandible and appears to potentially cross midline across the mandibular symphysis. (b) Intraoral dental radiographic image of the caudal left mandible of a domestic long-hair cat diagnosed with an oral squamous cell carcinoma. Note the proliferative periosteal reaction of the ventral mandibular cortex and the loss of distinction between the mandibular cortex and the affected bone. Also note the absence of the left mandibular 4th premolar tooth. (c) Intraoral dental radiographic image of the rostral aspect of the left mandible of a domestic long-hair cat diagnosed with an oral squamous cell carcinoma. Note the lack of distinction between the mandibular cortex, mandibular body, and the alveolar crest due to the disease process. *Source:* Courtesy of Brenda Mulherin, DVM, DAVDC, Iowa State University, College of Veterinary Medicine.

surrounding boney lysis or invasion [32, 61]. On CT, tumors are generally found to be well-marginated, contrast-enhancing, round masses with heterogenous, granular bone proliferation [60] (Figure 6.22a and b).

Radiographic Indications of Cystic Conditions

Odontogenic cysts are considered benign lesions composed of epithelium-lined structures or concavities in the bone of the maxilla or mandible that contain fluid or semisolid material [62]. Histopathology demonstrates that the tissues are lined by stratified squamous epithelium and kerati-nized material [63]. Odontogenic cysts are thought to be rare in veterinary medicine [64], with a reported incidence of 1.4% in a study evaluating patients over 15 years at an academic dentistry practice [65]. Types of cysts commonly reported in veterinary medicine include dentigerous cysts, radicular cysts, lateral periodontal cysts, odontogenic keratocysts (OKCs), and furcation cysts [65–67]. Cysts can be considered developmental or inflammatory in ori-gin [62]. Forty-four percent of the time, cysts were reported to be discovered incidentally [65]. Brachycephalic dogs, such as pugs and boxers, are predisposed to develop these lesions [65].

Most commonly, lesions are described radiographically as distinct, well-marginated lucencies. A periapical lesion with well-defined borders is usually thought to represent a chronic lesion such as a granuloma or a cyst [21]. It is important to establish the distinction between a cystic lesion and a potential malignancy. Treatment for a cystic lesion can be successful with enucleation and curettage of the cystic lining with or without tooth extraction, while wide surgical margins may be needed for a potential malig-nant neoplasm. Repeat imaging should be performed for comparison if concerns arise clinically or if local recur-rence is observed or suspected.

Dentigerous Cyst

Dentigerous cysts, previously called follicular cysts [64], are benign cysts composed of odontogenic epithelium associated with the crown of an unerupted adult tooth. They are considered the most common type of oral cyst in dogs, comprising 71% [65] of all oral cysts. Clinically, they are commonly found in young (two- to three-year-old) dogs with reports of an oral fluctuant swelling with a bluish-hue observed clinically. Brachycephalic breeds are predisposed, and lesions can be multiple or bilateral in nature [65]. A reported predilection exists for the mandibular first premo-lar in 83% of cases [65], but they are also commonly reported in unerupted canine teeth [65] (Figure 6.23a1 and a2). Patients are oftentimes asymptomatic but may present with hypodontia. Dentigerous cysts are slow-growing and cause thinning of the surrounding cortical bone with increasing expansion in size [68]. With continued thinning of the alveolar bone, a blue-tinged appearance has been

(a)

(b)

(c)

(d)

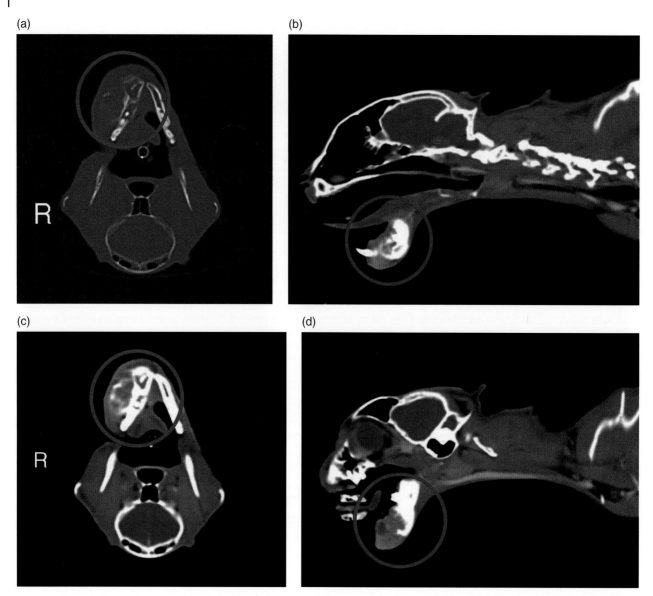

Figure 6.14 (a) Computed tomography scan from the cat pictured in Figure 6.11 diagnosed with a right-sided mandibular squamous cell carcinoma (red circle). Note the large caudal mandibular soft tissue mass with contrast enhancement, mineral attenuation, osteolysis, and proliferation of the mandible extending to the level of the ramus. The patient is positioned in dorsal recumbency for radiation therapy planning. Positioning the patient in dorsal recumbency was chosen to allow improved imaging of the mandible for therapeutic treatment planning. Traditional computed tomography scanning positioning would position the patient in ventral recumbency with a bite block obscuring imaging of a portion of the area of interest. Coronal/dorsal bone window, of the squamous cell carcinoma of the right mandible. Note the proliferation of bone with mineral attenuation and underlying cortical bone lysis. (b) Coronal/dorsal soft tissue post-contrast image of a squamous cell carcinoma of a right mandible. Note the proliferation of bone, soft tissue expansion, and contrast enhancement of the affected tissues. (c) Sagittal reconstruction, soft tissue post-contrast window of the squamous cell carcinoma at a more rostral level depicting the mandibular canine tooth. Note the osteolysis and proliferation of bone as well as the mineral attenuation and contrast enhancement, with expansion ventrally. (d) Sagittal reconstruction of the squamous cell carcinoma imaged with a soft tissue window at a more caudal level compared to the more rostral depiction of Figure (c). The osteolysis of the bone is much more prominent at this level.

(a)

(b)

(c)

(d)

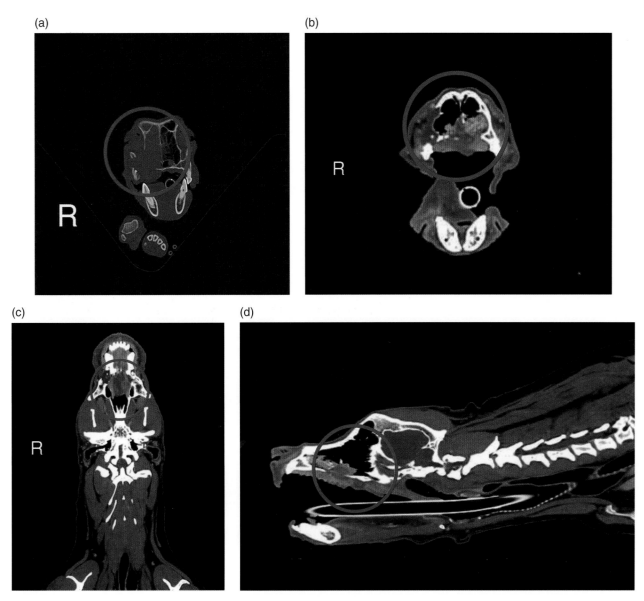

Figure 6.15 (a) Computed tomography scan of the dog pictured in Figure 6.12 with a large caudal maxillary squamous cell carcinoma (red circle). The computed tomography scan shows a large, heterogenous, soft tissue attenuating mass extending from the incisive bone to the level of the soft palate with extensive intranasal invasion and destruction. Axial/transverse bone window, of a dog with a caudal maxillary squamous cell carcinoma. Note the destruction of the hard palate as well as the maxillary bone. (b) Axial/transverse soft tissue post-contrast image of a dog with a caudal maxillary squamous cell carcinoma. Note the bony destruction of the maxillary bone and hard palate as well as the invasion of the soft tissue into the nasal cavity with a mild amount of contrast enhancement. (c) Coronal/dorsal reconstruction soft tissue post-contrast image of a dog with a caudal maxillary squamous cell carcinoma. Note the bony destruction of the right maxillary bone and extension of the soft tissue mass invading into the area of the soft palate. (d) Sagittal reconstruction soft tissue post-contrast image of a dog with a caudal maxillary squamous cell carcinoma. Note the heterogenous, soft tissue attenuating mass extending from the incisive bone to the area of the soft palate. The extension of soft tissues into the nasal cavity and underlying lysis of the hard palate can be seen.

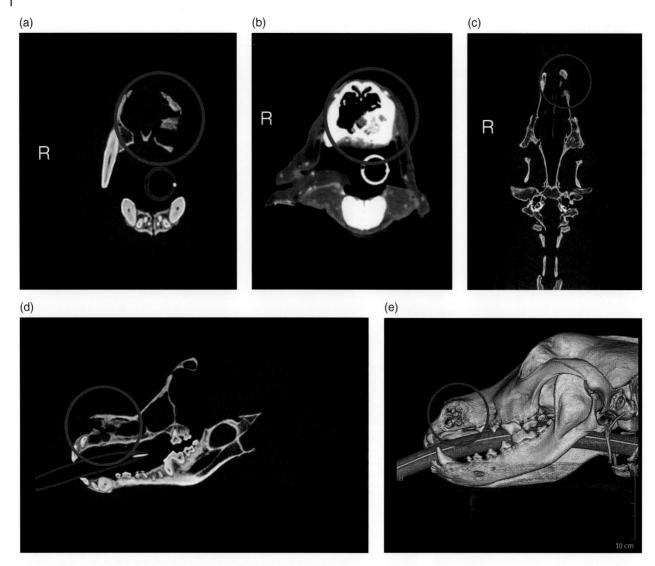

Figure 6.16 (a) Computed tomography images of a six-year-old female spayed Golden retriever with a left rostral maxillary papillary squamous cell carcinoma (red circle). The mass is mineral-attenuating and contrast- enhancing with osteolysis and proliferation. Axial/ transverse bone window image of a Golden retriever with a left rostral maxillary papillary squamous cell carcinoma. Note the osteolysis of the maxillary bone associated with the tumor and absence of the left maxillary canine tooth. (b) Axial/transverse soft tissue window post-contrast image of the dog with a left rostral maxillary papillary squamous cell carcinoma. Note the contrast enhancement of the affected tissues and extension of the soft tissues within the nasal cavity on the left. (c) Coronal/dorsal bone window image of a maxillary papillary squamous cell carcinoma. Note the lysis of the underlying maxillary bone in the affected region. (d) Sagittal bone window image of a dog with a left rostral maxillary papillary squamous cell carcinoma. Note the cavitated appearance of the rostral maxilla in the area affected by the papillary squamous cell carcinoma. (e) Sagittal view of a 3D reconstruction of a dog diagnosed with a papillary squamous cell carcinoma of the left maxilla. Note the extensive area of bone lysis and proliferation in the region of the left maxillary canine depicted in the sagittal image.

noted orally on clinical examination [69]. Local recurrence is considered rare but has been reported; therefore, re-evaluation with dental radiographs is recommended for follow-up of these lesions annually [65].

There is a classic pathopneumonic appearance radiographically, where the crown of an unerupted tooth is displaced from its normal eruption location and is surrounded by a uni- or multilocular radiolucency arising from the cementoenamel junction [65]. As the lesion size increases, it can cause cortical bone expansion [21] and present with a well-defined radiopaque line of cortex consistent with sclerosis radiographically [70] (Figure 6.23b1 and b2).

Radicular Cyst

Radicular cysts, previously called periapical cysts [64], are considered inflammatory lesions originating from necrotic pulp that forms secondary to a prior granuloma of a

(a) (b) (c)

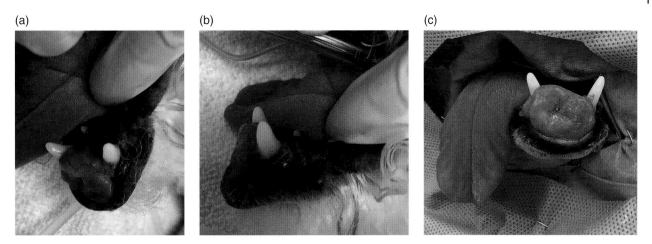

Figure 6.17 (a) Fourteen-year-old, male castrated Miniature Poodle diagnosed with an oral melanoma of the rostral mandible. Intraoral clinical image of an oral melanoma in the rostral mandible of a canine patient. Note the left and right mandibular 1st, 2nd, and 3rd mandibular incisors appear to be clinically missing. (b) Lateral clinical image of the oral melanoma in the rostral mandible. Note the proliferative nature of the affected tissue. (c) Clinical image of the rostral mandible affected by an oral melanoma of the patient as seen in (a) and (b). Note how the affected tissue is not pigmented.

nonvital tooth [62, 69]. They arise from the cells of Malassez within the periodontal ligament [62, 64] at the root apex [71]. On presentation, lesions are described as smooth, non-painful, raised lesions below the gingiva, coronal to the mucogingival line, specifically within the premaxilla [71–73].

Radiographically, lesions are most commonly <1 cm in diameter and are observed as having a unilocular periapical radiolucent appearance [21]. Secondary tooth resorption, tooth displacement, and root resorption have also been reported with these lesions [20, 69, 74]. A soft tissue density within the cystic lesion itself has also been described [71] (Figures 6.24a1, a2, b1, b2, c1, c2, and 6.25a–d).

Canine Furcation Cyst

Canine furcation cysts are described as fluctuant swellings over the buccal gingiva and mucosa, apical to the mucogingival line, overlying the furcational area of a multi-rooted tooth [66]. There is no tooth displacement associated with these lesions. The mean age at presentation is eight years old [66]. No obvious cause or trauma has been linked to the development of the lesion [66]. In dogs, there is a predilection for the maxillary fourth premolar furcational area to be affected [66] (Figure 6.26a and b).

On radiographic evaluation, there is a radiolucent region in the furcation area of the tooth roots with no cortical bone expansion [66]. Rarely root resorption mid-root, not within the apex, has been reported [66] (Figures 6.27a1, a2, 6.28a, b, and 6.29).

Surgical Ciliated Cyst

In humans, surgical ciliated cysts have been referred to as postoperative maxillary cysts (POMC) [75]. These cysts are located within the maxilla and histopathologically are lined by respiratory epithelium. They are considered inflammatory cysts, secondary to a prior surgical nidus. This type of cyst appears to afflict patients with a historical maxillary or sinus surgery [75, 76]. The development of these cysts appears to be caused by entrapment of respiratory mucosa in the iatrogenic surgical defect [75, 76]. Patients commonly present with swelling of the maxilla and occasionally the palate, along with secondary infection or pain [77, 78]. The development of these cysts is typically reported years after the original procedure [77, 78], so it is thought that this may be the reason it is uncommonly reported in dogs and cats.

Radiographically, surgical ciliated cysts appear as well-defined, unilocular radiolucencies closely associated with the maxillary sinus in people [77, 78]. As they expand, a sclerotic rim develops between the sinus and oral cavity, which thins over time and can rupture [78]. Therefore, the lesions are considered locally aggressive and expansile (Figures 6.30a–e and 6.31a–d).

Lateral Periodontal Cyst

Lateral periodontal cysts are considered developmental cysts that arise from the odontogenic epithelial rests of dental lamina [62, 79]. These cysts are most commonly found laterally between tooth roots of vital, erupted teeth

(a)

(b)

(c)

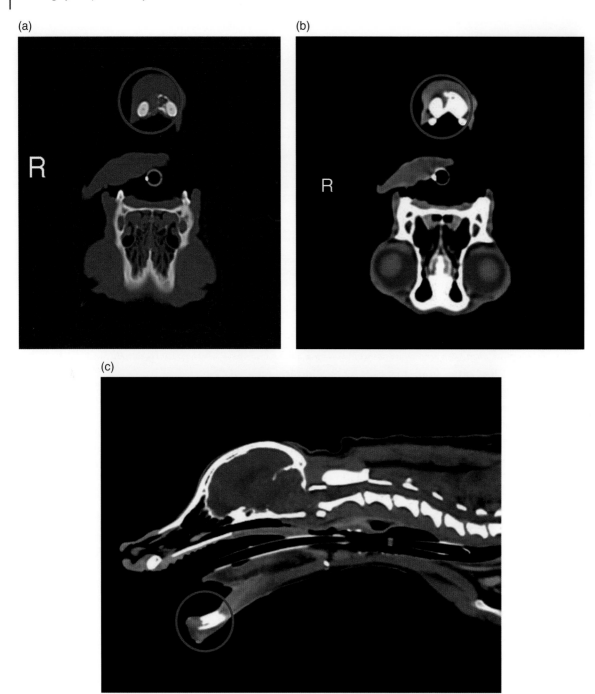

Figure 6.18 (a) Computed tomographic images of the fourteen-year-old, male castrated Miniature Poodle pictured in Figure 6.17a–c diagnosed with a rostral mandibular oral melanoma (red circle). Note the soft tissue- attenuating and contrast- enhancing mass at the rostral mandible with associated boney lysis. The patient is positioned in dorsal recumbency for radiation therapy planning. Positioning the patient in dorsal recumbency was chosen to allow improved imaging of the mandible for therapeutic treatment planning. Axial/transverse bone window image of an oral melanoma of the rostral mandible in a Miniature Poodle. Note the significant bone lysis at the root of the right mandibular canine tooth that is extending across midline. (b) Axial/transverse soft tissue post-contrast image of an oral melanoma of the rostral mandible. Note the contrast enhancement of the affected tissues and focal expansion of the soft tissues. (c) Sagittal reconstruction soft tissue post-contrast image of an oral melanoma of the rostral mandible. Note the proliferation of soft tissue in the area of the rostral mandible affected by the oral melanoma.

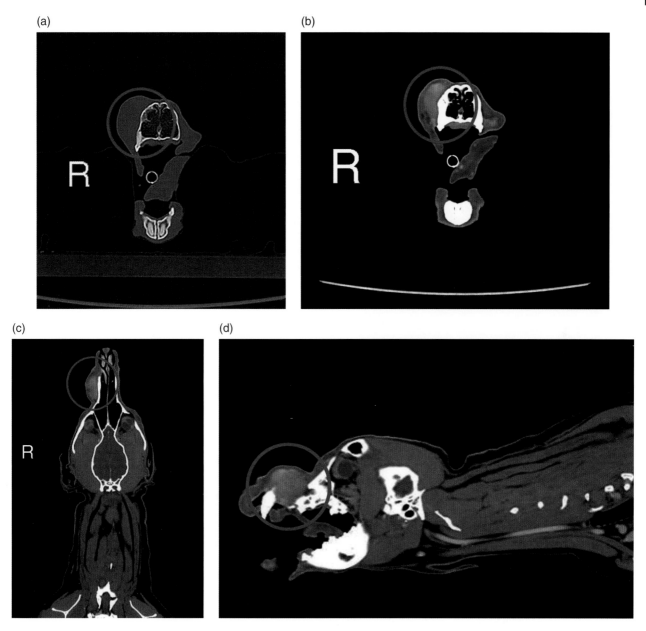

Figure 6.19 (a) Computed tomographic images of an eight-year-old female spayed Golden retriever with a right maxillary fibrosarcoma (red circle). Note the mass is heterogeneously soft tissue attenuating with no underlying osteolysis or proliferation. Axial/transverse bone window image of a right maxillary fibrosarcoma in a Golden retriever. Note the smooth margin of cortical bone associated with the maxillary bone and lack of lysis. (b) Axial/transverse soft tissue post-contrast image of a right maxillary fibrosarcoma in a Golden retriever. Note the soft tissue attenuation and expansion of the affected tissue and lack of bony destruction or proliferation. (c) Coronal/dorsal reconstruction soft tissue post-contrast image of a right maxillary fibrosarcoma in a Golden retriever. Note the soft tissue attenuation of the affected area and lack of involvement of the underlying bone. (d) Sagittal reconstruction soft tissue post-contrast image of a right maxillary fibrosarcoma in a Golden retriever. Note the soft tissue attenuation of the affected tissues as well as the expansile appearance of the soft tissues within the maxilla.

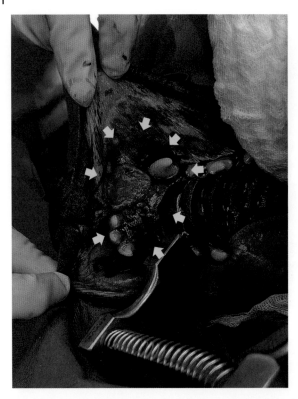

Figure 6.20 Clinical image of a three-year old male castrated Weimaraner with an oral osteosarcoma of the left rostral maxilla. The surgical margin in the buccal and palatal mucosa (yellow arrows) is inked with a sterile marking pen (purple) surrounding the mass. Surgical bone margins would likely extend caudal to the left maxillary canine tooth. Note the clinical absence of the left maxillary 1st, 2nd, and 3rd incisors.

within the alveolar bone [62, 79]. They have also been referred to as lateral radicular cysts [70]. They are often associated with the maxillary canine teeth [70]; however, a mandibular location, primarily between premolars has been noted in people and reported in a single veterinary case [65, 79]. These lateral cysts can cause root divergence but do not typically cause root resorption [79]. In veterinary patients, these cysts are typically asymptomatic and found incidentally or present as nonpainful swellings.

Radiographs reveal a well-defined, radiolucent region with a sclerotic margin of bone, typically between the apex and cervical margin of the tooth [21]. Lesions are distinct on histopathology with a plaque-like thickening of the epithelium [66].

Odontogenic Keratocyst (OKC)/Canine Odontogenic Parakeratinized Cyst (COPC)

OKCs are considered developmental cysts not associated with teeth but rather the body or ramus of the mandible or maxilla itself in people [20, 80]. In people, they have been

reported to contain a viscous or caseous material in the center. It has been proposed to rename them canine odontogenic parakeratinized (COPC) cysts in veterinary medicine because the histopathologic findings do not perfectly match that of human OKCs [65]. The cysts do span multiple tooth roots of fully erupted, normally developed teeth within the maxilla [65, 69]. Miniature Schnauzers appear overrepresented within the cases that are affected [65]. Patients may be asymptomatic aside from facial deformity [65, 80]. Clinically, these cysts are characterized as aggressive lesions with a high risk of local recurrence in humans [80]; however, no recurrence was noted in a single veterinary study following cystic enucleation [65].

Radiographically, these cysts are more likely to be multilocular and expansile with interradicular expansion, adjacent tooth displacement, root resorption, and surrounding cortical bone thinning [20, 21, 81] (Figures 6.32a1, a2, b1, b2, and 6.33a–c).

Compound and Complex Odontomas

Compound and complex odontomas are considered benign tumors that arise from the dental follicle during development [63, 67, 82]. Complex odontomas have multiple odontogenic tissue precursors and do not resemble normal tissues [63, 82], while compound odontomas form denticles resembling tooth-like structures [63]. Characteristically, these are found in young patients, typically 6–18 months of age, with altered numbers of teeth [63, 67, 82]. They are associated with a firm, nodular swelling in the affected area [63, 67, 82] (Figure 6.34a–c).

The two types of odontomas look different radiographically. Complex odontomas contain irregular, mineralized, or calcified material within a radiolucent lining (Figures 6.35a–d and 6.36a–d). Compound odontomas contain tooth-like structures throughout the lesion, which is considered pathognomonic [83] (Figure 6.37). Odontomas commonly displace surrounding teeth [21].

Limitations of Dental Radiography for Neoplasia

Despite potential pathognomonic radiographic descriptions and location predilections for various oral lesions and tumors, oral abnormalities cannot be diagnosed or distinguished from one another without histopathologic confirmation. While cysts oftentimes contain a fluid-filled center, tumors oftentimes develop necrotic centers as well and should be differentiated using histopathology [67]. Thus,

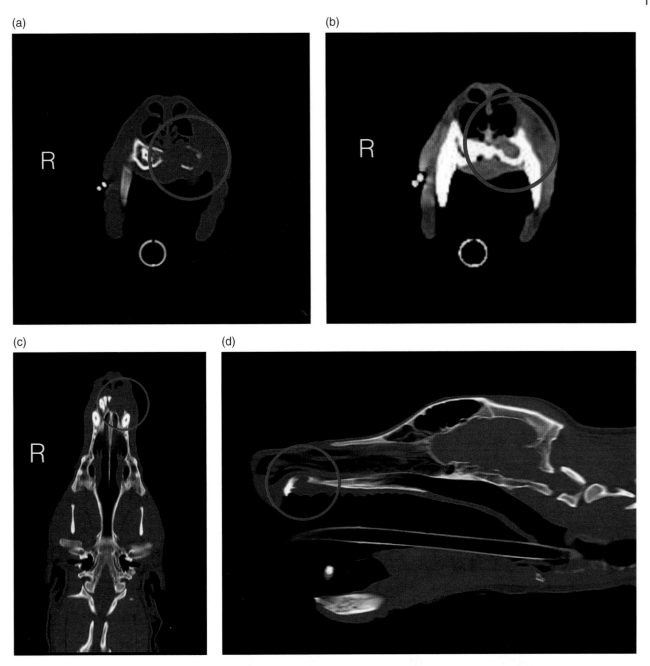

Figure 6.21 (a) Computed tomography images from the three-year-old male castrated Weimaraner diagnosed with a maxillary osteosarcoma pictured in Figure 6.20. Note the left rostral maxillary bone osteolysis (red circle). Axial/transverse bone window image of an osteosarcoma in a dog. Note the extensive osteolysis of the left maxilla. (b) Axial/transverse soft tissue post-contrast image of a maxillary osteosarcoma in a dog. Note the soft tissue contrast enhancement of the affected tissues at the level of the maxillary canine teeth. (c) Coronal/dorsal bone window image of a rostral maxillary osteosarcoma in a dog. Note the loss of architecture of the bone associated with the left rostral maxilla and the absence of the left maxillary 1st, 2nd, and 3rd incisor teeth. (d) Sagittal reconstruction bone window image of a maxillary osteosarcoma in a dog. Note the osteolysis of the bone of the rostral maxilla.

an oral incisional biopsy is still considered standard of care for the diagnosis of an oral lesion. All lesions addressed should have tissue submitted at the time of the procedure to verify whether an underlying neoplastic process exists. The biopsy should not interfere with a possible future surgical approach and should not alter surgical margins [1]. Biopsies should be performed intraorally rather than through the lip, as an extraoral approach could seed tumor cells and create difficulty when it comes to definitive surgical treatment later [1].

(a)   (b)

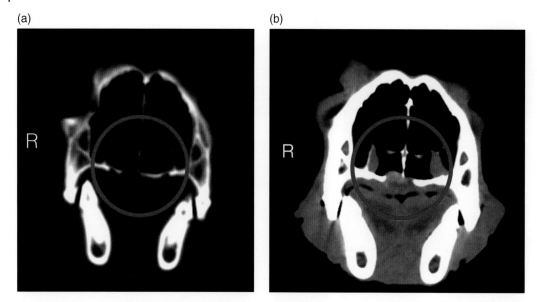

Figure 6.22 (a) Computed tomography image from a seven-year-old, female spayed German Shorthair Pointer with a caudal hard palate multilobular osteochondrosarcoma. Axial/transverse pre-contrast image of a multilobular osteochondrosarcoma in a German Shorthair Pointer. Note the lysis of the hard palate just to the right of midline. (b) Axial/transverse post-contrast soft tissue image of a Multilobular Osteochondrosarcoma in a German Shorthair Pointer. Images demonstrate mild contrast uptake of a soft tissue attenuating mass on midline of the caudal hard palate with focal osteolysis (red circle).

It is imperative that medical records be complete with photographic documentation and dental examination notes and oral charting [1, 11]. This is especially important when lesions are small, as the oral mucosa heals quickly. In these cases, scars may be difficult to locate at a later time for definitive, curative-intent surgery or radiation therapy [1] if needed.

For detailed evaluation of the lesions themselves, proper radiographic technique must be observed, and the appropriate radiographic views obtained in order to best assess the lesion at hand. For underlying boney invasion and for lysis to be detected using dental radiography, 40% or more of the cortex must be destroyed [3]; therefore, routine dental radiographs do not always rule out the extent of boney involvement. Dental radiography alone cannot assess the extent of soft tissue involvement and may not provide as much detail regarding underlying boney changes or the extent of disease [1, 65, 83, 84]. CT with contrast enhancement is especially important for lesions arising from the maxilla, palate, and caudal aspects of the mandible [1, 65, 83, 84]. Greater detail regarding bone and adjacent structure invasion found on a CT aids in planning for definitive surgery and further assessment of surgical margins [1, 60]. Historically, magnetic resonance imaging (MRI) has been shown to provide more information regarding size,

delineation of oral masses, adjacent structure invasion, and extension into underlying bone, compared to a CT scan [85]. However, CT remains superior for assessment of intra-tumoral calcification and underlying cortical bone erosion [85]. This is due to the smaller slice thickness [85] available for imaging with this modality, which is important when determining surgical margins. The use of sedation or brief anesthetic events combined with the increased availability of this advanced imaging modality, especially for assessment of smaller oral lesions, make CT evaluation a viable diagnostic option [85].

Radiographic assessment alone cannot provide all the information necessary to fully stage a patient with a neoplasm. With respect to oral tumors, staging includes evaluation of locoregional draining lymph nodes and the lungs for evidence of metastasis [3]. A head and neck CT extending through the chest should be considered for a thorough evaluation of the patient. CT also allows the patient to be positioned and assessed for radiation therapy planning at many institutions when advanced imaging capabilities and therapies are available. Since many oral tumors can be treated with a combination of surgery and radiation therapy or by radiation therapy alone, it is important to consider this modality when exploring treatment options with owners. Sentinel lymph node mapping, including ICTL, is

(a1)

(a2)

(b1)

(b2)

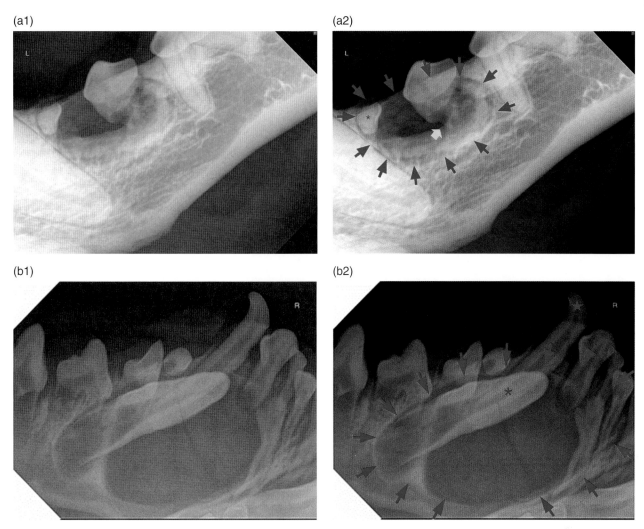

Figure 6.23 (a1) (unlabeled) Dental radiographic image of the left mandible of a dog diagnosed with a dentigerous cyst. There is a radiolucency surrounding the classic location of the mandibular first premolar tooth. (a2) (labeled) Note the area of mineralization adjacent to the distal aspect of the mandibular canine tooth which is the crown of the unerupted left mandibular 1st premolar tooth (asterisk). There is the appearance of a radiolucency associated with the mesial aspect of the left mandibular 2nd premolar tooth. The lucency appears to extend from the crown to the roots of this tooth. There appears to be resorption of the roots of the left mandibular 2nd premolar tooth (yellow arrowhead). There is a loss of mineralization to the bone associated with the distal aspect of the left mandibular 2nd premolar tooth. (b1) (unlabeled) Radiographic image of the right mandible of a dog diagnosed with a dentigerous cyst. Cortical expansion with a radiopaque rim of sclerosis around a unilocular swelling is present. (b2) (labeled) There is the presence of an unerupted right mandibular canine tooth present (asterisk). There is also the presence of a persistent deciduous right mandibular canine tooth (star). The cystic structure appears to be displacing the mandibular canine tooth as well (arrowheads).
Source: Courtesy of Brenda Mulherin, DVM, DAVDC, Iowa State University, College of Veterinary Medicine.

being further utilized within veterinary medicine for staging oral neoplasms and identifying the lymph node(s) of interest for sampling via cytology and/or histopathology.

Proper assessment of oral lesions and identifying treatment options is imperative. Equally as important is clinical follow-up after treatment. This could include repeat dental radiography and/or CT scans to monitor for recurrence of

disease following treatment. Any time oral surgery is performed, it is important to obtain immediate postoperative radiographs to evaluate for any potential retained tooth roots that could later cause clinical problems. Problems including pain or abscess in the patient may necessitate future surgery and extractions. Additionally post-procedure imaging can be used to document the radiographic

(a1)

(a2)

(b1)

(b2)

(c1)

(c2)

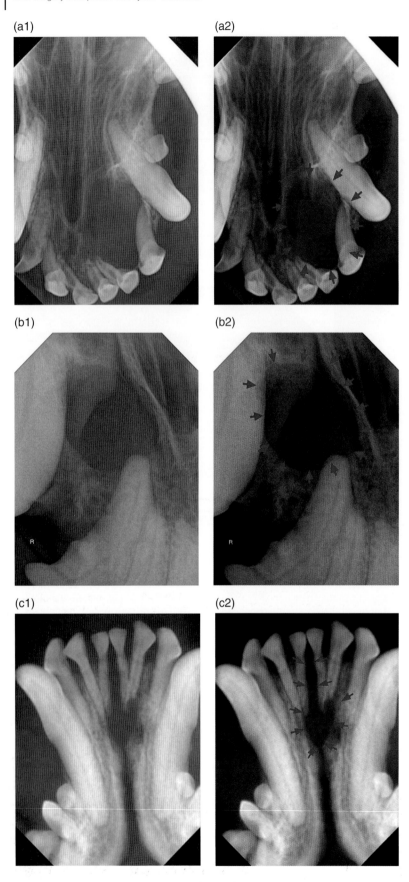

Figure 6.24 (a1) Dental radiographs of presumptive radicular cysts. (unlabeled): Classic premaxillary location for a radicular cyst with focal radiolucency and tooth displacement in a canine patient. (a2) (labeled) The arrows depict the extent of the cystic swelling of the radicular cyst. (b1) (unlabeled) Classic premaxillary region for a radicular cyst with focal radiolucency associated with the apical extent of the right maxillary 3rd incisor in a canine patient. (b2) (labeled) The arrows depict the extent of the cystic swelling associated with the apex of the right maxillary 3rd incisor tooth. (c1) (unlabeled) Dental radiographic image of the mandible of a dog diagnosed with a radicular cyst. (c2) (labeled) The image shows a focal radiolucency of the left and right mandibular 1st and 2nd incisors as well as tooth displacement and root resorption (circled). *Source:* Courtesy of Brenda Mulherin, DVM, DAVDC, Iowa State University, College of Veterinary Medicine.

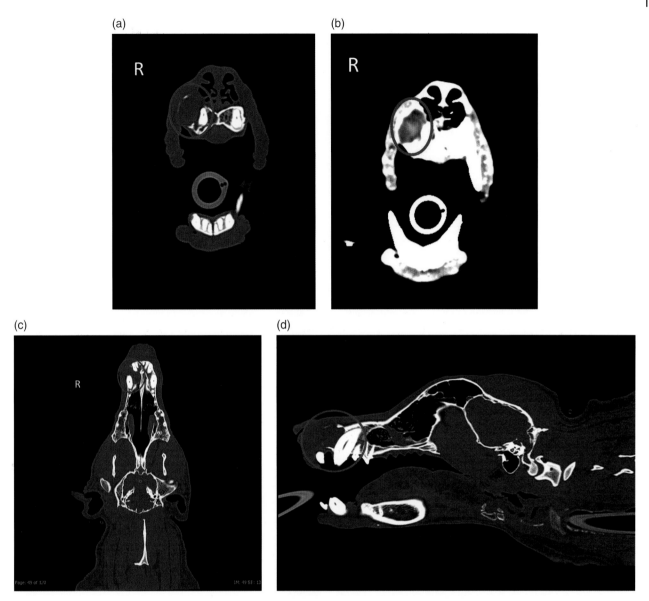

Figure 6.25 (a) Computed tomography images of a dog with a presumptive radicular cyst in the premaxilla. Note the tooth displacement and unilocular, focal expansion of surrounding tissue, and bone with soft-tissue attenuation (red circle). Axial/transverse bone window image of a suspected radicular cyst in the premaxilla of a dog. Note the expansion of the soft tissue associated with the right maxilla. (b) Axial/transverse soft- tissue window, post-contrast image of a dog with a suspected radicular cyst in the premaxilla of a dog. Note the contrast enhancement of the affected tissues in the right maxilla. (c) Coronal/dorsal reconstruction, bone window image of a suspected radicular cyst in the premaxilla of a dog. Note the soft tissue enhancement of the soft tissues in the right maxilla and the loss of bone present within the rostral maxilla. (d) Sagittal reconstruction, bone window image a of a suspected radicular cyst in the premaxilla of a dog. Note the soft tissue expansion of the rostral maxilla and displacement of the teeth associated with the affected area. *Source:* Courtesy of Brenda Mulherin, DVM, DAVDC, Iowa State University, College of Veterinary Medicine.

(a)   (b)

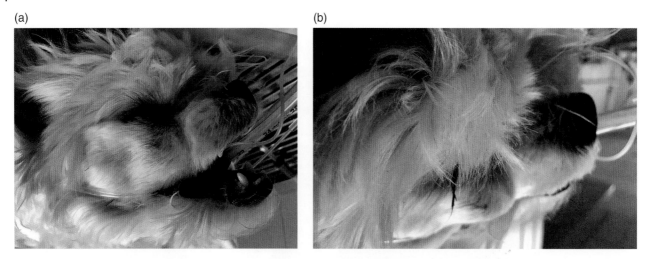

Figure 6.26 (a) Five-year old, female spayed Lhasa Apso with a right maxillary canine furcation cyst. This is a lateral view of the patient demonstrating the swelling of the right caudal maxilla. (b) Clinical image of a patient with a canine furcation cyst. This is a dorsal view of the patient depicting the swelling associated with the right maxilla. Both images demonstrate significant swelling and external expansion on the right side of the maxilla ventral to the eye that was fixed and mildly fluctuant on palpation.

(a1)   (a2)

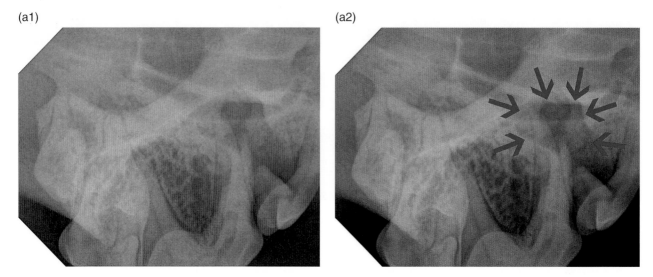

Figure 6.27 (a1) Dental radiographs of the dog pictured in Figure 6.26a, b with a right maxillary canine furcation cyst. Note the radiolucency at the furcation of the maxillary 4th premolar. (unlabeled): Dental radiographic image of the right maxillary 4th premolar, 1st molar, and 2nd molar teeth in a dog with a canine furcation cyst. Note the radiolucency associated with the mesiobuccal and mesiopalatal roots of the right maxillary 4th premolar tooth. (a2) (labeled) Dental radiographic image of the right maxillary 4th premolar, 1st molar, and 2nd molar teeth in a dog with a canine furcation cyst. The red arrows outline the radiolucency associated with the mesiobuccal and mesiopalatal roots of the maxillary 4th premolar tooth indicating the area affected by the cystic lesion.

(a)

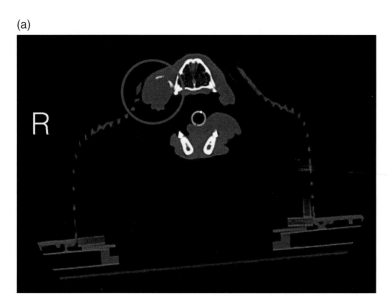

(b)

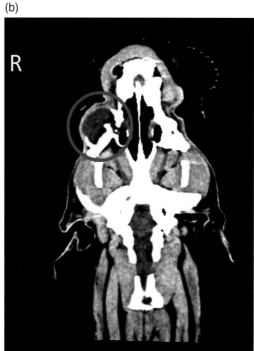

Figure 6.28   (a) Computed tomography images of the dog pictured in Figures 6.26a, b and 6.27a1, a2 with a right maxillary canine furcation cyst (red circle). Axial/transverse bone window image of a dog with a right maxillary canine furcation cyst. Note the soft tissue expansion associated with the right maxillary 4th premolar tooth. (b) Coronal/dorsal reconstruction soft tissue window image of a dog with a right maxillary canine furcation cyst. The image demonstrates the soft tissue expansion at the location of the furcation of tooth 108 (right maxillary 4th premolar). Notice the radiolucency and fluid filled cyst associated with the right maxillary 4th premolar tooth.

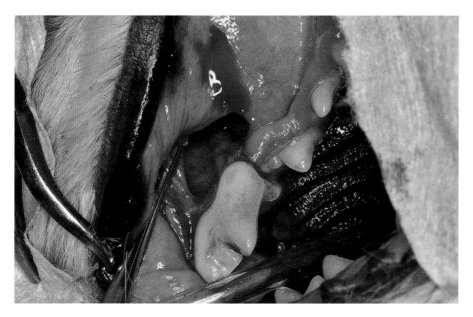

Figure 6.29   Intraoperative image of the affected area associated with a right maxillary canine furcation cyst associated with the right maxillary 4th premolar tooth (108) in the dog pictured in Figures 6.26–6.28.

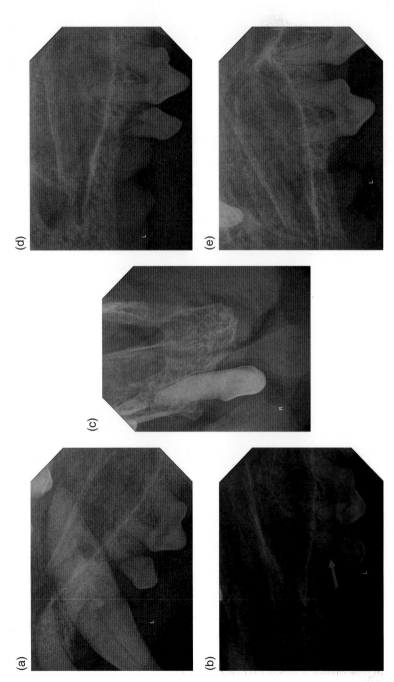

Figure 6.30 (a) Dental radiographs from a dog with a surgical ciliated cyst. Dental radiographic image of the left maxilla of a dog on initial presentation for extraction of the left maxillary canine tooth due to periodontal disease and excessive periodontal probing. (b) Immediate post-extraction dental radiograph of the left maxillary canine tooth (204) extraction site. There is no obvious evidence of retained tooth roots present in the radiographic image. Note there does appear to be evidence of a focal area of tooth resorption associated with the left maxillary 1st premolar tooth 205 (arrow). There is also evidence of replacement resorption of the apical extent of this tooth. (c) Dental radiographic image of the rostral maxilla of a canine patient presenting one-year following the initial presentation for extraction of the left maxillary canine tooth. Note the remodeling of bone in the area of the previously extracted left maxillary canine tooth (204). The bone remodeling indicates no obvious radiographic evidence of disease present in this area. (d) Bisecting angle radiographic view of the left maxillary region one-year following the initial presentation for extraction of the left maxillary canine tooth. Note the remodeling of the bone in the location of the previously extracted left maxillary canine tooth (204). Note the progressive tooth resorption associated with the left maxillary 1st premolar tooth (205). (e) Post-extraction dental radiographic image of the left maxillary 1st premolar tooth (205) and the previous extraction site of 204 that occurred one-year previously.
Source: Courtesy of Brenda Mulherin, DVM, DAVDC, Iowa State University, College of Veterinary Medicine.

(a)

(b)

(c)

(d)

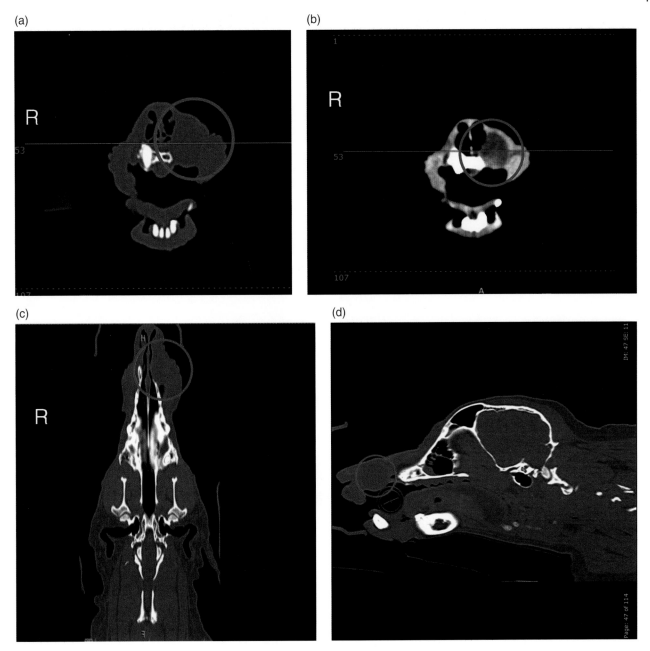

Figure 6.31 (a) Computed tomography images of a surgical ciliated cyst that developed following the extraction of the left maxillary canine tooth. The images are of the same dog pictured in Figure 6.30a–e, taken two years following the initial extraction of the left maxillary canine tooth. The computed tomography image depicts a unilocular, hypoattenuating lesion at the location of the previous tooth extraction. The hypoattenuating lesion expands into the nasal passage (red circle) and extends extraorally. Axial/transverse bone window image of a surgical ciliated cyst that developed two years following surgical extraction of the left maxillary canine tooth. Note the swelling associated with the left maxilla with a mildly hypoechoic appearance. (b) Axial/transverse soft tissue window post-contrast image of a surgical ciliated cyst of the left maxilla following a left maxillary canine tooth extraction which occurred two years previously. Note the appearance of soft tissue contrast-enhancing attenuation of the affected tissues. (c) Coronal/dorsal reconstruction bone window image of a surgical ciliated cyst in a canine patient, two years following extraction of the left maxillary canine tooth. Note the soft tissue swelling associated with the left maxilla affected by the surgical ciliated cyst. (d) Sagittal reconstruction soft tissue window image of a surgical ciliated cyst that developed two years following extraction of the left maxillary canine tooth. Note the mildly radiolucent appearance of the surgical ciliated cyst of the left maxilla. *Source:* Courtesy of Brenda Mulherin, DVM, DAVDC, Iowa State University, College of Veterinary Medicine.

(a1) (a2)

(b1) (b2)

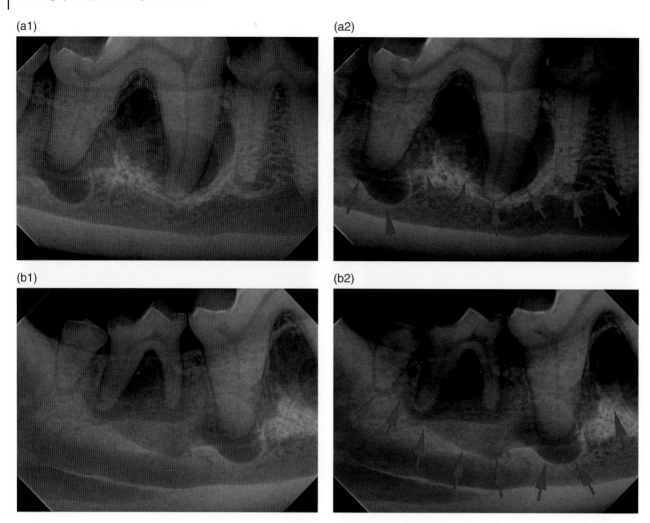

Figure 6.32 (a1) (unlabeled): Dental radiographic image of the right mandible of a dog diagnosed with an odontogenic keratocyst. Note the radiographic presence of a multilocular, radiolucency that spans multiple roots of fully erupted and developed teeth. (a2) (labeled) Dental radiographic image of the right mandible of a dog diagnosed with an odontogenic keratocyst. Note the red arrows depicting the radiographic appearance of the lesion. (b1) (unlabeled) Dental radiographic image of the right mandible of the same dog in Figure (a1) and (a2) diagnosed with an odontogenic keratocyst. Note the continued presence of a multilocular radiolucency that surrounds additional tooth roots as the lesion extends caudally. (b2) (labeled) Dental radiographic image of the right mandible of the same dog in Figure (a1) and (a2) diagnosed with an odontogenic keratocyst. Note the red arrows surrounding the radiolucency depicting the extent of the lesion. *Source:* Courtesy of Christopher J. Snyder, DVM, DAVDC, Founding Fellow, AVDC Oral and Maxillofacial Surgery, University of Wisconsin-Madison, School of Veterinary Medicine.

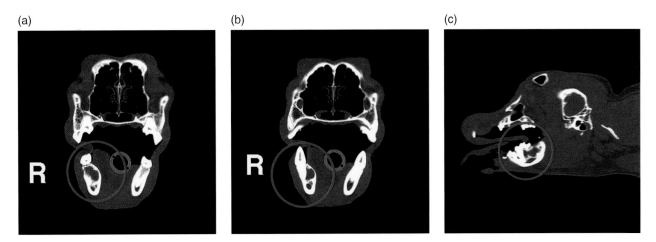

Figure 6.33 (a) Computed tomography scans of the dog pictured in Figure 6.32a1, a2, b1, b2 diagnosed with an odontogenic keratocyst in the right mandible. Axial/transverse bone window of a dog diagnosed with an odontogenic keratocyst of the right mandible. The red circle denotes the lytic and expansile region within the mandible at the level of the tooth root of the right mandibular first molar (409). (b) Axial/transverse bone window of a dog diagnosed with an odontogenic keratocyst. The red circle denotes the lytic and expansile region within the mandible at the level of a different, adjacent tooth root. Note the smooth cortical bone and lack of periosteal bone reaction. (c) Sagittal reconstruction CT of a dog diagnosed with an odontogenic keratocyst. The red circle denotes the multilocular and expansile region bridging multiple tooth roots within the right mandible at the level of the right mandibular first molar tooth (409). Note the lack of periosteal bone reaction and the smooth appearance of the cortical bone.
Source: Courtesy of Christopher J. Snyder, DVM, DAVDC, Founding Fellow, AVDC Oral and Maxillofacial Surgery, University of Wisconsin-Madison, School of Veterinary Medicine.

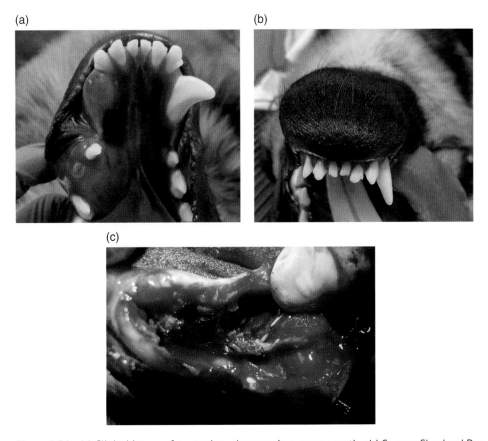

Figure 6.34 (a) Clinical image of a complex odontoma in a seven-month-old German Shepherd Dog. Note the clinically missing left mandibular canine tooth as well as the lingual swelling of the mandible on the left side. Also note the ulceration of the gingiva distal to the left mandibular 1st premolar as well as the displacement of these teeth causing a very large diastema between the left mandibular 1st and 2nd premolar teeth. (b) Extraoral clinical image of the rostral mandible depicting the swelling extraorally associated with the complex odontoma. Upon palpation the swelling was firm and nonfluctuant. (c) Intraoperative clinical image of a rostral complex odontoma of a seven-month-old German Shepherd Dog. Note the appearance of multiple spiculated fragments that are representative of denticles or small tooth-like structures. *Source:* Courtesy of Brenda Mulherin, DVM, DAVDC, Iowa State University, College of Veterinary Medicine.

(a)

(b)

(c)

(d)

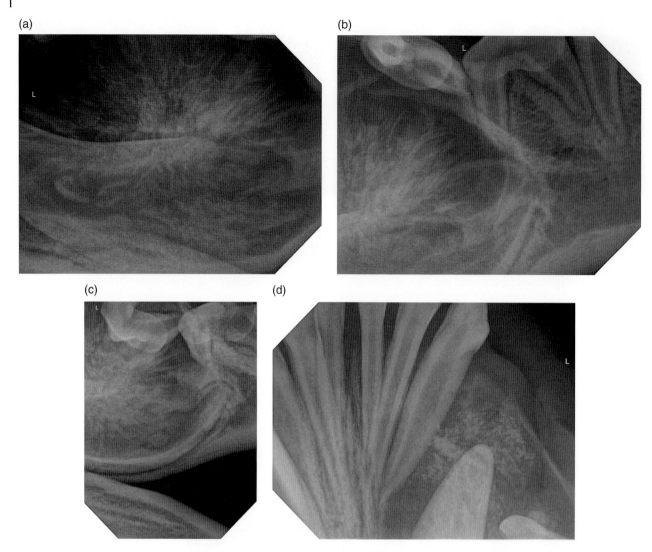

Figure 6.35 (a) Dental radiographs of the dog pictured in Figure 6.34a–c with a complex odontoma of the left ventral mandible. Dental radiographic image of the left rostral mandible of a seven-month-old German Shepherd Dog diagnosed with a complex odontoma. Note the irregular mineralization and calcification of the area. Also note the presence of the body of the unerupted left mandibular canine tooth. (b) Dental radiographic image of a dog diagnosed with a complex odontoma of the left mandible. Note the spiculated mineralization and calcification of the surrounding cystic structures and the displacement of the associated teeth. Also note the appearance of a thick, sclerotic rim of bone that appears to encapsulate the cystic structure. (c) Dental radiographic image of a German Shepherd Dog diagnosed with a complex odontoma. Note the tooth displacement and areas of mineralization and calcification encased in a sclerotic rim of bone. (d) Dental radiographic image of a German Shepherd Dog diagnosed with a complex odontoma of the left rostral mandible. Note the appearance of the cusp tip of the unerupted left mandibular canine tooth surrounded by a mineralized and calcified area of soft tissue. *Source:* Courtesy of Brenda Mulherin, DVM, DAVDC, Iowa State University, College of Veterinary Medicine.

(a)

(b)

(c)

(d)

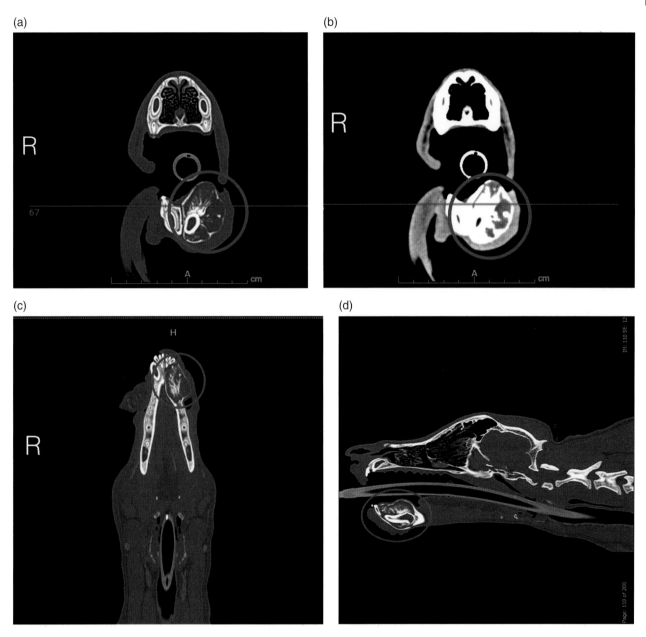

Figure 6.36 (a) Computed tomography scan of the dog pictured in Figures 6.34a–c and 6.35a–d diagnosed with a complex odontoma of the left ventral mandible (red circle). Axial/transverse bone window image of a dog with a complex odontoma of the left mandible. Note the expansile mass with calcified material in the center. Also, note the thin rim of cortical bone on the buccal aspect of the left mandible. (b) Axial/transverse soft tissue window post-contrast image of a dog with a complex odontoma of the left mandible. Note the increased contrast enhancement associated with the affected area and the hypoattenuating areas of affected tissue void of contrast enhancement. (c) Coronal/dorsal reconstruction bone window image of a dog with a complex odontoma of the left mandible. Note the expansile nature of the lesion. There is a thin rim of alveolar bone present on the buccal aspect of the left mandible. (d) Sagittal reconstruction bone window image of a dog with a complex odontoma of the left mandible. Note the presence of the unerupted left mandibular canine tooth surrounded by the areas of increased mineralization and spiculated calcified tissue. *Source:* Courtesy of Brenda Mulherin, DVM, DAVDC, Iowa State University, College of Veterinary Medicine.

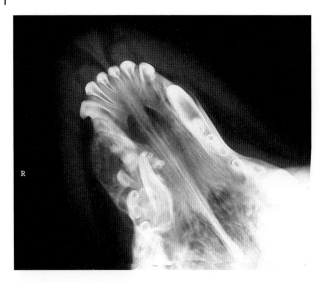

Figure 6.37 Dental radiograph of a dog with a compound odontoma. Note the denticles in the center of the expansile mass with surrounding sclerotic rim. There is the presence of normally appearing teeth within the area of affected tissue. *Source:* Courtesy of Christopher J. Snyder, DVM, DAVDC, Founding Fellow, AVDC Oral and Maxillofacial Surgery, University of Wisconsin-Madison, School of Veterinary Medicine.

margins following surgical treatment. Furthermore, malignant transformation of benign cysts to malignant tumors has been reported to occur rarely in people [86] and dogs [67], making clinical follow-up oral examinations standard of care.

Conclusion

Diagnostic imaging of oral lesions including conventional radiography to advanced imaging modalities, such as CT and MRI, is imperative to evaluate the extent of disease present within the oral cavity of canine and feline patients. While histopathology is necessary for a definitive diagnosis, diagnostic imaging can assist the surgeon in treatment planning and surgical margin preparation, as well as for patient follow-up postoperatively.

References

1 Liptak, J.M. and Lascelles, D.X. (2012). Oral tumors. In: *Veterinary Surgical Oncology*, 1e (ed. S.T. Kudnig and B. Seguin), 119–177. Ames: Wiley.

2 Reeves, N.C., Turrel, J.M., and Withrow, S.J. (1993). Oral squamous cell carcinoma in the cat. *J. Am. Anim. Hosp. Assoc.* 29: 438–441.

3 Liptak, J.M. (2020). Cancer of the gastrointestinal tract: oral tumors. In: *Withrow & MacEwen's Small Animal Clinical Oncology*, 6e (ed. D.M. Vail, D.H. Thamm, and J.M. Liptak), 432–338. St. Louis: Elsevier.

4 Verstraete, F.J.M. (2005). Mandibulectomy and maxillectomy. *Vet. Clin. North Am. Small Anim. Pract.* 35: 1009–1039.

5 Hoyt, R.F. and Withrow, S.J. (1984). Oral malignancy in the dog. *J. Am. Anim. Hosp. Assoc.* 20: 83–92.

6 Kosovsky, J.K., Matthiesen, D.T., Marretta, S.M. et al. (1991). Results of partial mandibulectomy for the treatment of oral tumors in 142 dogs. *Vet. Surg.* 20: 397–401.

7 Wallace, J., Matthiesen, D.T., and Patnaik, A.K. (1992). Hemimaxillectomy for the treatment of oral tumors in 69 dogs. *Vet. Surg.* 21: 337–341.

8 Berg, J. (2003). Surgical therapy. In: *Textbook of Small Animal Surgery*, 3e (ed. D.C. Slatter), 2324–2328. Philadelphia: Saunders.

9 Salisbury, S.K. (2003). Maxillectomy and mandibulectomy. In: *Textbook of Small Animal Surgery*, 3e (ed. D.C. Slatter), 561–572. Philadelphia: Saunders.

10 Sarowitz, B.N., Davis, G.J., and Kim, S. (2017). Outcome and prognostic factors following curative-intent surgery for oral tumours in dogs: 234 cases (2004 to 2014). *J. Small Anim. Pract.* 58: 146–153.

11 Bellows, J., Berg, M.L., Dennis, S. et al. (2019). 2019 AAHA dental care guidelines for dogs and cats. *J. Am. Anim. Hosp. Assoc.* 55: 49–69.

12 Wingo, K. (2018). Histopathologic diagnoses from biopsies of the oral cavity in 403 dogs and 73 cats. *J. Vet. Dent.* 35: 7–17.

13 Bell, C.M. and Soukup, J.W. (2014). Nomenclature and classification of odontogenic tumors – part II: clarification of specific nomenclature. *J. Vet. Dent.* 31: 234–243.

14 Chamberlain, T.P. and Lommer, M.J. (2012). Clinical behavior of odontogenic tumors. In: *Oral Maxillofacial Surgery in Dogs and Cats*, 1e (ed. F.J.M. Verstraete, M.J. Lommer, and A.J. Bezuidenhout), 403–410. Edinburgh: Elsevier.

15 Goldschmidt, S.L., Bell, C.M., Hetzel, S., and Soukup, J. (2017). Clinical characterization of canine acanthomatous ameloblastoma (CAA) in 263 dogs and

the influence of postsurgical histopathological margin on local recurrence. *J. Vet. Dent.* 34 (4): 241–247.

16 White, R.A.S. and Gorman, N.T. (1989). Wide local excision of acanthomatous epulides in the dog. *Vet. Surg.* 18 (1): 12–14.

17 Yoshida, K., Yanai, T., Iwasaki, T. et al. (1999). Clinicopathological study of canine oral epulides. *J. Vet. Med. Sci.* 61: 897–902.

18 Fiani, N., Verstraete, F.J.M., Kass, P.H., and Cox, D.P. (2011). Clinicopathologic characterization of odontogenic tumors and focal fibrous hyperplasia in dogs: 152 cases (1995–2005). *J. Am. Vet. Med. Assoc.* 238: 495–500.

19 Schmidt, A., Kessler, M., and Tassani-Prell, M. (2011). Computed tomographic characteristics of canine acanthomatous ameloblastoma – a retrospective study in 52 dogs. *Tierarztl. Prax.* 40: 155–160.

20 Scholl, R.J., Kellet, H.M., Neumann, D.P., and Lurie, A.G. (1999). Cysts and cystic lesions of the mandible: clinical and radiologic-histopathologic review [Scientific exhibit]. *RadioGraphics* 19 (5): 1107–1124.

21 Roy, C.G. (2018). Canine and feline dental disease. In: *Textbook of Veterinary Diagnostic Radiology*, 7e (ed. D.E. Thrall), 153–182. St. Louis: Elsevier.

22 Goldschmidt, S.L., Bell, C., Waller, K. et al. (2020). Biological behavior of canine acanthomatous ameloblastoma assessed with computed tomography an histopathology: a comparative study. *J. Vet. Dent.* 37 (3): 126–132.

23 Amory, J.T., Reetz, J.A., Sanchez, M.D. et al. (2013). Computed tomographic characteristics of odontogenic neoplasms in dogs. *Vet. Radiol. Ultrasound* 55 (2): 147–158.

24 Colgin, L.M.A., Schulman, F.Y., and Dubielzig, R.R. (2001). Multiple epulides in 13 cats. *Vet. Pathol.* 38: 227–220.

25 Gardner, D.G. and Dubielzig, R.R. (1995). Feline inductive odontogenic tumor (inductive fibroameloblastoma) – a tumor unique to cats. *J. Oral Pathol. Med.* 24: 185–190.

26 Beatty, J.A., Charles, J.A., Malik, R. et al. (2000). Feline inductive odontogenic tumour in a burmese cat. *Aust. Vet. J.* 78: 452–455.

27 Patnaik, A.K., Liu, S.K., Hurvitz, A.I. et al. (1975). Nonhematopoietic neoplasms in cats. *J. Natl. Cancer Inst.* 54: 855–860.

28 Dorn, C.R. and Priester, W.A. (1976). Epidemiologic analysis of oral and pharyngeal cancer in dogs, cats, horses, and cattle. *J. Am. Vet. Med. Assoc.* 169: 1202–1206.

29 Stebbins, K.E., Morse, C.C., and Goldschmidt, M.H. (1989). Feline oral neoplasia: a ten-year survey. *Vet. Pathol.* 26: 121–128.

30 Mikiewicz, M., Pazdzior-Czapula, K., Gesek, M. et al. (2019). Canine and feline oral cavity tumours and tumour-like lesions: a retrospective study of 486 cases (2015–2017). *J. Comp. Pathol.* 172: 80–87.

31 Brodey, R.S. (1960). A clinical and pathologic study of 130 neoplasms of the mouth and pharynx in the dog. *Am. J. Vet. Res.* 21: 787–812.

32 Todoroff, R.J. and Brodey, R.S. (1979). Oral and pharyngeal neoplasia in the dog: a retrospective survey of 361 cases. *J. Am. Vet. Med. Assoc.* 175: 567–571.

33 Forrest, L. (2018). The cranial nasal cavities: canine and feline. In: *Textbook of Veterinary Diagnostic Radiology*, 7e (ed. D.E. Thrall), 183–203. St. Louis: Elsevier.

34 Fulton, A.J., Nemec, A., Murphy, B.G. et al. (2013). Risk factors associated with survival in dogs with nontonsillar oral squamous cell carcinoma: 31 cases (1990–2010). *J. Am. Vet. Med. Assoc.* 243: 696–702.

35 Gendler, A., Lewis, J.R., Reetz, J.A., and Schwarz, T. (2010). Computed tomographic features of oral squamous cell carcinoma in cats: 18 cases (2002–2008). *J. Am. Vet. Med. Assoc.* 236: 319–325.

36 Bilgic, O., Duda, L., Sanchez, M.D., and Lewis, J.R. (2015). Feline oral squamous cell carcinoma: clinical manifestations and literature review. *J. Vet. Dent.* 32: 30–40.

37 Frew, D.G. and Dobson, J.M. (1992). Radiological assessment of cases of incisive or maxillary neoplasia in the dog. *J. Small Anim. Pract.* 33: 11–18.

38 Strohmayer, C., Klang, A., and Kneissl, S. (2020). Computed tomographic and histopathological characteristics of 13 equine and 10 feline oral and sinonasal squamous cell carcinomas. *Front. Vet. Sci.* 7: 591437.

39 Stapleton, B.L. and Barrus, J.M. (1996). Papillary squamous cell carcinoma in a young dog. *J. Vet. Dent.* 13: 65–68.

40 Ogilvie, G.K., Sundberg, J.P., O'Banion, M.K. et al. (1988). Papillary squamous cell carcinoma in three young dogs. *J. Am. Vet. Med. Assoc.* 192: 933–936.

41 Nemec, A., Murphy, B.G., Jordan, R.C. et al. (2014). Oral papillary squamous cell carcinoma in twelve dogs. *J. Comp. Pathol.* 150: 155–161.

42 Soukup, J.W., Synder, C.J., Simmons, B.T. et al. (2013). Clinical, histologic, and computed tomographic features of oral papillary squamous cell carcinoma in dogs: 9 cases (2008–2011). *J. Vet. Dent.* 30: 18–24.

43 Thaiwong, T., Sledge, D.G., Collins-Webb, A. et al. (2018). Immunohistochemical characterization of canine oral papillary squamous cell carcinoma. *Vet. Pathol.* 55: 224–232.

44 McEntee, M.C. (2012). Clinical behavior of nonodontogenic tumors. In: *Oral Maxillofacial Surgery in*

Dogs and Cats, 1e (ed. F.J.M. Verstraete, M.J. Lommer, and A.J. Bezuidenhout), 387–402. Edinburgh: Elsevier.

45 Ramos-Vara, J.A., Beissenherz, M.E., Miller, M.A. et al. (2000). Retrospective study of 338 canine oral melanomas with clinical, histologic, and immunohistochemical review of 129 cases. *Vet. Pathol.* 37: 597–608.

46 Patnaik, A.K. and Mooney, S. (1988). Feline melanoma: a comparative study of ocular, oral, and dermal neoplasms. *Vet. Pathol.* 25: 105–112.

47 Chamel, G., Abadie, J., Albaric, O. et al. (2017). Non-ocular melanoma in cats: a retrospective study of 30 cases. *J. Feline Med. Surg.* 19: 351–357.

48 Farrelly, J., Denman, D.L., Hohenhaus, A.E. et al. (2004). Hyopofractionated radiation therapy in five cats. *Vet. Radiol. Ultrasound* 45: 91–93.

49 Martano, M., Lussich, S., Morello, E., and Buracco, P. (2018). Canine oral fibrosarcoma: changes in prognosis over the last 30 years? *Vet. J.* 241: 1–7.

50 Gardner, H., Fidel, J., Haldorson, G. et al. (2013). Canine oral fibrosarcomas: a retrospective analysis of 65 cases (1998–2010). *Vet. Comp. Oncol.* 13: 40–47.

51 Ciekot, P.A., Powers, B.E., Withrow, S.J. et al. (1994). Histologically low-grade, yet biologically high-grade, fibrosarcomas of the mandible and maxilla in dogs: 25 cases (1982–1991). *J. Am. Vet. Med. Assoc.* 204: 610–615.

52 Frazier, S.A., Johns, S.M., Ortega, J. et al. (2011). Outcome in dogs with surgically resected oral fibrosarcoma (1997–2008). *Vet. Comp. Oncol.* 10: 33–43.

53 Northrup, N.C., Selting, K.A., Rassnick, K.M. et al. (2006). Outcomes of cats with oral tumors treated with mandibulectomy: 42 cases. *J. Am. Anim. Hosp. Assoc.* 42: 350–360.

54 Heldmann, E., Anderson, M.A., and Wagner-Mann, C. (2000). Feline osteosarcoma: 145 cases (1990–1995). *J. Am. Anim. Hosp. Assoc.* 36: 518–521.

55 Heyman, S.J., Diefenderfer, D.L., Goldschmidt, M.H. et al. (1992). Canine axial skeletal osteosarcoma: a retrospective study of 116 cases (1986 to 1989). *Vet. Surg.* 21: 304–410.

56 Bitteto, W.V., Patnaik, A.K., Schrader, S.C. et al. (1987). Osteosarcoma in cats: 22 cases (1974–1984). *J. Am. Vet. Med. Assoc.* 190: 91–93.

57 Farcas, N., Arzi, B., and Verstraete, F.J.M. (2012). Oral and maxillofacial osteosarcoma in dogs: a review. *Vet. Comp. Oncol.* 12: 169–180.

58 Pool, R.R. (1990). Tumors of bone and cartilage. In: *Tumors of Domestic Animals* (ed. J.E. Moulton), 159–213. Berkley: University of California Press.

59 Dernell, W.S., Straw, R.C., Cooper, M.F. et al. (1998). Multilobular osteochondrosarcoma in 39 dogs: 1979–1993. *J. Am. Anim. Hosp. Assoc.* 34: 11–18.

60 Hathcock, J.T. and Newton, J.C. (2000). Computed tomographic characteristics of multilobular tumor of bone involving the cranium in 7 dogs and zygomatic arch in 2 dogs. *Vet. Radiol. Ultrasound* 41: 214–217.

61 Straw, R.C., LeCouteur, R.A., Powers, B.E. et al. (1989). Multilobular osteochondrosarcoma of the canine skull: 16 cases (1978–1988). *J. Am. Vet. Med. Assoc.* 195: 1764–1769.

62 Gardner, D.G. (1992). An orderly approach to the study of odontogenic tumours in animals. *J. Comp. Pathol.* 107: 427–438.

63 Reichart, P.A. and Philipsen, H.P. (2000). *Oral Pathology*. New York: Georg Thieme Verlag.

64 El-Naggar, A.K., Chan, J.K.C., Grandis, J.R. et al. (2017). WHO classification of head and neck tumors. In: *WHO Classification of Tumours*, 4e (ed. A.K. El-Naggar, J.K.C. Chan, J.R. Grandis, et al.), 232–242. Lyon: International Agency for Research on Cancer.

65 Verstraete, F.J.M., Zin, B.P., Kass, P.H. et al. (2011). Clinical signs and histologic findings in dogs with odontogenic cysts: 41 cases (1995–2010). *J. Am. Vet. Med. Assoc.* 239: 1470–1476.

66 Soukup, J.W. and Bell, C.M. (2020). The canine furcation cyst, a newly defined odontogenic cyst in dogs: 20 cases (2013–2017). *J. Am. Vet. Med. Assoc.* 256: 1359–1367.

67 Poulet, F.M., Valentine, B.A., and Summers, B.A. (1992). A survey of epithelial odontogenic tumors and cysts in dogs and cats. *Vet. Pathol.* 29: 369–380.

68 D'Astous, J. (2011). An overview of dentigerous cysts in dogs and cats. *Can. Vet. J.* 52: 905–907.

69 Chamberlain, T.P. and Verstraete, F.J.M. (2012). Clinical behavior and management of odontogenic cysts. In: *Oral Maxillofacial Surgery in Dogs and Cats*, 1e (ed. F.J.M. Verstraete, M.J. Lommer, and A.J. Bezuidenhout), 481–486. Edinburgh: Elsevier.

70 DuPont, G.A. and DeBowes, L.J. (2009). Swelling and neoplasia. In: *Atlas of Dental Radiography in Dogs and Cats*, 1e (ed. G.A. DuPont and L.J. DeBowes), 182–194. St. Louis: Saunders/Elsevier.

71 Beckman, B.W. (2003). Radicular cyst of the premaxilla in a dog. *J. Vet. Dent.* 20: 213–217.

72 French, S.L. and Anthony, J.M.G. (1996). Surgical removal of a radicular odontogenic cyst in a four year old dalmation dog. *J. Vet. Dent.* 13: 149–151.

73 Reiter, A.M. (2001). Periapical cyst formation of the left maxillary third incisor in an adult standard poodle. In: *Proceedings 15th Annual Dental Forum*, vol. 1, 149–150.

74 Lommer, M.J. (2007). Diagnostic imaging in veterinary dental practice: periapical cyst. *J. Am. Vet. Med. Assoc.* 230: 997–999.

75 Kubo, I. (1927). A buccal cyst occurred after a radical operation of the maxillary sinus. *Z F Otol Tokyo* 3: 896–897.

76 Kaneshiro, S., Nakajima, T., Yoshikawa, Y. et al. (1981). The postoperative maxillary cyst: report of 71 cases. *J. Oral Surg.* 39 (3): 191–198.

77 Amin, M., Withrow, H., Lee, R., and Blenkinsopp, P. (2003). Surgical ciliated cyst after maxillary orthognathic surgery: report of a case. *J. Oral Maxillofac. Surg.* 61 (1): 138–141.

78 Bulut, A.S., Sehlaver, C., and Percin, A.K. (2010). Postoperative maxillary cyst: a case report. *Pathol. Res. Int.* 10: 810835.

79 De Andrade, M., Silva, A.P., de Moraes Ramos-Perez, F.M. et al. (2012). Lateral periodontal cyst: report of case and review of the literature. *Oral Maxillofac. Surg.* 16 (1): 83–87.

80 Regezi, J.A. (2002). Odontogenic cysts, odontogenic tumors, fibroosseous, and giant cell lesions of the jaws. *Mod. Pathol.* 15: 331–341.

81 Weber, A.L. (1993). Imaging of cysts and odontogenic tumors of the jaw. *Radiol. Clin. N. Am.* 31: 101–120.

82 Figueiredo, C., Barros, H.M., Alvares, L.C., and Damante, J.H. (1974). Composed complex odontoma in a dog. *Vet. Med. Small Anim. Clin.* 69: 268–270.

83 Ghirelli, C.O., Villamizar, L.A., Carolina, A. et al. (2013). Comparison of standard radiography and computed tomography in 21 dogs with maxillary masses. *J. Vet. Dent.* 30: 72–76.

84 Kafka, U.C.M., Carstens, A., Steenkamp, G. et al. (2004). Diagnostic value of magnetic resonance imaging for oral masses in dogs. *J. South Afr. Vet. Assoc.* 75: 163–168.

85 Anderson, J.G. and Harvey, C.E. (1993). Odontogenic cysts. *J. Vet. Dent.* 10: 5–9.

86 Borras-Ferreres, J., Sanchez-Torres, A., and Gay-Escoda, C. (2016). Malignant changes developing from odontogenic cysts: A systematic review. *J Clin. Exp. Dent.* 8 (5): e622–e628.

7

Interpretation of Uncommon Pathology in the Canine and Feline Patient

Brenda Mulherin[1], Chanda Miles[2], and Michael Congiusta[3]

[1] Lloyd Veterinary Medical Center, Iowa State University College of Veterinary Medicine, Ames, IA, USA
[2] Veterinary Dentistry Specialists, Katy, TX, USA
[3] Veterinary Dentistry and Oromaxillofacial Surgery, School of Veterinary Medicine, University of Wisconsin-Madison, Madison, WI, USA

CONTENTS

Introduction

The most common oral pathologies found in canine and feline patients have been demonstrated and discussed in detail in Chapters 4 and 5, respectively. While most oral pathologies previously discussed are observed in a general practice setting on a daily basis, there are a few uncommon conditions that have radiographic evidence that can be useful in their diagnosis and management. The conditions found in this chapter, while uncommon, should be considered if the more common diseases have been ruled out either through clinical presentation, radiographic interpretation, or biopsy.

Uncommon Conditions with Predilection for Canine Patients

Craniomandibular Osteopathy (CMO)

In dogs, craniomandibular osteopathy (CMO) occurs most commonly in dogs three to eight months of age and can result in substantial oral pain [1–4]. CMO is a nonneoplastic, noninflammatory condition which results in inappetence, pyrexia, inability to open the mouth, and palpably enlarged mandibles [1–5] (Figure 7.1a–d). This bone

disease most commonly occurs in West Highland White Terriers and may have an autosomal recessive mode of inheritance [6]. While it is frequently seen in this breed, any breed of dog can be affected. Patients affected with CMO usually have lesions that result in symmetrical, diffuse, irregular thickening of the mandible(s), occipital, temporal, and other bones of the skull [7].

Histopathology along with advanced diagnostic imaging (computed tomography) confirms a diagnosis of CMO [3, 4]. Computed tomography may reveal a severe amount of spiculated to amorphous and smoothly marginated periosteal proliferation along the affected mandible(s) (Figure 7.2). Histopathologic analysis reveals resorption of lamellar bone, periosteal proliferation, immature coarse woven bone, and poorly mineralized bony trabeculae interspersed with fibrous tissue [5]. Radiographically, severe mandibular swelling, obliteration of the intermandibular space, and dense periosteal proliferations are noted [3–5] (Figure 7.3a–c). Alkaline phosphatase may be the only abnormal change seen on a full bloodwork database (complete blood count, chemistry profile, and urinalysis) [3, 5].

CMO may present aberrantly as well. The appendicular skeleton can occasionally be affected [8, 9]. Once skeletal maturity is reached (10–11 months of age), the disease typically regresses [5]. CMO can present as a waxing and

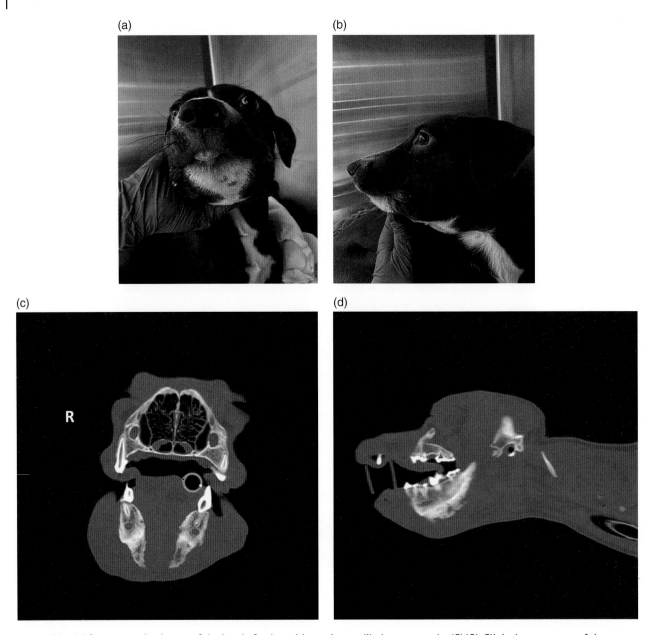

Figure 7.1 (a) Representative image of the head of a dog with craniomandibular osteopathy (CMO). Clinical appearance of the prominent enlarged mandibles in a rostrocaudal view. Observe the bulging appearance of the eyes which can be consistent with this disease. (b) Representative image of the head of a dog with craniomandibular osteopathy (CMO). Clinical appearance of the prominent enlarged mandibles in a left lateral view. (c) Representative image of the head of a dog with craniomandibular osteopathy (CMO). Transverse computed tomographic (CT) images of the head of the dog. Note the proliferative appearance of the right and left mandibles. (d) Representative image of the head of a dog with craniomandibular osteopathy (CMO). Sagittal computed tomographic (CT) images of the head of the dog. Note the proliferative appearance of the ventral mandibular cortex. *Source:* Courtesy of Michael Congiusta, DVM and the University of Wisconsin-Madison, School of Veterinary Medicine.

waning disease which can be frustrating for owners. The disease is generally self-limiting and can be managed with corticosteroids, nonsteroidal anti-inflammatories, opioids, and anticonvulsants [4]. Even with medical management relapses may occur. Treatment may be required until skeletal maturity is reached.

Prognosis is dependent on the severity of disease, the ability to control refractory chronic pain, and the involvement of anatomical structures such as, but not limited to the temporomandibular joint (TMJ), tympanic bullae, and the temporal petrous bone [10, 11].

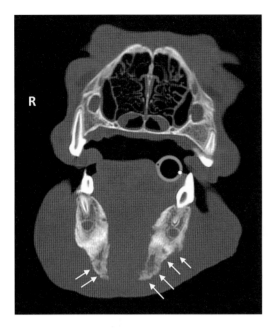

Figure 7.2 Representative transverse computed tomographic image of the head of the dog with craniomandibular osteopathy (CMO). Note the severe amount of spiculated to amorphous, and smoothly marginated periosteal proliferation (white arrows). *Source:* Courtesy of Michael Congiusta, DVM and the University of Wisconsin-Madison, School of Veterinary Medicine.

Idiopathic Calvarial Hyperostosis

Idiopathic calvarial hyperostosis (ICH) is a rare condition that is predominately seen in juvenile dogs, frequently under nine months of age [11–16]. It is a disease that has commonly been reported in Bullmastiffs but has also been reported in other breeds [11–16]. The condition is characterized by the proliferation of the bones associated with the skull, including the frontal, parietal, and temporal bones [12, 17] (Figures 7.4a–f, 7.5a, and b). Occasionally, involvement of the appendicular skeleton can be observed [16].

While found to be a nonneoplastic disease, the swelling associated with the skull has been reported to be extremely painful and result in the loss of appetite, lethargy, and pyrexia [12]. Nonsteroidal and steroidal medications have been suggested to help control the pain associated with the swelling [12]. Administration of nonsteroidal and steroid medications have yielded reduction in edema and pain but have not demonstrated any benefit in regression of the bony swelling [12]. Frequently the lesions may continue to grow causing pain and discomfort for the animal [12]. Most cases of ICH appear to be self-limiting, with potential regression of the lesions once the patient reaches skeletal maturity [12].

Radiographically, diffuse thickening of the frontal and parietal bones may be observed, along with increased bony opacity [12]. In many cases, the thickened calvaria will have an irregular appearance of chronic, yet active, bony proliferation [17]. It frequently is found to affect the frontal sinus and occipital bones [17] (Figure 7.6). The bone may have a smoothly irregular, cavitated appearance that is expansile in nature [14]. With the disease being self-limiting, once the lesions begin to regress, the thickness of the frontal bones may decrease, along with resolution of the cavitated areas [14]. In the end, only mild thickening of the affected bones may remain [14].

There are radiographic and clinical similarities between cranial mandibular osteopathy and ICH. In patients affected with ICH, the thickening of the frontal bones is almost identical to those patients diagnosed with cranial mandibular osteopathy (Figure 7.7a–d). ICH can appear as a focal osteopathy and may only present unilaterally [17]. Lack of involvement of the mandible appears to be a distinguishing factor in differentiating ICH from cranial mandibular osteopathy [16].

Periostitis Ossificans (PO)

Periostitis ossificans (PO) occurs most commonly in large breed dogs three to five months of age [18–22]. This disease can result in a nonpainful mandibular swelling that may be associated with an unerupted tooth, an incompletely erupted tooth with subsequent secondary pericoronitis, a reactive dental follicle or for a variety of other reasons [18–22] (Figure 7.8a–d). This self-limiting, proliferative bone disease has been reported in large breed dogs, such as the Labrador retriever, Dogue de Bordeaux, as well as others, with no specific breed predilection noted. Extraorally, PO results in a unilateral or bilateral firm swelling between the third and fourth premolars and molar teeth with variable lymph node involvement. Intraorally, PO may be observed as a fluctuant swelling [3, 4, 18] (Figure 7.9a and b).

Characteristic radiographic findings and histopathological analysis confirms a diagnosis of PO. Radiographic changes involve a double cortex formation along the ventral or lingual mandibular border with a linear radiolucent space between the two cortices. This change extends from the third or fourth premolar to beyond the first molar [3, 4, 18, 23, 24] (Figure 7.10a and b). Histopathological analysis reveals a pseudocystic wall of excessive periosteal new bone formation and marked hyperostosis with areas of well-differentiated lamellar bone indicative of chronicity [3, 4, 18, 23, 24]. Leukocytosis may be the only abnormal change seen on a full minimum database (complete blood count, chemistry profile, and urinalysis) [3, 18].

(a)

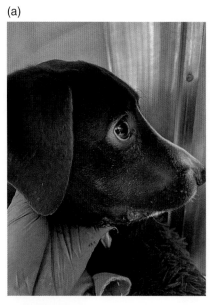

(b)   (c)

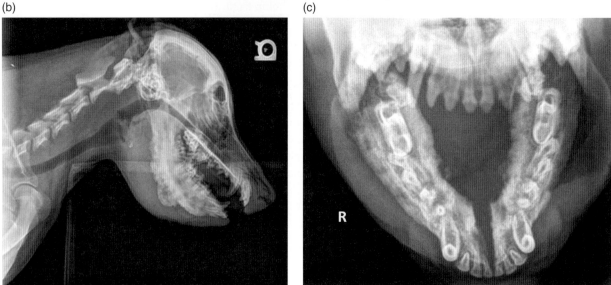

Figure 7.3 (a) Representative image of the head of a dog with craniomandibular osteopathy (CMO). Clinical appearance of the prominent enlarged mandible in a right lateral view. Note the bulging appearance of the eyes, consistent with this disease. (b) Representative image of the head of a dog with craniomandibular osteopathy (CMO). Lateral skull radiograph of a six-month-old Labrador mixed breed dog with CMO. Note the periosteal bone proliferation observed on the skull radiograph. (c) Representative image of the head of a dog with craniomandibular osteopathy (CMO). Dorsoventral skull radiograph of the same dog with CMO. Note the periosteal bone proliferation associated with both mandibles in this open mouth view. The proliferation appears to affect both sides with a symmetrical proliferation of the alveolar bone. *Source:* Courtesy of Michael Congiusta, DVM and the University of Wisconsin-Madison, School of Veterinary Medicine.

Most cases of PO resolve, but bony changes can be permanent [4, 18]. The core of the swelling contains necrotic bone, inflammatory cells, and immature granulation tissue [4, 18]. Other cells can also be present. If infection is suspected, a culture and susceptibility panel may be appropriate.

Generally, treatment for PO involves debridement of fluid filled lesions, as well as medical management with nonsteroidal anti-inflammatory medications, opioids, or anticonvulsants to manage post-operative pain [3].

Malformed Roots/Root Hypoplasia

The clinical appearance of teeth in the dog can be deceiving. Frequently, what lurks below the gumline can only be appreciated with diagnostic imaging. Root hypoplasia frequently has been found with patients who have also been diagnosed with enamel hypoplasia and infection with distemper [25] (Figure 7.11a and b). Many times these teeth are not mobile and do not yield any obvious

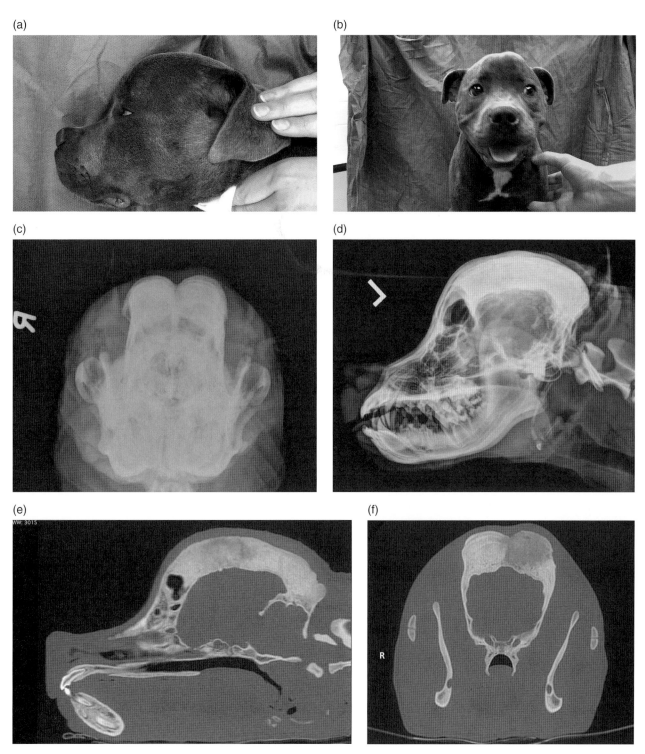

Figure 7.4 (a) Representative image of the head of a dog with idiopathic calvarial hyperostosis (ICH). Clinical appearance of this disease is an enlargement of the skull. The disease frequently affects the frontal, parietal, temporal, and occipital bones. In this image, there is suspicion of enlargement of both the frontal and parietal bones. (b) Representative image of the head of a dog with idiopathic calvarial hyperostosis (ICH). Note the asymmetry of the left side of the skull with enlargement and swelling of the frontal and parietal bones. (c) Rostrocaudal skull radiograph of the canine frontal sinus in a dog seen in Figure (a) and (b) affected with idiopathic calvarial hyperostosis (ICH). Note the increased mineral opacity on the region of the frontal sinus bilaterally. The left side appears to be mildly more affected. (d) Mediolateral projection of the skull of a dog affected by idiopathic calvarial hyperostosis. This is the same dog as seen in Figure (a)–(c). Note the diffuse thickening and sclerosis of the calvarium. (e) Sagittal plane computed tomographic image of the same dog in Figure (a)–(d) affected with idiopathic calvarial hyperostosis. Diffuse thickening and sclerosis of the calvarium is more clearly evident in the computed tomographic image than in the skull radiograph in Figure (d). (f) Transverse plane tomographic image of same dog in Figure (a)–(e) affected with idiopathic calvarial hyperostosis. Note the right side of the frontal bone is more sclerotic compared to the seemingly more clinically affected left side as seen in Figure (b). Appreciate how there is subjectively more soft tissue swelling associated with the left side when compared to the right side. *Source:* Courtesy of Bart Van Goethem, DVM, PhD, Diplomate ECVS, Ghent University.

(a) (b)

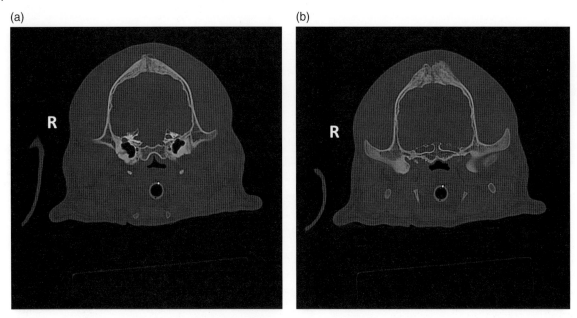

Figure 7.5 (a) Transverse plane computed tomographic image of a dog diagnosed with idiopathic calvarial hyperostosis. Note the thickening of the parietal bone at the level of the tympanic bulla. While both sides are affected, the left side is subjectively more thickened. (b) Transverse plane computed tomographic image of the same dog in Figure (a) affected with idiopathic calvarial hyperostosis. This slice is taken at the caudal aspect of the temporomandibular joint. Note the thickening of the parietal bone of both the right and left side, with obvious bony proliferation and hyperattenuation of the affected bone. *Source:* Courtesy of Julius M. Liptak, BVSc, MVetClinStud, FANZCVSc, DACVS-SA, DECVS, ACVS Founding Fellow, Surgical Oncology, ACVS Founding Fellow, Oral and Maxillofacial Surgery, RCVS Specialist in Surgical Oncology, Capital City Specialty & Emergency Animal Hospital.

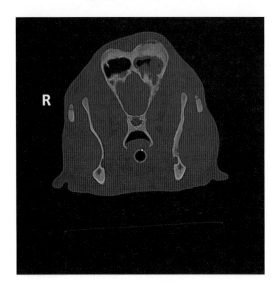

Figure 7.6 Transverse plane computed tomographic image of the same dog as seen in Figure 7.5 (a) and (b) affected with idiopathic calvarial hyperostosis. Note the bilateral thickening of the frontal bone. There is asymmetry of the thickening with the left side more affected than the right. Also note the thickening of the sinus mucosa associated with the left side, consistent with a concurrent sinusitis in this patient. *Source:* Courtesy of Julius M. Liptak, BVSc, MVetClinStud, FANZCVSc, DACVS-SA, DECVS, ACVS Founding Fellow, Surgical Oncology, ACVS Founding Fellow, Oral and Maxillofacial Surgery, RCVS Specialist in Surgical Oncology, Capital City Specialty & Emergency Animal Hospital.

signs of disease. Once there becomes radiographic or clinical evidence of disease, extraction is the recommended treatment.

Dens Invaginatus/Dens in Dente

Dens invaginatus also known as dens in dente, or tooth within a tooth, is a developmental abnormality of the tooth that is characterized by multiple invaginations of the tooth structure into the pulp of the tooth [26]. These invaginations result in a malformed tooth by creating infoldings of the enamel within the dentin with a formation of an area of dead space [27] (Figure 7.12a–c). While the exact etiology for this condition is unknown, there is suspicion pulp pathology may be a contributing factor [28, 29]. Both the crown and/or the root can be affected [27].

Radiographically, dens invaginatus may have the appearance of grooving of the enamel that coincides with the entrance into an invagination in the dentin [30]. A more complex appearing pulp morphology, infoldings of tooth structure appearing separate from the pulp, or an abrupt shift in the border of a pulp chamber or horn may also be observed [30] (Figure 7.13a and b). Lesions may also be barely noticeable, necessitating multiple radiographic views [30].

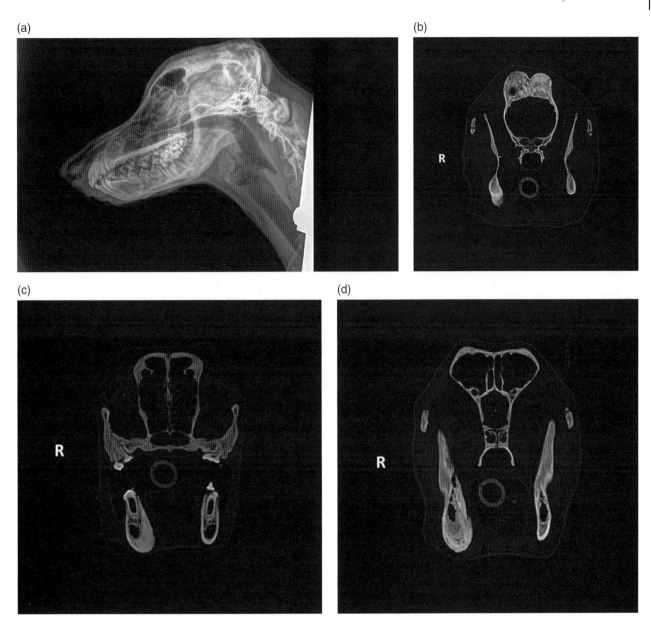

Figure 7.7 (a) Lateral skull radiograph of a 6.5-month-old intact German Shepherd dog who presented for a waxing and waning firm bony mass present on his head. Note the swelling associated with the parietal and occipital bones/regions of the skull. There also appears to be thickening of the mandibular cortex in this image as well, although it is difficult to ascertain which mandible may be affected. Because this patient had both the calvarium and the mandible affected, it was difficult to distinguish if it was affected with both idiopathic calvarial hyperostosis and/or craniomandibular osteopathy. Since treatment for both conditions are similar, a definitive diagnosis may not be required. (b) Transverse plane computed tomographic image of the juvenile dog with a swelling associated with the head as seen in Figure (a). Note on this image there appears to be thickening of the caudal aspect of the ventral mandibular cortex on the right side. There is also smooth osseous proliferation along the dorsum of the right frontal bone and calvarium. The osseous proliferation is overall heterogenous with regions of patchy decrease in mineral attenuation. (c) Transverse plane computed tomographic image of the juvenile dog with a swelling associated with the head as seen in Figure (a) and (b). Note on this image there appears to be significant thickening of the caudal aspect of the ventral mandibular cortex. The smoothly marginated dense osseous proliferation is present along the ventral mandibular cortex of the caudal right mandible. The proliferation is most prominent ventrally and medially. The left mandible is normal. (d) Transverse plane computed tomographic image of the juvenile dog with a swelling associated with the head as seen in Figure (a)–(c). There is smoothly marginated dense osseous proliferation which is present focally along the margins of the caudal right mandible, at the level of the ramus.

(a) (b)

(c) (d)

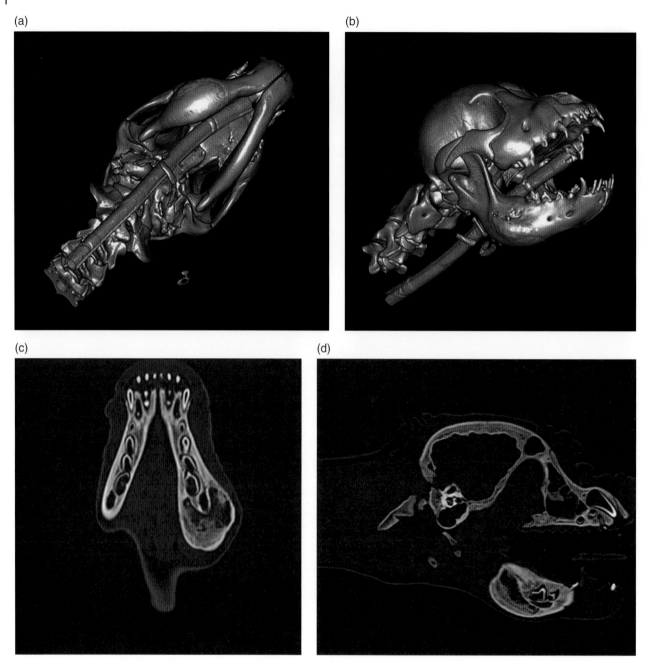

Figure 7.8 (a) Tridimensional (3D) reconstructed computed tomographic image of the right mandible from a dog diagnosed with periostitis ossificans. Note the increased thickness of the right mandible as observed from the ventrodorsal view. (b) Tridimensional (3D) reconstructed computed tomographic image of a dog diagnosed with periostitis ossificans (PO). Note the thickening of the right mandible observed from a right lateral view. (c) Representative computed tomographic image of the head of a dog diagnosed with periostitis ossificans from a dorsoventral view. Note the expansile nature of the right mandible with a smooth cortical margin. (d) Computed tomographic image of the head of a dog diagnosed with periostitis ossificans from a sagittal view. Note the expansile nature of the right mandible with a smooth cortical margin. In this sagittal view you can also appreciate the unerupted teeth and the expansile nature of this condition.

(a)

(b)

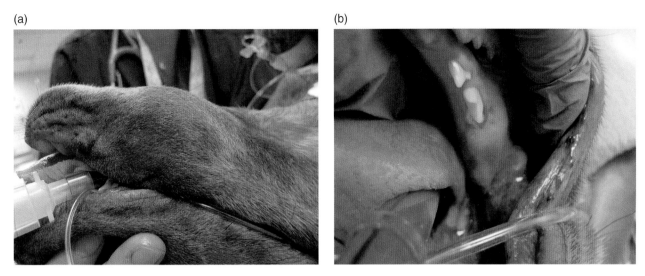

Figure 7.9   (a) Clinical image of a dog in dorsal recumbency diagnosed with periostitis ossificans. Observe the presence of swelling associated with the ventral mandible. The patient is intubated in the image. (b) Clinical image of the right mandible of a dog diagnosed with periostitis ossificans. Note the presence of a flocculent intraoral swelling within the area of the unerupted mandibular first molar. The blue gloved fingers in the image represent the thickness of the affected mandible.

(a)

(b)

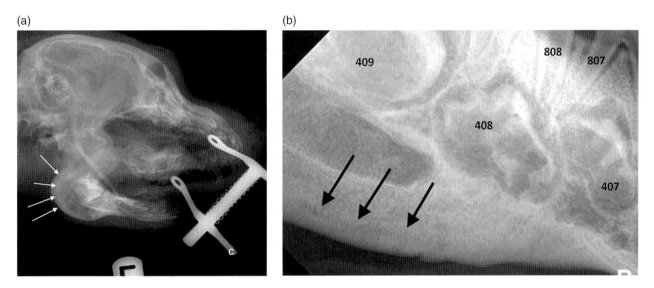

Figure 7.10   (a) Radiographic images of the skull of a dog diagnosed with periostitis ossificans (PO). Oblique skull radiograph demonstrating the mandibular swelling and radiolucent line (white arrows) illustrating the double cortex ventrally extending from the third or fourth premolars to beyond the last molar commonly associated with a patient diagnosed with periostitis ossificans. (b) Intraoral parallel dental radiograph of a dog diagnosed with periostitis ossificans demonstrating the double cortex at the ventral aspect of the mandible (black arrows) frequently observed in a juvenile patient diagnosed with periostitis ossificans. Note the unerupted permanent right mandibular 3rd and 4th premolars and 1st molar teeth labeled, 407, 408, and 409, respectively. Also note the distal root of the right mandibular deciduous 3rd premolar and mesial root of the deciduous right mandibular 4th premolar tooth, 807 and 808, respectively.

(a)

(b)

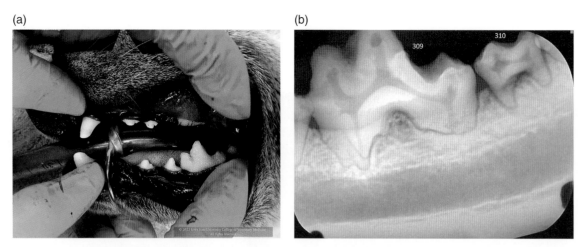

Figure 7.11 (a) Clinical image of the left maxilla of a five-year-old Australian cattle dog who presented for a history of enamel fractures that did not extend into the pulp. The dog was reluctant to chew on toys. (b) Intraoral radiographic image of the same five-year-old Australian Cattle dog seen in Figure (a). Note the malformation of the roots of both the left mandibular 1st and 2nd molar teeth (309, 310). The left mandibular 2nd molar tooth has an increased periodontal ligament space; therefore, this tooth warrants extraction. The left mandibular 1st molar tooth radiographically shows an irregular surface, but a somewhat normal appearing periodontal ligament space around the irregularly formed roots. Neither tooth was mobile. Recommendations for serial diagnostic and clinical monitoring of the affected teeth was given. *Source:* Courtesy of Dr. S. Kobiela, Casselton Veterinary Services Inc.

(a)

(b)

(c)

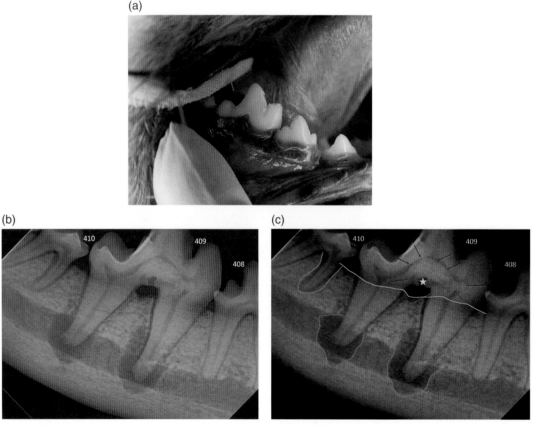

Figure 7.12 (a) Clinical image of the right mandible of a dog with evidence of an abnormality associated with the crown of the right mandibular first molar tooth. Note the area of suspected enamel loss near the furcation of this tooth. The patient was suspected to have dens invaginatus. (b) Intraoral radiographic image of the right mandible of a dog. Note the appearance of bone loss within the furcation area of this tooth. Also appreciate the increased complexity of the pulp chamber of this tooth. There are areas of increased mineralization present within the pulp chamber as well as an area of suspected tooth resorption. Additionally, both the mesial and distal roots of this tooth have evidence of periapical lucencies suspected to be endodontic disease from pulpitis associated with dens invaginatus. The mesial root of the right mandibular 2nd molar (410) has an increased periodontal ligament space as well. An additional image would need to be taken of this tooth, combined with the oral examination to identify whether this tooth may need to be addressed. (c) Intraoral radiographic image of the right mandible of a dog. Note the increased complexity of the pulp chamber of this tooth and areas of increased mineralization present within the pulp chamber (red arrows) as well as an area of suspected tooth resorption (yellow star). Both the mesial and distal roots of this tooth have evidence of periapical lucencies (blue outline) suspected to be endodontic disease from pulpitis associated with dens invaginatus. The orange line depicts the alveolar crest of bone, identifying the appearance of bone loss within the furcation area of this tooth. The mesial root of the right mandibular 2nd molar (410) has an increased periodontal ligament space (green outline).

Figure 7.13 (a) Intraoral radiographic image of the right mandible of a dog diagnosed with dens invaginatus. Note the multiple mineralized convolutions within the pulp chamber of the right mandibular 1st molar tooth (409). The right mandibular 2nd molar appears to be missing. (b) Intraoral radiographic image of the right mandible of a dog diagnosed with dens invaginatus. This is the same patient as seen in Figure (a). Note the multiple mineralized convolutions within the pulp chamber of the right mandibular 1st molar tooth (409), identified by the red arrows.

(a)

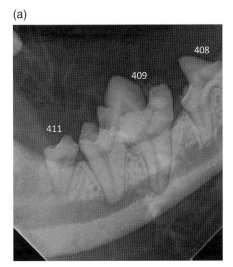

(b)

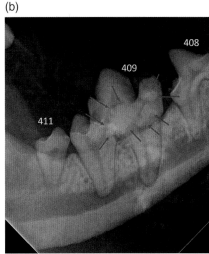

Diagnosis of this condition is based on the gross appearance, diagnostic imaging findings and ultimately, histopathology of the affected tooth/teeth. Histologically, enamel and cementum can be found within the pulp chamber [27]. The observance of irregular dentinal tubules as well as fewer dentinal tubules has also been observed [27].

Affected teeth are at increased risk of developing caries, periodontal disease, and endodontic disease [27] (Figures 7.14a–c and 7.15a–c). Treatment options for teeth affected with dens invaginatus commonly include extraction or endodontic therapy [27], although it has been speculated that the nature of the condition may complicate the success of root canal therapy if performed [29].

Uncommon Conditions Observed in both Canine and Feline Patients

Masticatory Myositis

Masticatory myositis is thought to be an autoimmune disorder in which the masticatory muscles swell and become painful. The masticatory muscles affected include the masseter, temporalis, and pterygoid muscles which are innervated by the mandibular branch of the trigeminal nerve. Patients affected with this condition typically present with an inability to open the mouth, swelling of the masticatory muscles, and extreme pain (Figure 7.16). Frequently, the clinical signs are present bilaterally, but if one side is more affected, there can be the appearance of unilateral disease [31]. Masticatory myositis can occur in any breed, but there is a predilection for large-breed dogs, including German shepherds and Labrador and Golden retrievers [31].

There are typically two phases of the disease characterized by an acute phase and a chronic phase. In the dog, during the acute phase, patients present with swelling of the masticatory muscles, pain in the jaw, and restricted range of jaw motion [32]. The restricted range of motion can also be seen as an overall inability to open the mouth, even when sedated or anesthetized [32]. This condition, left untreated, can progress to a chronic phase in which affected patients will present with significant atrophy of the masticatory muscles and fibrosis of the tissues. The fibrosis and atrophy restrict the range of motion even more dramatically. Additionally, there is also the description of a more slowly progressive myositis which does not present with an obviously acute, painful phase [32].

Diagnosis of masticatory myositis is frequently confirmed with a 2M antibody test which measures the circulating antibodies found within the blood. The myofibers found in masticatory muscles are primarily comprised of type 2M (masticatory) fibers [33]. Clinical signs that are consistent with masticatory myositis along with a positive 2M antibody test are confirmatory for a diagnosis of the disease. If immunosuppressive doses of corticosteroids have been administered to patients prior to 2M antibody testing, false-negative results can occur [31]. Additionally, patients in end-stage masticatory myositis who have significant fibrosis to the muscles and loss of myofibers may also have a false-negative 2M antibody result [31]. Biopsy and histopathology of the muscles of mastication is the best way to confirm a patient is affected by masticatory myositis [34].

Radiographic imaging of patients affected with masticatory myositis commonly includes use of computed tomography. The phase of the disease distinguishes whether there will be atrophy or swelling of the masticatory

(a)

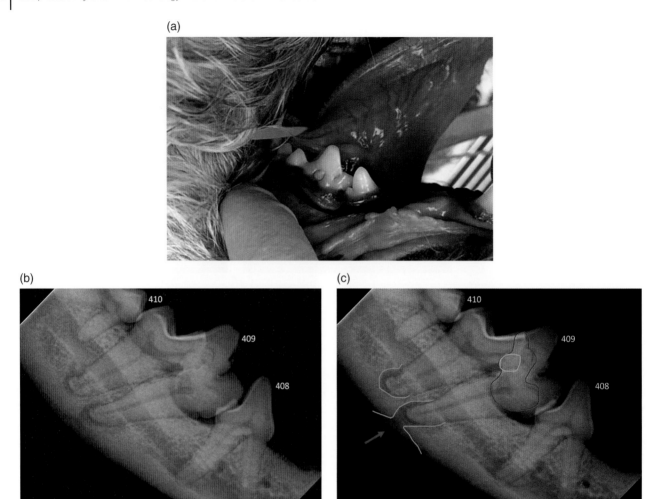

(b)

(c)

Figure 7.14 (a) Clinical image of the right mandible of a dog diagnosed with dens invaginatus. Note the circular area of depression within the crown at the level of the furcation. This is an enfolding of the enamel into the dentin. (b) Intraoral radiographic image of the right mandible of a dog diagnosed with dens invaginatus. This is the same patient as seen in Figure (a). The circular depression seen in Figure (a) can be observed within the pulp chamber of this tooth in the radiographic image. Note the periapical lucencies associated with the mesial and distal roots of this tooth as well as the disease extending to the ventral cortex of the mandible. There is mild horizontal bone loss associated with the mesial root of this tooth. (c) Intraoral radiographic image of the right mandible of a dog diagnosed with dens invaginatus. The circular depression seen in Figure 7.14a can be observed within the pulp chamber of the right mandibular 1st molar tooth in the radiographic image (yellow outline), along with the multiple mineralized convolutions (red outline). Note the periapical lucencies associated with the mesial and distal roots of this tooth (blue outlines) as well as the disease extending to the ventral cortex of the mandible (red arrow).

muscles [35] (Figure 7.17a and b). Frequently all masticatory muscles except for the digastricus show some evidence of change when affected with this condition [35]. Contrast enhancement of the temporalis, masseter, and pterygoid muscles with an heterogenous pattern can be observed [35] (Figures 7.18a, b, 7.19a, and b). Biopsy samples should be collected from areas with the greatest contrast enhancement for the best chance at an accurate diagnosis.

Treatment of this condition is aimed at aggressive immunosuppressive therapy [31]. Early recognition is paramount in diagnosing the disease, and aggressive immunosuppressive therapies are needed to help prevent irreversible jaw

dysfunction and muscle atrophy [31]. While this condition is predominately recognized in dogs, it has also been identified in cats [32].

Pulp Stones and Denticles

In the literature, there have been two different types of mineralized structures within the dental pulp of humans: denticles and pulp stones [36]. Denticles are thought to be a developmental abnormality in which an area of mineralization forms after an interaction between the pulp tissue and the epithelium [36]. Denticles are larger areas of

(a)

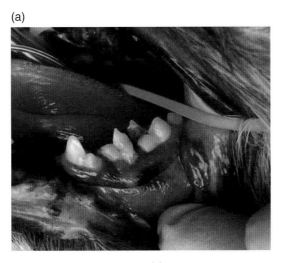

(b)

(c)

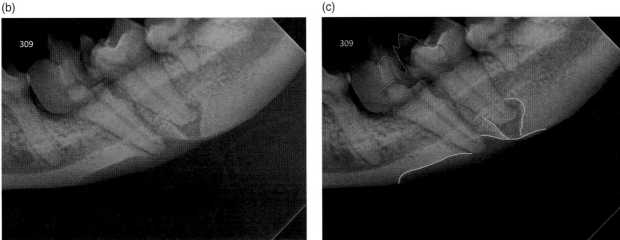

Figure 7.15 (a) Clinical image of the left mandible of a dog diagnosed with dens invaginatus. Note the significant resorption and decay of the left mandibular 1st molar tooth (309), which gives the appearance that the tooth is split. (b) Intraoral dental radiographic image of the left mandible of a dog diagnosed with dens invaginatus. This is the same patient as seen in Figure (a). Note the increased complexity and convolutions within the pulp chamber of the left mandibular 1st molar tooth (309). Also note the periapical lucency associated with both the mesial and distal roots affecting the ventral mandibular cortex. (c) Intraoral dental radiographic image of the left mandible of a dog diagnosed with dens invaginatus. This is the same patient as seen in Figure (a) and (b). Note the increased complexity and convolutions within the pulp chamber of the left mandibular 1st molar tooth (309) depicted by the red outline. The radiographically affected area of the periapical lucencies associated with the mesial and distal roots of the left mandibular 1st molar and the affected area of the ventral cortex leading to a draining tract of the ventral mandible are outlined by the yellow lines.

calcification within the pulp of the tooth. True denticles are rare calcifications that are composed of dentin, lined by odontoblasts [37].

Pulp stones are thought to be discrete areas of calcification or mineralization that form around a foci of calcified pulp components found within the pulp chamber or canal of a tooth [36, 37] (Figure 7.20a–d). Pulp stones are usually found in mature teeth. A pulp stone may form in response to chronic irritation within the pulp canal or chamber, depending on its location [37].

The clinical significance of a pulp stone or denticle is the alteration of the internal anatomy of the tooth. When endodontic therapy is necessary, navigation of the instruments, chemicals, and obturation materials around the calcification may make endodontic treatment more difficult or potentially impossible, depending on the size and location of the obstruction.

Osteosclerosis

Osteosclerosis is a developmental variant of the normal bony architecture that forms within the jaw [38]. Lesions can be associated with a specific root or be a distinct entity away from the root [39] (Figures 7.21a, b, 7.22a, and b).

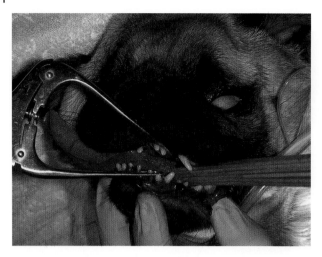

Figure 7.16 Clinical image of a three-year-old, castrated male Pug who presented with progressive increased difficulty upon opening his mouth. Upon sedated examination, the extent in which the mouth could be opened is demonstrated in the photograph. This can present a challenge especially in brachycephalic patients. Note the stacked tongue depressors in the photograph which have been historically used in attempt to increase the extent to which the mouth can be opened. Caution must be used when using the rodent mouth gag so as not to damage or fracture the teeth.

Radiographically, a well-circumscribed lesion within the bone is observed [40]. The lesions are commonly seen near the compact bone of the ventral mandible. Their appearance is frequently found to vary from round to elliptical or irregular in shape [40]. The formation of these radiodense areas appear to be unrelated to any local stimulus or inflammation [38]. Lesions can form at any point in an animal's life. The mineralized lesions can persist for many years or even indefinitely but rarely require treatment. Generally, they are asymptomatic, and no etiological agent is found [40]. If there is no evidence of endodontic disease or periodontal disease, a presumptive diagnosis of osteosclerosis can be considered [39]. Conservative monitoring with serial diagnostic images is recommended to evaluate whether changes occur over time (Figure 7.23a–c).

Renal Secondary Hyperparathyroidism

Renal secondary hyperparathyroidism is an endocrinopathy that is frequently associated with dogs and cats diagnosed with chronic kidney disease [41]. Renal insufficiency or impairment can result in phosphate accumulation, a reduction of vitamin D, and a reduction in calcium [42]. When this occurs, it leads to

(a)

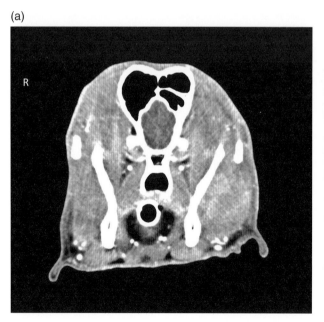

(b)

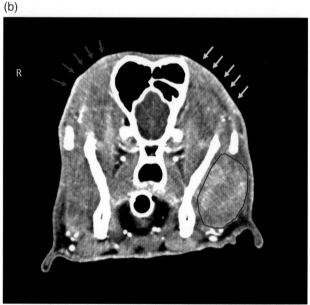

Figure 7.17 (a) Transverse computed tomographic image of an 11-month-old mixed breed dog with a four-week history of a painful jaw and inability to grip a tennis ball. Note the heterogenous contrast enhancement identified throughout the temporalis musculature bilaterally. The enhancement is more prominent on the masseter muscle of the left side and extends through the muscle fibers at the level of the caudal ramus. (b) Transverse computed tomographic image of an 11-month-old mixed breed dog with a four-week history of a painful jaw and inability to grip a tennis ball. Note the heterogenous contrast enhancement identified throughout the temporalis musculature bilaterally. The left side (yellow arrows) demonstrate the increased contrast enhancement and the muscle atrophy that is present. The right-side temporalis muscle appears to have mild swelling (red arrows). The heterogenous contrast enhancement is more prominent on the left masseter muscle outlined in red. There also appears to be swelling associated with this muscle.

(a)

(b)

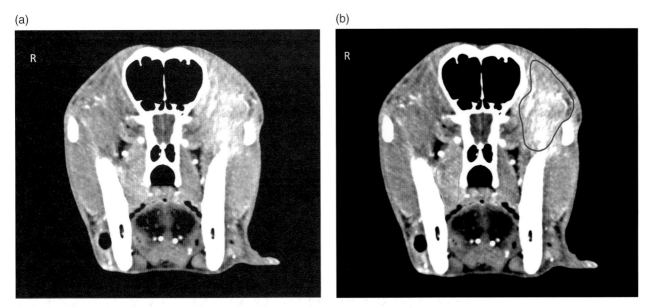

Figure 7.18 (a) Transverse computed tomographic image of the same 11-month-old mixed breed dog with a four-week history of a painful jaw and inability to grip a tennis ball as seen a few slices more caudally than seen in Figure 7.17 (a) and (b). Note the heterogenous, streaking contrast enhancement identified in the right medial pterygoid musculature. The left temporalis exhibits marked streaking enhancement. (b) Transverse computed tomographic image of the same 11-month-old mixed breed dog with a four-week history of a painful jaw and inability to grip a tennis ball taken a few slices caudally from the images in Figure 7.17 (a) and (b). The affected right medial pterygoid muscle is identified with the yellow outline. The left temporalis exhibits marked streaking enhancement, outlined in red.

(a)

(b)

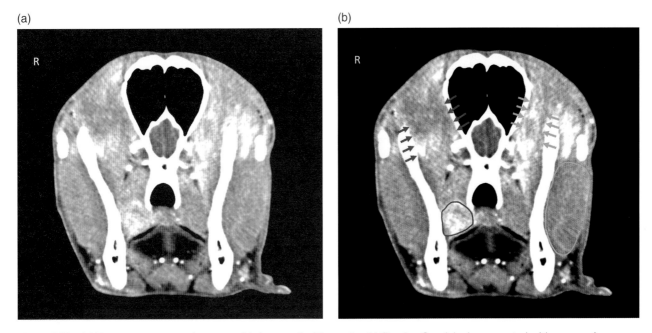

Figure 7.19 (a) Transverse computed tomographic image of a 10-month-old Clumber Spaniel who presented with progressive trismus. The image demonstrates the temporalis muscles are moderately asymmetrical with the right side being mildly larger than the left side. Similarly, the masseter muscles are also asymmetric with the left side being mildly larger than the right side. The right medial pterygoid muscle is also moderately heterogeneously contrast enhancing. (b) Transverse computed tomographic image of a 10-month-old Clumber Spaniel who presented with progressive trismus. The image demonstrates the temporalis muscles are moderately asymmetrical with the right side (between red arrows) being mildly larger than the left side (between green arrows). Similarly, the masseter muscles are also asymmetric with the left side (outlined in yellow) being mildly larger than the right side. The right medial pterygoid muscle is also moderately heterogeneously contrast enhancing outlined in red.

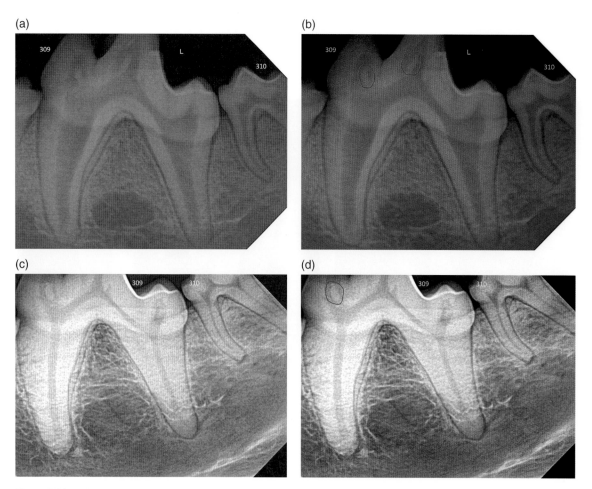

Figure 7.20 (a) Intraoral radiographic image of the left mandible of a 12-month-old English Springer Spaniel. Note the areas of increased mineralization within the mesial and middle pulp horns of the left mandibular 1st molar tooth (309). These calcifications are consistent with pulp stones. (b) Intraoral radiographic image of the left mandible of a 12-month-old English Springer Spaniel. Note the areas of increased mineralization within the mesial and middle pulp horns of the left mandibular 1st molar tooth (309), consistent with pulp stones (outlined in red). (c) Intraoral radiograph of the same dog as seen in Figure (a) and (b), five years later. Note how the size of the pulp stones within the pulp horns have not increased or decreased in size. The pulp chamber of the tooth has continued to decrease in size as would be expected in the normal aging process in a vital tooth. (d) Intraoral radiograph of the same dog as seen in Figure (a) and (b), five years later. Note how the size of the pulp stones within the pulp horns have not increased or decreased in size (pulp stone in mesial pulp horn outlined in red).

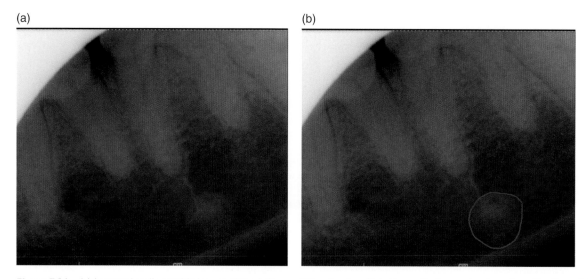

Figure 7.21 (a) Intraoral radiographic image of the left mandible of a dog. Note the radiodense circular mineralization within the mandibular canal just dorsal to compact bone of the mandible. The bony lesion is not associated with a tooth root. While there is some suspicion of replacement resorption associated with the mesial and distal roots of the left mandibular 4th premolar tooth, the circumscribed lesion does not appear to be associated with any of the roots, making it more likely to be diagnosed as osteosclerosis. (b) Intraoral radiographic image of the left mandible of a dog. Note the radiodense circular mineralization within the mandibular canal just dorsal to compact bone of the mandible, outlined in red. The circumscribed lesion does not appear to be associated with any of the roots, making it more likely to be diagnosed as osteosclerosis.

Figure 7.22 (a) Intraoral radiographic image of the left mandible of a dog. Note the radiodense irregular mineralization associated with the mesial surface of the distal root of the left mandibular 4th premolar tooth (308). While this bony lesion appears to be directly connected to the distal root, note how a clear periodontal ligament space can be appreciated between the lesion and the root of the tooth, making this less likely to be associated with inflammation of the tooth, and more likely to be diagnosed as osteosclerosis. (b) Intraoral radiographic image of the left mandible of a dog. Note the radiodense irregular mineralization associated with the mesial surface of the distal root of the left mandibular 4th premolar tooth (308), outlined in red.

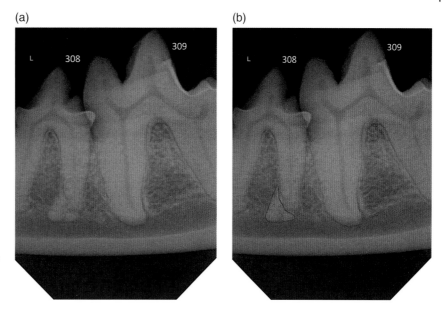

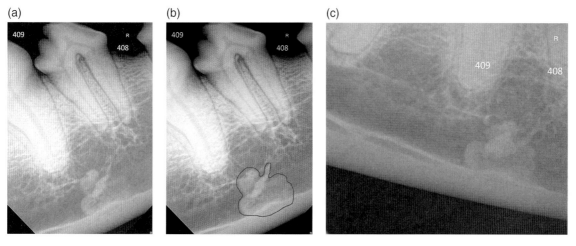

Figure 7.23 (a) Intraoral radiographic image of the right mandible of a dog. Note the very irregular radiodense area closely associated with the dorsal surface of the compact bone of the mandible. The lesion does not appear to be associated with any of the roots present within the image. Note the smooth ventral mandibular cortex of the mandible. (b) Intraoral radiographic image of the right mandible of a dog. Note the very irregular radiodense area closely associated with the dorsal surface of the compact bone of the mandible outlined in red. (c) Intraoral radiographic image of the right mandible of a dog. Note the very irregular radiodense area closely associated with the dorsal surface of the compact bone of the mandible. This image was taken three years following the initial images seen in Figure (a) and (b). Note there is no change in the appearance of the lesion and the ventral mandibular cortex is still smooth.

hyperparathyroidism with subsequent renal osteodystrophy [41]. The osteodystrophy results in weakening of the bones from the abnormal calcium and phosphorus concentrations related to the loss of kidney function. Clinically and radiographically, demineralization of the bones of the maxilla and mandible can be seen as well as pathologic jaw fractures and mobile teeth [41]. Exfoliation of the teeth due to excessive bone loss can also be observed [42], along with jaw and facial enlargement [43].

When bone is affected by renal hyperparathyroidism, there are two main presentations: hyperostotic osteodystrophy and isostotic osteodystrophy [42]. Hyperostotic osteodystrophy is more common in young dogs and presents as an abnormal increased growth or the appearance of swelling of the affected bones of the maxilla and mandible [42]. This is from fibrous osteodystrophy, a condition in which the bone becomes demineralized and is replaced by fibrous tissue [41]. Isostotic osteodystrophy is more frequently seen in older animals and is referred to as "rubber jaw" [42]. Due to the slow onset of disease progression in older animals, the size of the affected bones is normal although the bones themselves palpate more softened and pliable, giving the appearance of rubber.

The alveolar bone and cancellous bone of the mandible are more predisposed to demineralization than other bones of the body [44]. Abnormalities in these bones are appreciated earlier than abnormalities in the appendicular skeleton [44].

Radiographically, focal or generalized bone loss can be observed [41]. Fibrous osteodystrophy can appear radiographically as an expansion of the bone and replacement of the bone with a "homogenous, ground glass" density [41]. Additionally, the normal dentoalveolar structures including but not limited to the alveolar bone, lamina dura, and cortical bone of the ventral mandible are indistinct [41] (Figure 7.24a–c). The description of floating teeth has been used to depict the appearance of teeth within the bone of affected patients [41]. Decreased mineralization of the alveolar bone is frequently observed.

Clinically, periodontal probing depths do not appear to be excessive, although there is generally excessive mobility of the teeth in the affected jaws. Tooth resorption can also be seen with patients affected with renal secondary hyperparathyroidism [45] (Figure 7.25a–c).

Treatment of renal secondary hyperparathyroidism is aimed at controlling or treating the secondary hyperparathyroidism as well as treating the renal disease. Unfortunately, patients who have kidneys that are severely damaged can

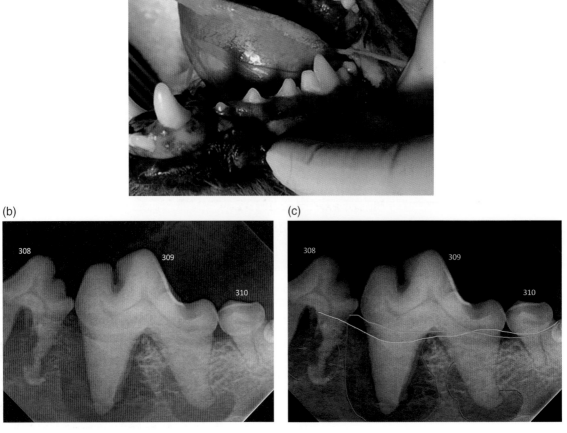

Figure 7.24 (a) Clinical image of the left mandible of a dog diagnosed with renal secondary hyperparathyroidism. Note the presence of all mandibular premolar teeth and the lack of inflammation and gross evidence of attachment loss associated with the teeth in the image. (b) Intraoral radiographic image of the left mandible of the patient seen in Figure (a) diagnosed with renal secondary hyperparathyroidism. Note how the left mandibular 1st molar tooth appears to have a relatively normal appearing alveolar margin height on both the lingual and buccal surfaces. Observe the lucency surrounding both the mesial and distal apices of the left mandibular first molar tooth (309) and the distal root of the left mandibular 4th premolar tooth (308). Also note the significant appearance of resorption associated with the distal root of 308. (c) Intraoral radiographic image of the left mandible of the patient seen in Figure (a) and (b). The left mandibular 1st molar tooth (309) appears to have a relatively normal appearing alveolar margin height on both the lingual and buccal surfaces (yellow and green lines). Observe the lucency (red outlines) surrounding both the mesial and distal surfaces of the left mandibular first molar tooth (309) and the distal root of the left mandibular 4th premolar tooth (308) (red outlines). Also note the appearance of resorption associated with the distal root of 308 (red arrows).

(a)

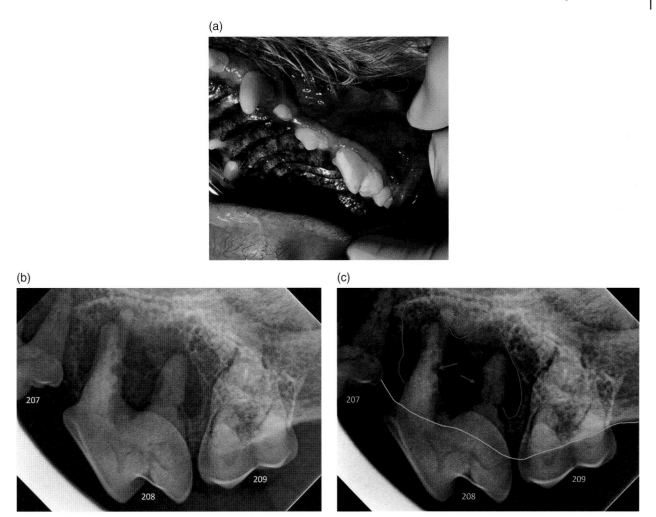

(b)   (c)

Figure 7.25 (a) Clinical image of the left maxilla of a dog diagnosed with renal secondary hyperparathyroidism. This is the same patient as seen in Figure 7.24 (a)–(c). Again, appreciate how there is no obvious inflammation or gross evidence of attachment loss associated with the teeth in the image. (b) Intraoral radiographic image of the left maxilla of a dog diagnosed with renal secondary hyperparathyroidism. Note the periapical lucency associated with the mesial and distal roots of the left maxillary 4th premolar tooth (208). There is also radiographic evidence of tooth resorption associated with the mesial and distal roots. Most appreciable is the normal appearing alveolar margin height of bone. (c) Intraoral radiographic image of the left maxilla of a dog diagnosed with renal secondary hyperparathyroidism. The periapical lucencies associated with the mesial and distal roots of the left maxillary 4th premolar (208) are outlined in red. There is also radiographic evidence of tooth resorption associated with the mesial and distal roots (red arrows). Most appreciable is the normal appearing alveolar margin height of bone (yellow line).

have a poor prognosis as returning them to normal function can be difficult. Management of affected teeth is based on response to treatment and resolution of the primary disease.

Enamel Pearls

A focal area of excess enamel on the surface of a tooth is described as an enamel pearl. While a fairly rare occurrence, it is a developmental abnormality that is most commonly appreciated in the furcation area of a multirooted tooth [46] (Figure 7.26). Frequently, the excess enamel deposition surrounds a core of dentin, and occasionally pulp tissue as well [47]. Depending on the location of the enamel pearl, local

periodontal destruction can be observed, predisposing the tooth to plaque retention, inflammation, and attachment loss.

Uncommon Conditions with Predilection for Feline Patients

Dentition Abnormalities

Abnormalities of the dentition in cats can include size and shape of the tooth, absence of a tooth, and position of the tooth within the jaw, all of which can affect occlusion. Dentition abnormalities are a rare occurrence in cats, with the absence of the maxillary second premolar teeth being

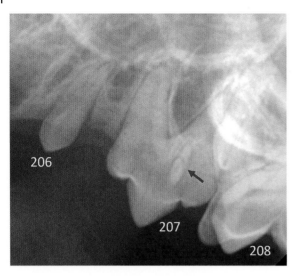

Figure 7.26 Intraoral radiographic image of the left maxilla of a cat. There is a focal area of increased mineralization within the crown of the left maxillary 3rd premolar tooth (207). The location of this mineralization and its position near the furcation would make the mineralization consistent with an enamel pearl.

cats found the maxillary second premolar to be bilaterally absent in only five of 155 cats [49]. It is worth mentioning that even though a tooth is missing, it may not be from a congenital abnormality. The tooth may be clinically missing for other reasons such as extraction or end-stage tooth resorption. However, end-stage tooth resorption can typically be recognized as such on radiographs (Figure 7.27a and b).

The size of teeth in cats typically remains uniform from patient to patient. Larger teeth may be present in larger patients and vice versa; the size of the teeth coincide with the size of the patient. More commonly seen are variations in sizes of the maxillary second premolar.

Other abnormalities such as fused roots (Figure 7.28a and b), supernumerary roots and teeth (Figures 3.55e, 7.29a, and b), and abnormal eruption or position of teeth are also rare findings in cat dentition when comparing these findings to dogs (Figures 3.55a–d, 3.56a, b, 3.57a, b, 3.58c, d, and 7.30).

one of the more common abnormalities that can arise. Two studies have shown the maxillary second premolar to be absent in 7.9% of one population and 16.8% of another population of cats that were evaluated [48, 49]. If a tooth is missing from a congenital disorder, either side (left or right) may be affected. A study that examined domestic

Fused Roots

Fused roots in cats are rare, but when seen, the most common teeth to exhibit fusion are the maxillary second premolars and first molars. The maxillary second premolar is typically known to be a one-rooted tooth, but occasionally fusion of a primary and supernumerary root will be present. This can be difficult to see radiographically, but when

(a)

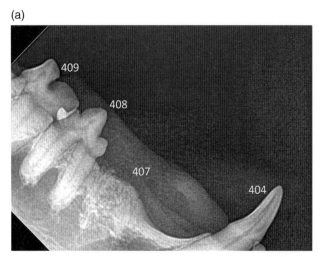

(b)

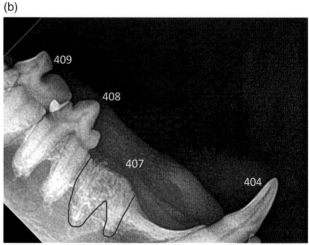

Figure 7.27 (a) Intraoral radiograph of the right mandible of a cat. Note the missing crown of the right mandibular 3rd premolar tooth (407). On conscious and anesthetized oral examination, this tooth would appear to be clinically missing. Only when dental radiographs are taken does there appear to be evidence of a tooth present below the gumline. This tooth was affected by end stage tooth resorption. Note the lack of a periodontal ligament space as well as the indistinct root structure associated with this tooth. (b) Intraoral radiograph of the right mandible of a cat. Note the missing crown of the right mandibular 3rd premolar tooth (407). This is the same image as in Figure (a). The red line depicts the mesial and distal roots of the right mandibular 3rd premolar tooth affected by end stage tooth resorption.

(a)

(b)

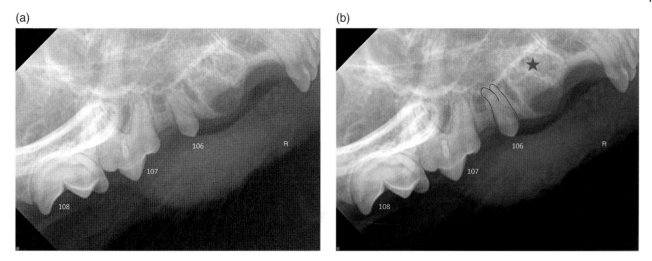

Figure 7.28 (a) Intraoral radiograph of the right maxilla of a cat. Note the right maxillary 2nd premolar tooth (106) has the appearance of a wider root. There is a separation of the roots at the very apical aspect of the tooth. Also note the mineralized opacity associated with the crown of the right maxillary 3rd premolar tooth (107). This is suspected to be an enamel pearl. (b) Intraoral radiograph of the right maxilla of a cat. Note the right maxillary 2nd premolar tooth (106) has the appearance of a wider root. The separation of the two roots is outlined in red. The mineralized opacity within the crown of the right maxillary 3rd premolar tooth is suspected to be an enamel pearl (outlined in yellow). A red star indicates a missing right maxillary canine tooth.

(a)

(b)

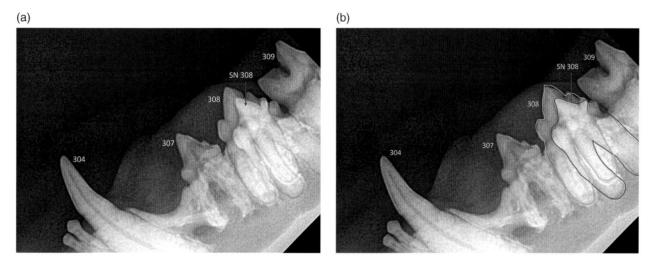

Figure 7.29 (a) Intraoral radiograph of the left mandible of a cat. Note the superimposition of two teeth in the location of the left mandibular 4th premolar tooth (308). Also note the evidence of tooth resorption associated with the left mandibular 3rd premolar tooth (307). (b) Intraoral radiograph of the left mandible of a cat. Note the superimposition of two teeth in the location of the left mandibular 4th premolar tooth (308). One tooth is outlined in yellow as it appears to be in alignment with the surrounding teeth within the arcade. This tooth is thought to be the left mandibular 4th premolar tooth (308). An additional tooth is outlined in red. This tooth, based on the radiograph, is thought to be the supernumerary left mandibular 4th premolar tooth (SN 308).

present, the tooth will appear to have a wider root. Fusion would likely only be seen when clinically looking at the tooth, in the event of an extraction for example. The maxillary first molar tooth is very small and considered to be two-rooted. A study found this tooth to have partially fused roots in 34.7% of the examined cat population [49].

Radiographically, fused roots will appear as one larger root. There may also be a separation of the roots at the root tips giving the appearance of two root tips (Figure 7.28a and b). Radiographically, it can be difficult to appreciate either fused roots or two separate roots of the maxillary first molar tooth. This is due to the position of the tooth

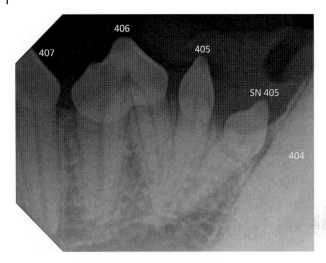

Figure 7.30 Intraoral radiograph of the right mandible of a dog. Note the two, identical, single rooted teeth just distal to the mandibular canine tooth. Both teeth have the clinical appearance of mandibular 1st premolar teeth.

and angulation that is necessary to acquire the image. Additionally, endodontic disease or bone loss of this particular tooth can be very difficult to discern at times because the tooth is so small (Figure 7.31a–c). Clinical findings on oral examination are necessary to aid in formulating an appropriate treatment plan.

Supernumerary Roots

The maxillary third premolar is the most common tooth to exhibit a supernumerary root but is still an uncommon finding in cats (Figure 7.32a and b). A study examining a population of domestic cats showed 10.3% of cats to have a supernumerary root associated with this tooth [49]. The supernumerary root usually lies between the normal mesial and distal root and can be much smaller (Figure 7.33a and b). Occasionally, the cusp of the additional tooth can be seen clinically.

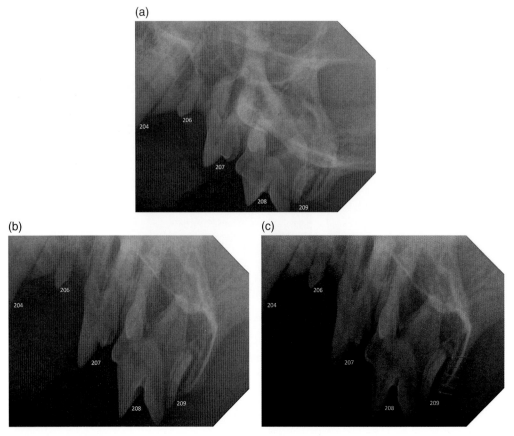

Figure 7.31 (a) Intraoral radiograph of the left maxilla of a cat. Note how the zygomatic arch is superimposed over the maxillary 1st molar tooth making it difficult to assess if there is any disease present. The small size of this tooth and the superimposition of the overlying bone and distal root of the maxillary 4th premolar tooth make it difficult to interpret if there is disease present. Clinical observation and assessment of this tooth is necessary as well as variation of the bisecting angle trying to reduce superimposition of overlying structures on this tooth. (b) Intraoral radiograph of the left maxilla of a cat. Variation of the bisecting angle trying to reduce superimposition of overlying structures on this tooth may be necessary to assist in interpretation of disease. Note in this image how elongation of the image moves the zygomatic arch off the distoapical aspect of the tooth, allowing the increased periodontal ligament space to be better appreciated. (c) Intraoral radiograph of the left maxilla of a cat. Variation of the bisecting angle trying to reduce superimposition of overlying structures on this tooth was necessary to assist in interpretation of disease. The red arrows identify the increased periodontal ligament space associated with the left maxillary 1st molar tooth (209).

(a) (b)

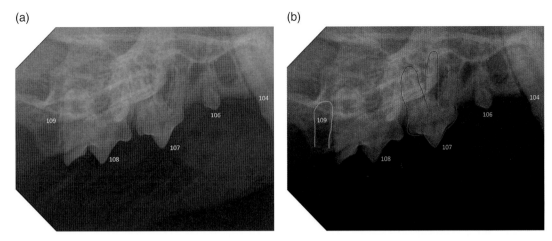

Figure 7.32 (a) Intraoral radiograph of the right maxilla of a cat. Note the presence of a 3rd root extending from the furcation of the right maxillary 3rd premolar tooth (107). There is also an empty alveolus of the right maxillary 1st molar tooth (109). (b) Intraoral radiograph of the right maxilla of a cat. Note the presence of a 3rd root extending from the furcation of the right maxillary 3rd premolar tooth (107) outlined in red. Also note the empty alveolus of the right maxillary 1st molar tooth (109) outlined in yellow.

(a) (b)

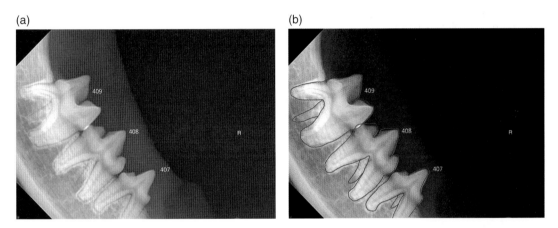

Figure 7.33 (a) Intraoral radiographic image of the right mandible of a cat. Note how all teeth in the image appear to have a supernumerary root. (b) Intraoral radiographic image of the right mandible of a cat. All three teeth in the image have evidence of a smaller supernumerary root extending from the furcation area of the tooth. This cat had multiple arcades with supernumerary roots present.

Supernumerary Teeth

Supernumerary teeth are additional teeth that have developed beyond the normal dental formula. This is rare in cats, but if observed, there will likely be crowding of the associated teeth (Figures 7.34, 7.35a, and b).

Abnormal Eruption

Abnormal eruption of teeth in cats is rare, but when seen it is frequently associated with the maxillary canine teeth being in a mesioverted position (Figure 7.36). This means the cusp of the tooth is deviated toward the cat's nose or toward midline. This abnormality causes a malocclusion, whereby the mesioverted tooth creates abnormal contact with another tooth. The teeth typically have a normal structure; however, the roots may be in a different location. This information is important if extraction is the anticipated treatment for the abnormally positioned tooth causing trauma.

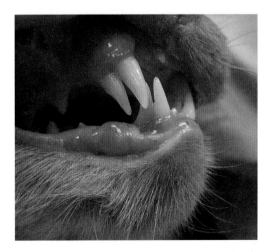

Figure 7.34 Clinical image of an adult cat with both supernumerary maxillary and mandibular canine teeth bilaterally. Note how the teeth are identical in size, shape, and color, indicating no evidence the teeth are deciduous in nature. (See Figure 3.16e for comparison.)

(a)

(b)

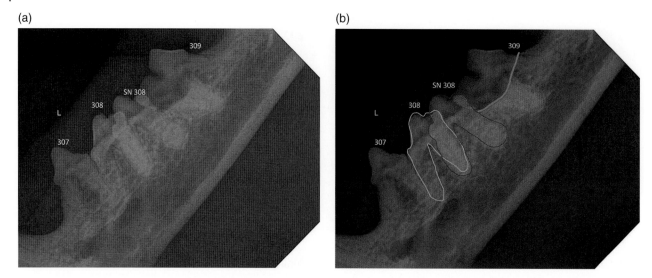

Figure 7.35 (a) Intraoral radiographic image of the left mandible of a cat. Note how there are two teeth superimposed or telescoped on each other in the region of the left mandibular 4th premolar tooth (308). Also appreciate the loss of the periodontal ligament space associated with the left mandibular 3rd premolar tooth (307). Additionally, there is horizontal bone loss associated with the mesial root of the left mandibular 1st molar tooth (309). (b) Intraoral radiographic image of the left mandible of a cat. Note how there are two teeth superimposed or telescoped on each other in the region of the left mandibular 4th premolar tooth (308). The left mandibular 4th premolar tooth is outlined in yellow (308), while the supernumerary left mandibular 4th premolar is outlined in red (SN 308). This image also demonstrates horizontal bone loss associated with the mesial root of the left mandibular 1st molar tooth (409) identified by the blue lines.

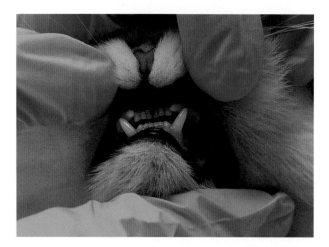

Figure 7.36 Mesioversion of the right and left maxillary canine teeth (104, 204) causing the mandibular canine teeth to be in an abnormal position. When the cat's mouth is completely closed the mandibular canine teeth will make slight contact with the maxillary canine on either side.

Unerupted Teeth

Unerupted teeth are much less common in cats than in dogs. This abnormality arises from a defect in the eruption process and can occur as a natural event, from trauma, or infection that may have occurred in the area of the unerupted tooth. Any tooth can be affected, as there is no predilection for certain teeth to be affected as is seen in the dog. Radiographically, the tooth will be completely encased within the bone and clinically no crown will be visible. There may be evidence of resorption of the tooth depending on how old the animal is and how long the tooth has been encased within the bone (Figure 7.37a and b).

Patellar Fracture and Dental Anomaly Syndrome (PADS) or Knees and Teeth Syndrome

Knees and Teeth Syndrome or Patellar Fracture and Dental Anomaly Syndrome (PADS) is a rare condition that affects young adult cats. The syndrome is described as cats who present with transverse fractures of the proximal aspect or base of the patella with no evidence of trauma to this region [50]. The condition commonly affects both patellas with a mean interval of only three months between the fractures [50]. The radiographic features of the patella fracture appear to demonstrate evidence of sclerosis with a loss of trabecular structure and lack of definition between the cortex and the medulla of the bones [50].

(a)

(b)

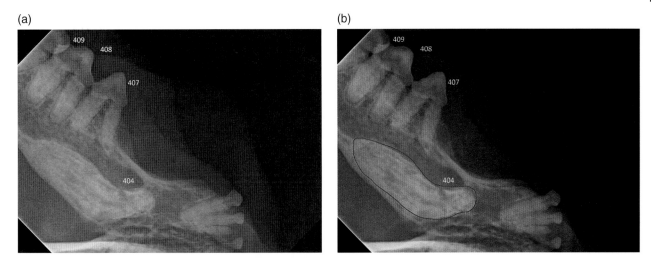

Figure 7.37   (a) Intraoral radiographic image of the right mandible of a cat. This image demonstrates an unerupted right mandibular canine tooth (404). Notice the abnormal shape of the tooth and evidence of resorption as indicated by the moth-eaten appearance of the tooth. (b) Intraoral radiographic image of the right mandible of a cat. This image demonstrates an unerupted right mandibular canine tooth (404) outlined in red.

Interestingly, this condition also frequently affects the oral cavity of the cat. Oral manifestations commonly seen with this syndrome include the presence of persistent deciduous teeth and missing teeth both clinically and radiographically because of a developmental abnormality [51]. Other oral abnormalities observed include malformation of the root structures and unerupted permanent teeth [51]. Affected cats also frequently have swelling associated with the skull. Lesions can appear as solid periosteal proliferations without the radiographic appearance of an aggressive process [51].

Clinically, cats present with the dental abnormalities previously noted, swelling of the maxilla or mandible and lameness associated with the fracture(s) of the patella. Histopathology of the swellings associated with the skull frequently are consistent with a diagnosis of osteomyelitis [51]. The majority of cases are treated with antibiotics and nonsteroidal pain medication. While initial improvement can be seen with symptomatic treatment of the clinical signs of osteomyelitis and pain, resolution of signs with medical management of the condition is uncommon [51]. Histopathology is recommended to differentiate this disease from other more aggressive neoplastic processes [51]. Treatment with antimicrobials is recommended for addressing the osteomyelitis [51]. Surgical debridement of the proliferative lesions and extraction of any persistent deciduous and/or unerupted permanent teeth is associated with a better clinical outcome for these patients [51] (Figures 7.38a–f, 7.39a, b, and 7.40a–c).

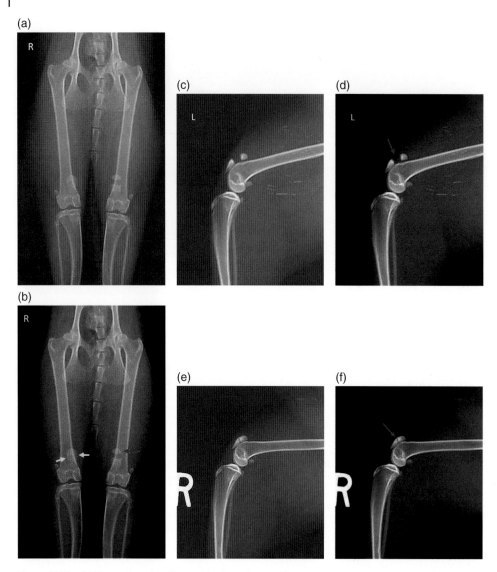

Figure 7.38 (a) Ventrodorsal radiographic view of a cat affected with Patellar Fracture and Dental Anomaly Syndrome (PADS). There is a transverse fracture of the left patella with proximal displacement of the proximal fragment. There is also a radiolucent transverse line associated with the right patella. (b) Ventrodorsal radiographic view of a cat affected with Patellar Fracture and Dental Anomaly Syndrome (PADS). There is a transverse fracture of the left patella with proximal displacement of the proximal fragment (red arrow). There is also a radiolucent transverse line associated with the right patella (yellow arrows). This lucency within the patella represents a concurrent nondisplaced right patellar fracture. (c) Mediolateral radiographic view of the left stifle region of a cat affected with PADS. There is a transverse fracture of the patella with proximal displacement of the proximal fragment. (d) Mediolateral radiographic view of the left stifle region of a cat affected with PADS. There is a transverse fracture of the patella with proximal displacement of the proximal fragment (red arrow). (e) Mediolateral radiographic view of the right stifle region of a cat affected with PADS. There is a radiolucent line within the patella which represents a nondisplaced right patellar fracture. (f) Mediolateral radiographic view of the right stifle region of a cat affected with PADS. There is a radiolucent line within the patella which likely represents a nondisplaced right patellar fracture. *Source:* Courtesy of Steven Bailey, DVM, DABVP (Feline), Exclusively Cats Veterinary Hospital, Waterford, Michigan.

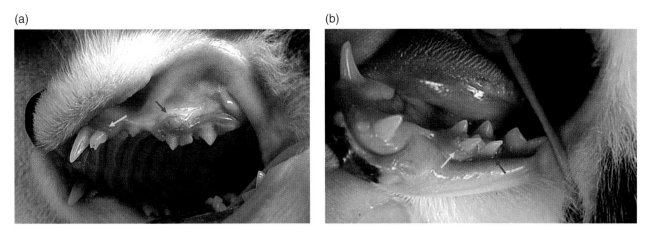

Figure 7.39 (a) Clinical image of the left maxilla of a cat affected with PADS. Note the presence of a persistent deciduous left maxillary canine tooth (604) (yellow arrow) and the left maxillary 3rd premolar tooth (607) (red arrow). Image courtesy of Steven Bailey DVM, DABVP (Feline), Exclusively Cats Veterinary Hospital, Waterford, Michigan. (b) Clinical image of the left mandible of a cat affected with PADS. Note the presence of a persistent deciduous left mandibular 3rd (yellow arrow) and 4th premolar (red arrow) (707 and 708, respectively). *Source:* Courtesy of Steven Bailey, DVM, DABVP (Feline), Exclusively Cats Veterinary Hospital, Waterford, Michigan.

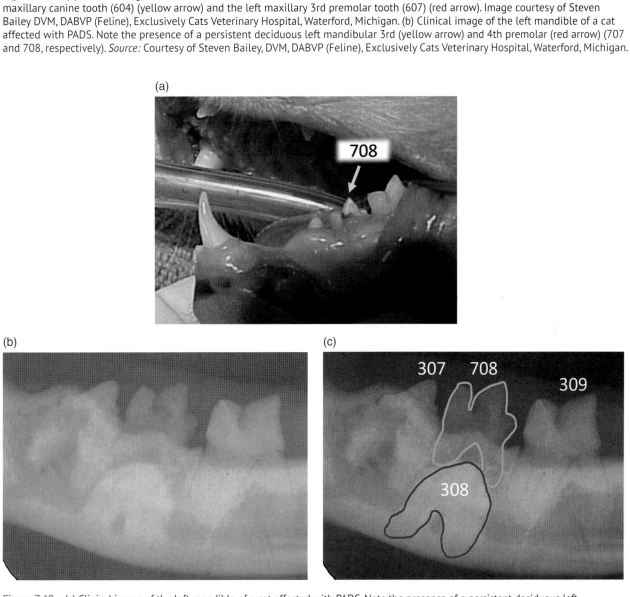

Figure 7.40 (a) Clinical image of the left mandible of a cat affected with PADS. Note the presence of a persistent deciduous left mandibular 4th premolar tooth indicated by the yellow arrow. (b) Intraoral radiographic image of a cat affected with PADS. This is the same cat as seen in Figure (a). Note the presence of a persistent deciduous left mandibular 4th premolar tooth (708) in the image and the presence of an unerupted permanent left mandibular 4th premolar tooth (308), both of which are frequently found in combination with fractures of the patella when affected with this condition. There also appears to be infraeruption of the left mandibular 3rd premolar tooth (307). (c) Intraoral radiographic image of a cat affected with PADS. This is the same cat as seen in Figure (a). Note the presence of a persistent deciduous left mandibular 4th premolar tooth (708), outlined in yellow in the image and the presence of an unerupted permanent left mandibular 4th premolar tooth (308), outlined in red. There also appears to be infraeruption of the left mandibular 3rd premolar tooth (307). *Source:* Courtesy of Steven Bailey, DVM, DABVP (Feline), Exclusively Cats Veterinary Hospital, Waterford, Michigan.

Conclusion

While most canine and feline patients present with oral abnormalities that are frequently observed in a general practice setting, unique manifestations of disease can be appreciated. Ruling out commonly identified oral abnormalities will help guide practitioners in identifying the more uncommon manifestations of disease presented in this chapter. Awareness of the different conditions, the diagnostic imaging findings observed, and potential treatment options available will help guide practitioners with developing a more effective and efficient treatment plan for their patient.

Acknowledgment

The authors would like to give a special acknowledgment to Kristina Miles, DVM, DACVR, and Robin White, DVM, DACVR for assistance in interpretation of several diagnostic images in this chapter.

References

1 Dobson, H. and Friedman, L. (2002). Radiologic interpretation of bone. In: *Bone in Clinical Orthopedics*, 2e (ed. G. Sumner-Smith), 175–202. New York: Thieme.

2 Pool, R.R. and Leighton, R.L. (1969). Craniomandibular osteopathy in a dog. *J. Am. Vet. Med. Assoc.* 154: 657–660.

3 Bonello, D., Roy, C.G., and Verstraete, F.J.M. (2019). Non-neoplastic proliferative oral lesions. In: *Oral and Maxillofacial Surgery in Dogs and Cats* (ed. F.J.M. Verstraete, M.J. Lommer, and B. Arzi), 411–421. Edinburgh: Elsevier Health Sciences.

4 Shope, B.H., Mitchell, P.Q., and Carle, D. (2019). Developmental pathology and pedodontology. In: *Wiggs's Veterinary Dentistry: Principles and Practice* (ed. H.B. Lobprise and J.R. Dodd), 63–79. Hoboken, NJ: Wiley.

5 Alexander, J.W. (1983). Selected skeletal dysplasias: craniomandibular osteopathy, multiple cartilaginous exostoses, and hypertrophic osteodystrophy. *Vet. Clin. North Am. Small Anim. Pract.* 13: 55–70.

6 Padgett, G.A. and Mostosky, U.V. (1986). The mode of inheritance of craniomandibular osteopathy in West Highland White terrier dogs. *Am. J. Med. Genet.* 25: 9–13.

7 Olson, E.J. and Carlson, C.S. (2017). Bone, joints, tendons, and ligaments. In: *Pathologic Basis of Veterinary Disease*, 6e (ed. J.F. Zachary), 954–1008.e2. Amsterdam: Elsevier.

8 Pettitt, R., Fox, R., Comerford, E.J. et al. (2012). Bilateral angular limb deformity in a dog with craniomandibular osteopathy. *Vet. Comp. Orthop. Traumatol.* 25: 149–154.

9 Riser, W.H., Parkes, L.J., and Shirer, J.F. (1967). Canine craniomandibular osteopathy. *Am. Vet. Radiol. Soc.* 8: 23–30.

10 Schulz, S. (1978). A case of craniomandibular osteopathy in a Boxer. *J. Small Anim. Pract.* 19: 749–757.

11 Thompson, D.J., Rogers, W., Owen, M.C., and Thompson, K.G. (2011). Idiopathic canine juvenile cranial hyperostosis in a Pit Bull Terrier. *N. Z. Vet. J.* 59: 201–205.

12 Haktanir, D., Yalin, E.E., Devecioğlu, Y. et al. (2018). Calvarial hyperostosis syndrome in an American Pit Bull Terrier. *Acta Vet. Eurasia* 44: 49–52.

13 Fischetti, A.J., Lara-Garcia, A., and Gross, S. (2006). What is your diagnosis? Idiopathic calvarial hyperostosis. *J. Am. Vet. Med. Assoc.* 229 (2): 211–212.

14 Mathes, R.L., Holmes, S.P., Coleman, K.D. et al. (2012). Calvarial hyperostosis presenting as unilateral exophthalmos is a female English Springer Spaniel. *Vet. Ophthalmol.* 15 (4): 263–270.

15 Slovak, J.E., Gilmour, L.J., and Miles, K.G. (2015). What is your diagnosis? Idiopathic calvarial hyperostosis. *J. Am. Vet. Med. Assoc.* 246 (11): 1187–1189.

16 McConnell, J.F., Hayes, A., Platt, S.R., and Smith, K.C. (2006). Calvarial hyperostosis syndrome in two Bullmastiffs. *Vet. Radiol. Ultrasound* 47 (1): 72–77.

17 Pastor, K.F., Boulay, J.P., Schelling, S.H., and Carpenter, J.L. (2000). Idiopathic hyperostosis of the calvaria in five young Bullmastiffs. *J. Am. Anim. Hosp. Assoc.* 36: 439–445.

18 Blazjewski, S.W. III, Lewis, J.R., Gracis, M. et al. (2010). Mandibular periostitis ossificans in immature large breed dogs: 5 cases (1999–2006). *J. Vet. Dent.* 27: 148–159.

19 Nortjé, C.J., Wood, R.E., and Grotepass, F. (1988). Periostitis ossificans versus Garrè's osteomyelitis. Part II: radiologic analysis of 93 cases in the jaws. *Oral Surg. Oral Med. Oral Pathol.* 66: 249–260.

20 Kannan, S.K., Sandhya, G., and Selvarani, R. (2006). Periostitis ossificans (*Garrè's osteomyelitis*) radiographic study of two cases. *Int. J. Paediatr. Dent.* 16: 59–64.

21 Kawai, T., Murakami, S., Sakuda, M., and Fuchihata, H. (1996). Radiographic investigation of mandibular periostitis ossificans in 55 cases. *Oral Surg. Oral Med. Oral Pathol. Oral Radiol. Endod.* 82: 704–712.

22 Kawai, T., Hiranuma, H., Kishino, M. et al. (1998). Gross periostitis ossificans in mandibular osteomyelitis: review of the English literature and radiographic variations. *Oral Surg. Oral Med. Oral Pathol. Oral Radiol. Endod.* 86: 376–381.

23 Gorman, J.M. (1957). Periostitis ossificans. *Oral Surg. Oral Med. Oral Pathol.* 10: 129–132.

24 Bellows, J. (2008). One swollen puppy jaw. *Vet. Forum* (June) 44–50.

25 Bittegeko, S.B., Arnbjerg, J., Nkya, R., and Tevik, A. (1995). Multiple dental developmental abnormalities following canine distemper infection. *J. Am. Anim. Hosp. Assoc.* 31 (1) (January–February): 42–45.

26 Assuncao, G.S.M., Ocarino, N.M., Sofal, L.C., and Serakides, R. (2020). A rare case of radicular dens invaginatus (dens in dente) in a dog. *J. Comp. Pathol.* 178: 46–49.

27 Eden, E.K., Koca, H., and Sen, B.H. (2002). Dens invaginatus in a primary molar: report of case. *ASDC J. Dent. Child.* 69 (1) (January–April): 49–53.

28 Stein, K.E., Marretta, S.M., and Eurell, J.C. (2005). Dens invaginatus of the mandibular first molars in a dog. *J. Vet. Dent.* 22 (1): 21–30.

29 Alani, A. and Bishop, K. (2008). Dens invaginatus. Part 1: classification, prevalence and aetology. *Int. Endod. J.* 41: 1123–1136.

30 Bishop, K. and Alani, A. (2008). Dens invaginatus. Part 2: clinical, radiographic features and management options. *Int. Endod. J.* 41: 1137–1154.

31 Melmed, C., Shelton, G.D., Bergman, R., and Barton, C. (2004). Masticatory muscle myositis: pathogenesis, diagnosis, and treatment. *Compendium* 26 (8): 590–604.

32 Blazejewski, S.W. and Shelton, G.D. (2018). Trismus, masticatory myositis and antibodies against type 2M fibers in a mixed breed cat. *JFMS Open Rep.* 4 (1): 2055116918764993.

33 Anderson, J.G. and Harvey, C.E. (1993). Masticatory myositis. *J. Vet. Dent.* 10 (1): 6–8.

34 Bishop, T.M., Glass, E.N., De Lahunta, A., and Shelton, G.D. (2008). Imaging diagnosis-masticatory muscle myositis in a young dog. *Vet. Radiol. Ultrasound* 49 (3): 270–272.

35 Reiter, A.M. and Schwarz, T. (2007). Computed tomographic appearance of masticatory myositis in dogs: 7 cases (1999–2006). *J. Am. Vet. Med. Assoc.* 231: 924–930.

36 Moss-Salentjn, L. and Klyvert, M.H. (1983). Epithelially induced denticles in the pulps of recently erupted, noncarious human premolars. *J. Endod.* 9 (12): 554–560.

37 Garg, N. and Garg, A. (2019). Pulp and periradicular tissue. In: *Textbook of Endodontics*, 4e. New Delhi: Jaypee Brothers Medical Publishers.

38 Sisman, Y., Ertas, E.T., Ertas, H., and Sekerci, A.E. (2011). The frequency and distribution of idiopathic osteosclerosis of the jaw. *Eur. J. Dent.* 5: 409–414.

39 Carle, D.S. and Shope, B.H. (2012). Diagnostic imaging in veterinary dental practice. *J. Am. Vet. Med. Assoc.* 241 (10): 1283–1285.

40 Halse, A. and Molven, O. (2002). Idiopathic osteosclerosis of the jaws followed through a period of 20–27 years. *Int. Endod. J.* 35 (9): 747–751.

41 Davis, E.M. (2015). Oral manifestations of chronic kidney disease and renal secondary hyperparathyroidism: a comparative review. *J. Vet. Dent.* 32 (2): 87–98.

42 Hazewinkel, H.A.W. (1989). Nutrition in relation to skeletal growth deformities. *J. Small Anim. Pract.* 30: 625–630.

43 Sarkiala, E.M., Dambach, D., and Harvey, C.E. (1994). Jaw lesions resulting from renal hyperparathyroidism in a young dog – a case report. *J. Vet. Dent.* 11 (4): 121–124.

44 Svanberg, G. (1973). Effect of nutritional hyperparathyroidism on experimental periodontitis in the dog. *Scand. J. Dent. Res.* 81 (2): 155–162.

45 Kwak, E.J. (2021). Internal resorption of multiple posterior teeth in a patient diagnosed with hyperparathyroidism: a case report. *J. Endod.* 47 (8): 1321–1327.

46 Pavlica, Z., Erjavec, V., and Petelin, M. (2001). Teeth abnormalities in the dog. *Acta Vet. Brno* 70: 65–72.

47 Moscow, B.S. (1990). Studies on root enamel: (2) Enamel pearls. A review of their morphology, localization, nomenclature, occurrence, classification, histogenesis, and incidence. *J. Clin. Periodontol.* 17 (5): 275–281.

48 Verstraete, F.J., van Aarde, R.J., Nieuwoud, B.A. et al. (1996). The dental pathology of feral cats on Marion Island, part I: congenital, developmental and traumatic abnormalities. *J. Comp. Pathol.* 115: 265–282.

49 Verstraete, F.J. and Terpak, C.H. (1997). Anatomical variations in the dentition of the domestic cat. *J. Vet. Dent.* 14 (4): 137–140.

50 Langley-Hobbs, S.J. (2009). Survey of 52 fractures of the patella in 34 cats. *Vet. Rec.* 164: 80–86.

51 Howes, C., Longley, M., Reyes, N. et al. (2019). Skull pathology in 10 cats with patellar fracture and dental anomaly syndrome. *J. Feline Med. Surg.* 21 (8): 793–800.

8

Diagnostic Imaging of Exotic Pet Mammals and Zoo Animals

June Olds

Lloyd Veterinary Medical Center, Iowa State University College of Veterinary Medicine, Ames, IA, USA

CONTENTS

Dental Diagnostic Imaging for Nontraditional (Exotic) Animals

Diagnosing and addressing oral and dental conditions in pet exotic mammals and other nondomestic species that may be housed within zoos or private animal collections can present unique challenges to the veterinary practitioner. Many nondomestic species have a small oral aperture (gape), making intraoral visualization and radiographic procurement challenging, if not impossible. In some species, whole-skull or extraoral dental radiographs may be the only techniques available to allow for an accurate diagnosis and to guide the veterinarian in approaches to treatment. For small species, acquiring detailed images can be challenging with the equipment available in a general practice setting. For species managed within zoos and private curated exotic animal collections, clinicians are also challenged to determine what may be normal anatomy or abnormal pathology in an image due to the scant amount of scientific literature available and the wide breadth of species that can be encountered. Many nondomestic species kept within curated collections are stoic and will not show external signs of disease until the ailment has progressed significantly [1]. Clinicians working with zoo animals must also balance the risks of prolonged anesthetic events with the necessity for acquisition of adequate and useful diagnostic images. Although dental disease topics might be discussed in various texts on exotic small mammals commonly kept as pets, publications and research regarding dental diseases, diagnostic imaging, and therapies for nondomestic animals housed within zoos and private collections are quite limited [2].

There is a high prevalence of dental abnormalities in exotic pet mammals; therefore, diagnostic imaging and dentistry techniques for commonly kept small pet mammals have been published and are often mentioned within veterinary conference proceedings [3–8]. The size and anatomic differences of these various species require a veterinarian working with exotic pet mammals to utilize unique techniques which creatively allow visualization of

---

Veterinary Oral Diagnostic Imaging, First Edition. Edited by Brenda L. Mulherin.
© 2024 John Wiley & Sons, Inc. Published 2024 by John Wiley & Sons, Inc.

the normal anatomic structures to be able to identify pathology within their patients. This chapter reintroduces topics relevant to the oral cavities of small exotic pet mammal species, yet also provides a review of diagnostic imaging techniques for conditions seen in species housed within zoos which may be unfamiliar to many veterinary practitioners.

General Considerations for Exotic Companion Mammals

Restraint

Rabbits and other small mammals should be heavily sedated or under general anesthesia for the acquisition of appropriate and diagnostic dental radiographs and skull views. For most, if not all these species, heavy sedation or general anesthesia is required to perform a thorough oral examination as well. Manual restraint of conscious exotic animal species for radiographic positioning is not advised. Manual restraint not only exposes the veterinary professional to unnecessary excess radiation exposure and

potential injury, but also is stressful and can result in injury to the patient. General anesthesia or heavy sedation will allow accurate patient positioning and avoid potential motion artifacts. While positioning the patient, appropriate personal radiation protective measures should be employed (lead aprons, lead gloves, thyroid shields, and radiation dosimetry monitoring devices) (For more information on radiation safety, see Chapter 1). When the animal is sedated, equipment and devices can be used to improve positioning (i.e. minimally sticky tape, sandbags, and foam pads), which will avoid the need for personnel to manually restrain and position the patient for imaging.

Knowledge of Normal Anatomy

Knowledge of the expected dental formula and the type of teeth present for each species treated will help the practitioner formulate an appropriate therapeutic plan and assist with an accurate diagnosis for the patient. Dental formulas and types of dentitions for common exotic pet mammals are summarized in Table 8.1. Common terms used to describe the different tooth types and root structures is described in Box 8.1.

Table 8.1 Dental formulas and tooth classifications of commonly kept exotic pet mammals.

	Incisors Maxillary/mandibular	Canines Maxillary/ mandibular	Premolars Maxillary/mandibular	Molars Maxillary/Mandibular	Total #
Lagomorphs (rabbits, hares, pikas)	2/1 Aradicular hypsodont	0/0	3/2 Aradicular hypsodont	3/3 Aradicular hypsodont	28
Hystricomorph rodents (guinea pigs, chinchilla, degu)	1/1 Aradicular hypsodont	0/0	1/1 Aradicular hypsodont	3/3 Aradicular hypsodont	20
Rat-like rodents (rats, mouse, hamster, gerbil)	1/1 Aradicular hypsodont	0/0	0/0 Anelodont brachyodont	2–3/2–3 Anelodont brachyodont	12–16
Squirrel-like rodents (squirrels, prairie dogs, chipmunks)	1/1 Aradicular, hypsodont	0/0	1–2/1 Anelodont brachyodont	3/3 Anelodont brachyodont	20–22
African pygmy hedgehogs*	2–3/2 Anelodont brachyodont	1/1 Anelodont brachyodont	3/2 Anelodont brachyodont	3/3 Anelodont brachyodont	34–36
Sugar gilders	3/2 Anelodont brachyodont	1/0 Anelodont brachyodont	3/3 Anelodont brachyodont	4/4 Anelodont brachyodont	40
Domestic ferrets*	3/3 Anelodont brachyodont	1/1 Anelodont brachyodont	3/3 Anelodont brachyodont	1/2 Anelodont brachyodont	34

* Hedgehogs and ferrets have diphyodont dentition – they develop both deciduous and permanent sets of teeth. Rabbits and guinea pigs are also considered diphyodont, although they are thought to shed their deciduous teeth in utero. The tooth count listed in this table represents expected adult dentition, but these formulas may vary in individual animals.

Box 8.1   Definition of terms used to classify teeth in exotic animal species.

Term	Definition
Anelodont	Teeth with a limited growth period and a clear line distinguishing the crown from the root (cementoenamel junction)
Aradicular/ Elodont	Continuously growing teeth that do not develop anatomical roots or "open rooted"
Brachydont/ Brachyodont	Short-crowned teeth with well developed roots, or the length of the crown is smaller than the length of the root
Diphyodont	Two successive sets of teeth (deciduous and permanent)
Heterodont	An animal that possesses teeth that are functionally and anatomically different (e.g. incisors, canines, premolars, molars)
Homodont	An animal that possesses teeth that are all functionally and anatomically similar
Hypsodont	Long-crowned teeth, or the length of the crown is greater than the length of the root
Radicular	Root systems that form a closed end, or "closed-rooted"

Table 8.2   Radiographic exposure settings for skull radiographs in rodents, rabbits, and ferrets using tabletop techniques and focal film distances of 38 inches.

Species	Approximate body size (g)	mAs	kVp
Mouse	30	7.5	49
Hamster	150	7.5	52
Rat	300	6.0	52–53
Chinchilla	500	6.0	54–56
Guinea pig	1200	7.5	54
Ferret	1200	6.0	54
Rabbit (small)	1200	7.5	54
Rabbit (medium)	2200	6.0	55
Rabbit (large)	4000	6.0	56–58

Source: Adapted from Ref. [10].

These settings are based on recommendations for 3M (3M Animal Care Products, 3M Center, St. Paul, Minn. 55144-1000) using an Asymetrix Detail Intensifying Screen with SE+ radiographic film. These settings may differ depending on different film and screens used, different imaging equipment, or digital systems. Body sizes are included to help guide settings for species not listed – i.e. settings for imaging a sugar glider may be closer to settings for mouse/hamster, while settings for an African pygmy hedgehog may be closer to those used in a rat. These settings are provided to support the notion that individual machine settings will vary dependent on the equipment used and are only given as a guide.

General Positioning and Projection Recommendations

Standard Radiography

Skull radiographs for most species can yield good quality images for the assessment of small mammal dentition with standard diagnostic radiographic equipment; however, multiple views are necessary to fully evaluate the dental and bony anatomy [9].

As an aid, generalized recommended settings of mAs and kVp for skull radiography for a variety of small exotic companion mammal species are listed in Table 8.2. As noted in the table, settings will vary depending on the type of equipment used at each facility, and the settings provided are offered only as a reference.

Standard Radiographic Positions

A clinician should not base a diagnosis, treatment, or prognosis on any single radiographic image. Best practices for skull radiography in small mammal patients should include four standard views – lateral (Figure 8.1a and b), dorsoventral (Figure 8.1c and d), and right and left oblique views (Figure 8.1e–j). For appropriate imaging of the skull, the first two planes – lateral (also called latero-lateral) and dorsoventral views – should be used *in all patients*. In rabbits and rodents, respiration may be impaired during ventrodorsal

recumbency positioning; therefore, dorsoventral positioning is preferred. If used, ventrodorsal positioning should be maintained only for brief periods of time. In some small mammals, slightly raising the nose with a foam wedge will allow proper lateral projection positioning [10–12].

A perfectly positioned lateral projection will give valuable information in herbivorous animals that frequently develop malocclusions, because according to Bohmer and Crossly, reference lines can be drawn [13] (Figure 8.2). This lateral projection may be used as a guide for prognosis and treatment [13]. Unfortunately, using the lateral and DV views alone will superimpose the structures of the jaw which can obscure pathological changes for a specific quadrant or side. For this reason, additional views of the skull are required for accurate assessment of the oral cavity.

Right and left oblique views with the head tilted 30–40° will allow the apical areas of each quadrant, and most of the intra-alveolar sections of the mandibular cheek teeth to be viewed [13] (Figures 8.3a, b, 8.4a, and b). Oblique projections are described by the direction that the central ray of the primary beam penetrates the body part of interest, from the point of entrance to point of exit [10, 14]. Even with oblique skull projections, radiographic examination of the maxillary premolar and molar teeth can still be limited [13].

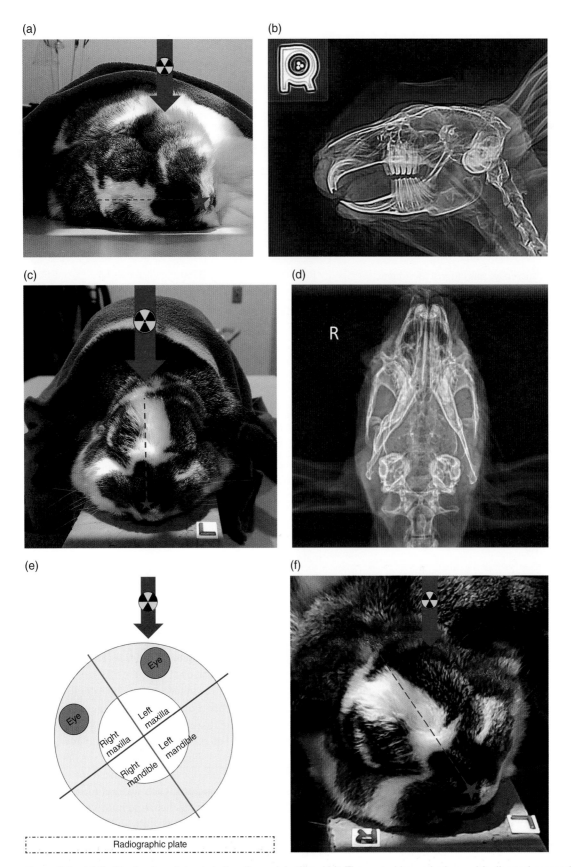

Figure 8.1 (a) Positioning for a lateral skull radiograph in the rabbit. The central beam (red arrow) is directed perpendicular to the film, centered on the premolars and molars (hereafter referred to as the "cheek teeth"). In some rabbits, the nose may need to be slightly elevated so that the sagittal plane of the head is parallel to the film. The red star indicates the nose, with the dashed line indicating the plane of the nasal bone in relation to the radiographic plate. (b) Lateral skull radiograph of an adult rabbit. The lateral projection is useful for the evaluation of the occlusal plane of the cheek teeth and the occlusion of the maxillary and mandibular incisor teeth.

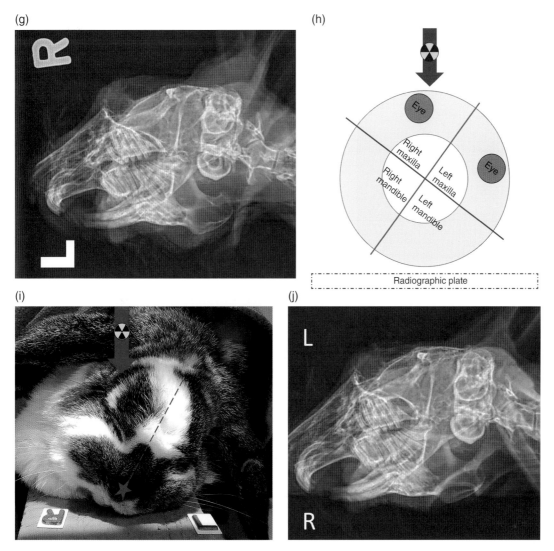

Figure 8.1 (Continued) However, superimposition of both tooth arcades will impede localization of pathology in the tooth roots. (c) Positioning an adult rabbit in sternal recumbency for dorsoventral projection of the skull. The X-ray beam is directed on the midsagittal plane (red arrow), midway along the mandible, or just rostral to a line drawn between the medial canthus of each eye. The red star indicates the center of the nose, and the red dashed line indicates the sagittal plane. The dorsoventral view is preferred for rabbits and rodents to avoid the respiratory impairment that may occur when they are placed in dorsal recumbency for a ventrodorsal position. In this image, a foam block is used to elevate the nose for patient positioning. (d) Dorsoventral skull radiograph of a normal adult rabbit. (e) Graphic drawing depicting the dental arcade quadrants that can be imaged using oblique views of the skull. The blue line indicates the sagittal plane, and the red line indicates the dorsal plane. In this example, the animal is in sternal recumbency, and you are looking at the animal from head on. To create the oblique shown, the head is rotated ~30° counterclockwise. The X-ray beam enters the left dorsal maxilla and exits the right ventral mandible. This produces a left dorsal-right ventral oblique (LD-RVO) radiographic projection, which will allow isolation of the right maxilla and the left mandible. This technique is demonstrated in a patient in Figure (f). (f) Photograph depicting positioning for left dorsal-right ventral oblique (LD-RVO) radiograph of the rabbit skull. The red arrow indicates the direction of the X-ray beam. The red star indicates the location of the patient's nose and the red dashed line the sagittal plane of the head. With this view, the right maxilla and left mandible will be isolated, but the left maxilla and right mandible will superimpose. It is important to include both right and left markers when performing this view, to help with image interpretation. (g) Left dorsal to right ventral oblique radiograph of the adult rabbit skull. In this view, the apical areas of the left mandible and right maxilla intra-alveolar sections may be viewed. Radiographic examination of the maxillary cheek teeth is limited to some extent but does allow some perception of the apical areas of the left maxillary arcade. (h) Graphic drawing depicting the dental arcade quadrants that can be imaged using oblique views. The blue line indicates the sagittal plane, and the red line indicates the dorsal plane. In this example, the animal is in sternal recumbency, and you are looking at the animal from head on. To create the oblique shown, the head is rotated ~30° clockwise. The X-ray beam enters the right dorsal maxilla and exits the left ventral mandible. This produces a right dorsal-left ventral oblique (RD-LVO) radiographic projection, which will allow isolation of the left maxilla and the right mandible. This technique is demonstrated in a patient in Figure (i). (i) Photograph demonstrating positioning for right dorsal-left ventral oblique (RD-LVO) radiograph of the rabbit skull. The rabbit is laying in sternal recumbency, and the head is rotated clockwise. The red arrow indicates the direction of the X-ray beam. The red star indicates the nose, and the dashed line indicates the sagittal plane. In this image, a foam block is used to elevate the chin for proper positioning. (j) Right dorsal-left ventral oblique (RD-LVO) radiograph of the rabbit skull. In this view, the apical areas and the majority of the intra-alveolar sections of the left maxillary and right mandibular cheek teeth are isolated. Radiographic examination of the right maxillary and left mandibular cheek teeth is limited due to superimposition.

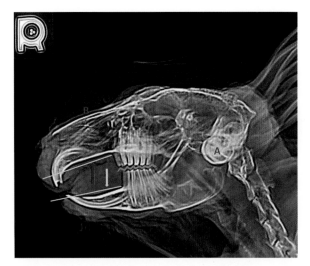

Figure 8.2 Lateral radiograph of an adult rabbit skull. In a well-positioned lateral view, there is exact superimposition of the right and left tympanic bullae (red A). Note that the hard palate in the diastema between the incisors and premolars appears as a single radiopaque line (red arrow). The radiopaque lines of the maxillary (red arrow) and mandibular (yellow arrow) diastemas should normally be slightly angled (yellow lines). If these lines are more parallel than normal, cheek tooth overgrowth should be suspected. The normal appearance of the occlusal plane of the cheek teeth is a zigzag (light blue line), with a slight rostrodorsal-caudoventral slope when compared with the dorsal aspect of the nasal bone (red B).

(a)   (b)

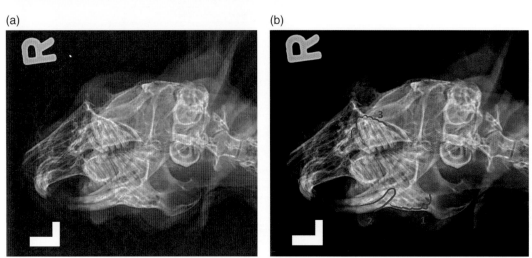

Figure 8.3 (a) Left dorsal to right ventral oblique radiograph of the adult rabbit skull. In this view, the apical areas of the left mandible and right maxilla intra-alveolar sections may be viewed. (b) Annotated left dorsal-right ventral oblique radiograph of the adult rabbit skull as shown in Figure (a). The right side of the patient's head is rotated toward the film. (1) The apices of the left mandibular cheek teeth. (2) The left mandibular incisor is visible ventrally. (3) Apices of the right maxillary cheek teeth. The right mandible and left maxillary teeth superimpose in this view and cannot provide reliable diagnostic information for these quadrants.

(a)   (b)

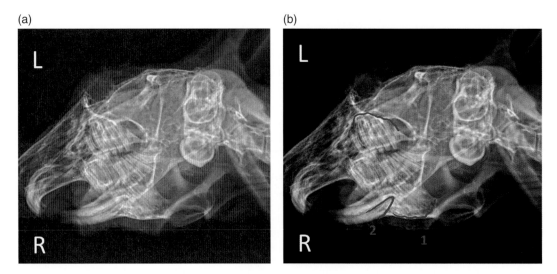

Figure 8.4 (a) Right dorsal-left ventral oblique (RD-LVO) radiograph of a rabbit skull. In this view, the apical areas of the cheek teeth, and the majority of the intra-alveolar sections of the left maxillary and right mandibular cheek teeth are isolated. (b) Annotated right dorsal-left ventral oblique (RD-LVO) radiograph as shown in Figure (a). (1) The apices of the right mandibular cheek teeth. (2) Right mandibular incisor is visible ventrally. (3) The apices of the left maxillary cheek teeth are isolated.

After the four standard projections have been obtained (lateral, dorsoventral, and right and left oblique views), positioning for additional views can be used on a case-by-case basis to provide additional information if needed. The rostrocaudal view is frequently used in herbivorous rodents (rabbits, guinea pigs, and chinchillas) (Figures 8.5a–c and 8.6a–d) which will allow visualization of specific changes in the caudal area of the head [13]. This technique allows for good imaging of the temporomandibular joint and the tympanic bulla. Using this technique, species-specific angulation of the molar occlusal planes may be verified [13]. The ventrolateral margin of the mandible can also be evaluated with the rostrocaudal projection [13].

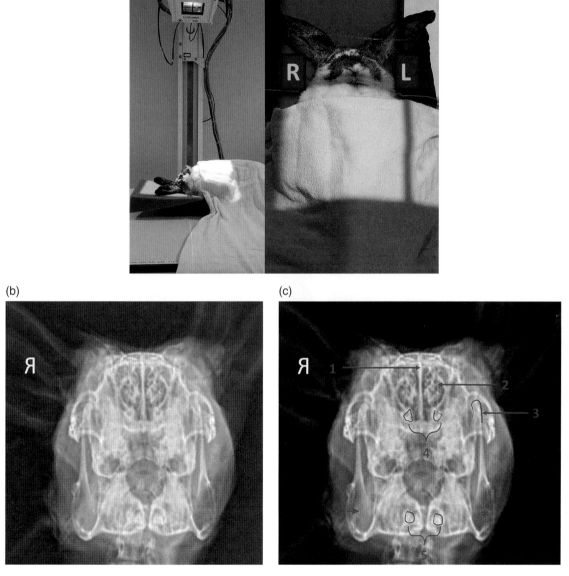

Figure 8.5 (a) Rostrocaudal radiographic positioning in the rabbit. The rostrocaudal projection is only possible with the patient heavily sedated or under general anesthesia. To avoid artifact, it is best if the patient is not intubated. To produce this projection, the patient is placed in dorsal recumbency with the nose pointing vertically. Right and left markers should be placed for proper image interpretation. (b) Rostrocaudal image of a normal rabbit. The rostrocaudal view is indicated if there is reason to suspect a pathologic change in the temporomandibular joints. This view also helps evaluate the maxillary sinuses for symmetry. (c) Annotated rostrocaudal image of a normal adult rabbit. (1) Nasal septum visible as a radiopaque line. (2) Nasal cavity and maxillary sinus. (3) Condyloid process of the left mandible. (4) The maxillary incisors are visible in transection. (5) The mandibular incisors are visible in transection. The left masseteric fossa (red asterisk) is more radiolucent than the right (red arrowhead) due to the head being slightly angled with towel placement, resulting in soft tissue asymmetry. This should not be misinterpreted as potential bone lysis or bone loss. Bilateral symmetry is evident in this view and the mandibular cortices appear smooth bilaterally.

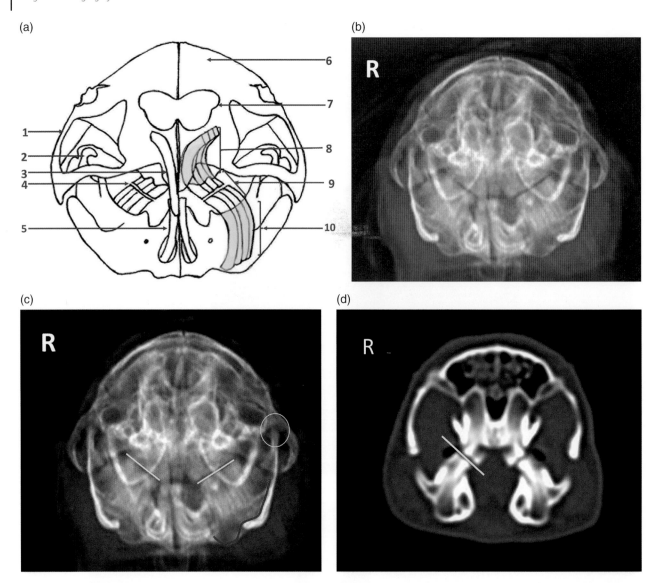

Figure 8.6 (a) Annotated drawing of the rostrocaudal view of the guinea pig skull. *Source:* Adapted from Crossley [15]. (1) Zygomatic bone. (2) Condylar process of the mandible. (3) Maxillary incisor tooth and apex. (4) Occlusal plane of the "cheek teeth." (5) Mandibular incisor tooth. (6) Parietal bone. (7) Nasal cavity/sinuses. (8) Apices of the maxillary cheek teeth within the skull (yellow highlights). (9) Clinical crowns of the cheek teeth. (10) Mandibular cheek teeth apices within the mandible (yellow highlights). (b) Rostrocaudal radiographic skull view of a normal guinea pig. The rostrocaudal view is the most challenging to obtain. This is the only radiographic projection that allows evaluation of the occlusal plane of the cheek teeth in guinea pigs. This view gives information on the cheek teeth including the occlusal plane angle, presence of spikes and spurs, coronal and apical elongation, and cortical perforation by the tooth apices. The temporomandibular joint and the mandibular symphysis are also clearly visible in this view. (c) Annotated rostrocaudal radiographic skull view of the normal guinea pig as shown in Figure (b). Although this image is very slightly oblique, it allows clear visualization of the occlusal plane of the cheek teeth, which, in guinea pigs, slopes approximately 30° dorsal to ventral from the buccal to lingual side (yellow lines). Because of the occlusal angle, the occlusal plane cannot be evaluated in the lateral view for guinea pigs. The mandibular cheek teeth apices reach close to the mandibular cortices, which should appear smooth (red line). The temporomandibular joint can also be evaluated (yellow circle). (d) Transverse computed tomography (CT) image of the rostro-caudal view in a normal guinea pig. The CT image is superior for visualization of the shape and orientation of the teeth and apices. The occlusal angle of the right cheek teeth is indicated by the yellow line.

Intraoral Radiographs

The intraoral technique is usually preferred over the extraoral technique because it produces images of optimal resolution and diagnostic quality [11]. Correct placement of intraoral films or digital dental sensors within the small oral cavity of rabbits and pet rodents is difficult, if not impossible, due to the small sizes of the patients (Figures 8.7a–c and 8.8a–c). In most small patients, intraoral techniques may only allow visualization of the incisors and the very rostral premolars of the maxilla and mandible. It may also be beneficial for the evaluation of the

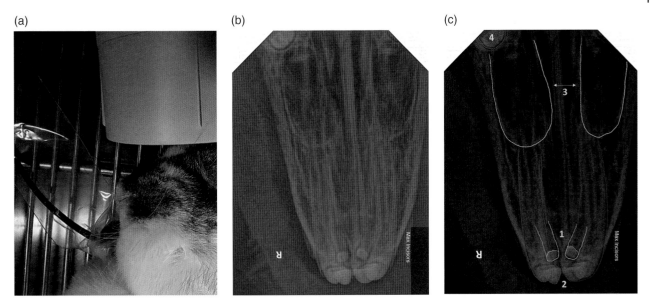

Figure 8.7   (a) Photograph demonstrating intraoral placement of a Size 2 dental sensor for radiographs of the maxillary incisors in an adult rabbit. The sensor should be gently introduced between the mandibular and maxillary dental arcades as far into the mouth as possible, and the beam directed perpendicular to the bisecting angle between the long axis of the film and the long axis of the incisor roots. Intraoral techniques may be useful not only for the study of the maxillary and mandibular incisor teeth but also for detecting changes in the nasal passages. (b) Rostral intraoral maxillary radiograph of a normal rabbit using a Size 2 dental sensor. In larger patients, the cheek teeth may also be evaluated with intraoral film. Depending on the size of the rabbit, part or all of one or more maxillary cheek teeth may be included. (c) Annotated intraoral radiograph of the rostral maxilla in a normal rabbit. (1) Peg teeth (2nd maxillary incisors) (yellow lines). (2) First maxillary incisors and apices (red lines). (3) Nasal cavity (yellow lines). (4) First maxillary premolar tooth (red line). Depending upon rabbit and film size, part or all of one or more maxillary cheek teeth may be included on the image.

Figure 8.8   (a) Positioning an intraoral dental sensor for radiographs of the mandibular incisors in a rabbit. The sensor is gently introduced between the mandibular and maxillary dental arcades as far into the mouth as possible, and the beam directed perpendicular to the bisecting angle between the long axis of the sensor and the long axis of the mandibular incisor roots.
(b) Intraoral dental radiograph of the rabbit mandible as shown in Figure (a). Both mandibular incisor apices and mandibular first premolars can be viewed in this image. The small size of this patient's mouth does not permit visualization of the remaining mandibular cheek teeth with this technique, and the crowns of the incisors are also excluded. (c) Annotated intraoral ventrodorsal radiograph of the rostral mandible of the rabbit as shown in Figure (b). (1) Mandibular incisor apices. (2) Mandibular first premolars.

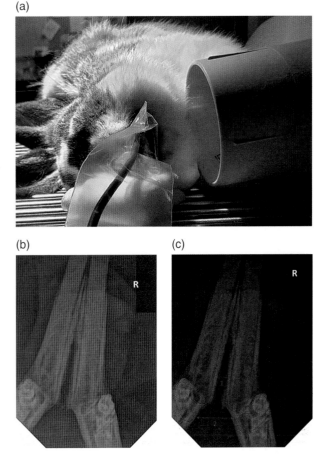

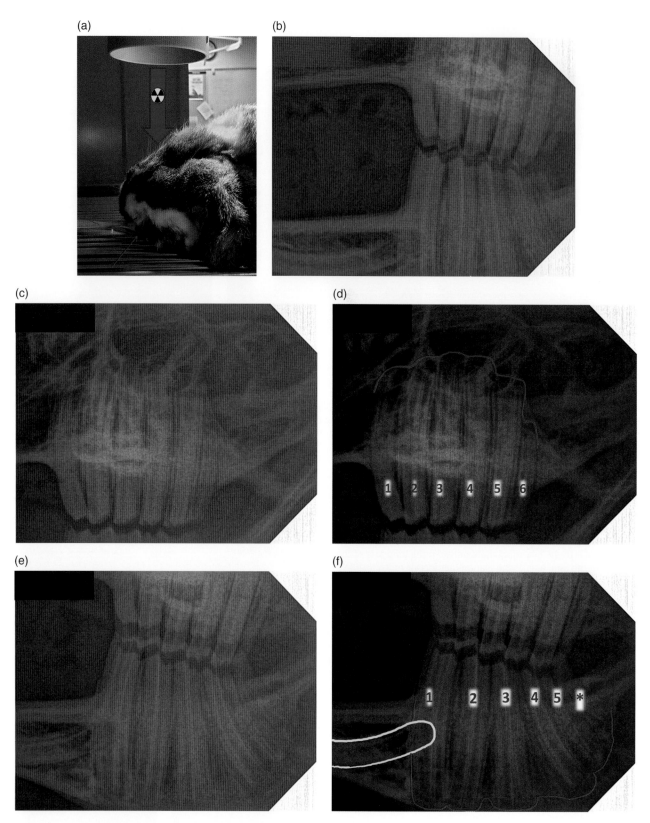

Figure 8.9 (a) Positioning the rabbit for extraoral views using intraoral dental sensor to obtain high-quality images. The dental sensor is parallel with the arcade to be evaluated, and the X-ray beam (thick red arrow) is centered perpendicular to the sensor. In this photo, the rabbit is in left lateral recumbency, and the dental sensor (thin red arrow) is placed parallel to the cheek teeth. (b) Lateral view of the cheek teeth of a rabbit obtained with an extraoral positioned dental sensor. The positioning of the sensor in the image is intended to demonstrate the occlusal plane of the cheek teeth. The normal zigzag apposition is evident with slight oblique offset positioning of the arcades. The periapical roots of the mandibular incisor teeth are visible. However, the small size of the dental sensor and the positioning excludes the apices of the cheek teeth roots. (c) Lateral view of the maxillary cheek teeth of the same rabbit as shown in Figure (b), obtained by repositioning the extraoral sensor more caudal and dorsal to the teeth to allow visualization

rostral sinuses. A dental radiographic generator is preferred, as it can be easily positioned in proper angles to obtain appropriate views.

Intraoral Films Used Extraorally

Due to the difficulties with obtaining good quality intraoral images in small species, extraoral techniques may be used with intraoral films or digital dental sensors. The resulting images may still require multiple views to avoid superimposition of bony structures. For larger patients, these techniques should not be used in place of skull radiography but may enhance the information gathered by gaining more detailed views of specific structures (Figure 8.9a–f). For some small mammal species, whole-skull radiographs can be obtained on digital dental sensors or dental films alone, as demonstrated in the hamster (Figures 8.10a–c and 8.11a–c).

Magnification Techniques

Because of the small size of many pet mammals, magnification radiographic techniques have been described [10] (Figure 8.12a–c). The magnification technique may be useful when dental sensors, dental films, or digital images are not available, or sensors are too large to fit into the oral cavity of the patient. For this technique, an ultrasmall focal spot X-ray tube and an increased object–film (OFD) distance is used instead of standard radiograph OFD techniques. The result is an enlarged image of the object being radiographed. These enlarged images may be useful for critically examining small patients or small body parts [10]. This is especially useful when using standard film radiography where digital manipulation and magnification of images are not possible. While this technique creates an enlarged image of the object being radiographed, image quality is decreased, especially when compared to the high-quality digital images created using standard techniques (compare guinea pig images in Figure 8.12b and c using the magnification technique with Figure 8.12d and e using standard digital radiography). Alternatively, when examining film radiographs of a small patient, the clinician may consider viewing standard radiographs with a magnifying glass to enhance the visibility of structures.

Anatomical Variations

Rabbits

Many textbooks and continuing education presentations have been dedicated to the radiology and dentistry of pet rabbits [9–12, 16–19], as dental disease is a common cause of morbidity and mortality in these popular pets. The enamel of rabbits is white. The incisors, molars, and premolars of rabbits are all aradicular and grow continuously. Premolar and molar teeth are anatomically indistinguishable and may be simply identified as "cheek teeth" [9]. In rabbits, elongation of the cheek teeth will prevent the mouth from closing fully, which may separate the incisor teeth, further reducing their occlusal wear. This could cause elongation of the crown and potentially the roots of these teeth. Beyond a certain level of elongation, the incisors will no longer function adequately enough to prehend food. Whole-skull radiography remains a valuable tool for the assessment of dental disease in rabbits. Figure 8.13 is an illustration of the important anatomical landmarks in the rabbit skull. Slightly raising the nose of the rabbit will allow proper lateral projection positioning [12]. In the lateral view, the hard palate in the diastema between incisor and cheek teeth appears as

Figure 8.9 (Continued) of the roots of the maxillary arcade. This image is annotated in Figure (d). Although there is superimposition using the lateral extraoral technique, the dental sensor is a detail film which allows more clear visualization of the maxillary premolar and molar apices than the standard film (or nondental) lateral skull radiograph. (d) Annotated extraoral lateral radiograph of the maxillary cheek teeth of an adult rabbit using an intraoral dental sensor. The maxillary cheek teeth apices (red line) are more clearly visualized using this extraoral film technique than previously noted on skull radiographs. The teeth are numbered cranially to caudally in this image. Maxillary cheek tooth 1 is slightly curved, and the remaining maxillary cheek teeth are almost straight, with slight convergence of the apices. The reserve crowns of maxillary cheek tooth 3 to cheek tooth 5 are located inside the alveolar bulla, which lies cranial, ventral, and medial to the orbital fossa. Periapical infection in these maxillary teeth plays an important role in the formation of retrobulbar and peribulbar abscesses. The apex of maxillary cheek tooth 3 is slightly dorsal to the apices of the other cheek teeth radiographically, following the dome of the alveolar bulla. (e) Extraoral lateral dental radiograph of a rabbit mandible using an intraoral dental sensor in an extraoral position. In this view, there is superimposition of both right and left arcades and mild oblique positioning. The apices of the mandibular incisors are visible underlying the mandibular first premolar. This image is annotated in Figure (f). (f) Annotated lateral extraoral radiograph of the mandible of a rabbit using an intraoral dental sensor positioned extraorally. There is mild oblique rotation in this image. The mandibular cheek tooth roots (red line) are more clearly visualized using the high-detail dental sensor than previously noted on standard skull radiographs. The roots of the mandibular incisors are outlined in yellow in this image and extend medially to the apices of the cheek teeth. There should be space between the mandibular cheek teeth apices and the ventral cortex of the mandible, which is not included in this film. The expected dentition in rabbits is five mandibular cheek teeth. The mild cranial-caudal obliquity of this image gives the impression of a sixth molar (red asterisk).

(a)

(b)

(c)

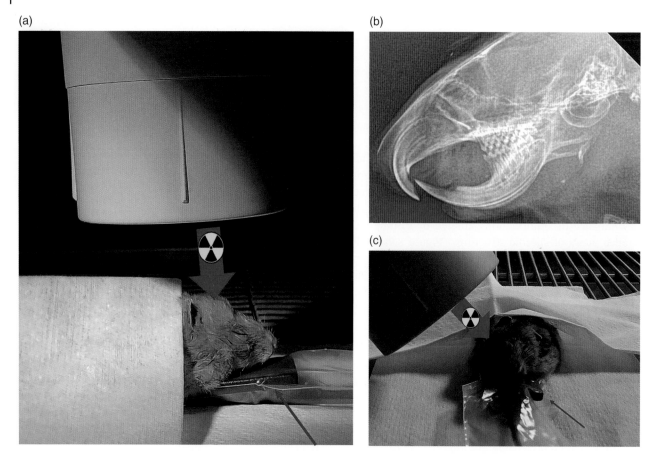

Figure 8.10 (a) Positioning a hamster for an extraoral DV skull radiograph using a Size 2 intraoral dental sensor (thin red arrow) positioned extraorally. The small size of the rodent skull and ability to center the beam on the small skull makes this an ideal method for obtaining high-quality detailed views of smaller patients like rodents. (b) Right lateral skull radiograph of a normal hamster obtained using extraoral positioning of an intraoral Size 2 dental sensor. (c) Positioning a hamster for an extraoral right dorsal-left ventral oblique skull radiograph using a dental generator and a Size 2 intraoral dental sensor (thin red arrow) placed extraorally.

a single radiopaque line when properly positioned. The radiopaque lines of the maxillary and mandibular diastemas should normally be slightly angled, converging rostrally to the incisor teeth [12] (Figure 8.14a and b). Normal rabbit positioning and radiographs are shown in Figure 8.1a–j. The dorsoventral skull radiograph of the rabbit is also very useful to evaluate for evidence of disease (Figure 8.15a and b). Diagnostic images of rabbit oral and dental disease are shown in Figures 8.16a–d, 8.17a–g, and 8.18a–f.

Guinea Pigs and Chinchillas

Grossly, the enamel of guinea pigs is white in color. The length of the mandibular incisors is normally triple the length of the maxillary incisors in this species [9]. The incisors, molars, and premolars of guinea pigs are all considered aradicular hypsodont teeth that grow continuously. Premolar and molar teeth are anatomically indistinguishable and may be simply called "cheek teeth" [9]. As true

herbivores, the occlusal surface of the cheek teeth is rough and uneven due to enamel crests and dentinal grooves. Unlike rabbits, the occlusal surfaces are smooth in guinea pigs and do not present a zigzag pattern. The cheek teeth should maintain a 30° oblique occlusal plane that slopes from dorsobuccal to ventrolingual/palatal [11] (see Figure 8.6a–d). The cheek teeth are curved with the mandibular teeth having a buccal (lateral) convexity and the maxillary teeth exhibiting a palatal (medial) convexity [9]. Overgrowth of teeth and associated malocclusions are relatively common in guinea pigs. The mandibular cheek teeth are directed slightly inward toward the tongue, such that any small spurs on the lingual aspect of these teeth will rapidly cause pain. Tongue entrapment is also possible if the condition goes untreated [20]. The underlying cause of malocclusions in guinea pigs may be congenital or acquired due to lack of fiber in the diet and other husbandry conditions that do not allow the teeth to wear at an appropriate rate. Chronic hypovitaminosis C (scurvy) can cause

(a)

(b)

(c)

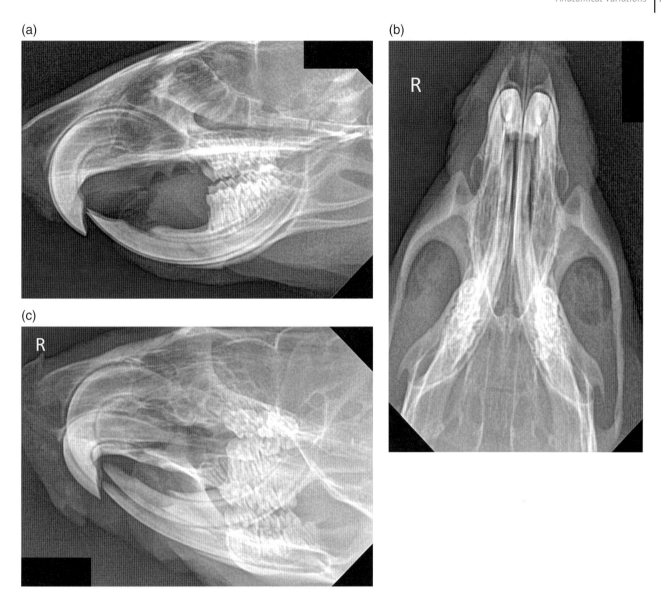

Figure 8.11 (a) Lateral skull radiograph of an adult rat using an intraoral Size 2 dental sensor placed extraorally. (b) Dorsoventral skull radiograph of an adult rat, taken on a Size 2 intraoral dental sensor placed extraorally. The high-quality sensors give nicely detailed views of incisors in such a small patient. (c) Left dorsal-right ventral lateral oblique (LD-RVO) skull radiograph of a rat taken on an intraoral radiographic plate using extraoral positioning.

irregular dentin formation and has also been associated with dental disease in the guinea pig [9, 21]. Periodontal ligament integrity is compromised by defective collagen synthesis in hypovitaminosis C, which leads to teeth loosening and progressive malocclusion development [21]. Normal guinea pig radiographs can be found in Figures 8.6b–d, 8.19a–d, 8.20a, and b. Images of abnormal guinea pig dental pathology are shown in Figure 8.21a–k.

In chinchillas, the facial surfaces of the incisor enamel have superficial yellow to orange pigmentation which is normal for this species. Chinchillas have prominent strongly curved incisor teeth, with one incisor in each

quadrant of the mouth. Like the guinea pig and rabbit, all teeth grow continuously. There is also a single premolar and three molar teeth in each quadrant. The reserve crown is embedded in the alveolus with the exposed crown visible in the oral cavity. The clinical crowns of chinchilla teeth are much shorter than those of rabbits [9]. The cheek teeth wear to form a continuous horizontal occlusal surface that should be contiguous with the gingiva except at the mesial surface of the mandibular premolar teeth (Figure 8.22a and b). Tooth elongation and resulting tooth curvature can reduce chewing efficiency and will exacerbate a malocclusion if one is present [20]. Many dental lesions are difficult to find

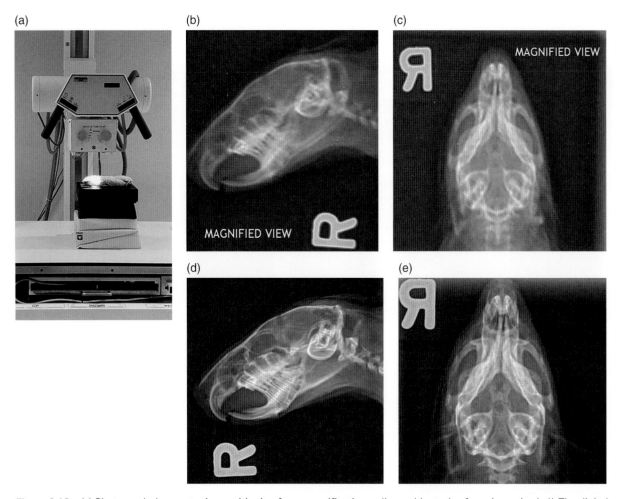

Figure 8.12 (a) Photograph demonstrating positioning for a magnification radiographic study of a guinea pig skull. The digital cassette (sensor) is located below the top of the radiology table. The object–film distance (OFD) is increased by elevating the patient above the cassette with radiolucent foam sponges. The focal–film distance is decreased by lowering the tube housing closer to the cassette. (b) Right lateral skull radiograph of a guinea pig using the "magnified radiographic study" technique as shown in Figure (a). Although this technique creates an enlarged image of the object being radiographed, image quality decreases, especially when compared to the high-quality digital images created using standard techniques in the guinea pig (Figure (d) and (e)). Examining magnified images for small patients or small body parts may make sense in some circumstances, especially if using standard film radiographs where digital refinement of images is not possible. As seen in these images, the foam used to elevate the patient above the cassette created small artifacts (gray spots) and shows decreased contrast as opposed to the digital images of the same guinea pig in Figure (d) and (e). (c) Dorsoventral skull radiograph of a guinea pig using the "magnified radiographic study" technique as shown in Figure (a). (d) Right lateral digital skull radiograph of a guinea pig utilizing a standard technique as previously demonstrated in the rabbit in Figure 8.1a. (e) Dorsoventral digital skull radiograph of a guinea pig using a standard radiographic technique as demonstrated in the rabbit in Figure 8.1c.

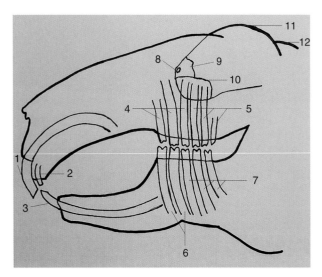

Figure 8.13 Line drawing of the lateral rabbit skull showing dentition and important clinical anatomical reference points. (1) Maxillary first incisor. (2) Maxillary second incisor ("peg tooth"). (3) Mandibular incisor. (4) Maxillary premolars*. (5) Maxillary molars*. (6) Mandibular premolars*. (7) Mandibular molars*. (8) Lacrimal foramen. (9) Lacrimal bone. (10) Alveolar bulla. (11) Supraorbital margin/zygomatic process of the frontal bone. (12) Frontal bone*. In rabbits and other herbivorous exotic pets, the premolars and molars are referred to as "cheek teeth."

(a)

(b)

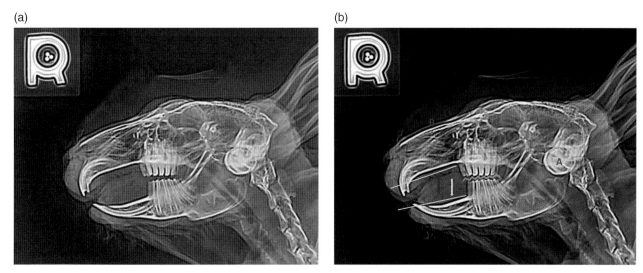

Figure 8.14 (a) Lateral skull radiograph of an adult rabbit. The lateral projection is useful for evaluation of the occlusal plane of the cheek teeth and the occlusion of the maxillary and mandibular incisor teeth. (b) Annotated lateral radiograph of an adult rabbit skull. In a well-positioned lateral view, there is exact superimposition of the right and left tympanic bullae (red A). Note that the hard palate in the diastema between the incisors and premolars appears as a single radiopaque line (red arrow). The radiopaque lines of the maxillary (red arrow) and mandibular (yellow arrow) diastemas should normally be slightly angled (yellow lines). If these lines are more parallel than normal, cheek tooth overgrowth should be suspected. The normal appearance of the occlusal plane of the cheek teeth is a zigzag (light blue line), with a slight rostrodorsal-caudoventral slope when compared with the dorsal aspect of the nasal bone (red B).

(a)

(b)

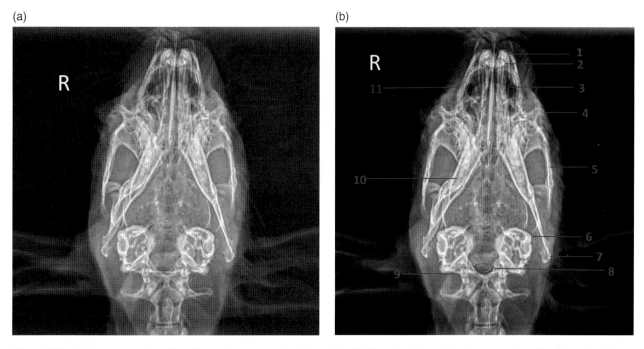

Figure 8.15 (a) Dorsoventral skull radiograph of a normal adult rabbit. (b) Normal adult rabbit dorsoventral skull radiograph with annotations of anatomical structures. (1) Maxillary incisor tooth. (2) 2nd maxillary incisor tooth ("peg tooth"). (3) Nasal cavity. (4) Facial tuberosity of the maxilla. (5) Zygomatic bone. (6) Tympanic bulla. (7) Angular process of the mandible. (8) Foramen magnum. (9) Occipital condyle. (10) Mandible. (11) Maxilla.

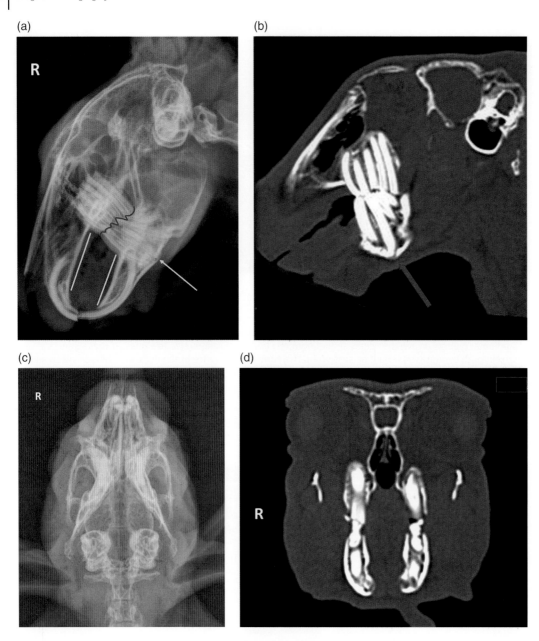

Figure 8.16 (a) Lateral radiograph of a rabbit with chronic dental disease. The cheek teeth are variable in length and apposition. The radiopaque lines of the maxillary and mandibular diastemas are nearly parallel as opposed to the normal oblique orientation (yellow lines). The mandible is roughened, and there is evidence of osteomyelitis of the mandible at the molar roots (yellow arrow). The normal zigzag pattern of the occlusal surfaces of the cheek teeth is lost and irregular (red lines). (b) Left parasagittal computed tomographic image of the same rabbit shown in Figure (a). With the slice locations centered at the maxillary and mandibular cheek teeth, severe malocclusion is observed, and variable length of the cheek teeth is demonstrated. The occlusal surfaces of the upper and lower arcade are uneven throughout the entire dental arcade. Multiple teeth exhibit retrograde apical root elongation which appear to penetrate the mandibular cortex causing focal thinning of the bone. This finding was most apparent at the left and right 2nd and 3rd mandibular cheek teeth (red arrow). (c) Dorsoventral radiograph of the same rabbit shown in Figure (a) and (b). Superimposition of the facial structures, maxilla, and mandible make visualization of dental structures challenging in this view. For this patient, a rostro-caudal radiograph may have been beneficial. (d) Transverse CT image of the same rabbit shown in Figure (a)–(c). The left and right 2nd and 3rd mandibular cheek teeth are overgrown. The 3rd left mandibular crown is shortened. At the occlusal surface, the maxillary crowns are displaced laterally, and the mandibular crowns are displaced medially.

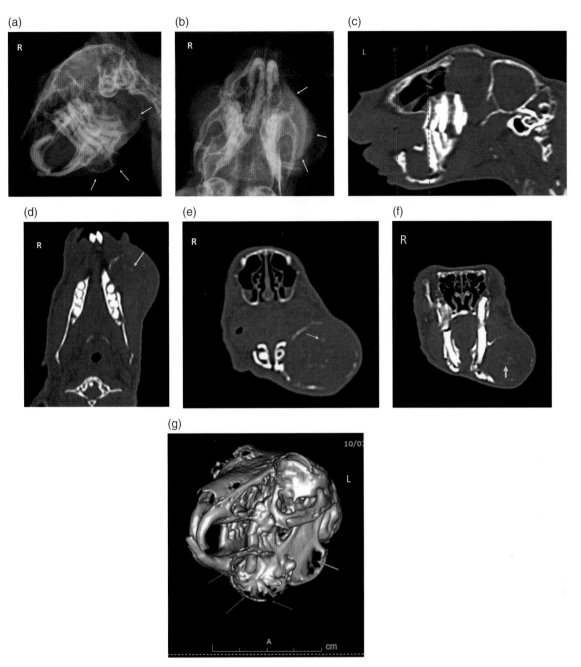

Figure 8.17 (a) Lateral radiograph of a rabbit with a left mandibular abscess. The ventral cortex of the mandible from the level of the incisor apex extending caudally to the first molar has a large ventrolateral expanding periapical osteolytic lesion (yellow arrows). The lesion is centered at the premolars. The ventral margin is mildly irregular with multifocal defects in the cortex. The lesion extends ventrally from the mandible and the soft tissue contours demonstrate soft tissue thickening. Incisor malocclusion from inappropriate attrition is also evident. (b) Dorsoventral radiograph of the rabbit with a left mandibular abscess as shown in Figure (a). A large lateral expanding periapical osteolytic lesion is observed (yellow arrows). The lesion is centered at the premolars. The lateral margin of the bony wall is not well defined in the DV view. The lesion extends laterally from the mandible and the soft tissue contours demonstrate soft tissue thickening. (c) Left parasagittal CT of the same rabbit shown in Figure (a) and (b). The parasagittal image shows the expansion and bony lysis of the ventral mandible identified in the radiographic images. Slice locations indicated by the red dashed lines "e" and "f" indicate the location of the images shown in Figure (e) and (f). (d) Dorsal CT of the mandible of the same rabbit shown in Figure (a)–(c), showing lysis of periapical bone and lateral cortical bone adjacent to the second premolar. The cavity created by the abscess is primarily filled with soft tissue/fluid attenuating material with several mineral attenuating foci (yellow arrow). In this slice, the root of the first molar is the in the caudal portion of the abscess cavity. (e) Transverse CT image of the rabbit shown in Figure (a)–(d). This image is located at the mandibular incisor roots just cranial to the premolars (red dashed line labeled "e" in Figure (c)). The expansile lesion displaces the skin of the left mandible laterally. The thin bony rim of the expansile lesion is disrupted by multiple small lytic foci (yellow arrow), indicating mineralization of some of the abscess contents. (f) Transverse CT image of the rabbit shown in Figure (a)–(e), with the image located at the level of the first premolars (red dashed-line labeled "f" in Figure (c)). The expansile lesion displaces the skin of the left mandible laterally. The thin bony rim of the expansile lesion is disrupted by multiple small lytic foci (yellow arrow), indicating mineralization of some of the abscess contents. The lesion cavity incorporates the roots of the incisor, first and second premolars and mesial border of the first molar. (g) Three-dimensional (3D) reconstruction of mineralized tissues of the rabbit shown in Figure (a)–(f). This is a viewer's rostral left lateral oblique perspective of the skull. Osteolytic interruptions in the expanded left lateral mandibular wall of the abscess cavity are demonstrated (red arrows). The root of the left mandibular first premolar (yellow asterisk) is isolated in the cavity. Soft tissues including the contents of the abscess cavity and normally very thin bone (caudal portion of the mandible – blue arrow) appear as voids in this reconstruction. Severe incisor malocclusion from inappropriate attrition is easily identified.

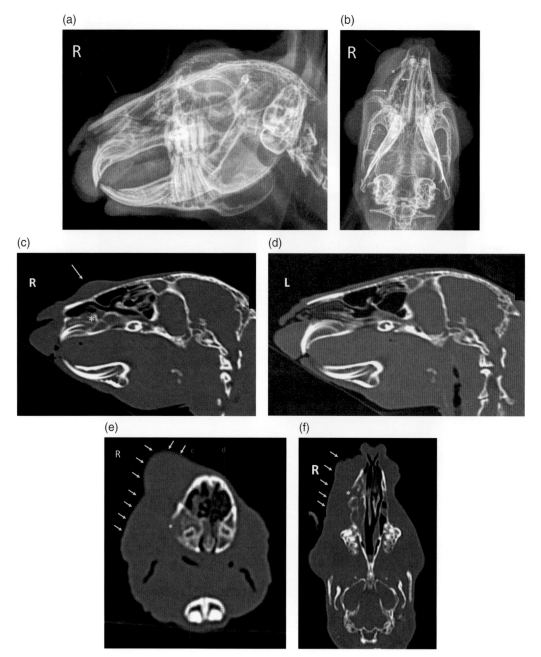

Figure 8.18 (a) Mildly oblique right lateral radiograph of a rabbit who presented with a swelling of the right cranial dorsolateral face. At the rostral maxillary region, a broad-based soft tissue swelling bulges dorsally (red arrow). Maxillary incisor or cheek teeth abnormalities are not identified in these views. (b) Dorsoventral radiograph of a rabbit who presented with a swelling of the right cranial dorsolateral face. At the rostral maxillary region, a broad-based soft tissue swelling bulges laterally (red arrow). The right incisive and maxillary bones are thicker than the left (yellow arrows), and lysis is suspected at the lateral margin (yellow asterisk). Maxillary incisor or cheek teeth abnormalities are not identified in this view. (c) Parasagittal conventional CT images of the same rabbit shown in Figure (a) and (b). The right parasagittal CT image of the rostral maxillary nasal region shows part of the dorsally bulging soft tissue mass (yellow arrow) and increased soft tissue extending from the dorsal periapical incisor region into the rostral nasal cavity (yellow asterisk). (d) The left parasagittal image of the same rabbit as in Figure (a)–(c) is shown to demonstrate the difference between the right and left sides. This side appears normal. (e) Transverse CT image of the rabbit shown in Figure (a)–(d). This transverse image is close to the apices of the maxillary incisor roots. Right lateral facial soft tissue swelling is evident (yellow arrows). Right incisor periapical expansion of the incisive bone is present medially, dorsally, and laterally with disruption of the lateral incisive/maxillary bone (yellow asterisk). The nasal conchal pattern is asymmetrical with loss of small conchal opacities in the right side and the presence of a vertically oriented region of soft tissue attenuation in the ventral nasal meatus. In this image, "c" indicates the position the slice was taken from that corresponds to Figure (c) demonstrating the disease process, while "d" corresponds to the position the slice was taken from in Figure (d), representing the normal left side of the patient. (f) Dorsal CT image of the rabbit shown in Figure (a)–(e). This slice is located dorsal to the plane of the maxillary incisors. There is lateral and dorsal facial soft tissue swelling evident (yellow arrows) on the image. Right incisor periapical expansion of the incisive bone is present medially, dorsally, and laterally with disruption of the lateral incisive bone (yellow asterisk). The nasal conchal pattern is asymmetrical with loss of small conchal opacities in the right side and the presence of a region of soft tissue attenuation in the ventral nasal meatus.

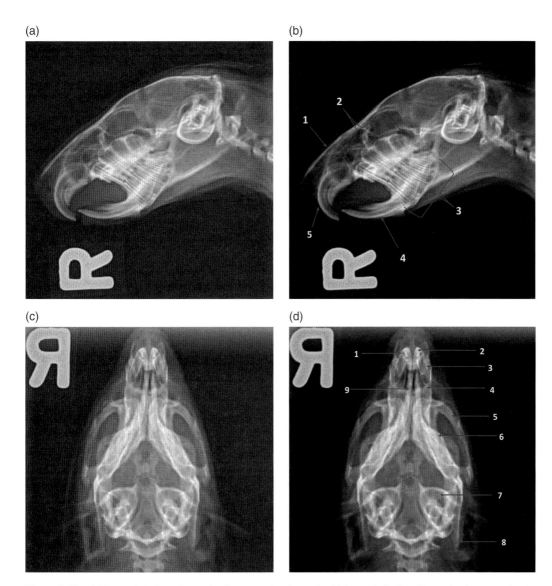

Figure 8.19 (a) Lateral skull radiograph of a normal guinea pig. (b) Lateral skull radiograph of a normal guinea pig with annotation of important anatomy. (1) Nasal bone. (2) Maxillary cheek teeth apices. (3) Apices of the mandibular cheek teeth. (4) Mandibular incisor teeth (superimposed). (5) Maxillary incisor teeth (superimposed). [Both the occlusal plane of the cheek teeth and the apices of the incisors are difficult to evaluate in this view. The apices of the mandibular incisors extend lingual to the second cheek teeth, which obscure them on a true lateral projection. The apices of the maxillary incisor teeth are visible just mesial to the roots of the first cheek teeth. The mandibular cheek teeth apices are very close to the ventral cortices of the mandible. Unlike in rabbits and chinchillas, the occlusal plane is not visible in the lateral projection of the skull in the guinea pig.] (c) Dorsoventral skull radiograph of a normal guinea pig. (d) Annotated dorsoventral skull radiograph of a normal guinea pig. (1) Right maxillary incisor tooth. (2) Left maxillary incisor tooth. (3) Incisive bone. (4) Maxilla. (5) Zygomatic arch. (6) Mandible. (7) Tympanum. (8) Angular process of the mandible. (9) Mandibular incisor. Symmetry between right and left sides is critical for proper evaluation of VD or DV projections. This view allows visualization of the relationship between the mandible and the skull and the integrity of the margins of the mandibular and maxillary bones. This view is also useful for evaluation of the anterior nasal cavity. Individual molar teeth are not discernable in this view.

with oral examination of the conscious chinchilla, so anesthesia and diagnostic imaging including either radiography or computed tomography (CT) are required for a thorough assessment [22]. Most chinchillas will not display clinical signs of dental disease until there is significant oral dysfunction present [20, 22]. Normal chinchilla radiographs are shown in Figures 8.22a, b, 8.23a and b. Abnormal chinchilla images are shown in Figures 8.24a–d, 8.25a and b.

Rats, Mice, Hamsters, Gerbils, and Other Commonly Kept Rodent Pets

For rats, mice, and other pet rodents, the incisors are openrooted (aradicular) and can overgrow. The molar teeth are brachydont and do not grow continuously. All rodents lack canine teeth. A diastema is present between the incisors and molar teeth. The enamel is typically yellow in color. Incisor malocclusions can be congenital or acquired.

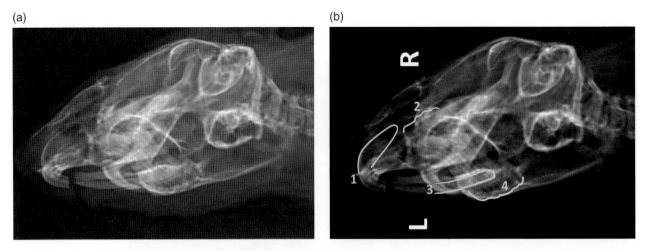

Figure 8.20 (a) Left dorsal-right lateral oblique (LD-RVO) radiograph of a normal guinea pig skull. The mandibular check teeth apices lie close to the ventral mandibular cortex, which should appear smooth. Performing oblique images allows visualization of each quadrant. Despite these high-quality images, visualization of the apices of the maxillary incisor teeth is still challenging. Right to left and left to right oblique views should always be obtained for comparison, even if dental disease is suspected only on one side. (b) Annotated left dorsal right ventral oblique radiograph of a guinea pig skull. (1) Right maxillary incisor root. (2) Right maxillary cheek teeth apices are still challenging to critically evaluate. (3) Left mandibular incisor root. (4) Apices of the left mandibular cheek teeth.

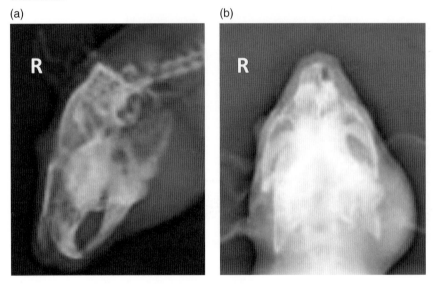

Figure 8.21 (a) Preliminary right lateral radiograph of a guinea pig with caudal left facial swelling. This image was taken with standard digital radiography. The image demonstrates poor detail of the dentoalveolar structures. (b) Preliminary right dorsoventral radiograph of the same guinea pig with caudal left facial swelling. This image was taken with standard digital radiography. The image demonstrates poor detail of the dentoalveolar structures. (c) Right lateral skull radiograph of the same guinea pig shown in Figure (a) and (b). Notice the improved clarity of the skull bones and increased detail which allows the identification of the molar apices extending below the cortices of the mandible, giving the mandibular margins an irregular appearance. (d) Annotated right lateral skull radiograph of the same guinea pig shown in Figure (a)–(c). This image is mildly oblique. The margins of both mandibles appear irregular compared to the expected normal smooth mandible as seen in Figure 8.19(a). The lateral positioning does not allow for identification of the affected quadrants. (e) Dorsoventral radiographs of the same guinea pig as shown in Figure (a)–(d). The improved technique allows for a clearer assessment of the changes in the left mandible. (f) Annotated dorsoventral radiograph of the same guinea pig shown in Figure (a)–(e). The yellow arrow points to the marked irregular margins of the left mandible, while the white asterisk indicates the soft tissue swelling associated with the abscess. When comparing the margins of the right and left mandibular profiles, it is obvious that the left side is irregular, thickened, and mottled in appearance. (g) Left parasagittal computed tomography image of the same guinea pig shown in Figure (a)–(f). Computed tomography allows better identification of the affected teeth, and the osteomyelitis associated with the abscess of the left third molar, with extension into the mandible and surrounding soft tissues. (h) Dorsal computed tomography image of the same guinea pig shown in Figure (a)–(g). (i) Transverse computed tomography image of the same guinea pig shown in Figure (a)–(h). (j) For the guinea pig in Figure (a)–(i), CT allowed 3D reconstruction of the skull to demonstrate the degree of bony changes present in the left mandible. This is a lateral view of the left side of the guinea pig skull, with the soft tissues removed, demonstrating the severe remodeling of the left mandible, with an open tract in the caudolateral mandible. (k) Computed tomography allowed 3D reconstruction of the skull of the guinea pig shown in Figure (a)–(j) to demonstrate the degree of bony changes present in the left mandible. This image represents a cranial to caudal view of the guinea pig with the soft tissues removed, demonstrating the degree of bony remodeling ventrally and laterally on the left mandible compared to the right.

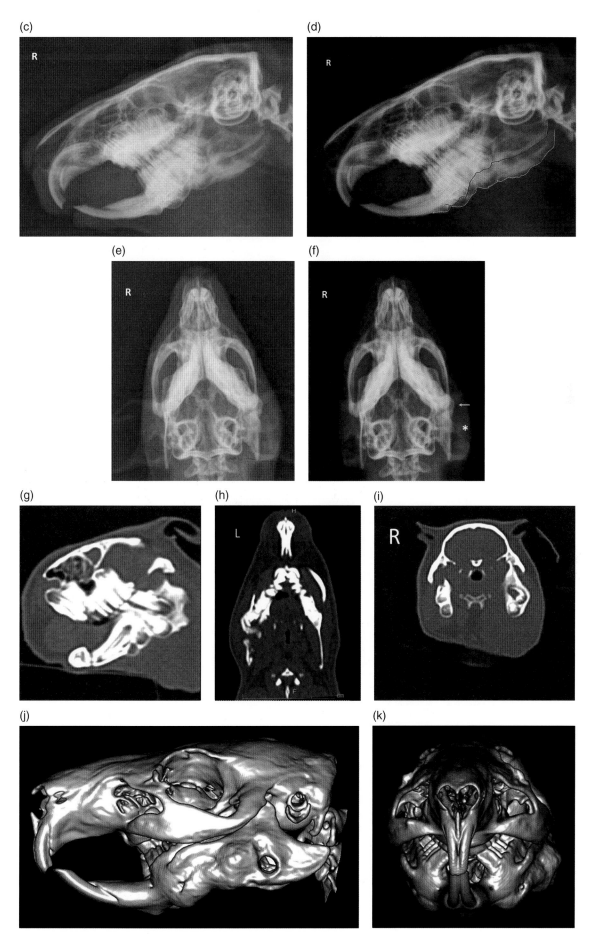

Figure 8.21 (Continued)

(a)

(b)

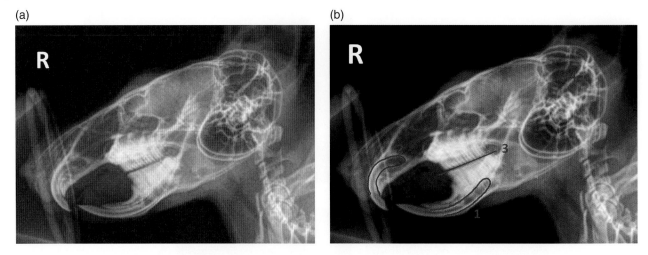

Figure 8.22 (a) Lateral radiograph of the normal chinchilla skull. The cheek teeth are in occlusion when the chinchilla is at rest. In the lateral view, the cheek teeth meet in a flat, horizontal occlusal plane, forming a regular, smooth palisade. The cheek teeth are relatively short. This is especially apparent in the last mandibular and maxillary molar teeth. The apices of the first three mandibular cheek teeth are close to the ventral cortices of the mandible. The mandibular incisor teeth are very long and slightly curved. The mandibular incisor roots are positioned lingually to the cheek teeth, and their apices reach the second or third cheek tooth. Maxillary incisors are even more curved, forming a nearly complete half-circle. The maxillary incisor apices are located near the palate, about 2/3 the distance of the maxillary diastema. The tympanic bullae occupy most of the caudal aspect of the skull. (b) Annotated lateral radiograph of the normal chinchilla skull. (1) Mandibular incisor teeth roots. (2) Maxillary incisor roots. (3) In the lateral view, the cheek teeth meet in a flat, horizontal occlusal plane, forming a regular, smooth palisade. (4) The tympanic bullae occupy most of the caudal aspect of the skull.

(a)

(b)

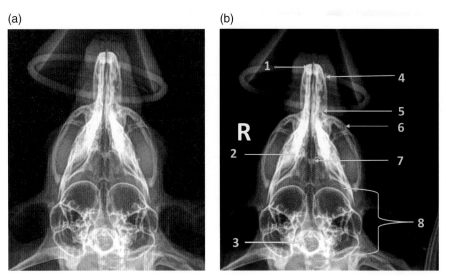

Figure 8.23 (a) Dorsoventral radiograph of a normal chinchilla skull. (b) Annotated dorsoventral radiograph of a normal chinchilla skull. (1) Maxillary incisor tooth. (2) Mandible. (3) Foramen magnum. (4) Incisive bone. (5) Maxilla. (6) Zygomatic bone. (7) Parietal bone. (8) Tympanic bulla.

Acquired malocclusions are generally due to trauma or from inappropriate chewing of surfaces within the habitat. In these small rodents, treatment of malocclusions pertaining to the overgrown incisor teeth requires regular trimming every four to five weeks [20]. Trimming teeth with a dental burr or rotary tool is best, as clipping with nail or dental clippers may shatter or splinter the teeth, causing pain and trauma to the roots. This will exacerbate dental disease already existing in these patients. Extraction of these teeth can be performed but is very difficult due to the length and location of the long incisor tooth roots [20] (Figures 8.26a, b, 8.27a, and b). As previously noted, because of the small size of the skull of most rodent exotic pets, whole-skull views may be possible with extraoral positioning of the skull on a standard intraoral dental film or digital dental radiographic sensor (see hamster Figures 8.26a, b, and 8.28a–d and rat Figures 8.27a, b, and 8.29a–d).

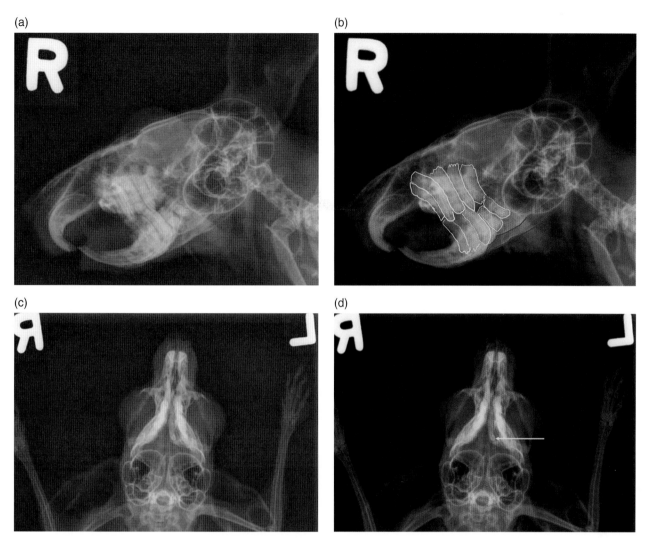

Figure 8.24 (a) Lateral radiograph of a chinchilla with significant malocclusion. This image is mildly oblique, as evident by the offset of the tympanic bullae. The maxillary and mandibular incisors appear normal. The tympanic bullae are normal in size and normally air-filled. (b) Annotated lateral skull radiograph of the chinchilla from Figure (a) depicting severe molar overgrowth. Yellow outlines the maxillary and mandibular cheek teeth. Note the curvature of the apices, with the rostral maxillary premolar apices extending into the nasal cavity. Red outlines the irregular ventral margins of the left mandible, and smoother margin of the right mandible. The malocclusion of the cheek teeth artificially obliques the orientation of the mandibles in this image. (c) Dorsoventral radiograph of the same chinchilla in Figure (a) and (b). This is a well-positioned DV with good symmetry of the bullae and the maxillary incisors. Abnormal deviation of the left mandibular incisor is visible medial to the left cheek tooth arcade. Molar malocclusion is not visible with this projection. (d) Annotated dorsoventral radiograph of the same chinchilla shown in Figure (a)–(c). Superimposition of the maxilla and mandible make visualization of individual teeth challenging, however, abnormal deviation of the apex of the left mandibular incisor tooth is evident (yellow arrow). This view does not display the degree of soft tissue enlargement that would be more evident in a computed tomographic image.

Ferrets

Ferrets have typical brachydont caniniform dentition similar to cats. Oral imaging and treatment for ferrets are similar to felines patients, although the small gape in some animals may prevent intraoral imaging and extraoral techniques may be necessary. Images of ferrets are not included in this chapter due to their radiographic positioning similarity to cats. Please see Chapter 2 for suggestions on radiographic techniques for the feline patient.

African Pygmy Hedgehogs

The teeth of the African pygmy hedgehog are all anelodont and brachydont, therefore closed-rooted teeth that do not grow continuously. In hedgehogs, the first maxillary incisors are long and widely spaced, projecting slightly forward [9]. The canine teeth are small and similar to the second or third pair of incisors and the first premolars. Hedgehog premolars have prominent cusps, more like those of a carnivore [23]. The third maxillary premolar

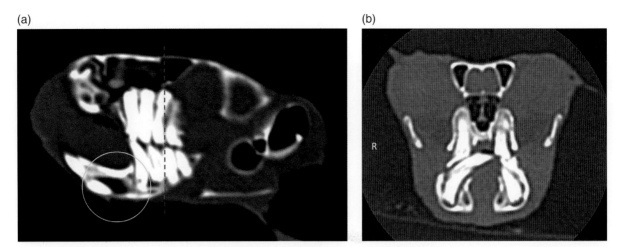

Figure 8.25 (a) Right parasagittal CT image of the same chinchilla as shown in Figure 8.24 (a)–(d). By removing superimposition, CT provides a better demonstration of the molar malocclusion. CT also identified gas attenuation lateral to the second mandibular molar indicating root infection in this area (yellow circle). These findings allowed for appropriate treatment, including extraction of the left mandibular incisor, in addition to occlusal equilibration of the left cheek teeth. (b) Transverse CT image of the same chinchilla shown in radiographs in Figure 8.24 (a)–(d). This image clearly shows the deviation of the cheek teeth, which would result in tongue entrapment and trauma to the oral mucosa. The slice was taken at the level of red dashed line in the transverse image in Figure (a).

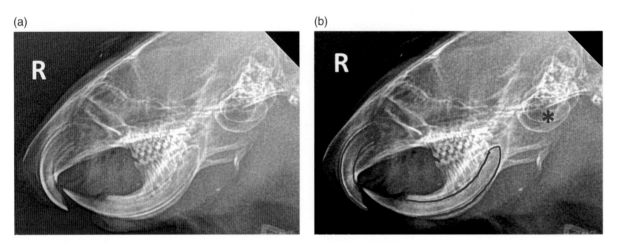

Figure 8.26 (a) Right lateral skull radiograph of a normal hamster obtained using extraoral positioning of an intraoral Size 2 dental sensor. (b) Annotated right lateral skull radiograph of a normal hamster as shown in Figure (a). The red outlines display the extensive mandibular incisor apices which extend lingual and caudal to the molars. The incisors are the only aradicular hypsodont teeth in these rodent patients. This image is slightly oblique, as is evidenced by the lack of overlap of the tympanic bullae (red asterisk).

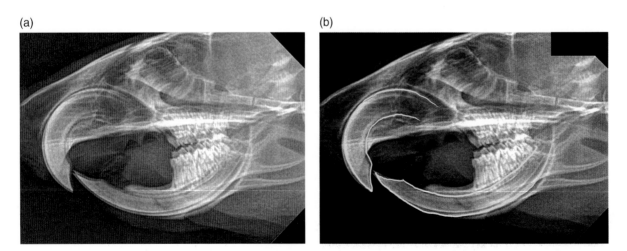

Figure 8.27 (a) Lateral skull radiograph of an adult rat using an intraoral Size 2 dental sensor placed extraorally. (b) Annotated lateral skull radiograph of the adult rat shown in Figure (a) using extraoral positioning of an intraoral Size 2 dental sensor. The yellow lines highlight the extent of the maxillary and mandibular incisors.

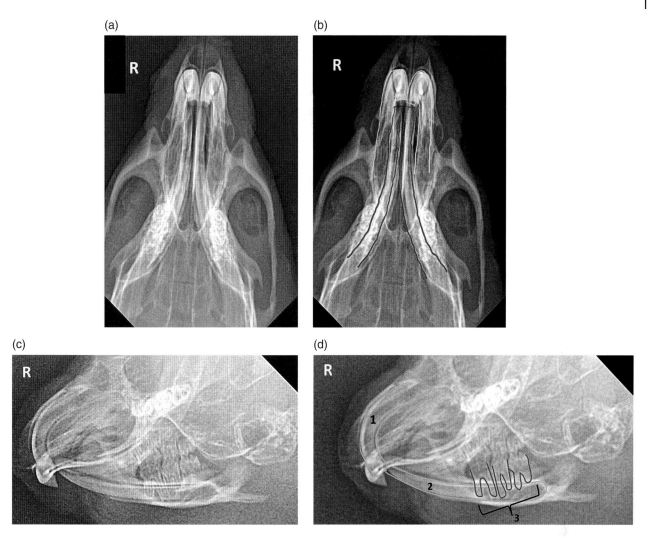

Figure 8.28 (a) Dorsoventral skull radiograph of a hamster as shown in Figure 8.26 (a) and (b). The small sensor size allows high resolution for skull and dental detail in these small rodent patients. (b) Annotated dorsoventral skull radiograph of a hamster as shown in Figures 8.26a, b, and 8.28a. Yellow outlines show the extent of the maxillary incisors. Red outlines the extent of the mandibular incisor apices. (c) Left dorsal-right ventral oblique (LD-RVO) skull radiograph of a normal hamster obtained using an extraoral technique with a Size 2 intraoral dental sensor. (d) Annotated left dorsal-right ventral oblique (LD-RVO) skull radiograph of a normal hamster obtained using an extraoral technique with a Size 2 intraoral dental sensor. In this image, the skull is mildly over-rotated, which obscures the apices of the right maxillary molars. (1) Right maxillary incisor. (2) Left mandibular incisor. (3) Left mandibular molar apices (red outlines).

tooth resembles the carnassial tooth of a carnivore as well. The first two maxillary premolars have four cusps, resembling the molars of primates [9] (Figure 8.30a and b). Diagnostic radiographs of hedgehogs can be taken with a conventional X-ray system (Figure 8.31a–f). Utilizing computed tomographic imaging can improve the diagnostic quality of images in small patients, but regardless, the smaller the patient, the more difficult it is to acquire crisp images with good detail. Normal hedgehog CT images are found in Figure 8.32a–c. Abnormalities in tooth numbers are frequent in hedgehogs, including supernumerary incisors or the absence of the second pair of mandibular incisors [9]. Dental disease is common in hedgehogs and includes periodontal disease and oral neoplasia

(Figure 8.33a–d). Odontogenic fibromas have also been described in hedgehogs [23]. Metabolic bone disease can also be observed in this species which can contribute to the development of a periodontal disease presentation (Figure 8.34a and b).

Sugar Gliders

Sugar glider teeth are small except for the mandibular first incisors, which are prominent, sharp, and specialized for gouging [9]. The dentition is anelodont and brachydont which does not grow continuously. Dental disorders found in sugar gliders include trauma, metabolic bone disease, periodontal disease, and dental calculus [8, 9, 20].

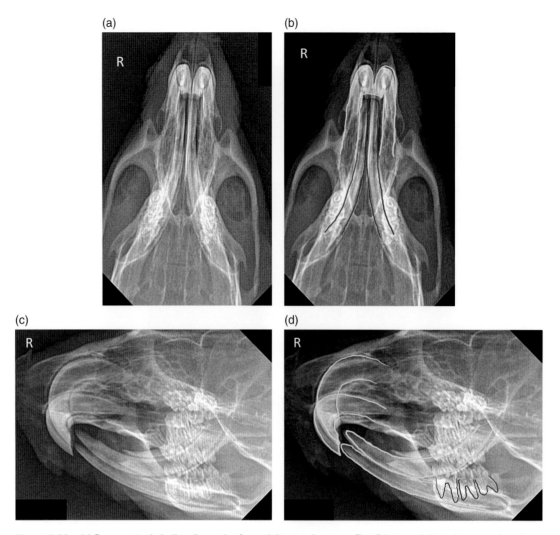

Figure 8.29   (a) Dorsoventral skull radiograph of an adult rat, taken on a Size 2 intraoral dental sensor placed extraorally. The high-quality sensors give nicely detailed views of incisors in such a small patient. (b) Annotated dorsoventral radiograph of a rat skull taken extraorally using a Size 2 intraoral dental sensor as seen in Figure (a). The yellow outlines the extent of the maxillary incisors, while the red lines note the extent of the mandibular incisors. The mandibular and maxillary premolars and molars are superimposed in this view. (c) Left dorsal-right ventral lateral oblique (LD-RVO) skull radiograph of a rat taken on an intraoral radiographic plate using extraoral positioning. (d) Annotated right lateral oblique skull radiograph of a rat obtained with an intraoral Size 2 dental sensor and extraoral positioning as seen in Figure (c). This view shows the extent of the aradicular hypsodont incisors (yellow lines) in relation to the apices of the mandibular molars (red lines). The oblique positioning allows observation of detail in each quadrant more clearly.

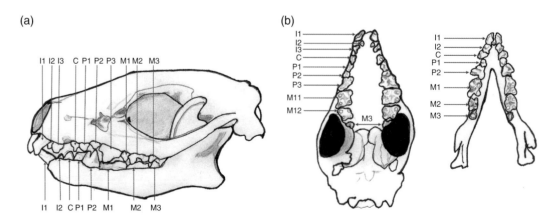

Figure 8.30   (a) Line drawing illustration of the expected normal dentition of an African pygmy hedgehog. As insectivores/omnivores, hedgehogs have brachydont dentition. Maxillary I2 is normally lingual to I1 and I3. (b) Line drawing of the expected dental anatomy of African pygmy hedgehog. This drawing better illustrates how Maxillary I2 is lingual to I1 and I3. Abnormalities in tooth numbers are frequent in hedgehogs, including supernumerary incisors or the absence of the second pair of mandibular incisors.

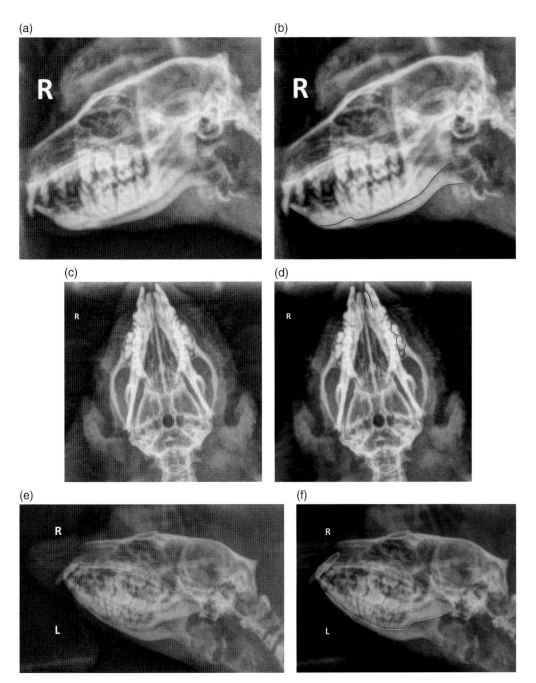

Figure 8.31   (a) Lateral skull radiograph of a normal African pygmy hedgehog showing the dentition. This radiograph is mildly oblique, making visualization of the roots of the maxillary arcade more easily visualized, but the mandibular apices are still superimposed making localization challenging. The small skull and teeth of the hedgehog can make visualization of individual teeth or dental disease challenging when using conventional X-ray machines. (b) Annotated lateral skull radiograph of a normal African pygmy hedgehog showing the dentition as shown in Figure (a). The red lines indicate the margins of the mandible for each arcade. More detail would be evident if an intraoral dental sensor were used extraorally for the skull in this species, similar to the images shown for the hamster in Figure 8.26a and b and rat in Figure 8.27a and b. (c) Dorsoventral skull radiograph of an African pygmy hedgehog skull. This hedgehog was determined to have normal dentition on physical examination and with CT. The small size of the hedgehog skull can make positioning and selection of radiographic settings challenging for such a small species. Similar to the hamster shown in Figure 8.26a and b, and rat in Figure 8.27a and b, use of an intraoral sensor extraorally would have given sharper detail to the skull images in a small mammal like the hedgehog. (d) Annotated dorsoventral skull radiograph of the African pygmy hedgehog shown in Figure (a)–(c). Yellow outlines the margins of the maxillary first incisor, blue outlines the margins of the mandibular first incisor, and red outlines some of the visible margins of the maxillary molars. Unfortunately, clear delineation of the mandibular molars is difficult due to superimposition of the maxilla and mandible with this view. (e) Left dorsal-right ventral oblique skull radiograph of an African pygmy hedgehog. This is the same patient as in Figure (a)–(d). (f) Annotated left dorsal-right ventral oblique skull radiograph of the African pygmy hedgehog as shown in Figure (a)–(e). The right maxillary incisor is outlined in yellow rostrally. Unfortunately, this image was under-rotated and possibly angled rostrally, such that the mandibles superimpose more toward the nose and less caudally. The left mandible is outlined in yellow, and the right mandible is outlined in red. The poor positioning makes it difficult to isolate the other maxillary and mandibular teeth that might be possible in a well-positioned image. This image could have been improved using a high detail film, such as a dental sensor placed extraorally.

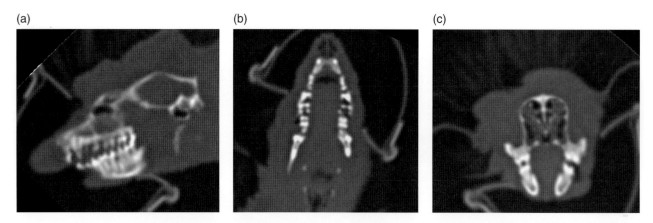

Figure 8.32 (a) Parasagittal conventional CT image of the normal skull and dentition of an African pygmy hedgehog. CT will give a better impression of soft tissue changes associated with the dental arcades for this small species. This is especially important in hedgehogs, as squamous cell carcinoma is a common condition for the species, and important to differentiate from dental disease. Even with this technology, the small tooth size of the hedgehog dentition makes crisp image detail challenging. (b) Dorsal maxilla conventional CT image of the normal skull and dentition of an African pygmy hedgehog. (c) Transverse image of the molars and sinuses of an African pygmy hedgehog.

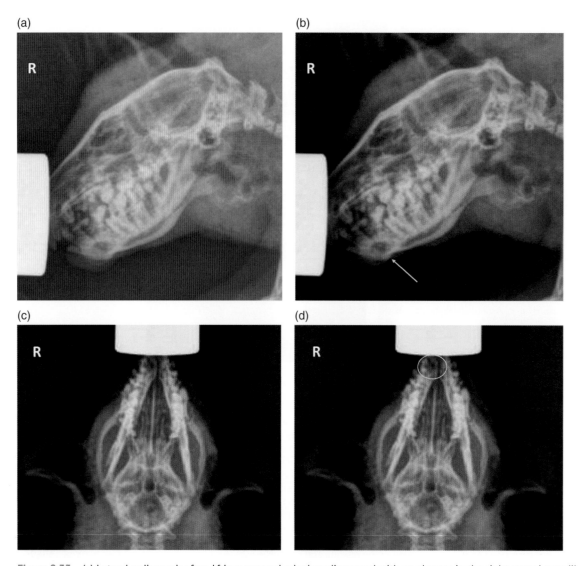

Figure 8.33 (a) Lateral radiograph of an African pygmy hedgehog diagnosed with an abscess in the right rostral mandible. (b) Annotated lateral radiograph of the African pygmy hedgehog shown in Figure (a). The expansile lytic lesion in the right rostral mandible is noted with the yellow arrow. Fine needle aspirate of this area identified an abscess. (c) Dorsoventral radiograph of the same African pygmy hedgehog shown in Figure (a) and (b), diagnosed with an abscess in the right rostral mandible. (d) Dorsoventral radiograph of the same African pygmy hedgehog shown in Figure (a)–(c), diagnosed with an abscess in the right rostral mandible. The lesion is circled in yellow, showing osteolysis of the rostral mandible near the mandibular symphysis.

Figure 8.34 (a) Lateral radiograph of an African pygmy hedgehog suffering from severe metabolic bone disease. All bone structures, except the petrous temporal bones, are more radiolucent than normal and have diminished contrast with the surrounding soft tissues. The teeth remain radiopaque. A pathologic fracture is present in the isolated radius/ulna (yellow arrow). Nutritional secondary hyperparathyroidism causing metabolic bone disease is unfortunately a common problem in pet exotic mammals fed an inappropriate diet. (b) Dorsoventral radiograph of the same hedgehog shown in Figure 8.33a. All bones of the skull, except the petrous temporal bones, are nearly translucent. The teeth remain radiopaque.

(a)

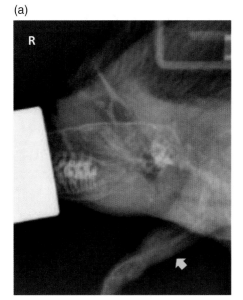

(b)

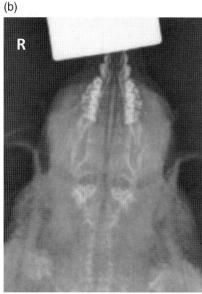

Prairie Dogs (*Cyomys ludovicianus*)

Prairie dogs have dentition similar to other rodents, with the incisors open-rooted (aradicular) and subject to overgrowth with inadequate wear. The molars are brachydont and do not grow continuously. Dental pathology is common in prairie dogs and includes fractured teeth, tooth root abscesses and malocclusions associated with loss or overgrowth of teeth. Maxillary teeth may abscess into the nasal cavities and sinuses, resulting in clinical signs of upper respiratory disease and dyspnea [24]. Odontomas in prairie dogs have been associated with chronic dental disease or trauma resulting from chewing on inappropriate objects such as the animals caging [5, 24]. Radiographs and thorough oral examination under general anesthesia are necessary to diagnose dental abnormalities in this species. When the jaw is at rest, the incisors and cheek teeth of prairie dogs are in occlusion [16]. The incisor teeth are very large. The apex of the maxillary incisor tooth in this species is apical to the first cheek tooth. The mandibular incisor teeth traverse below the cheek teeth, with the apex of the incisor tooth located distal to the last cheek tooth [16].

Captive Nondomestic or "Wild" Mammals

Dental disease is a common cause of morbidity in many species that might be housed within zoos or in private animal collections, as well as those animals that are considered free-ranging wildlife. In small zoologic species, whole-skull radiographs can be obtained using intraoral

dental sensors (tenrec Figure 8.35a–f) similar to techniques previously described in pet rodents (Figures 8.26a, b, 8.27a, b, 8.28a–d, and 8.29a–d).

Nonhuman Primates

Nonhuman primates may suffer from many forms of oral disease, including periodontal disease, gingivitis, tartar, calculus, caries, osteomyelitis, malocclusion, pulp exposure, fistulas, tumors, and tooth fractures (as seen in the baboon Figure 8.36a–g), abscesses (gorilla Figure 8.37a–e), and several other oral abnormalities [25]. Knowledge of all of the distinct dental characteristics and associated pathology for the large variety of nonhuman primates is extremely difficult [26]. A drawing representing the expected dentition of an Old World primate is shown in Figure 8.38. Like humans, nonhuman primates have brachydont dentition, composed of teeth that are adapted to a combination of protection, consumption of a wide range of foods, and sexual dimorphism [26]. In some veterinary literature, the canine teeth are referred to as cuspids. Many nonhuman primates have comparatively large canine teeth and adjacent anatomical diastemas. The diastema that is mesial to the maxillary canine tooth allows for lateral movement of the lower canines [26]. In male baboons (Figure 8.36a), the oversized maxillary canine tooth passes laterally to the mandibular first cheek tooth (third premolar) [26]. In the baboon, the mesial surface of the third premolar tooth is commonly long and drawn out which provides a specialized shearing action as the jaw closes and the maxillary canine moves past it. This may possibly replace the carnassial function that is seen in carnivores [26]. Several types of teeth are represented in primate dentition, including incisors, canine teeth

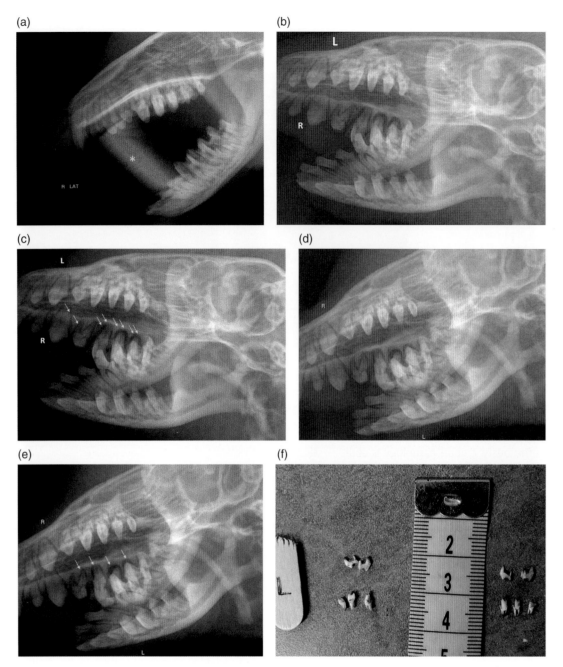

Figure 8.35 (a) Right lateral skull radiograph of a lesser Madagascar tenrec (*Echinops telfairi*) with visible periodontitis noted during the physical examination. A small section of a syringe is used as an oral wedge (yellow asterisk). This image was performed with extraoral positioning on an intraoral dental sensor for skull radiography. An adult tenrec of this species weighs approximately 200 g, and the feeding ecology is faunivorous. The dentition is brachydont. The small size of the lesser tenrec allows the skull to fit well on an intraoral sensor placed extraorally and can provide more detailed images for such a small species, similar to techniques demonstrated in the hamster Figures 8.26a, b, and 8.28a–d and rat Figures 8.27a, b, and 8.29a–d. Tenrecs are a species commonly housed in zoos, frequently used in outreach education programs. They may also be a privately owned exotic pet species as well. (b) Left dorsal-right ventral oblique radiograph of the same tenrec shown in Figure (a). Over-rotation of the skull makes assessment of the right mandible challenging, but in sections of the right maxilla, significant periapical lucency is present surrounding the right maxillary molar apices, as annotated in Figure (c). (c) Annotated left dorsal-right ventral oblique radiograph of the same tenrec shown in Figure (a) and (b). Significant periapical lucency is present surrounding the right maxillary premolars and molars (yellow arrows). Superimposition of the mandibles, and over-rotation of the left maxilla interferes with interpretation in these arcades. (d) Right dorsal-left ventral oblique radiograph of the same tenrec as shown in Figure (a)–(c). In this image, the skull is over-rotated, causing superimposition of the small mandibular apices. However, in the caudal left maxilla, significant periapical lucency is present surrounding the premolars and molars. (e) Annotated right dorsal-left ventral oblique radiograph of the same tenrec shown in Figure (a)–(d). The yellow arrows point to areas of periapical lucency surrounding the apices of the left maxillary premolar and molar teeth, indicating periodontal disease. Following the acquisition of these diagnostic radiographs, affected teeth were subsequently extracted from both the maxilla and mandibles, although the small tooth size in this species necessitated using an 18-gauge needle as a periodontal elevator for the extraction. (f) Post-extraction photograph demonstrating the tiny teeth of the lesser Madagascar tenrec shown in Figure (a)–(e). The teeth are laid out in this photograph to demonstrate the left and right maxillary and mandibular teeth extracted. *Source:* Courtesy of June Olds, DVM, DACZM, Iowa State University, College of Veterinary Medicine.

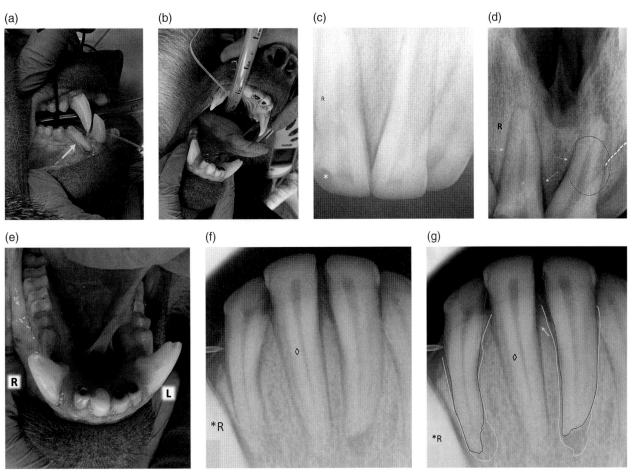

Figure 8.36 (a) Photograph of the dentition of an adult male Hamadryas baboon (*Papio hamadryas*), an Old-World primate, obtained during an anesthetized examination. In this baboon, the incisor teeth are blunted and there is attrition of the canine teeth and premolars, with visible caries present in the incisors, most evident in the following images. The elongated and angular first mandibular premolar (yellow arrow) is a normal species variation and should not be interpreted as pathology or attrition. Intraoral radiographs of this baboon are shown in the following images. (b) Rostral photograph of the adult male baboon shown in Figure (a). This baboon was rescued from a poor welfare situation. It has visible caries in the maxillary and mandibular incisors, with attrition of all teeth visible. *Source:* Photographs courtesy of Dana Foster. (c) Intraoral dental radiograph of the maxillary central incisor crowns of the baboon shown in Figure (a) and (b). The right maxillary central incisor has radiographic evidence of the carie (white asterisk) as shown in the clinical photo in Figure (b). (d) Intraoral dental radiograph of the maxillary central incisor apices of the same baboon as seen in Figure (a)–(c). There is widening of the periodontal ligament space surrounding the right and left central incisors (yellow arrows). Superimposition of the left lateral incisor (white dashed line) over the lateral aspect of the left central incisor could give the false impression of a fracture of the left central incisor body (red circle), unless you closely follow the outline of the lateral incisor and see the difference in opacity. These images are a good example of the challenges to obtaining whole-tooth images in nondomestic species when using dental sensors designed for the typical dentition of a dog or cat. Frequent repositioning for the "perfect" view will prolong anesthesia time and may increase complication risks for the animal being evaluated. (e) Occlusal photograph of the mandibular arcade of the same baboon shown in Figure (a)–(d). Incisor caries are more clearly seen in this view, with attrition and crown fractures of the canines, and attrition of the premolars and molars also visible. *Source:* Photograph courtesy of Dana Foster. (f) Intraoral radiograph of the mandibular incisors of the baboon shown in Figure (e). The needle indicates the right mandibular lateral incisor and the surrounding inflamed gingiva. The *R indicates the right mandibular canine tooth. The ◊ symbol indicates the right mandibular central incisor, which appears to be the only normal incisor grossly. (g) Annotated intraoral digital radiograph of the mandibular incisors of the baboon shown in Figure (a)–(f). The needle indicates the inflamed tissue near the right mandibular lateral incisor.
*R indicates the right mandibular canine tooth. The ◊ symbol identifies the right mandibular central incisor. The red lines indicate the tooth margins discernable, while the yellow lines indicate the areas of periapical lucency and widening of the periodontal ligament space around the visibly affected incisors. The right lateral incisor has a narrowed pulp canal, which can be an indication of an increased rate of dentin deposition due to pulpitis. The left central incisor also has evidence of tooth nonvitality due to an increased width of pulp canal size, which is also suspicious for pulpitis.

(a)   (b)   (c)

(d)   (e)

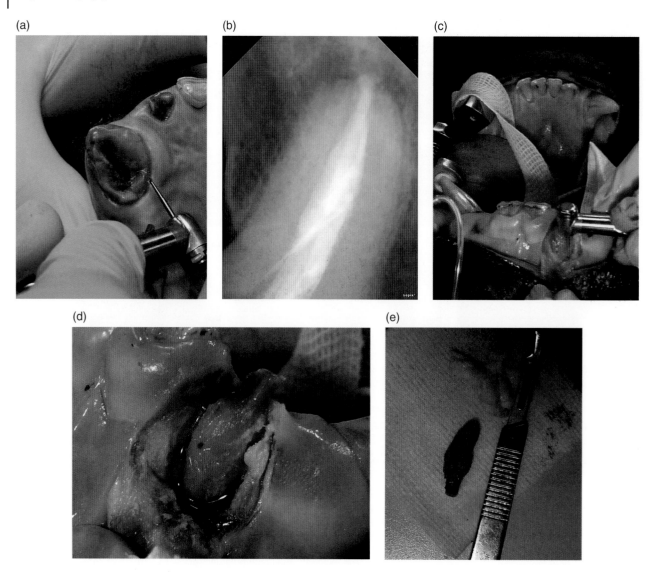

Figure 8.37 (a) Intraoperative photograph of the maxilla of a silverback Western lowland gorilla (*Gorilla gorilla*) undergoing a dental procedure to address disease in the right maxillary canine tooth and right lateral incisor. The pulp canal of the maxillary canine tooth is exposed and necrotic. The lateral maxillary incisor is fractured and has evidence of a carie and abscessation. This gorilla underwent endodontic therapy (root canal) for the canine tooth, and extraction of the affected incisor. (b) Postprocedural intraoral dental radiograph of the apex of the right maxillary canine tooth of the same gorilla shown in Figure (a) following root canal therapy. Note how only the apex of the tooth can be imaged on the dental sensor due to the large size of the teeth in this species. There is suspicion of periapical lucency associated with this tooth, although additional imaging would be necessary to confirm.
(c) Intraoperative photograph of the silverback gorilla shown in Figure (a) and (b) undergoing right maxillary incisor extraction. In this image, the gorilla is in dorsal recumbency, with the maxilla in the ventral position and the mandible positioned dorsal. This image demonstrates how deep the roots of the incisor teeth extend into the bone. Removal of these teeth requires competency in surgical extraction techniques. (d) Close-up intraoperative photograph of the right lateral maxillary incisor of the silverback gorilla shown in Figure (a)–(c), demonstrating the amount of bone removal that may be necessary to extract a diseased tooth in this species. *Source:* Courtesy of Utah's Hogle Zoo. (e) Post-extraction photograph of the right lateral maxillary incisor of the silverback gorilla shown in Figure (c) and (d). This photograph demonstrates how long the roots are compared to the visible crowns in this species, and why a major surgical extraction was necessary.

(cuspids), premolars, and molars [26]. Canine tooth extraction in nonhuman primates was previously considered an acceptable practice to protect human handlers; however, this procedure is no longer considered ethical. Defanging primates (and nondomestic carnivores) is no longer considered acceptable under the US Animal Welfare Act (AWA) and is also deemed unacceptable in a position statement issued by the American Veterinary Medical Association in 2006. In laboratory primates, canine tooth crown reduction techniques are still considered acceptable

Figure 8.38 Annotated drawing of the average Old World (OW) primate and great ape dentition. Most New World (NW) primate dental formulas differ only in that NW primate species typically have three maxillary and mandibular premolars as opposed to the two premolars found in humans, OW primates, and great apes.

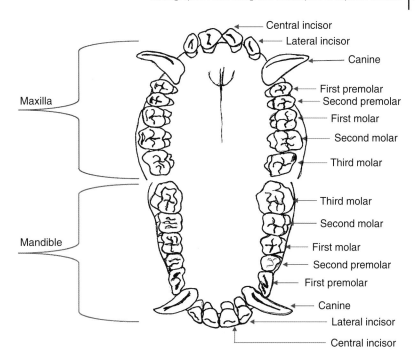

Maxilla

Central incisor
Lateral incisor
Canine
First premolar
Second premolar
First molar
Second molar
Third molar

Mandible

Third molar
Second molar
First molar
Second premolar
First premolar
Canine
Lateral incisor
Central incisor

procedures to reduce the severity of harm to humans or other monkeys; however, complications such as periapical abscess requiring extraction of the diseased canine tooth secondary to coronal reduction have been documented [27].

Carnivores

In small carnivores like meerkats (*Suricata suricatta*), fractures and attrition to the tooth surface have been identified as affecting the animal's ability to eat [28] (Figure 8.39a–e). In coatimundi (*Nasua nasua*), plaque, gingivitis, periodontitis, dental staining, dental abrasion, dental fracture, pulp exposure, malocclusion, and supernumerary teeth have all been identified [29] (Figures 8.40a–g, 8.41a–g, and 8.42a–d).

Some studies have suggested that the captive diet fed to carnivores in North American zoos might contribute to an increase in cranial deformation and is correlated to an increased incidence in periodontal disease and calculus accumulation for these species [30]. Complicated crown fractures are commonly encountered in captive carnivores, including bears [31] (Figure 8.43a–c) and large felids such as tigers (Figure 8.44a–i), cheetah, jaguars, lions [32–36] and snow leopards (Figure 8.45) as well as other small carnivores such as skunks (Figures 8.46a–h, 8.47a–c, and 8.48a–c), and marine mammals such as sea lions and seals [37] (Figure 8.49a–i). Periodontal disease with resultant osteomyelitis can also be seen in other marine mammals such as dolphins (Figure 8.50a–d).

In an older survey of dental disease conditions in exotic and zoo animals housed under human care, malocclusion,

periodontal disease, and trauma (specifically tooth fractures) were the most common clinical conditions documented to affect zoo-housed animals [38]. This survey also conveyed that primates and carnivores appear to be the most common taxonomic groups affected by these conditions [38]. In a more recent survey of zoos in North and South America, skull radiography was the most common diagnostic imaging modality available for acquiring dental images of zoo animals (Powers/Olds/Mulherin 2020 publication pending). For this reason, utilizing the positioning described for skull radiography of small mammals, including at least four views – lateral, dorsoventral or ventrodorsal, and right and left lateral oblique views, are recommended to give the most complete assessment of all four quadrants. Less than half of the zoos responding to the survey indicated that intraoral dental radiography is available within the zoo facility. If intraoral images are possible, the practitioner may find that the size and length of the teeth may not fit on normally sized intraoral plates or dental sensors used for companion animals or humans (see gorilla Figure 8.37b and tiger Figure 8.44g–i).

Radiographic Positioning and Techniques in Captive Animals

Techniques described for equine patients in Chapter 9 can be used in large zoo species to help facilitate acquiring diagnostic images (as shown in the dolphin Figure 8.50a–c and camel Figure 8.51a–e). However, an important difference is that while most equine techniques can be

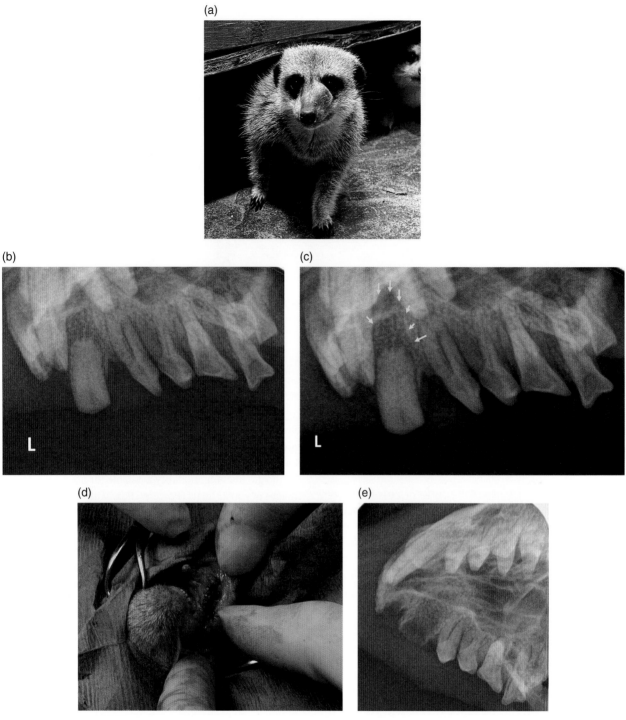

Figure 8.39 (a) Photograph of a meerkat (*Suricata suricatta*) showing left side facial swelling suggestive of a maxillary tooth root abscess. *Source:* Courtesy of Henry Vilas Zoo. (b) Extraoral dental radiograph of the meerkat shown in Figure (a), obtained with use of an intraoral dental sensor placed extraorally, showing significant periapical lucency surrounding the fractured left maxillary canine tooth. This was suspected to be the cause of the facial swelling noted in the clinical photograph as seen in Figure (a). (c) Annotated extraoral dental radiograph of the meerkat shown in Figure (a) and (b). The yellow arrows demonstrate the significant periapical lucency surrounding the fractured left maxillary canine tooth. This was suspected to be the cause of the facial swelling noted in the clinical photograph (Figure (a)). (d) Postoperative photograph of the meerkat shown in Figure (a)–(c), following canine tooth removal for abscess treatment. This photograph demonstrates the small size of the meerkat oral cavity in relation to the dentist's fingers in this view. This small oral cavity interfered with intraoral sensor positioning, which caused the oblique appearance of the radiographic images in Figure (b) and (c). (e) Postoperative intraoral radiograph of the left maxillary dental arcade of the meerkat shown in Figure (a)–(d), following extraction of the affected canine tooth. *Source:* Courtesy of Jill Medenwaldt, RVT, VTS-Dentistry, University of Wisconsin.

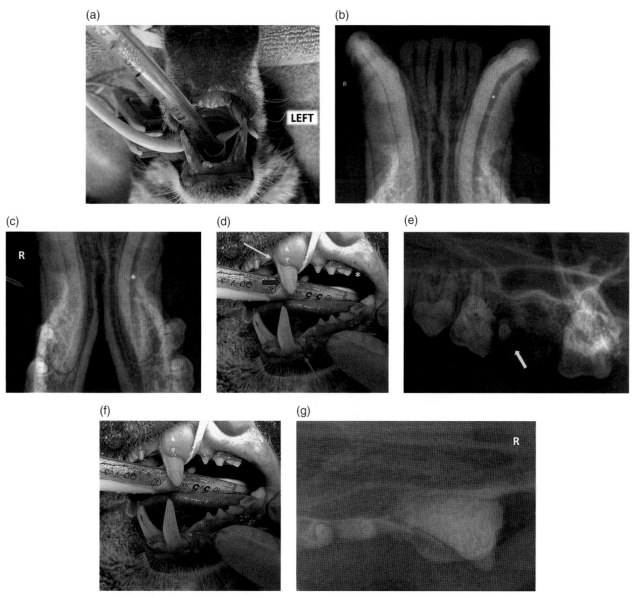

Figure 8.40 (a) Rostral photograph of an adult white-nosed coatimundi (*Nasua narica*) with chronic periodontal disease, severe dental calculus, and attrition. This photograph was taken during an anesthetized examination. *Source:* Photograph courtesy of Dana Foster. (b) Intraoral rostral mandibular radiograph of the mandibular canine teeth and incisors of the adult male coatimundi shown in Figure (a). The left mandibular canine tooth has increased width of the pulp canal (yellow asterisk) consistent with a nonvital tooth with arrested tooth development. Both teeth show irregular and mottled enamel margins and chronic wear. (c) Intraoral dental radiograph of the rostral mandible of the coatimundi shown in Figure (a) and (b) demonstrating the mandibular canine teeth apices. The left mandibular canine tooth root is shorter compared to right, which may indicate this tooth has arrested development. Additionally, the left canine tooth pulp canal is widened (yellow asterisk). The needle on the right of the image was inserted as a marker for the right side and is also pointing to an area of significant gingivitis visible grossly. (d) Lateral photograph of the left side of the oral cavity of the same coatimundi following dental scaling and polishing of the teeth. The left mandibular canine tooth displays an area of significant gingival recession (red arrow), which is also present at the mesial aspect of the left maxillary canine tooth (yellow arrow). Prominent dental grooves are common in the lingual and buccal aspects of the canine teeth of this species (purple arrows). The molars visible in this photo show attrition with gingivitis present at the free gingival margin throughout the oral cavity. The dental formula for the coatimundi is I3/3, C1/1, P3–4/3–4, and M2/2. In this photograph there is a space present where the left maxillary M1 should be visible (yellow asterisk). (e) Intraoral radiograph of the mid-maxilla of the same coatimundi shown in Figure (a)–(d). This radiograph demonstrates a retained tooth root (yellow arrow) present at the location of the left molar which appears grossly absent in the clinical photograph seen in Figure (d). (f) Photograph of the right side of the oral cavity of the same coatimundi shown in Figure (a)–(e). This image was taken following scaling and polishing of the teeth. The right maxillary canine tooth is fractured, and there is gingival recession (yellow arrow) present on the mesial aspect of the tooth. Gingival recession is also present at the distal and buccal aspects of the right mandibular canine tooth (red arrow) and the prominent lingual dental groove is visible on the left mandibular canine tooth (purple arrow). *Source:* Photograph courtesy of Dana Foster. (g) Intraoral radiograph taken at an occlusal angle of the right maxillary canine tooth of the coatimundi shown in Figure (a)–(f).

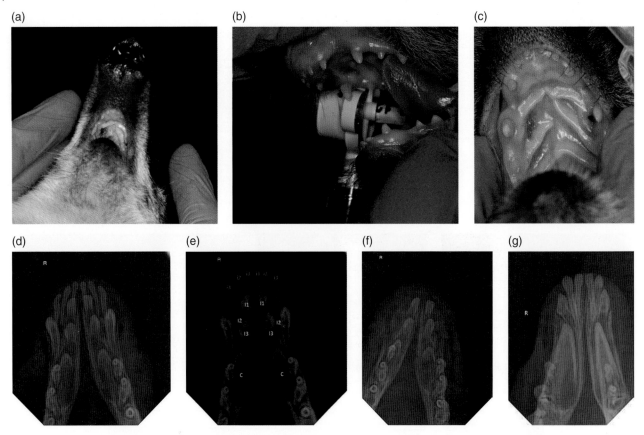

Figure 8.41 (a) Photograph demonstrating severe mandibular brachygnathism, malocclusion, and secondary mucosal trauma in a juvenile coatimundi. (b) Left lateral photograph of the same juvenile coatimundi shown in Figure (a), demonstrating the severe mandibular brachygnathism and Class 2 malocclusion. (c) Intraoral photograph of the maxilla and hard palate of the juvenile coatimundi shown in Figure (a) and (b) with severe mandibular brachygnathism. The yellow arrows point to the areas of trauma in the hard palate secondary to penetration from the deciduous mandibular canine teeth. *Source:* Courtesy of Brenda L. Mulherin, DVM, DAVDC, Iowa State University College of Veterinary Medicine. (d) Intraoral radiograph of the rostral mandible of the coatimundi shown in Figure (a)–(c). Note the presence of both the deciduous and unerupted permanent teeth. (e) Annotated pretreatment intraoral radiograph of the rostral mandible of the coatimundi in Figure (a)–(d). The deciduous teeth are numbered in red, while the unerupted permanent teeth are numbered in yellow. "I" identifies the permanent incisor teeth, while "i" identifies the deciduous incisor teeth. "C" identifies the permanent canine teeth while "c" identifies the deciduous canine teeth. (f) Postprocedure intraoral radiograph of the same coatimundi shown in Figure (a)–(e), following extraction of the deciduous teeth for treatment of the Class II malocclusion. (g) Intraoral radiograph of the same coatimundi shown in Figure (a)–(f), four months following extraction of the deciduous teeth for treatment of the Class II malocclusion, demonstrating eruption of the permanent incisors, but eruption of the permanent canine teeth has not yet occurred.

accomplished with standing sedation, most zoo species must be fully anesthetized prior to obtaining appropriate views due to the nature of the species. For many large zoo animals, the examination, immobilization, and anesthesia will occur in the animal's off-exhibit quarters, which necessitates bringing diagnostic equipment to the patient, rather than transporting the patient to the hospital. Portable radiography equipment has made diagnostic imaging much more attainable for many zoo animals. Unfortunately, the size of the skull, limitations of the kVP output of many portable X-ray generators, and the many challenges associated with anesthetizing and positioning large and potentially dangerous animals for diagnostic imaging can offer even more obstacles (grizzly bear Figure 8.52a–e and tapir

Figure 8.53a–i). Logistical challenges at locations outside of the zoo hospital, such as inadequate electrical access, Wi-Fi connectivity issues for wireless systems, and managing employee and animal safety throughout the procedure also exist.

Animal Training

Depending on the species, oral examinations and procurement of diagnostic images may be able to be obtained with training alone (see dolphin Figure 8.50a–d, rhinoceros Figure 8.54a–c, giraffe Figure 8.55a–g, seal Figure 8.56a, sea lion Figure 8.56b). Movement artifacts and superimposition of structures can interfere with image quality and the

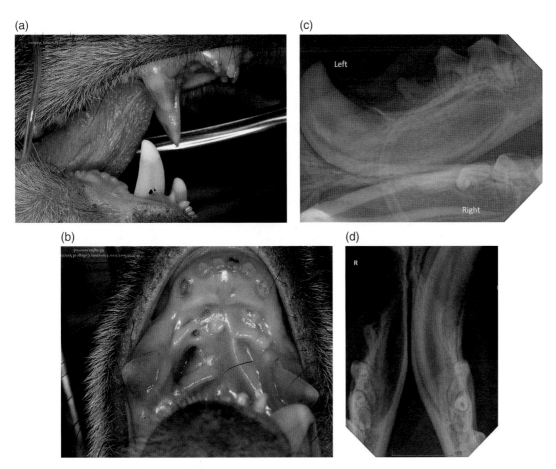

Figure 8.42 (a) Photograph of the same coatimundi shown in Figure 8.41 (a)–(g) two and a half years after the original dental procedure. Mandibular brachygnathism with a significant Class 2 malocclusion is still present. The permanent dentition appears to have erupted. In this image, the right maxillary canine tooth appears to be infra-erupted compared to the left maxillary canine tooth and right mandibular canine tooth. (b) Intraoral photograph of the rostral maxilla of the same adult coatimundi shown in Figure (a). There is significant occlusal trauma to the hard palate lingual to the right maxillary canine tooth from contact with the right mandibular canine tooth. There no longer appears to be occlusal contact with the hard palate lingual to the left maxillary canine tooth as was seen in Figure 8.41(c) when juvenile dentition was still present. (c) Intraoral dental radiograph of the rostral mandible in the adult coatimundi shown in Figure (a) and (b). Note the extreme but normal curvature of the canine teeth in this species. This image demonstrates the normal left mandibular canine tooth. The image was taken pre-extraction of the right mandibular canine tooth, as this tooth was causing trauma to the hard palate as was shown in Figure (b). (d) Intraoral rostral mandibular radiograph of the adult coatimundi shown in Figure (a)–(c) post-extraction of the right mandibular canine tooth, demonstrating an intact mandibular cortex following the surgical procedure.

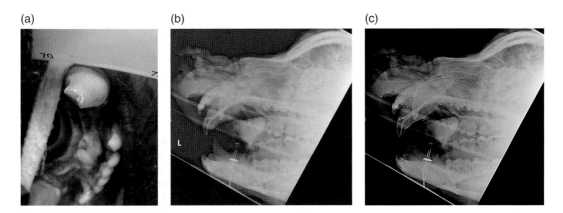

Figure 8.43 (a) Clinical photograph of the right maxillary canine tooth of a grizzly bear demonstrating the appearance of a crown fracture of the tooth. This patient previously had a root canal procedure performed. *Source:* Courtesy of Brenda L. Mulherin, DVM, DAVDC, Iowa State University College of Veterinary Medicine. (b) Right dorsal-left ventral oblique skull radiograph of the same grizzly bear shown in Figure (a). The beam was re-collimated to focus on the dentition in this view. (c) Annotated right dorsal-left ventral oblique skull radiograph of the same grizzly bear shown in Figure (a) and (b). The superimposition of the left maxillary canine tooth (white dashed lines) leads to distortion of the margins and apices of the right maxillary canine tooth, which has had a previous root canal performed. This image demonstrates how challenging it may be to get useful diagnostic radiographs in a timely manner during a zoo animal immobilization procedure. *Source:* Radiographs courtesy of Anne Rivas, DVM, DACZM, of the Minnesota Zoo.

(a) (b)

(c) (d)

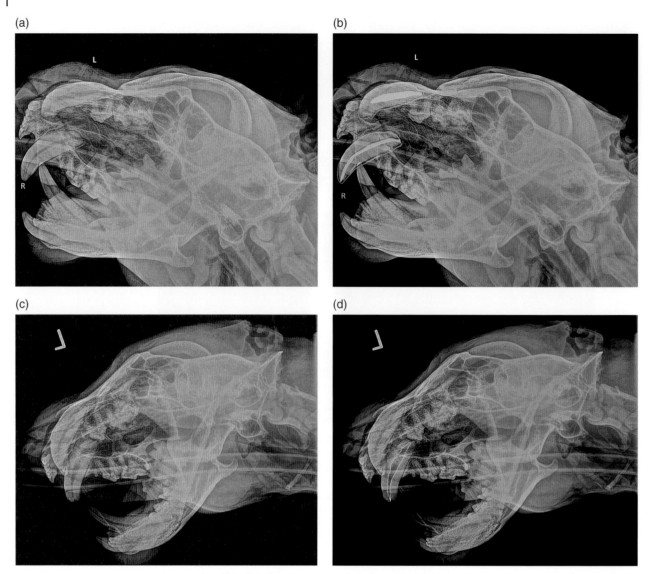

Figure 8.44 (a) Left dorsal-right ventral oblique (LD-RVO) skull radiograph of a three-year-old Amur tiger (*Panthera tigris altaica*) with a crown fracture of the left maxillary canine tooth. The pulp canal of the left maxillary canine tooth is wide compared to the right maxillary canine tooth. (b) Annotated left dorsal-right ventral oblique (RD-LVO) skull radiograph of the three-year-old Amur tiger in Figure (a). The yellow outline follows around the tooth and root margins as well as the pulp canals. The white filling within the pulp canals demonstrates the enlargement of the left maxillary canine tooth pulp canal compared to the right. (c) Right dorsal-left ventral oblique (RD-LVO) skull radiograph of the same tiger shown in Figure (a) and (b) with a crown fracture of the left maxillary canine tooth. The pulp cavity of the left maxillary canine tooth is discernibly wide compared to the right as a result of pulpitis in the fractured tooth. (d) Annotated right dorsal-left ventral oblique skull radiographs of the three-year-old Amur Tiger with coronal fracture of the left maxillary canine tooth as shown in Figure (a)–(c). The pulp cavity of the left maxillary canine tooth is outlined in yellow to demonstrate how it is expanded and irregular compared to the left. This oblique rotation separates the right and left maxilla well and allows for good detail of the left maxillary dentition. (e) Dorsoventral skull radiograph of the same Amur tiger shown in Figure (a)–(d). Superimposition of the mandibular and maxillary arcades obscures effective assessment of the affected tooth. The differences in the pulp cavity width between the right and left maxillary canine teeth is still evident, however. (f) Annotated dorsoventral radiograph of the skull of the same Amur tiger shown in Figure (e). Although the mandibular canine teeth partially overlay the maxillary canine teeth and obscure detail of the apices, the yellow lines highlighting the pulp cavities of both canine teeth illustrate the increased pulp canal width of the fractured right maxillary canine tooth. (g) Intraoral dental radiograph of the left maxillary canine tooth root of the tiger shown in Figure (a)–(f). The large size of the canine teeth of a tiger necessitates multiple images using a standard digital dental sensor. In this image, periapical lucency is present as indicated by the yellow arrows. (h) Postoperative intraoral radiograph of the same tiger's canine tooth apex as shown in Figure (a)–(h) at the end of the root canal procedure. (i) Intraoral dental radiograph of the crown of the same tiger canine tooth shown in Figure (a)–(h). The crown alone fills the entire dental sensor, requiring multiple images of the tooth to completely visualize the pathology or condition of the tooth and apex. This image demonstrates that both a coronal access site and mesial access site were necessary to complete the root canal procedure in this large, long tooth.

(e)

(g)

(f)

(h)

(i)

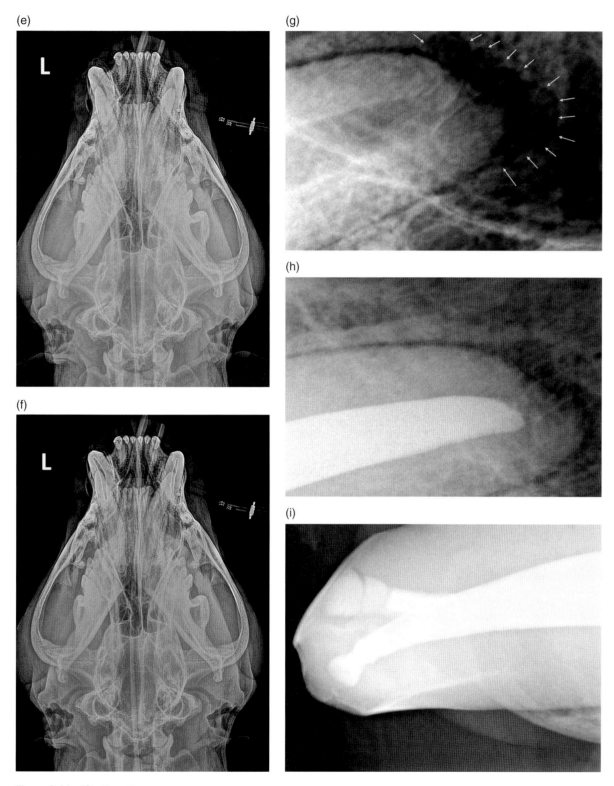

Figure 8.44   (Continued)

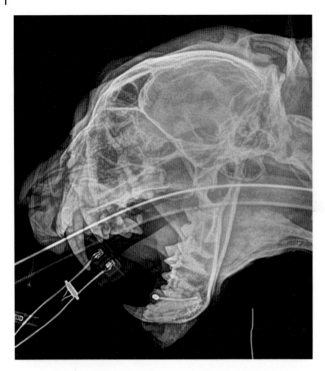

Figure 8.45 Right lateral oblique skull radiograph of a snow leopard (*Panthera uncia*) post root canal of the left mandibular canine tooth. The bright white radiopacity associated with the restoration in this snow leopard is consistent with use of an amalgam filling.

inability for accurate interpretation when images are obtained without sedation (Figure 8.54c, 8.55b, and c). Whole-skull radiographs are included within this chapter as reference for the grizzly bear (Figures 8.43b, c, and 8.52c–e),

tiger (Figure 8.44a–f), snow leopard (Figure 8.45), sea lion (Figure 8.49a and b), tapir (Figure 8.53c and d), and porcupines (Figure 8.57a, b, and 8.58).

Other Dental Conditions in Zoologic Animals

Trauma

Trauma is a common cause of dental abnormalities for many of zoological animals (lesser kudu Figure 8.59a–k, giraffe Figure 8.55b–g, and wallaby Figure 8.60a–l). Trauma may be caused by multiple factors, including conspecific interactions, falls or collisions, or chewing on objects within enclosures.

Attrition

Attrition can be observed in multiple zoologic species (opossum, Figure 8.61a–c). Attrition is tooth on tooth contact which can be considered normal wear in hypsodont teeth. In animals with brachydont teeth such as the opossum, the wear can lead to loss of the crown structure resulting in pain, pulp exposure, and eventual loss of the tooth.

Macropod Progressive Periodontal Disease (MPPD)

Oral disease is a common and frustrating problem for veterinarians caring for macropods (kangaroos and wallabies). Molar progression is a normal phenomenon exhibited by macropods but also occurs in elephants and

Figure 8.46 (a) Lateral photograph of the left mandibular arcade of a captive striped skunk (*Mephitis mephitis*) with significant periodontal disease, canine tooth fracture, and attrition of the premolars and molars. A fractured left mandibular canine tooth is visible, with marked gingival enlargement and inflammation around the remaining tooth. *Source:* Photograph courtesy of Dana Foster. (b) Intraoral rostral mandibular radiograph of the same skunk shown in Figure (a). Abnormalities observed in this image are annotated in Figure (c). (c) Annotated rostral mandibular intraoral radiograph of the skunk shown in Figure (a) and (b). The yellow arrow points to a fractured left incisor (I3) below the gumline that was not visible grossly. The red arrow points to the coronal fracture of the left mandibular canine tooth. The area around the fractured mandibular canine apex shows an indistinct and widened periodontal ligament space, with pocketing present at the apex of the tooth indicating abscessation (purple arrows). (d) Photograph of the right maxilla and mandible of the same skunk as shown in Figure (a)–(c). There is discoloration of the right maxillary canine tooth indicating suspicion of previous tooth death. *Source:* Photograph courtesy of Dana Foster. (e) Intraoral radiograph of the right maxillary canine tooth of the skunk shown in Figure (a)–(d). The pulp cavity of the canine tooth is irregular. There are artificially increased areas of opacity in this image due to placement of the endotracheal tube and tube tie within the radiograph. This can interfere with the interpretation of the film. (f) Annotated intraoral radiograph of the right maxillary canine tooth of the skunk shown in Figure (a)–(e). The pulp cavity of the canine tooth is irregular (dashed red line). The margins of the canine tooth (solid red lines) are superimposed by the endotracheal tube (yellow lines) and endotracheal tube cuff inflator (orange lines) as well as the tube tie (white lines), causing artifacts which interfere with the interpretation of the dental pathology. This image is a good example of why endotracheal tubes, oral monitors, and associated ties should be repositioned during intraoral or extraoral dental imaging to give the most diagnostic information possible. (g) Intraoral radiograph of the rostral maxilla of the same skunk shown in Figure (a)–(f). Because the endotracheal tube was positioned such that it was superimposed on the left maxillary second and third incisors, the pathology present in the right maxillary third incisor and the right maxillary canine tooth is more easily discernable. (h) Annotated intraoral radiograph of the rostral maxillary arcade of the same skunk shown in Figure (a)–(g). The right maxillary canine tooth has an irregular and widened pulp canal (dashed red lines), although superimposition by the first maxillary premolar interferes with discernment of the pulp canal of the canine tooth as it approaches the apex. The apices of the canine teeth were not included in this view. Interestingly, the grossly normal appearing right maxillary third incisor tooth as seen in Figure (a) also has pulp chamber widening (dashed red lines), irregular margins of the apex, and evidence of a periapical lucency (small yellow arrows), which is consistent with a nonvital tooth and periapical abscessation.

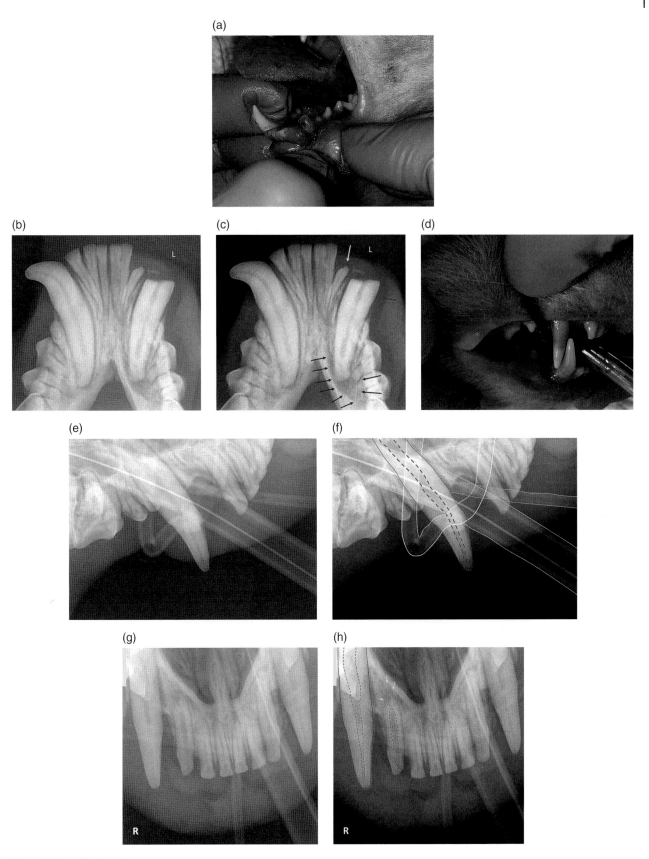

Figure 8.46 (Continued)

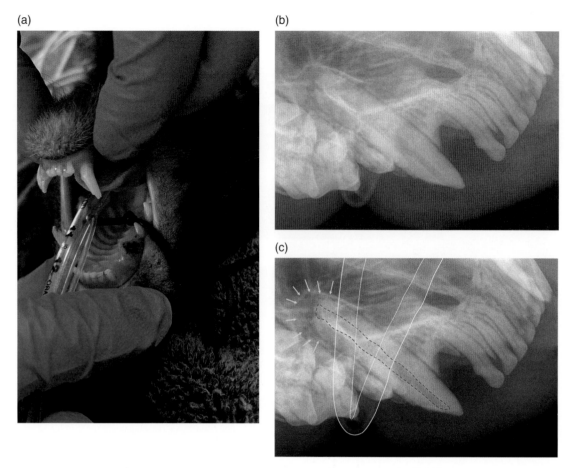

Figure 8.47 (a) Photograph of a pet striped skunk (*Mephitis mephitis*) during an anesthetized examination. There is a crown fracture with abscessation of the right maxillary canine tooth. *Source:* Photograph courtesy of Dana Foster. (b) Intraoral radiograph of the same skunk shown in Figure (a) demonstrating the radiographic appearance of the right maxillary canine tooth. Although this image is mildly oblique, the apex of the canine tooth is visible, and the right maxillary incisors are demonstrated without superimposition. (c) Annotated intraoral radiograph of the fractured right maxillary canine tooth of the skunk shown in Figure (a) and (b). In this view, you can appreciate the widened and irregular pulp canal (red dashed lines), although the margins of the pulp canal are obscured by superimposition of the endotracheal tube tie (white lines) and soft tissues. Periapical lucency (yellow arrows) is also visible.

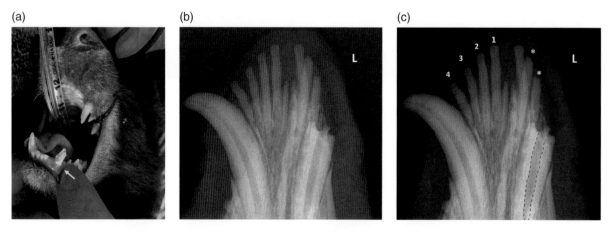

Figure 8.48 (a) Photograph of a striped skunk with significant oral disease. There is a fracture of the left mandibular canine tooth with mild gingival recession and gingivitis (yellow arrow). *Source:* Photograph courtesy of Dana Foster. (b) Intraoral rostral mandibular radiograph of the same skunk shown in Figure (a). A supernumerary incisor is present on the right mandible. In the left arcade, there are two incisor teeth present radiographically which are not observed clinically in Figure (a), and the fractured left mandibular canine tooth shows widening of the pulp canal. (c) Annotated intraoral rostral mandibular radiograph of the same skunk shown in Figure (a) and (b). A supernumerary incisor is present on the right (white numerals). In the left arcade, there are two incisor teeth present radiographically which are not observed clinically indicated by yellow asterisks. Compare these findings to the incisors visible in the photograph of the skunk in Figure (a). The fractured left mandibular canine tooth shows widening and irregular margins of the pulp canal (red dashed lines). Unfortunately, the apex of the left mandibular canine tooth is not visible in this view to assess the degree of periapical lucency associated with the fractured tooth.

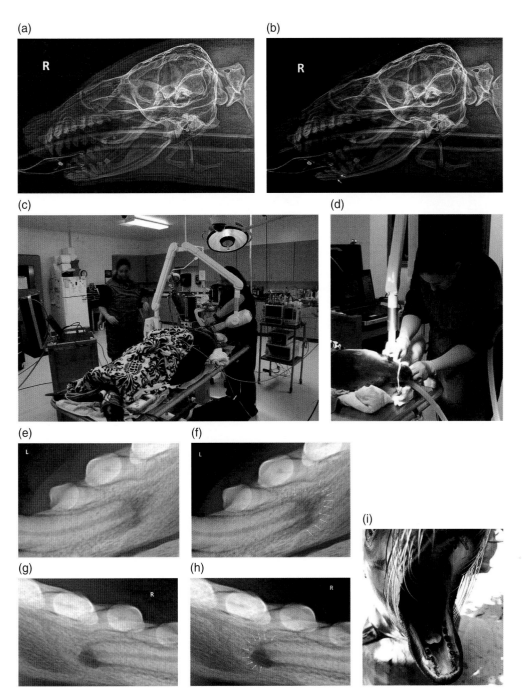

Figure 8.49 (a) Left dorsal-right ventral oblique skull radiograph of a California sea lion with bilateral mandibular canine tooth fractures identified during physical examination for another condition. In this view, the presence of the pulse-oximeter probe on the tongue and superimposition of the contralateral mandible obscures visibility of the left mandibular canine tooth. (b) Annotated left dorsal-right ventral oblique skull radiograph of the California sea lion with bilateral mandibular canine tooth fractures shown in Figure (a). The yellow arrows point to the presence of a periapical lucency surrounding the right mandibular canine tooth. The red arrow identifies the left mandibular canine tooth that is obscured by the pulse-oximetry probe and the superimposition of the right mandible. (c) Photograph demonstrating anesthesia and preoperative radiographic positioning of the California sea lion shown in Figure (a) and (b) for treatment of bilateral mandibular canine tooth fractures. Anesthetic procedures in marine mammals, like seals and sea lions, have increased risks of peri-anesthetic death. Clinicians working with these species should employ the assistance of experienced clinicians or anesthetists when planning a dental procedure or planning diagnostic imaging for the diagnosis and treatment of dental disease in these species to avoid potential life-threatening complications. *Source:* Courtesy of June Olds, DVM, DACZM, Iowa State University, College of Veterinary Medicine. (d) Photograph demonstrating preoperative radiographic positioning of the California sea lion shown in Figure (a)–(c) for the treatment of bilateral mandibular canine tooth fractures. *Source:* Courtesy of Brenda Mulherin DVM, DAVDC, Iowa State University, College of Veterinary Medicine. (e) Intraoral dental radiograph of the left mandibular canine tooth apex of the same sea lion shown in Figure (a)–(d), which demonstrate the periapical lucency affecting this tooth, which was obscured in the skull radiographs shown in Figure (a) and (b). (f) Annotated intraoral dental radiographic image of the left mandibular canine tooth apex of the same sea lion shown in Figure (a)–(e). Yellow arrows outline the periapical lucency surrounding the fractured left mandibular canine tooth. (g) Intraoral dental radiograph of the right mandibular canine tooth apex of the same sea lion shown in Figure (a)–(f), demonstrating the periapical lucency more clearly than noted in the skull radiographs shown in Figure (a) and (b). (h) Annotated intraoral dental radiograph of the right mandibular canine tooth apex of the same sea lion shown in Figure (a)–(g), with yellow arrows demonstrating the periapical lucency. (i) Open-mouth postoperative photograph of the California sea lion shown in Figure (a)–(h), taken during a training session. Note the sutures present at the sites of bilateral mandibular canine tooth extraction. This sea lion recovered and healed without complication. The enamel of sea lions is normally stained brown/black, which is not indicative of a pathologic condition.

(a)

(b)

(c)

(d)

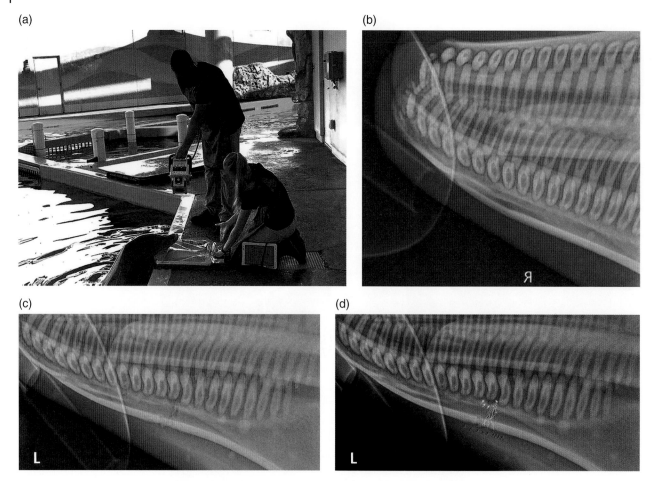

Figure 8.50 (a) Photograph demonstrating a training session with a bottlenosed dolphin (*Tursiops truncates*) to position for skull radiography. In this session, the dolphin was being introduced to the equipment for desensitization, but images were not acquired. In future sessions, trainers were wearing appropriate protective equipment to prevent unnecessary radiation exposure during image acquisition. (b) Oblique radiograph of the anterior mandible and maxilla in a bottlenose dolphin (*Tursiops truncatus*). Dolphins have homodont dentition, meaning that all teeth are alike in structure. The teeth are not used for chewing, but only used for grasping prey that are swallowed whole. (c) Lateral oblique radiograph of the middle left mandible of the same dolphin shown in Figure (a). There is evidence of osteomyelitis in the left mandible secondary to periodontal disease extending from the teeth. (d) Annotated lateral oblique radiograph of the left mandible of the dolphin shown in Figure (a)–(c). The yellow arrows point to periapical lucency surrounding the affected tooth. The yellow lines outline the tracts communicating with the ventral mandible, and the red arrows point to the irregular mandibular cortex with evidence of osteomyelitis. *Source:* Courtesy of Taylor Yaw, DVM, DACZM.

manatees (Figure 8.62a–c). Molar progression is the sequential eruption of molars, with the most worn-down molars shed from the front and the new molars erupting caudally and moving forward. Normal diagnostic images of the species that are being evaluated are also very useful to discern normal anatomy from potential pathology.

Molar Progression

Molar progression is a hypothesized risk factor for the development of macropod progressive periodontal disease (MPPD). Diseases such as endodontic disease and MPPD [39] can advance to chronic alveolar osteomyelitis

(CAO), which has been identified as a common source of morbidity and mortality in these species [40] (Figures 8.63a–f, 8.64a–e, 8.65a, and b).

Advanced Diagnostic Imaging in Exotic Pet Mammals and Zoo Animals

Standard Computed Tomography

As described in Chapter 10, CT overcomes the challenge of superimposition of structures that can occur with conventional radiographs of the skull. CT will generate multiple,

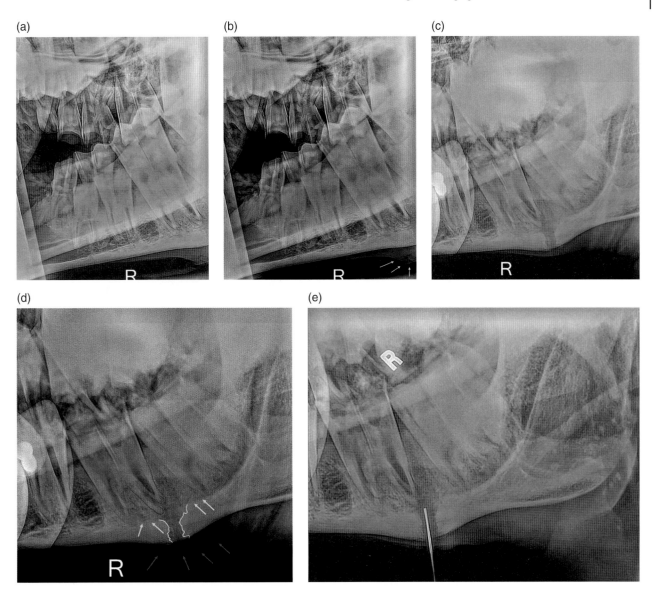

Figure 8.51 (a) Lateral oblique radiograph of a Bactrian camel (*Camelus bactrianus*) that presented with right ventral mandibular swelling and a draining abscess tract. In this radiograph, bony changes are present in the mandible in the caudal aspect of this view. *Source:* Courtesy of Joan Howard. (b) Annotated oblique radiograph of the right mandible of the Bactrian camel shown in Figure (a). The yellow arrows point to the thickened, irregular right mandible at the caudal ventral aspect of this image. (c) Oblique radiograph of the mid-caudal right mandible of the same Bactrian camel shown in Figure (a) and (b). In this image, a fissure is visible in the ventral mandible at the level of the caudal root of the last premolar tooth, with secondary osteomyelitis. (d) Annotated oblique radiograph of the mid-caudal right mandible of the same Bactrian camel shown in Figure (a)–(c). Margins of the fissure in the mandible are outlined in yellow. The red lines outline the jagged margins of the caudal root of the last premolar tooth indicating necrosis of the root associated with suspected periodontal disease. The margins of the increased density associated with the periodontitis are indicated by the yellow arrows. The red arrows point to the soft tissue swelling surrounding the bony changes in the mandible representing the abscess associated with the lesion. (e) Oblique radiograph of the mid-caudal right mandible of the same Bactrian camel shown in Figure (a)–(d). In this image, a metal probe has been inserted through the soft tissue swelling into the fissure in the mandible associated with the distal roots of the premolar tooth.

parallel, cross-sectional images of the skull that are elaborated and rendered by computer software [11]. When available, CT can provide superior diagnostic image assessment compared to conventional radiography. Within this chapter, computed tomographic images are shown to compare

the differences observed between conventional radiography and CT images of the same patient (guinea pig Figures 8.6b–d and 8.21c–i; domestic rabbit Figures 8.16a–d, 8.17a–f, and 8.18a–f; chinchilla Figures 8.22a, b, 8.25a, and b; African pygmy hedgehog Figures 8.31a–d and 8.32a–c;

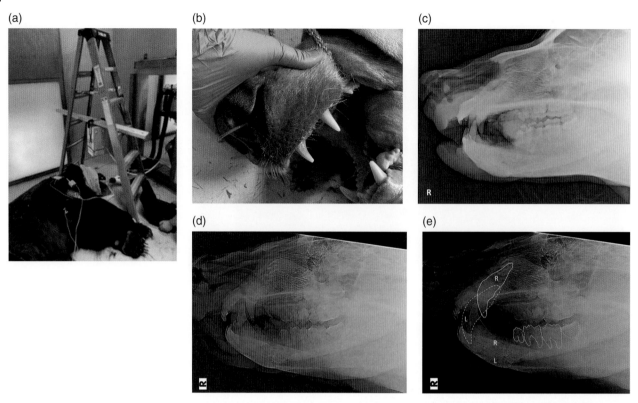

Figure 8.52 (a) Photograph demonstrating the challenges with positioning to obtain quality diagnostic dental radiographs for a zoo animal. Accurate positioning of an 1100 lb. grizzly bear (*Ursos arctos horribillis*) for skull radiographs is only one of the challenges. In most zoo animal examinations, the immobilization and anesthesia will occur in the animal's off-exhibit quarters, which necessitates bringing diagnostic equipment to the patient, rather than transporting the patient to the hospital. As shown in the figure, a ladder and 2X4 are used to position the portable X-ray generator above the digital radiograph sensor. (b) Photograph of the normal canine teeth and dentition of a female grizzly bear. Note the large size of the canine teeth in the patient. *Source:* Courtesy of Brenda Mulherin DVM, DAVDC, Iowa State University, College of Veterinary Medicine. (c) Lateral, mildly obliqued skull radiograph the female grizzly bear shown in Figure (b), obtained during a routine anesthetized examination. (d) Left dorsal-right ventral oblique (LD-RVO) radiograph of the same female grizzly bear shown in Figure (b) and (c), demonstrating normal dentition. A more obliqued image with adjusted kVp and MA settings was used compared to Figure (c). (e) Annotated left dorsal-right ventral oblique (LD-RVO) digital skull radiograph of the female grizzly bear as shown in Figure (b)–(d). The left maxillary canine (yellow dashed line), right maxillary canine (solid yellow line), left mandibular canine tooth (dashed red lines), and right mandibular canine tooth (solid red lines). The left mandibular molars are outlined in orange. In this view, the maxillary premolars and molars are indistinct and difficult to discern due to the superimposition of facial structures and the thick skull features of the bear. *Source:* Courtesy of Anne Rivas, DVM, DACZM, of the Minnesota Zoo.

Malayan tapir Figures 8.53c, d, and g–i; giraffe Figure 8.55b–e; wallaby Figures 8.63a, c–e, and 8.64a–d; and Patagonian mara Figure 8.66a–h). The capability of using CT to create 3D reconstructions may help with the assessment, treatment, and surgical planning for a patient. The reconstruction may also give the clinician a more comprehensive assessment of the clinical condition affecting the patient (domestic rabbit Figure 8.17g; guinea pig Figure 8.21j and k; giraffe Figure 8.55f and g; wallaby Figures 8.60k, l, 8.63f, and 8.64c; Patagonian mara Figure 8.66h). When advanced imaging technology is available, some clinicians will opt to perform a skull CT alone in lieu of skull radiographs due to the quality of the images, quick acquisition, and improved diagnostic capabilities. Most small animal patients can be imaged in a CT scanner with heavy

sedation alone. Compared to conventional radiography, CT images provide more details regarding the extent of the dental pathology present, which is likely to be important for establishing a more accurate diagnosis and prognosis as well as supporting a more informed decision-making process for the clinician and the client [17]. Computed tomographic scanning has been determined to be suitable for the detection of small changes in both hard and soft tissue structures in small mammals. It can be used to detect early evidence of root pathology, bony orbital changes, and occlusal abnormalities [22]. Computed tomographic scanning is suitable for noninvasive screening for cheek tooth abnormalities in animals with continuously growing teeth (rabbits, chinchillas, and guinea pigs), enabling detection of changes before they become clinically apparent. Early

(a) (b)

(c) (d)

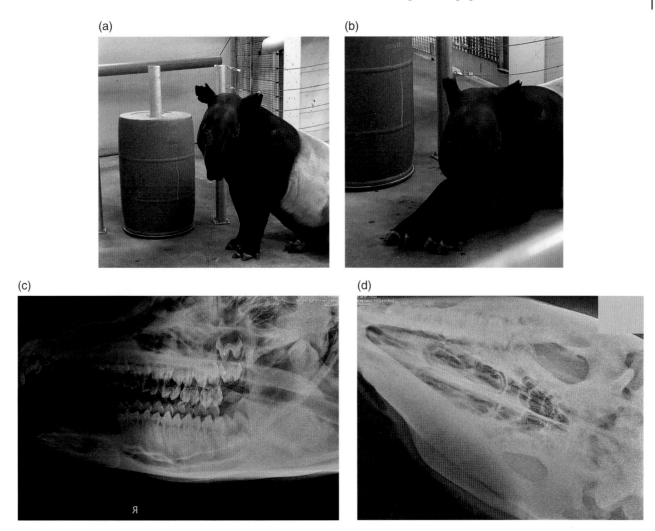

Figure 8.53 (a) Photograph of a Malayan tapir (*Tapirus indicus*) with right-sided facial swelling and perceived difficulty with prehension of food. (b) Closer clinical photograph of a Malayan tapir (*Tapirus indicus*) with right-sided facial swelling and perceived difficulty with prehension of food. (c) Right lateral mildly oblique radiograph of the same tapir shown in Figure (a) and (b). The large thick skull of the tapir makes it difficult to obtain diagnostic images, and the size of the tapir (300 kg) makes positioning challenging during an anesthetized examination. In this image, note the presence of bilateral unerupted maxillary molars (yellow asterisks), which were not suspected to be the cause of the clinical signs. (d) Dorsoventral radiograph of the skull of the tapir shown in Figure (a)–(c). Because of the large, thick skull of the tapir, there is lack of penetration of the X-ray beam to allow a diagnosis of the underlying cause of the right-sided facial swelling. *Source:* Courtesy of Omaha's Henry Doorly Zoo. (e) Photograph of the anesthetized tapir shown in Figure (a)–(d) being positioned for conventional computed tomography imaging of the skull to elucidate the cause of the right-sided facial swelling shown in Figure (a) and (b). (f) Photograph of the anesthetized tapir shown in Figure (a)–(d) being positioned for conventional computed tomography imaging of the skull to elucidate the cause of the right-sided facial swelling shown in Figure (a) and (b). *Source:* Courtesy of June Olds, DVM, DACZM, Iowa State University, College of Veterinary Medicine. (g) Transverse CT image of the tapir shown in Figure (a)–(f). There is temporal muscle swelling (yellow arrow) and loss of soft tissue symmetry, with a gas filled pocket under the right temporalis muscle. Increased opacity of the right sinus is suspected to be a positional artifact. (h) Right parasagittal CT image of the tapir shown in Figure (a)–(g). In this image, the undescended caudal maxillary molar is visible (yellow asterisk). (i) Transverse CT image of the mid-caudal skull of the tapir shown in Figure (a)–(h), taken at the level of the last mandibular molars. Mandibular bone remodeling is present in the right caudal mandible (yellow arrow) from a previously treated abscess secondary to dental disease. This image also demonstrates unerupted mandibular molars bilaterally (yellow asterisks). Right-sided soft tissue facial swelling is also evident. The underlying problem was believed to be secondary to temporal myositis caused by a foreign object penetration and not related to the resolving mandibular dental condition.

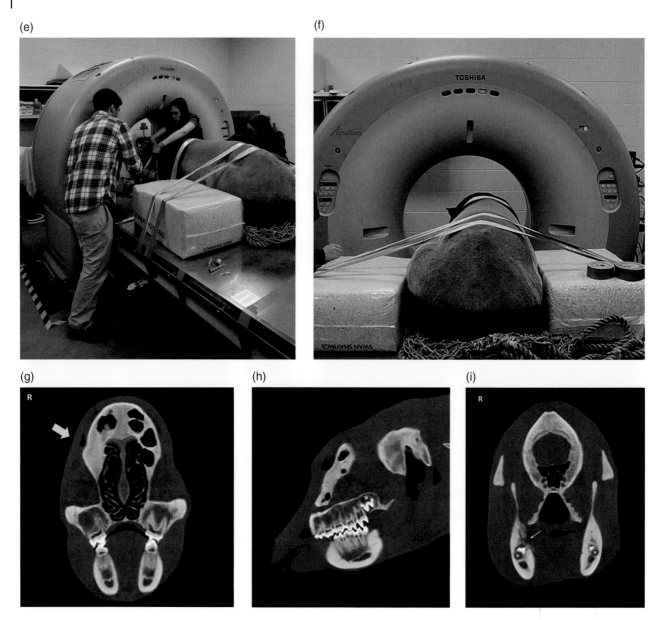

Figure 8.53 (Continued)

diagnosis will provide the opportunity of instituting treatment measures to control the abnormalities observed [22]. Removing crown abnormalities such as spikes, crown height reduction, and occlusal equilibration are examples of treatments that can be performed [22].

Cone Beam Computed Tomography

Cone beam computed tomography (CBCT) was introduced to the European market in 1998 and to the United States in 2001. Compared to conventional CT, the patient ionizing radiation dose levels can be reduced by as much as one-sixth. Scan times are typically only 5–40 seconds,

depending on the unit and protocol settings, allowing comparable or decreased time under anesthesia compared to standard computed tomographic scanning [41]. CBCT uses a divergent cone-shaped source of radiation to image the anatomy of interest [41]. CBCT has been used in imaged-based evaluation of dogs and cats and in anatomical studies on rabbits and guinea pigs [41]. Some small animal practitioners and a few zoological institutions have portable CBCT units, which can be moved through a standard-sized door and positioned with various procedure tables, depending on the size and shape of the patient. CBCT units are self-shielding, and radiation exposure is avoided by positioning the operator behind the device at an

(a)

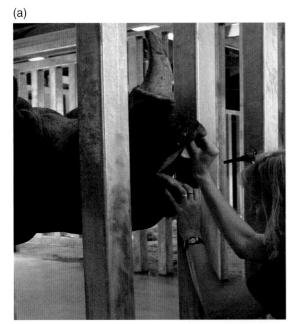

(b)

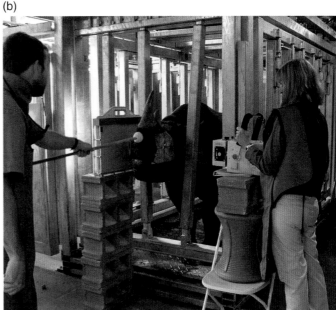

(c)

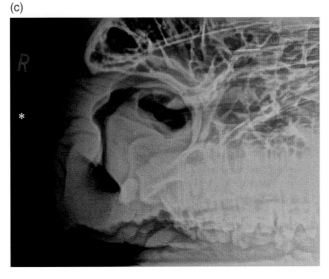

Figure 8.54 (a) Photograph of an Eastern black rhinoceros (*Diceros bicornis michaeli*) allowing oral examination. Many zoo animals can be trained for oral examination with the "open mouth" behavior. However, visualization may still be limited. Trainers spend countless hours developing behavioral training programs to allow zoo animals to participate willingly in veterinary procedures. This training can help avoid the use of anesthesia and sedation due to the inherent risks of immobilization and anesthesia in many mega-vertebrate species. (b) Photograph of skull radiography performed on the same black rhinoceros as shown in Figure (a). Training for veterinary procedures in zoos takes extensive time and patience and requires a trusting relationship between the animal, trainer, and veterinarian. Zoo veterinarians must get creative with the use of nontraditional tools to assist in their methods – hence the use of cement blocks, folding chairs, enrichment devices, duct tape and a tennis ball to acquire the images in this patient. (c) Slightly oblique lateral radiograph of the Eastern black rhinoceros (*Diceros bicornis michaeli*) taken as demonstrated Figure (a) and (b) with training alone. This image allows good visualization of the extensive sinuses of this species. The large size of the head, superimposition of the maxillary and mandibular molars, as well as the thick skull and facial structures, makes interpretation of the dentition for diagnostic purposes challenging. Note that there is motion artifact present, as these animals are given food rewards to participate in training. In this image, there is motion artifact from chewing during the radiograph acquisition. The tennis ball, used as a training target, is visualized rostrally (yellow asterisk).

(a)

(b)

(c)

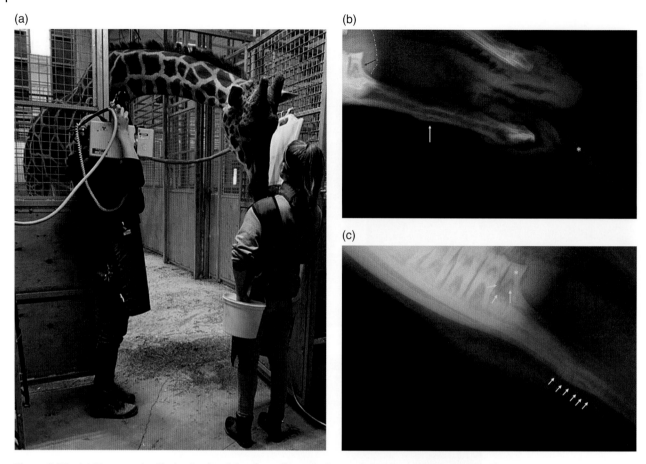

Figure 8.55 (a) Photograph of behavioral training for radiography in an adult reticulated giraffe (*Giraffa camelopardalis reticulata*). Radiographic positioning is opportunistic in these species, and motion artifacts are common. However, due to the high risk of morbidity and mortality in mega-vertebrate animals with sedation and anesthesia, training for radiographic positioning can help provide clues as to the underlying conditions that may be associated with subtle clinical signs. It may also allow for more accurate treatment and management planning. Note how the radiographic plate is affixed to the pen gate. This will reduce the risk to caretakers or technicians of unnecessary radiation exposure that may occur by manually positioning and holding the radiographic sensor. (b) Standing lateral radiograph of the rostral mandible and maxilla of the 21-year-old adult female reticulated giraffe shown in Figure (a). This radiograph was obtained with behavioral training and food rewards; therefore, there is motion artifact which can obscure interpretation of the image. In this view, the tongue (yellow asterisk) is extended as the animal reaches for its training reward. A bolus of food (white dashed line) is present, which gives contrast to the mandibular first premolar (red arrow). This image shows some evidence of a periapical lucency around the mandibular first premolar (red arrow) and shows an irregular margin of the anterior mandible (white arrow), but no definitive diagnosis could be made from this radiograph. Ideal radiographic positioning is challenging with images obtained via training alone. (c) Standing lateral oblique radiograph of the caudal mandible of the same giraffe shown in Figure (a) and (b), obtained during training. This image again demonstrates motion artifact, but there is more obvious periapical lucency and suspected root resorption (yellow arrows) surrounding the left mandibular premolar (yellow asterisk). The absent right premolar was extracted during an immobilization for the treatment of joint disease approximately nine months prior to this image. Also note the irregular appearance of the mid-rostral mandibular cortex (white arrows). (d) Postmortem coronal CT image of the same giraffe as shown in Figure (a)–(c). This giraffe was euthanized three months following the acquisition of the images in Figure (a)–(c), for comorbidities unrelated to the oral pathology noted. In this computed tomography image, a bony sequestrum is evident in the left mandible, at the location of the irregular appearance of the mid-rostral mandible in the radiographs in Figure (b) and (c). Despite the time that had passed, there was minimal evidence of bony callus formation. (e) Coronal postmortem CT image of the giraffe in Figure (a)–(d). In this view, the bony sequestrum and mandibular fracture is more evident (red arrow). Despite repeated lateral and lateral-oblique radiographs obtained with training, this lesion was only clearly visible on computed tomographic imaging three months after the initial clinical presentation of the giraffe. This case highlights the limitations of standard diagnostic imaging capabilities for mega-vertebrate animals. (f) Computed tomography 3D virtual reconstruction of the giraffe skull from the previous images. Note the deviation in the anterior left mandible at the site of the fracture and bony sequestrum (red arrow). (g) Computed tomography 3D virtual reconstruction of the giraffe skull shown in Figure (d)–(f). This lateral view of the skull demonstrates the length and extensive nature of the bony sequestrum present secondary to the mandibular fracture.

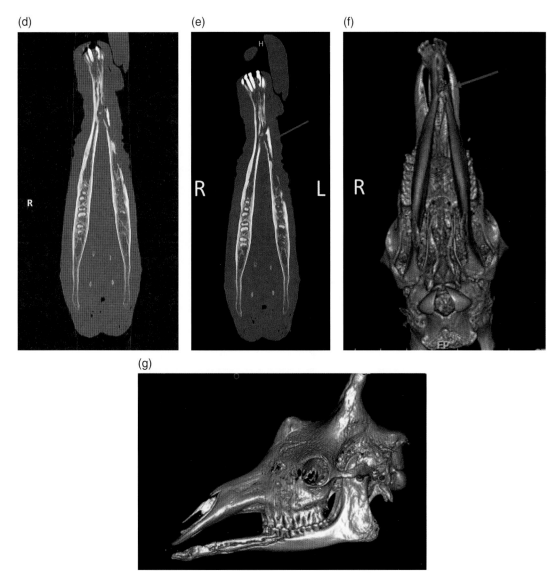

Figure 8.55   (Continued)

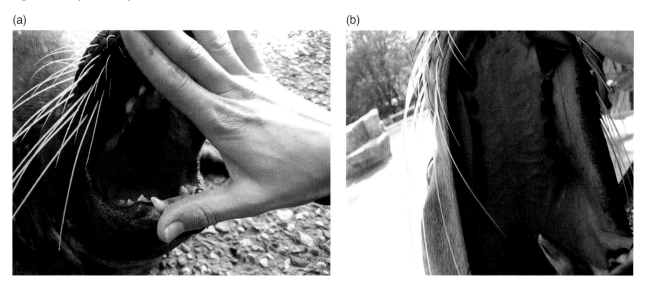

Figure 8.56   (a) Rostral open-mouth photograph demonstrating the normal dentition and enamel coloration of a pacific harbor seal (*Phoca vitulina*) allowing an oral examination to be performed. Many zoo animals can be trained for oral examination with the "open mouth" behavior. However, visualization may still be limited. Note, while both the seal and the sea lion are pinnipeds, the seal has an expected enamel coloration, and the sea lion has a normal brown-black discoloration (see comparison of sea lion in Figure (b)).
(b) Open-mouth photograph of the dentition of a California sea lion (*Zalophus californianus*). In this species, black/brown discoloration of the enamel is normal and should not be interpreted as pathological. See Figure 8.49i. *Source:* Courtesy of June Olds, DVM, DACZM, Iowa State University, College of Veterinary Medicine.

(a)

(b)

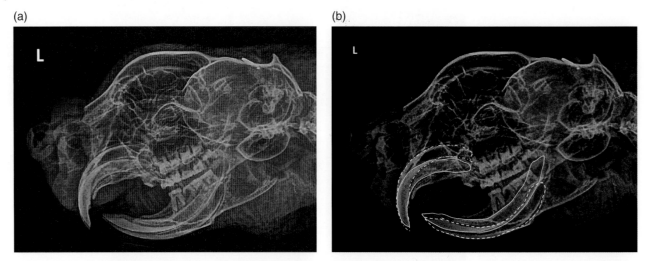

Figure 8.57 (a) Right dorsal-left ventral lateral oblique radiograph of a Brazilian prehensile-tailed porcupine (*Coendou prehensilis*). Note how the dentition of this rodent species is similar to that noted in the hamster and rat shown in Figures 8.10a, b, 8.11a, and b, with continuously growing maxillary and mandibular incisors and brachydont premolars and molars that do not grow continuously. (b) Annotated lateral mildly oblique radiograph of the Brazilian prehensile-tailed porcupine shown in Figure (a). The maxillary and mandibular incisors are outlined in yellow or white dashed lines to demonstrate how they are superimposed in this image rostrally. Note how the apices of the maxillary incisors terminate rostral to the apices of the maxillary premolars and molars, but the mandibular incisor apices traverse ventral and distal to the mandibular premolars and molars.

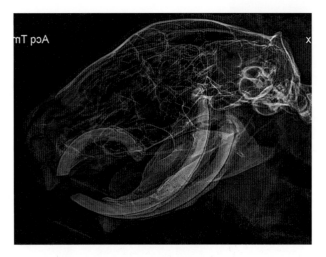

Figure 8.58 Lateral mildly oblique radiograph of a geriatric African crested porcupine (*Hystrix cristata*) demonstrating loss of all molars and premolars, as well as loss of one maxillary incisor tooth. *Source:* Courtesy of Utah's Hogle Zoo.

appropriate distance [41]. While CBCT may be a useful device for the examination of smaller mammal patients and has been used on animals up to the size of a chimpanzee, the opening is not large enough to obtain images in a large mammal [41]. CBCT has been used more recently to describe the dental morphology in a chimpanzee [42], giant panda [43], and orangutan [44] and has been used clinically for the diagnosis and management of dental pathology in an aardvark [45]. More information regarding the use of CBCT can be found in Chapter 10.

Micro-computed Tomography

Micro-computed tomography (micro-CT) is another technology that has been studied in small animal patients [18, 46]. Micro-CT has a shorter capture time than CBCT. Studies have found that micro-CT equipment facilitates the collection of accurate data, as well as having a rapid image

Figure 8.59 (a) Photograph demonstrating subtle right-sided facial swelling with loss of facial symmetry in a lesser kudu (*Tragelaphus imberbis*) following a suspected collision with fencing. (b) Photograph of the same kudu shown in Figure (a), taken two weeks after the original suspected injury, demonstrating more significant right ventral mandibular facial swelling. (As noted by the yellow arrows.) (c) Dorsoventral mildly obliqued skull radiograph of the kudu shown in Figure (a) and (b), taken after the observation of the significant right mandibular swelling shown in Figure (b). (d) Annotated dorsoventral mildly obliqued skull radiograph of the kudu shown in Figure (a)–(c). In this DV view, you can see a mildly displaced fracture in the rostral maxilla (red dashed lines) and an incomplete fracture callus at the level of the mandibular premolar (white dashed lines) with significant soft tissue swelling consistent with abscessation (yellow arrows). The red solid lines outline the margins of the right mandible until it is lost in the superimposed area of the maxilla and mandible at the level of the first premolar. (e) Left dorsal-right ventral oblique skull radiograph of the kudu shown in Figure (a)–(d). In this view, the right rostral maxillary fracture is more easily observed, while the fracture in the right mandible is more difficult to discern. (f) Annotated left dorsal-right ventral oblique skull radiographs of the kudu shown in Figure (a)–(e). The right rostral maxillary fracture is visible (red dashed lines) as a nonunion with the associated right maxilla (solid red lines). The fracture in the right mandible is more difficult to discern (white dashed lines) within the fracture callus and abscess (yellow arrows). (g) Left dorsal-right ventral oblique radiograph of the same kudu shown in Figure (a)–(f), taken six weeks after the original injury, following medical management of the right ventral mandibular abscess. Note the enlargement of the fracture callus on the right mandible, and the presence of the deciduous premolar with underlying adult molar present at the site of the callus. This radiograph was taken prior to extraction

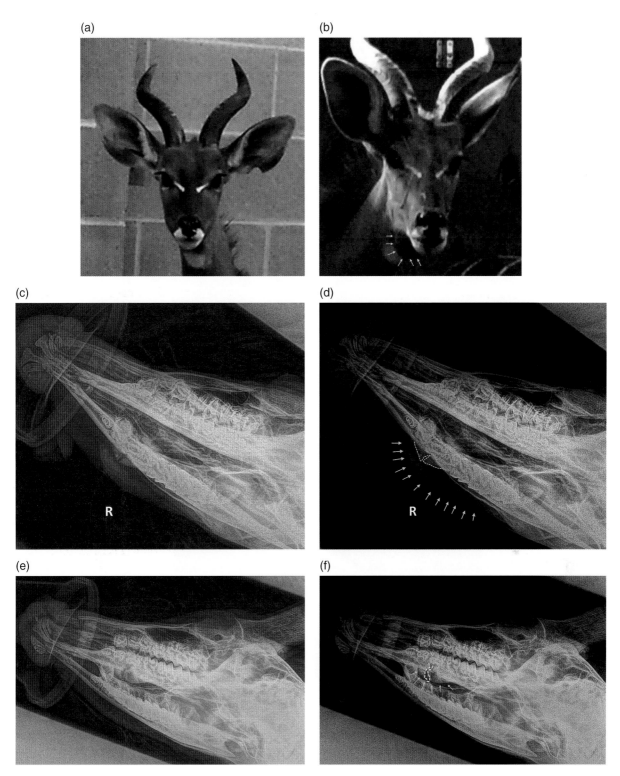

Figure 8.59 (Continued) of the teeth overlying the fracture callus site. (h) Annotated left dorsal-right ventral oblique radiograph of the same kudu shown in Figure (a)–(g), taken six weeks after the original injury. The right ventral mandibular abscess had been treated with medical management. There is enlargement and increased opacity of the fracture callus on the right mandible (yellow arrows), still showing incomplete ossification, and the presence of the deciduous premolar with an underlying adult molar present (yellow asterisk) at the site of the callus. The yellow circle demonstrates the previously identified maxillary fracture. This radiograph was taken prior to extraction of the teeth overlying the fracture callus to allow continued healing. (i) Postoperative photograph of the kudu shown in Figure (a)–(h). A buccotomy was performed to permit extraction of the deciduous premolar and nonerupted adult molar teeth that were present at the fracture site in the right mandible. The buccotomy was closed with buried continuous absorbable suture. In addition to systemic antibiotics to manage the ongoing abscess in the mandible, the abscess cavity was packed with silver-sulfadiazine cream (white cream on the ventral mandible) postoperatively for local treatment and to help prevent additional contamination of the draining abscess site. (j) Lateral radiograph of the same kudu shown in Figure (a)–(i) taken five months following extraction of the deciduous mandibular premolar and unerupted mandibular molar teeth that appeared to be interfering with the healing of the fracture of the right mandible. There is still a fracture callus present, but the fistula within the bone has healed, and union is complete. (k) The same kudu shown in Figure (a)–(j). In this right dorsal-left ventral oblique view, the right mandible displays complete healing with no evidence of residual active osteomyelitis at the fracture site (yellow arrow). The right maxilla is not easily discerned in this image due to superimposition. The kudu continued to eat and behave normally during the prolonged management of this case.

(g)

(h)

(i)

(j)

(k)

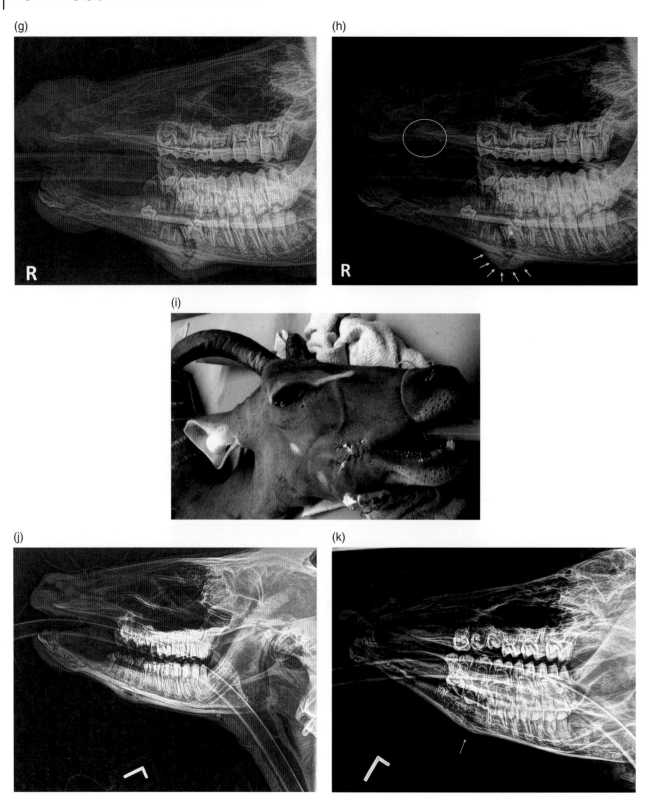

Figure 8.59 (Continued)

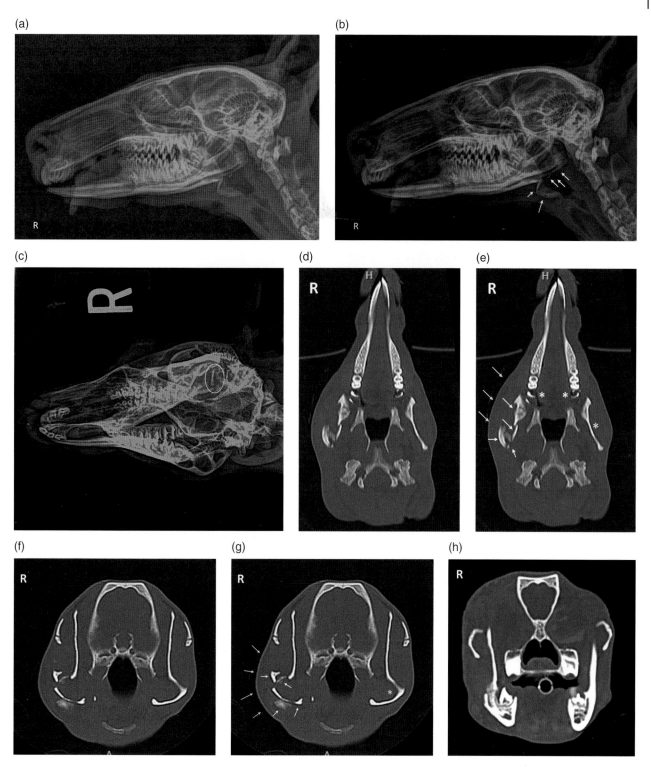

Figure 8.60 (a) Right lateral radiograph of a red-necked wallaby that presented with soft tissue swelling in the mid to caudal right mandible. (b) Annotated right lateral radiograph the red-necked wallaby shown in Figure (a). There is loss of congruence of the caudal mandible (white arrows) with small, ossified fragments visible ventrally (yellow arrows). (c) Right dorsal-left ventral lateral oblique radiograph of the same wallaby shown in Figure (a) and (b). Over-rotation of the skull in this image obscures visualization of the right mandibular anatomical abnormalities. A small bony fragment is visible at the location of the ramus of the right mandible (yellow circle). (d) Dorsal CT of the wallaby shown in Figure (a)–(c). This image captures the comminuted fracture of the right caudal mandible much more clearly than seen in the previous radiographic images. (e) Annotated dorsal CT of the wallaby shown in Figure (a)–(d). The normal ramus of the left mandible is indicated by the yellow asterisk. Marked soft tissue swelling is evident in the caudal mandible

(i)   (j)   (k)

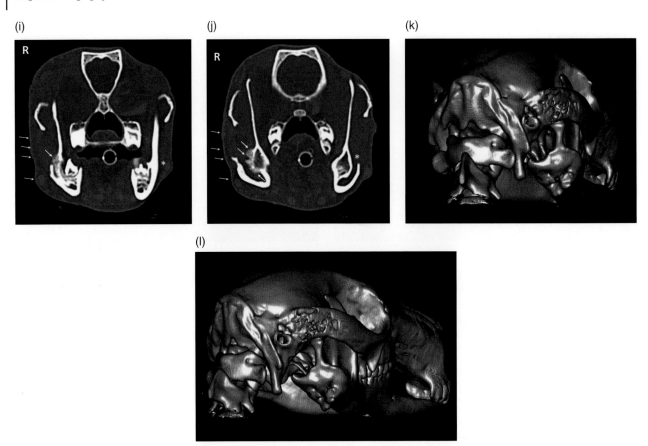

(l)

Figure 8.60 (Continued) (yellow arrows), with multiple fragments and abnormal shape of the ramus of the right mandible evident (white arrows). The normal unerupted caudal molars are also present (white asterisks). (f) Transverse CT of the same wallaby shown in Figure (a)–(e). This image demonstrates the displacement of the mandibular ramus fragments within the soft tissue swelling of the caudal mandible. (g) Annotated transverse CT of the same wallaby shown in Figure (f). The normal ramus of the left mandible is indicated by the yellow asterisk. White arrows point to the bone fragments of the ramus of the right mandible in various stages of displacement. The soft tissue swelling is designated by the yellow arrows. (h) Transverse CT of the same wallaby shown in Figure (a)–(g), taken one year after the initial injury. This image demonstrates the bone remodeling in the caudal mandible at the level of the last molar. There is still evidence of facial asymmetry, with a fracture callus still present. (i) Annotated transverse CT at the level of the last molar of the same wallaby shown in Figure (h). Facial asymmetry is still present, with a more rounded appearance and exaggerated right ventral swelling surrounding the remodeling mandible (yellow arrows). A fracture callus is present with evidence of active bone remodeling, due to the wispy appearance of the bone (white arrow) compared to the normal left mandible (yellow asterisk). (j) Annotated transverse CT of the caudal skull of the wallaby at the level of the ramus of the mandible. This is the same wallaby shown in Figure (a)–(i), taken one year after the original injury. The caudal head still exhibits soft tissue asymmetry with a more rounded appearance of the right side and exaggerated right ventral swelling surrounding the remodeling mandible (yellow arrows). The fracture callus has evidence of active bone remodeling, with the wispy appearance of the bone (white arrows) compared to the normal left mandible (yellow asterisk). (k) Computed tomography 3D virtual reconstruction of the wallaby skull demonstrating remodeling of the right mandible one year following the fracture shown in Figure (a)–(j). This view is concentrated on the caudal aspect of the mandible. This reconstruction demonstrates how the bony callus re-incorporated the bone fragments that were visible in the preceding images. (l) Computed tomography 3D virtual reconstruction of the wallaby skull demonstrating remodeling of the right mandible one-year following the fracture shown in Figure (a)–(j). The view of this image is slightly more lateral, showing the remodeling of the fracture site. This reconstruction demonstrates how the bony callus re-incorporated the bone fragments that were visible in the preceding images.

processing and reconstruction time (approximately one minute) [18]. Micro-CT also allows for the reconstruction of images, with the ability to assess overall dentition and occlusion and evaluate morphology of the upper and lower jaw and assess abnormalities regarding the length

and angle of teeth. Micro-CT allows evaluation of tooth malformations, excessive length, and occlusal abnormalities of the clinical crown, identify deformities of the dental apices, soft tissue, and bony proliferative lesions, as well as identify fractures of the tooth and bone. Changes identified

(a)

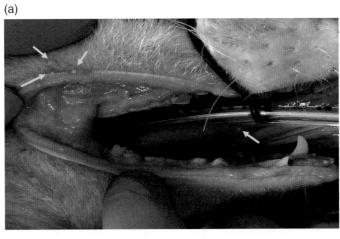

(b)   (c)

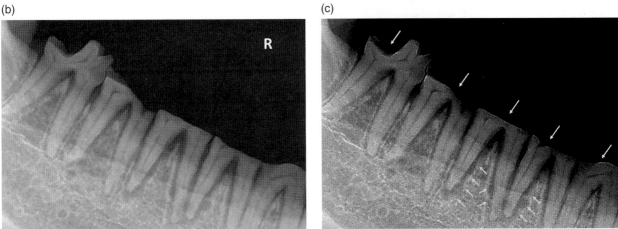

Figure 8.61　(a) Photograph of the dentition of an adult male North American Virginia opossum (*Didelphis virginiana*), demonstrating a fracture of the right mandibular canine tooth and severe attrition of the premolars and molars. Incidentally, the small white nodules seen on the margins of the lips and the underside of the tongue were diagnosed as Besnoitiosis caused by B. darlingi infection. *Source:* Photograph courtesy of Dana Foster. (b) Intraoral radiograph of the right mandible of the adult captive opossum shown in Figure (a). This animal was rescued from a poor welfare situation, so it cannot be determined if these teeth were worn down by attrition or abrasion. There is loss of the crowns of nearly all the premolars and molars in this view. (c) Annotated intraoral radiograph of the mid-caudal right mandible of the adult opossum shown in Figure (a) and (b). There is loss of the crowns on nearly all premolars and molars (white arrows) and periapical lucency surrounding several premolar and molar teeth (yellow arrows).

included dental, skeletal, anatomical, and pathologic abnormalities [18]. Another advantage of micro-CT is that most images may be obtained without anesthesia [18].

Considerations for Computed Tomography

When imaging any small mammal patient using any of the CT techniques, the patient is ideally placed in dorsoventral (sternal) recumbency to avoid the potential respiratory depression caused by ventrodorsal positioning.

When possible, CT of the skull will give more clarity to pathology affecting a zoologic patient. Unfortunately,

patient transportation to a facility in which CT is available, the risks associated with general anesthesia, and the overall size and potentially dangerous nature of zoo patients may cause additional challenges in acquiring diagnostic images (tapir, Figure 8.53e and f). For these reasons, many computed tomographic evaluations of the skulls of zoo animal species are performed on cadavers or museum specimens as a reference for morphologic anatomy [42–44] (Figure 8.55d–g). Very few zoologic institutions have in-house computed tomographic capabilities. Frequently, zoologic institutions must rely on specialty facilities nearby to facilitate diagnostic image acquisition.

(a)

(b)

(c)

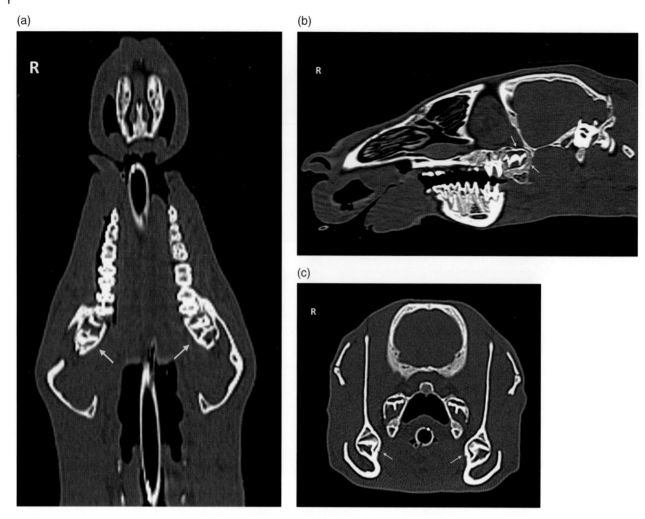

Figure 8.62   (a) Dorsal computed tomography image of the normal mandible in a red-necked wallaby (*Macropus rufogriseus*), which illustrates normal molar progression (yellow arrows). (b) Parasagittal CT of the normal skull of the same, red-necked wallaby shown in Figure (a), demonstrating normal molar progression in the maxilla (yellow arrows). (c) Transverse CT of a normal caudal wallaby skull, demonstrating nonerupted molars within the mandible (yellow arrows). The normal images in Figure (a)–(c) should be used as a references to compare to the abnormal wallaby images in Figures 8.63a–f, 8.64a–e, 8.65a, and b.

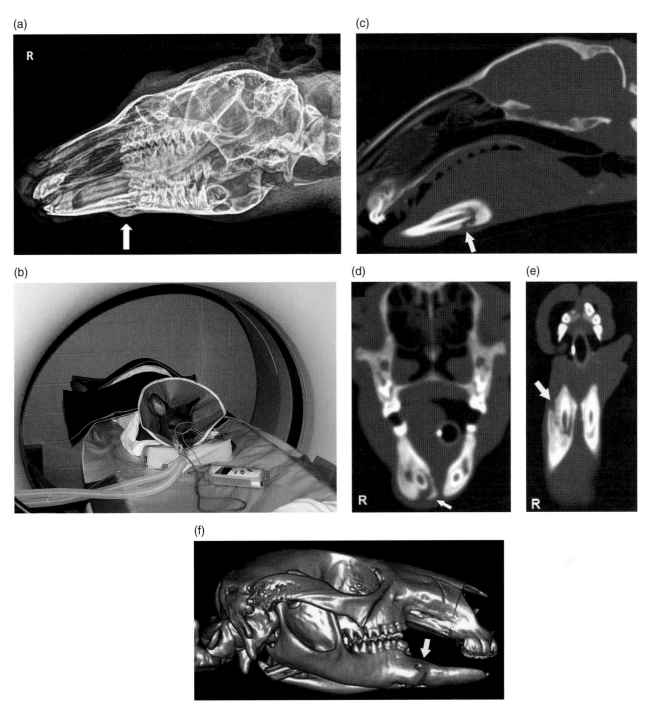

Figure 8.63 (a) Left dorsal–right ventral lateral oblique radiograph of a red-necked wallaby (*Macropus rufogriseus*) with right mandibular swelling and early evidence of macropod progressive periodontal disease (MPPD). The white arrow points to bony lysis and proliferation due to osteomyelitis surrounding the apex of the right mandibular incisor. (b) Photograph of the wallaby shown in Figure (a), undergoing computed tomography for the assessment of early MPPD identified via radiography. The smaller size of the wallaby (less than 35 lbs) makes CT evaluation a more manageable diagnostic option for these animals compared to other zoo species that are much larger or potentially more dangerous to transport to a facility with advanced diagnostic capabilities. (c) Right parasagittal CT of the same wallaby shown in Figure (a) and (b), demonstrating the extent of osteomyelitis surrounding the right mandibular incisor apex with a draining tract (white arrow) communicating with the soft tissue swelling, indicative of an abscess on the ventral mandible. Soft tissue swelling is the typical early presentation of MPPD in macropods. Unfortunately, most patients will not display signs of oral pain or appetite changes until the condition has become advanced. (d) Transverse CT of the same wallaby shown in Figure (a)–(c), again detailing the extent of osteomyelitis surrounding the right mandibular incisor apex with a draining tract (white arrow) communicating to the soft tissue and bony abscess on the ventral mandible. Note how the right mandibular incisor pulp canal is widened compared to the left, indicating active pulpitis, and nonvitality of this tooth. (e) Dorsal CT of the same wallaby shown in Figure (a)–(d), showing the extent of bone remodeling associated with the osteomyelitis in the right mandible secondary to MPPD. The white arrow indicates the draining tract in the bone communicating with the grossly visible soft tissue swelling and abscess. (f) Computed tomography 3D bony reconstruction of the wallaby shown in Figure (a)–(e), demonstrating the mandibular remodeling due to osteomyelitis associated with early to moderate macropod progressive periodontal disease (MPPD).

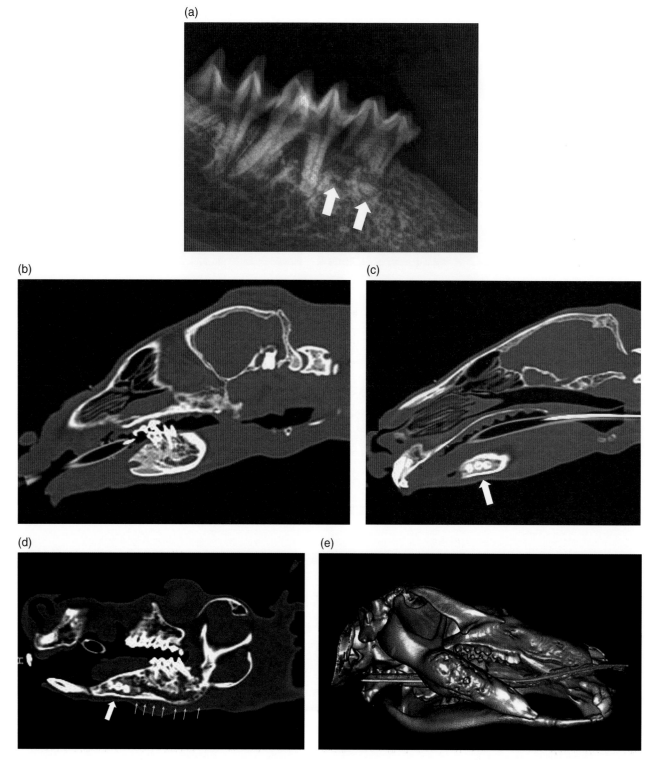

Figure 8.64 (a) Intraoral dental radiograph of a red-necked wallaby with more advanced chronic mandibular osteomyelitis secondary to macropod progressive periodontal disease. In this wallaby, the right mandibular incisor had previously been extracted to address the original infection. This image shows how periodontitis is beginning to cause lysis of the right mandibular first premolar apices (white arrows). (b) Right parasagittal CT of the same wallaby shown in Figure (a), demonstrating the degree of bony remodeling and osteomyelitis associated with a more advanced stage of MPPD compared to the wallaby shown in Figure 8.63 (a)–(f). As shown in this image, the right mandibular incisor tooth had previously been extracted to address the original presentation of the condition. This image demonstrates the osteomyelitis associated with the remaining premolars and molars more clearly than the intraoral dental radiograph shown in Figure (a). (c) Right parasagittal CT of the same, red-necked wallaby shown in Figure (a) and (b). This wallaby was previously treated with extraction of the right mandibular incisor tooth and insertion of commercially prepared antibiotic impregnated polymethylmethacrylate (PMMA) beads (white arrow) for the treatment of residual osteomyelitis. Because these beads do not degrade over time, their use has fallen out of favor, as they can often serve as a nidus for future infections. (d) Parasagittal CT of the same wallaby, taken two years after the images shown in Figure (a)–(c). In this image, you can see that the PMMA beads are still present (white arrow), and the progressive osteomyelitis has advanced despite ongoing systemic treatment and extraction of the affected premolars shown in Figure (a)–(c). In this image, the entire right mandible is now affected by the disease (yellow arrows). (e) Computed tomography 3D virtual reconstruction of the wallaby shown in Figure (d), demonstrating the extension of the osteomyelitis into the right caudal mandible, and the shortening of the mandible secondary to the extraction of the right mandibular incisor and bone remodeling.

(a) (b)

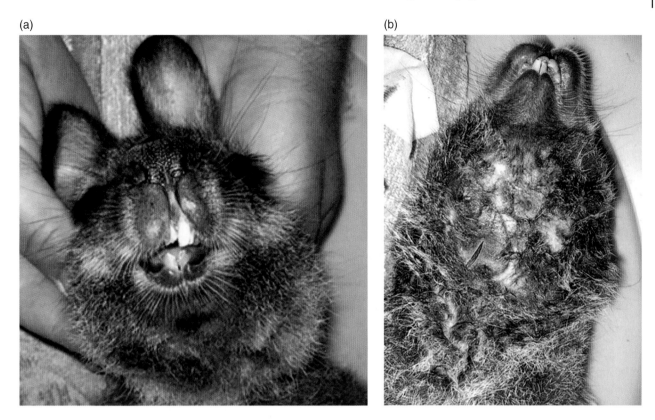

Figure 8.65 (a) Clinical photograph of an adult, red-necked wallaby (*Macropus rufogriseus*) with advanced, severe macropod progressive periodontal disease (MPPD) and chronic alveolar osteomyelitis (CAO). (b) Clinical photograph of the ventral mandibles in the same adult wallaby shown in Figure (a). This wallaby had undergone long-term systemic and local therapy for chronic mandibular osteomyelitis with little improvement and was euthanized due to the severity of the condition.

(a) (b) (c)

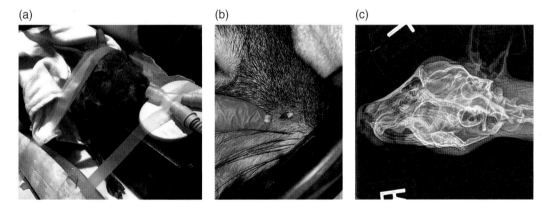

Figure 8.66 (a) Photograph of a Patagonian mara (*Dolichotis patagonum*) under anesthesia and being positioned for computed tomography to identify underlying dental disease. This mara had right-sided facial swelling with an abscess fistula in the rostral maxilla. (b) Close-up photograph of the right rostral maxilla of the same Patagonian mara shown in Figure (a), demonstrating thick caseous discharge from a fistula associated with the right maxillary arcade. *Source:* Courtesy of June Olds, DVM, DACZM, Iowa State University, College of Veterinary Medicine.

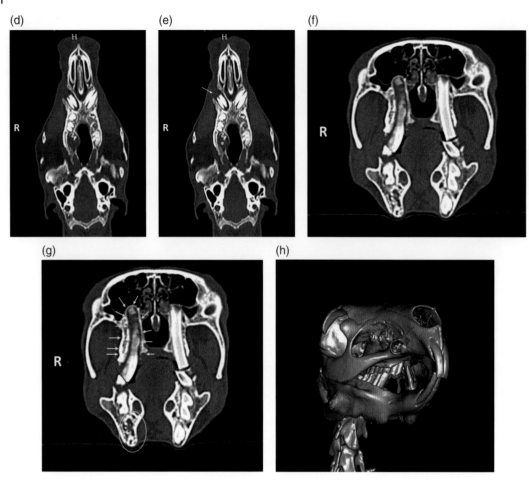

(d) (e) (f)

(g) (h)

Figure 8.66 (Continued) (c) Oblique skull radiograph of the Patagonian mara shown in Figure (a) and (b). Coronal and apical elongation of the cheek teeth is strongly suspected, but there is difficulty in interpretation of the skull radiograph due to the irregular occlusal angles in this animal, and the normal occlusal angle of this species. In general, the occlusal angle of the mara is similar to the guinea pig (see drawing in Figure 8.6a). It was also challenging to obtain diagnostic intraoral radiographs due to the small oral aperture of the mara. Because of these challenges, computed tomography was elected to identify the source of the abscess as shown in Figure (d)–(g). (d) Dorsal CT image of the Patagonian mara shown in Figure (a)–(c). In this image, the maxillary abscess is visible associated with the right first premolar. There also appears to be lysis and remodeling of the maxilla surrounding the right caudal molar. (e) Annotated dorsal CT image of the Patagonian mara shown in Figure (a)–(d). The maxillary abscess is associated with the right first premolar (yellow arrow) with visible soft tissue swelling in this region. There is osteomyelitis and remodeling of the maxilla surrounding the right caudal molar which appears to be resorbing (yellow asterisk). (f) Transverse CT image of the Patagonian mara shown in Figure (a)–(e). This image demonstrates the necrosis of the right maxillary first premolar and the significant malocclusion of the maxillary and mandibular cheek teeth. The right mandibular incisor appears necrotic, with remodeling of the right mandible surrounding the apices of the incisor and premolar teeth. (g) Annotated transverse CT image of the Patagonian mara shown in Figure (a)–(f). This image demonstrates the resorption of the apex of the right maxillary first premolar (yellow arrows) and significant malocclusion of the maxillary and mandibular cheek teeth (red lines and red arrows). The apex of the right mandibular incisor appears to be resorbed (red asterisk), with remodeling of the right mandible surrounding the apices of the incisor and premolar teeth (yellow circle). (h) Computed tomography 3D-reconstructed virtual image of the Patagonian mara skull shown in Figure (a)–(g). In this image, note the bony remodeling and fistula (red arrow) in the right rostral maxilla, and the malocclusion of all visible cheek teeth.

Conclusion

Dental disease has been documented in a variety of exotic felids [2, 32–35], canids [2, 38, 47, 48], great apes [2, 38, 49], other primates [2, 26, 50–52], lagomorphs [2, 38, 53], a wide variety of pet and wild rodents [2, 3, 9, 38, 54], lorises [55, 56], mustelids [2, 57], ursids [2, 31], hyenas [2, 58], aardvarks [38, 45, 59], elephants [2, 60, 61], hyrax [62], tapirs [63–66], suids [67], peccaries [67], hippos [68], giraffe [69], other ungulates [1, 70–72], koalas [2, 73–75], wombats [73, 76], and macropods [2, 39, 40, 77–81]. This chapter could not encompass all the potential species that might be encountered in a curated zoologic collection. Clinicians faced with dental disease issues in a captive wild animal are encouraged to search the references provided in this chapter for the diagnosis, treatment, and management of the specific species and are equally encouraged to consult with a board-certified veterinary dentist and zoo veterinarian to help with appropriate diagnosis and treatment of these patients.

Acknowledgment

The author would like to give a special acknowledgment to Elizabeth Riedesel DVM, DACVR, for assistance in interpretation of several diagnostic images and editing of figure legends within this chapter.

References

1 Knightly, F. and Emily, P. (2003). Oral disorders of exotic ungulates. *Vet. Clin. North Am. Exot. Anim. Pract.* 6 (3): 565–570. https://doi.org/10.1016/S1094-9194(03)00037-9.

2 Emily, P. and Eisner, E.R. (2021). *Zoo and Wild Animal Dentistry*. Hoboken: Wiley.

3 Legendre, L.F.J. (2003). Oral disorders of exotic rodents. *Vet. Clin. North Am. Exot. Anim. Pract.* 6 (3): 601–628. https://doi.org/10.1016/S1094-9194(03)00041-0.

4 Legendre, L. (2016). Anatomy and disorders of the oral cavity of guinea pigs. *Vet. Clin. North Am. Exot. Anim. Pract.* 19 (3): 825–842.

5 Mancinelli, E. and Capello, V. (2016). Anatomy and disorders of the oral cavity of rat-like and squirrel-like rodents. *Vet. Clin. North Am. Exot. Anim. Pract.* 19 (3): 871–900. https://doi.org/10.1016/j.cvex.2016.04.008.

6 Johnson-Delaney, C.A. (2016). Anatomy and disorders of the oral cavity of ferrets and other exotic companion carnivores. *Vet. Clin. North Am. Exot. Anim. Pract.* 19 (3): 901–928. https://doi.org/10.1016/j.cvex.2016.04.009.

7 Mans, C. and Jekl, V. (2016). Anatomy and disorders of the oral cavity of chinchillas and degus. *Vet. Clin. North Am. Exot. Anim. Pract.* 19 (3): 843–869. https://doi.org/10.1016/j.cvex.2016.04.007.

8 Lennox, A.M. and Miwa, Y. (2016). Anatomy and disorders of the oral cavity of miscellaneous exotic companion mammals. *Vet. Clin. North Am. Exot. Anim. Pract.* 19 (3): 929–945. https://doi.org/10.1016/j.cvex.2016.04.005.

9 Lennox, A.M., Capello, V., and Legendre, L.F. (2021). Chapter 36 – small mammal dentistry. In: *Ferrets, Rabbits, and Rodents*, 4e (ed. K. Quesenberry, C. Orcutt, C. Mans, and J. Carpenter), 514–535. St. Louis: Elsevier.

10 Silverman, S. and Tell, L.A. (2005). *Radiology of Rodents, Rabbits and Ferrets : An Atlas of Normal Anatomy and Positioning*. St. Louis: Elsevier/Sauders.

11 Capello, V. (2016). Diagnostic imaging of dental disease in pet rabbits and rodents. *Vet. Clin. North Am. Exot. Anim. Pract.* 19 (3): 757–782. https://doi.org/10.1016/j.cvex.2016.05.001.

12 Capello, V. (2008). *Clinical Radiology of Exotic Companion Mammals*. Hoboken: Wiley.

13 Bohmer, E. (2015). Radiographic examination. In: *Dentistry in Rabbits and Rodents* (ed. E. Bohmer), 49–87. Chichester: Wiley.

14 Smallwood, J.E., Shively, M.J., Rendano, V.T., and Habel, R.E. (1985). A standardized nomenclature for radiographic projections used in veterinary medicine. *Vet. Radiol.* 26 (1): 2–9.

15 Crossley, D.A. (1995). Clinical aspects of rodent dental anatomy. *J. Vet. Dent.* 12: 131–135.

16 Capello, V. and Gracis, M. (2005). *Rabbit and Rodent Dentistry Handbook* (ed. A.M. Lennox). Lake Worth: Zoological Education Network.

17 van Caelenberg, A.I., de Rycke, L.M., Hermans, K. et al. (2011). Comparison of radiography and CT to identify changes in the skulls of four rabbits with dental disease. *J. Vet. Dent.* 28 (3): 172–181.

18 Sasai, H., Iwai, H., Fujita, D. et al. (2014). The use of micro-computed tomography in the diagnosis of dental and oral disease in rabbits. *BMC Vet. Res.* 10 (1): 209. https://doi.org/10.1186/s12917-014-0209-4.

19 Crossley, D.A. (2003). Oral biology and disorders of lagomorphs. *Vet. Clin. North Am. Exot. Anim. Pract.* 6 (3): 629–659.

20 Meredith, A. and Johnson-Delaney, C. (2010). *BSAVA Manual of Exotic Pets: A Foundation Manual*. Quedgeley: British Small Animal Veterinary Association (BSAVA).

21 Mayer, J. and Donnelly, T.M. (2012). Clinical veterinary advisor: birds and exotic pets. In: *Clinical Veterinary Advisor: Birds and Exotic Pets* (ed. J. Mayer and T. Donnelly), 1–752. St. Louis: Elsevier https://doi.org/10.1016/C2009-0-36486-7.

22 Crossley, D.A., Jackson, A., Yates, J., and Boydell, I.P. (1998). Use of computed tomography to investigate cheek tooth abnormalities in chinchillas (*Chinchilla laniger*). *J. Small Anim. Pract.* 39 (8): 385–389.

23 Wozniak-Biel, A., Janeczek, M., Janus, I., and Nowak, M. (2015). Surgical resection of peripheral odontogenic fibromas in African pygmy hedgehog (*Atelerix albiventris*): a case study. *BMC Vet. Res.* 11 (1): https://doi.org/10.1186/s12917-015-0455-0.

24 Eshar, D. and Gardhouse, S.M. (2020). Prairie dogs. In: *Ferrets, Rabbits, and Rodents* (ed. K. Quesenbery, C. Orcutt, C. Mans, and J. Carpenter), 334–344. St. Louis, MO: Elsevier https://doi.org/10.1016/B978-0-323-48435-0.00024-1.

25 Dias Neto R das, N., Fecchio, R.S., Rahal, S.C. et al. (2016). Dental disorders in brown howler monkeys (*Alouatta guariba clamitans*) maintained in captivity. *J. Med. Primatol.* 45 (2): 79–84. https://doi.org/10.1111/jmp.12208.

26 Wiggs, R.B. and Hall, B. (2003). Nonhuman primate dentistry. *Vet. Clin. North Am. Exot. Anim. Pract.* 6 (3): 661–687. https://doi.org/10.1016/S1094-9194(03)00039-2.

27 Kim, S.M. and Kim, J.M. (2020). Evaluation of canine teeth crown reduction technique in macaques. *Lab. Anim. Res.* 36 (1): 16. https://doi.org/10.1186/s42826-020-00051-3.

28 Kvapil, P., Nemec, A., Zadravec, M., and Račnik, J. (2018). Oral and dental examination findings in a family of zoo suricates (*Suricata suricatta*). *J. Vet. Dent.* 35 (2): 114–120. https://doi.org/10.1177/0898756418776729.

29 Freitas, E.P., Rahal, S.C., Teixeira, C.R. et al. (2008). Oral cavity evaluation and dental chart registration of coati (*Nasua nasua*) in captivity. *J. Vet. Dent.* 25 (2): 110–117. https://doi.org/10.1177/089875640802500212.

30 Kapoor, V., Antonelli, T., Parkinson, J.A., and Hartstone-Rose, A. (2016). Oral health correlates of captivity. *Res. Vet. Sci.* 107: 213–219. https://doi.org/10.1016/j.rvsc.2016.06.009.

31 Collins, D.M. (2015). Chapter 50 – ursidae. In: *Fowler's Zoo and Wild Animal Medicine*, vol. 8 (ed. R.E. Miller and M.E. Fowler), 498–508. Philadelphia: W.B. Saunders https://doi.org/10.1016/B978-1-4557-7397-8.00050-5.

32 Lamberski, N. (2015). Chapter 47 – felidae. In: *Fowler's Zoo and Wild Animal Medicine*, vol. 8 (ed. R.E. Miller and M.E. Fowler), 467–476. Philadelphia: W.B. Saunders https://doi.org/10.1016/B978-1-4557-7397-8.00047-5.

33 Norton, B.B., Tunseth, D., Holder, K. et al. (2018). Causes of morbidity in captive African lions (*Panthera leo*) in North America, 2001–2016. *Zoo Biol.* 37 (5): 354–359. https://doi.org/10.1002/zoo.21435.

34 Schneider, L.A., Jimenez, I.A., Crouch, E.E.V. et al. (2021). Dental diseases and other oral pathologies of captive jaguars (*Panthera onca*) from Belize, Central America. *J. Zoo Wildl. Med.* 51 (4): 856–867.

35 Steenkamp, G., Boy, S.C., van Staden, P.J., and Bester, M.N. (2018). Oral, maxillofacial and dental diseases in captive cheetahs (*Acinonyx jubatus*). *J. Comp. Pathol.* 158: 77–89.

36 Longley, L. (2011). A review of ageing studies in captive felids. *Int. Zoo Yearbook* 45 (1): 91–98. https://doi.org/10.1111/j.1748-1090.2010.00125.x.

37 van Bonn, W.G. (2015). Chapter 44 – pinnipedia. In: *Fowler's Zoo and Wild Animal Medicine*, vol. 8 (ed. R.E. Miller and M.E. Fowler), 436–450. Philadelphia: W.B. Saunders https://doi.org/10.1016/B978-1-4557-7397-8.00044-x.

38 Glatt, S.E., Francl, K.E., and Scheels, J.L. (2008). A survey of current dental problems and treatments of zoo animals. *Int. Zoo Yearbook* 42 (1): 206–213. https://doi.org/10.1111/j.1748-1090.2007.00032.x.

39 Kane, L.P., Langan, J.N., Adkesson, M.J. et al. (2017). Treatment of mandibular osteomyelitis in two red-necked wallabies (*Macropus rufogriseus*) by means of intensive long-term parenteral drug administration and serial computed tomographic monitoring. *J. Am. Vet. Med. Assoc.* 251 (9): 1070–1077. https://doi.org/10.2460/javma.251.9.1070.

40 Hoyer, N., Rawlinson, J., and Klaphake, E. (2020). Treatment of oral disease in eight captive Bennett's wallabies (*Macropus rufogriseus*) between 2011 and 2019: a case series. *J. Zoo Wildl. Med.* 51 (3): 705–719.

41 Duncan, A.E. (2021). A cost effective portable option for computed tomography imaging in a zoological setting. In: *2021 Joint AAZV/EAZWV Conference*, Jacksonville, FL, 45.

42 Al-Amery, S.M., Nambiar, P., John, J. et al. (2018). Unusual dental morphology in a chimpanzee: a case report utilizing cone-beam computed tomography. *J. Vet. Dent.* 35 (2): 96–102. https://doi.org/10.1177/0898756418776448.

43 Endo, H., Komiya, T., Narushima, E., and Suzuki, N. (2002). Three-dimensional image analysis of a head of the giant panda by the cone-beam type CT. *J. Vet. Med. Sci.* 64 (12): 1153–1155. https://doi.org/10.1292/jvms.64.1153.

44 Nambiar, P., John, J., Al-Amery, S.M. et al. (2013). Quantification of the dental morphology of orangutans. *Sci. World J.* 2013: 1–10. https://doi.org/10.1155/2013/213757.

45 Christman, J.E., VanderHart, D., Colmery, B. et al. (2022). Management of dental disease in aardvarks (*Orycteropus afer*) and potential use of cone-beam computed tomography. *Animals* 12 (7): 845. https://doi.org/10.3390/ani12070845.

46 de Rycke, L.M., Boone, M.N., van Caelenberg, A.I. et al. (2012). Micro-computed tomography of the head and dentition in cadavers of clinically normal rabbits. *Am. J. Vet. Res.* 73 (2): 227–232.

47 Padilla, L.R. and Hilton, C.D. (2015). Chapter 46 – canidae. In: *Fowler's Zoo and Wild Animal Medicine*, vol. 8 (ed. R.E. Miller and M.E. Fowler), 457–467. Philadelphia: W.B. Saunders https://doi.org/10.1016/B978-1-4557-7397-8.00046-3.

48 Pires, A., Caldeira, I., Petrucci-Fonseca, F. et al. (2020). Dental pathology of the wild Iberian wolf (*Canis lupus signatus*): the study of a 20th century Portuguese museum collection. *Vet. Anim. Sci.* 9: 100100. https://doi.org/10.1016/j.vas.2020.10010.

49 Murphy, H.W. (2015). Chapter 38 – great apes. In: *Fowler's Zoo and Wild Animal Medicine*, vol. 8 (ed. R.E. Miller and M.E. Fowler), 336–354. Philadelphia: W.B. Saunders https://doi.org/10.1016/B978-1-4557-7397-8.00038-4.

50 Calle, P.P. and Ott Joslin, J. (2015). Chapter 37 – new world and old world monkeys. In: *Fowler's Zoo and Wild Animal Medicine*, vol. 8 (ed. R.E. Miller and M.E. Fowler), 301–335. Philadelphia: W.B. Saunders https://doi.org/10.1016/B978-1-4557-7397-8.00037-2.

51 Przydzimirski, A.C., Correia, A.M., Scalise, V.P. et al. (2022). Prevalence and description of dental disorders in skulls of free-living wild primates from Paraná State, Brazil. *J. Med. Primatol.* 51 (1): 3–19. https://doi.org/10.1111/jmp.12548.

52 Johnson-Delaney, C.A. (2008). Nonhuman primate dental care. *J. Exot. Pet. Med.* 17 (2): 138–143.

53 Graham, J.E. (2015). Chapter 41 – lagomorpha (pikas, rabbits, and hares). In: *Fowler's Zoo and Wild Animal Medicine*, vol. 8 (ed. R.E. Miller and M.E. Fowler), 375–384. Philadelphia: W.B. Saunders https://doi.org/10.1016/B978-1-4557-7397-8.00041-4.

54 Yarto-Jaramillo, E. (2015). Chapter 42 – rodentia. In: *Fowler's Zoo and Wild Animal Medicine*, vol. 8 (ed. R.E. Miller and M.E. Fowler), 384–422. Philadelphia: W.B. Saunders https://doi.org/10.1016/B978-1-4557-7397-8.00042-6.

55 Cabana, F. and Nekaris, K.A.I. (2015). Diets high in fruits and low in gum exudates promote the occurrence and development of dental disease in pygmy slow loris (*Nycticebus pygmaeus*). *Zoo Biol.* 34 (6): 547–553. https://doi.org/10.1002/zoo.21245.

56 Simpson, G.M., Fuller, G., Lukas, K.E. et al. (2018). Sources of morbidity in lorises and pottos in North American zoos: a retrospective review, 1980–2010. *Zoo Biol.* 37 (4): 245–257. https://doi.org/10.1002/zoo.21429.

57 Kollias, G.V. and Fernandez-Moran, J. (2015). Chapter 48 – mustelidae. In: *Fowler's Zoo and Wild Animal Medicine*, vol. 8 (ed. R.E. Miller and M.E. Fowler), 476–491. Philadelphia: W.B. Saunders https://doi.org/10.1016/B978-1-4557-7397-8.00048-7.

58 Suedmeyer, W.K. (2015). Chapter 51 – hyaenidae. In: *Fowler's Zoo and Wild Animal Medicine*, vol. 8 (ed. R.E. Miller and M.E. Fowler), 509–514. Philadelphia: W.B. Saunders https://doi.org/10.1016/B978-1-4557-7397-8.00051-7.

59 Buss, P.E. and Meyer, L.C.R. (2015). Chapter 52 – tubulidentata (aardvark). In: *Fowler's Zoo and Wild Animal Medicine*, vol. 8 (ed. R.E. Miller and M.E. Fowler), 514–516. Philadelphia: W.B. Saunders https://doi.org/10.1016/B978-1-4557-7397-8.00052-9.

60 Wiedner, E. (2015). Chapter 53 – proboscidea. In: *Fowler's Zoo and Wild Animal Medicine*, vol. 8 (ed. R.E. Miller and M.E. Fowler), 517–532. Philadelphia: W.B. Saunders https://doi.org/10.1016/B978-1-4557-7397-8.00053-0.

61 Steenkamp, G. (2003). Oral biology and disorders of tusked mammals. *Vet. Clin. North Am. Exot. Anim. Pract.* 6 (3): 689–725. https://doi.org/10.1016/S1094-9194(03)00035-5.

62 Napier, J.E. (2015). Chapter 54 – hyrocoidea (hyraxes). In: *Fowler's Zoo and Wild Animal Medicine*, vol. 8 (ed. R.E. Miller and M.E. Fowler), 532–538. Philadelphia: W.B. Saunders https://doi.org/10.1016/B978-1-4557-7397-8.00054-2.

63 Zimmerman, D.M. and Hernandez, S. (2015). Chapter 56 – tapiridae. In: *Fowler's Zoo and Wild Animal Medicine*, vol. 8 (ed. R.E. Miller and M.E. Fowler), 547–559. Philadelphia: W.B. Saunders https://doi.org/10.1016/B978-1-4557-7397-8.00056-6.

64 Fernandes-Santos, R.C., Medici, E.P., Testa-José, C., and Micheletti, T. (2020). Health assessment of wild lowland tapirs (*Tapirus terrestris*) in the highly threatened Cerrado biome, Brazil. *J. Wildl. Dis.* 56 (1): 34. https://doi.org/10.7589/2018-10-24.

65 Tjørnelund, K.B., Jonsson, L.M., Kortegaard, H. et al. (2015). Dental lesions in the lowland tapir (*Tapirus terrestris*). *J. Zoo Wildl. Med.* 46 (2): 363–366.

66 da Silva, M.A.O., Kortegaard, H.E., Choong, S.S. et al. (2011). Resorptive tooth root lesions in the Malayan tapir (*Tapirus indicus*). *J. Zoo Wildl. Med.* 42 (1): 40–43. https://doi.org/10.1638/2009-0247.1.

67 Sutherland-Smith, M. (2015). Chapter 58 – suidae and tayassuidae (wild pigs, peccaries). In: *Fowler's Zoo and Wild Animal Medicine*, vol. 8 (ed. R.E. Miller and M.E. Fowler), 568–584. Philadelphia: W.B. Saunders https://doi.org/10.1016/B978-1-4557-7397-8.00058-x.

68 Walzer, C. and Stalder, G. (2015). Chapter 59 – hippopotamidae (hippopotamus). In: *Fowler's Zoo and Wild Animal Medicine*, vol. 8 (ed. R.E. Miller and M.E. Fowler), 584–592. Philadelphia: W.B. Saunders https://doi.org/10.1016/B978-1-4557-7397-8.00059-1.

69 Bertelsen, M.F. (2015). Chapter 61 – giraffidae. In: *Fowler's Zoo and Wild Animal Medicine*, vol. 8 (ed. R.E. Miller and M.E. Fowler), 602–610. Philadelphia: W.B. Saunders https://doi.org/10.1016/B978-1-4557-7397-8.00061-x.

70 Wolfe, B.A. (2015). Chapter 63 – bovidae (except sheep and goats) and antilocapridae. In: *Fowler's Zoo and Wild Animal Medicine*, vol. 8 (ed. R.E. Miller and M.E. Fowler), 626–645. Philadelphia: W.B. Saunders https://doi.org/10.1016/B978-1-4557-7397-8.00063-3.

71 Weber, M.A. (2015). Chapter 64 – sheep, goats, and goat-like animals. In: *Fowler's Zoo and Wild Animal Medicine*, vol. 8 (ed. R.E. Miller and M.E. Fowler), 645–649. Philadelphia: W.B. Saunders https://doi.org/10.1016/B978-1-4557-7397-8.00064-5.

72 Kertesz, P. and Gulland, F.M.D. (1987). The surgical and restorative dental treatment of a Bactrian camel (*Camelus bactrianus*). *J. Zoo Anim. Med.* 18 (2/3): 73. https://doi.org/10.2307/20460243.

73 Vogelnest, L. (2015). Chapter 33 – marsupialia (marsupials). In: *Fowler's Zoo and Wild Animal Medicine*, vol. 8 (ed. R.E. Miller and M.E. Fowler), 255–274. Philadelphia: W.B. Saunders https://doi.org/10.1016/B978-1-4557-7397-8.00033-5.

74 Pettett, L., Wilson, G., Nicolson, V. et al. (2019). Malocclusions in the koala (*Phascolarctos cinereus*). *Aust. Vet. J.* 97 (11): 473–481. https://doi.org/10.1111/avj.12863.

75 Butcher, R.G., Pettett, L.M., Fabijan, J. et al. (2020). Periodontal disease in free-ranging koalas (*Phascolarctos cinereus*) from the Mount Lofty Ranges, South Australia, and its association with koala retrovirus infection. *Aust. Vet. J.* 98 (5): 200–206.

76 Wilson, G. and Gillett, A. (2010). Commissurotomy for improving access to the oral cavity of the wombat. *Aust. Vet. J.* 88 (7): 277–279. https://doi.org/10.1111/j.1751-0813.2010.00586.x.

77 Rendle, J., Jackson, B., vander Hoorn, S. et al. (2020). A retrospective study of macropod progressive periodontal disease ("lumpy jaw") in captive macropods across Australia and Europe: using data from the past to inform future macropod management. *Animals* 10 (11): 1954. https://doi.org/10.3390/ani10111954.

78 Watson, M.K., Papich, M.G., and Chinnadurai, S.K. (2017). Pharmacokinetics of intravenous clindamycin phosphate in captive Bennett's wallabies (*Macropus rufogriseus*). *J. Vet. Pharmacol. Ther.* 40 (6): 682–686.

79 Kido, N., Chikuan, A., Omiya, T. et al. (2013). Retrospective study of oral necrobacillosis in 54 swamp wallabies. *Vet. Rec.* 173 (5): 118. https://doi.org/10.1136/vr.101694.

80 Hartley, M.P. and Sanderson, S. (2003). Use of antibiotic impregnated polymethylmethacrylate beads for the treatment of chronic mandibular osteomyelitis in a Bennett's wallaby (*Macropus rufogriseus rufogriseus*). *Aust. Vet. J.* 81 (12): 742–744. https://doi.org/10.1111/j.1751-0813.2003.tb14604.x.

81 Brookins, M.D., Rajeev, S., Thornhill, T.D. et al. (2008). Mandibular and maxillary osteomyelitis and myositis in a captive herd of red kangaroos (*Macropus rufus*). *J. Vet. Diagn. Investig.* 20 (6): 846–849. https://doi.org/10.1177/104063870802000627.

9

Diagnostic Imaging and Interpretation of the Equine Patient

Joan Howard[1], Molly Rice[2], Kara Frerichs[1], and Beatrice Sponseller[1]

[1] *Lloyd Veterinary Medical Center, Iowa State University College of Veterinary Medicine, Ames, IA, USA*
[2] *Midwest Veterinary Dental Services, Elkhorn, WI, USA*

CONTENTS

Introduction to Equine Dental Radiographs

The equine practitioner may experience trepidation when taking dental radiographs of the equine patient. Clinicians performing diagnostic imaging of this species need to consider the amount of time it takes to set up the radiographic equipment and provide effective, extended sedation during routine dental examinations and procedures. This often leads to difficulty in the scheduling of field appointments. The time it takes to perform a thorough oral evaluation and acquire diagnostic images of an equine patient makes it difficult to add another procedure or appointment into the schedule. In addition, capturing diagnostic images can be technically difficult. Despite these challenges, equine practitioners should consider the benefits of diagnostic imaging and the information it provides for the identification and diagnosis of abnormalities within the equine oral cavity. The ability to take diagnostic radiographs of the equine oral cavity is a valuable service that practitioners can provide to their clients and patients within their veterinary practice. Dedicating the time and effort to understand how to procure a diagnostic, quality image can offer clients a better understanding of a disease process and provide a visual representation of their horses' dental abnormalities. A dental radiograph can reveal valuable information that may not be visible on oral examination. For example, if a diastema and periodontal pocket are noted on oral examination, a radiograph can help the clinician decide whether cleaning and lavage of the pocket or extraction of the tooth is the best treatment option.

This chapter can be a useful guide to the equine practitioner in obtaining diagnostic radiographs of the equine oral cavity in a clinical setting or in the field. It will also discuss radiographic anatomy and guidelines for interpretation of dental radiographs in the equine patient as well as common disease processes that can be observed.

Veterinary Oral Diagnostic Imaging, First Edition. Edited by Brenda L. Mulherin.
© 2024 John Wiley & Sons, Inc. Published 2024 by John Wiley & Sons, Inc.

Radiation Safety

Equine veterinarians should follow the basic rules of radiation safety when taking radiographs in the field. Adequate restraint of the patient is important to minimize the need for repeated radiographs as well as reduce excessive radiation exposure. Care should be taken so the assistant does not have a hand or an arm that is exposed to the primary beam. Clinicians and assistants should also use protective gowns, thyroid shields, and dosimetry badges [1]. For more information on radiation safety, see Chapter 1.

Radiographic Systems

Direct Digital Radiographic System (DR)

This chapter will focus on radiographic techniques for direct digital radiographic (DR) systems. A DR system provides radiographic images that are digitally transferred to a computer for assessment and manipulation. Direct digital radiographic systems have algorithm settings which can allow single views that are diagnostic for multiple areas of the skull [2].

Computed Tomography

Computed tomography is a valuable tool for imaging of the equine dentition when it is available. However, this chapter is focused on radiographic imaging for the mobile equine veterinary practice.

Standard Radiographic System

The standard radiographic imaging system for procuring radiographic images in a field practice utilizes a generator that has up to 90 kilovoltage peak (kVp) and 15 milliamps (mA). Standard film would be developed with an automatic processor or in dip tanks utilizing developing techniques that are discussed in Chapter 1. Standard film radiographs necessitate markedly different settings to acquire images of the different areas of the head (teeth versus sinus).

Radiographic Technique

Most digital radiographic systems provide suggested techniques for dental radiograph procurement of the horse. If settings for an area of interest are not available, it can be useful to compare the area of interest to an area that has an established technique. For example, to take an occlusal intraoral view of the maxillary incisors, the same technique used for a 60° dorsoproximal-palmarodistal oblique image of the distal phalanx could suffice. When an effective technique is established, it is helpful to record it for future use to keep as a reference.

Lateral radiographs are used to evaluate the sinuses. The sinuses are largely composed of air; therefore, lower generator settings are needed to take a lateral view of the skull compared to procuring oblique views of the maxillary and mandibular cheek teeth. On intraoral views of the incisors, only the maxillary or mandibular incisors are being viewed, thus a lower kVP and shorter exposure time would be required for those views.

If adjustments need to be made to a radiographic image, a few basic concepts of radiographic procurement should be considered. The contrast of a radiographic image is affected by the opacity of the objects in the radiographic field. Increasing the milliampere per seconds (mAs) increases the number of photons which reach the radiographic detector, thus increasing the contrast of the image. Increasing the kilovoltage peak (kVp) will increase the energy of the photon, allowing greater penetration of the energy through the tooth and bone, but will provide less contrast at higher settings. If an image has an acceptable opacity but needs more contrast, the kVp can be lowered by 15% and the mAs can be doubled. To decrease the contrast of an image, mAs can be decreased by half and the kVp can be increased by 15% [1]. Sometimes moving the generator closer to the horse's head or object to be radiographed can also increase the number of photons which reach the sensor, thus increasing the contrast of an image.

Guidelines for Radiographic Views

The following are guidelines that can be used to obtain diagnostic dental radiographic images in the equine patient. These views should be taken with adequate sedation and careful attention to the radiation and physical safety of the equipment, patient, and assistants.

When obtaining oblique dental radiographic projections, it should be noted that the primary beam will NOT be perpendicular to the sensor, contrary to traditional radiographic guidelines regarding projections.

Concepts to Understand

Two key positioning concepts to understand when taking dental radiographs of the cheek teeth of the horse:

1) The importance of directing the primary beam through the interproximal spaces to prevent superimposition of neighboring teeth
2) An understanding of how open-mouth oblique projections of the mandible and maxilla will minimize superimposition of the opposite quadrant of cheek teeth

Directing the Primary Beam Through the Interproximal Spaces

The horse's head is triangular, with narrowing of the maxilla and mandible toward the rostral aspect of the skull. The interdental spaces are not perpendicular to the midline of the skull, so if the primary beam is directed perpendicular to midline, the diagnostic quality of the radiograph will be subpar. With the detector placed flush against the lateral aspect of the skull, the plane of the detector will be parallel to the cheek teeth quadrant nearest the detector. It is easiest when learning to obtain oblique cheek teeth projections, to first position the generator perpendicular to the detector as this will direct the primary beam through the interproximal spaces (Figure 9.1a and b). Once that angle has been determined, raise or lower the generator to achieve the appropriate obliquity for the desired projection (Figure 9.1c and d). If the primary beam is not perpendicular to the quadrant being imaged, the primary beam will

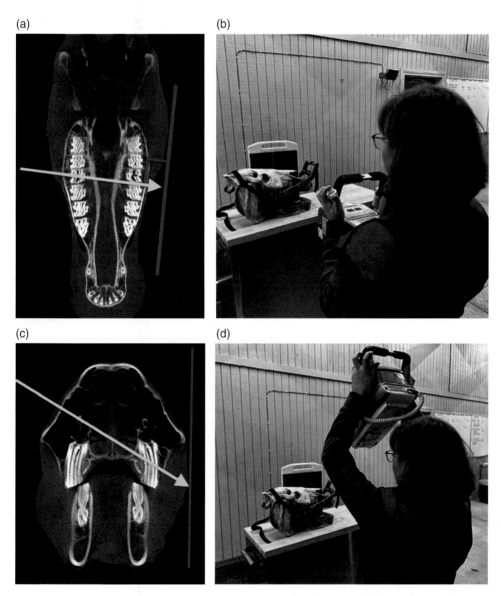

(a)   (b)   (c)   (d)

Figure 9.1 (a) This image illustrates the importance of positioning the detector against the horse's face then positioning the primary beam perpendicular to the detector. The computed tomographic (CT) image of the maxillary dental quadrants of a horse is used to illustrate that the detector (red line) when placed flush against the horse's head should be parallel to the maxillary cheek teeth so that if the primary beam (yellow line) is perpendicular to the detector it should penetrate the interproximal spaces of the teeth without creating overlap between the adjacent teeth. (b) The photograph demonstrates positioning the primary beam perpendicular to the detector to penetrate the interproximal spaces of the teeth. (c) This image illustrates that once the angle which directs the primary beam through the interproximal spaces has been determined, the generator can be raised or lowered for the appropriate obliquity of the desired projection. (d) This figure demonstrates positioning for a dorsal ventral oblique projection of the left maxillary quadrant. *Source:* Courtesy of Molly Rice, DVM, DAVDC-EQ, Midwest Veterinary Dental Services.

not be parallel to the interproximal spaces. This will result in the teeth appearing overlapped in the image, preventing maximum visualization of the structures of interest. If the detector is placed correctly against the quadrant of interest (ensuring that the primary beam is perpendicular to the plane of the detector), the correct radiographic angle should be established (Figure 9.2).

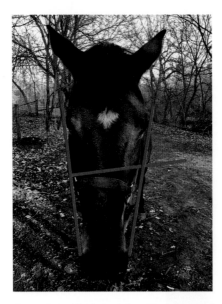

Figure 9.2 The horse's head has a triangular shape (red lines), so when taking dorsal ventral and ventral dorsal oblique projections of the cheek teeth, it is important that the primary beam is perpendicular to the detector. The blue line represents the primary beam in this photo for the right side of the horse.

Open Mouth Oblique Cheek Teeth Projections

The second key concept is that by opening the mouth for your oblique cheek teeth projections, space is created to allow for decreased superimposition of the cheek teeth on the right and left side of the head. Open-mouth projections of the maxillary and mandibular cheek teeth should allow clear visualization of the roots of the teeth, the surrounding alveolar bone, and the periodontal attachment of the target teeth. For open-mouth views, when the generator is raised in a dorsal direction and the central beam is directed in a ventral direction at the maxillary cheek teeth on the same side as the detector, the viewer will visualize the apex of the maxillary cheek teeth on the same side as the detector. If the generator is lowered ventrally, and the primary beam is directed in a dorsal direction at the maxillary cheek teeth closest to the detector, the viewer will be able to evaluate the clinical crown, palatal root, and interdental spaces of the cheek teeth next to the detector (Figures 9.3a, b, 9.4a, b, 9.5a, b, 9.6a, and b).

Radiographic Views

Lateral View

Digital Detector: The detector should be centered on the rostral aspect of the facial crest. The detector is positioned parallel to the dorsal contour of the skull [2]. The caudal aspect of the orbit marks the caudal border of the

(a)

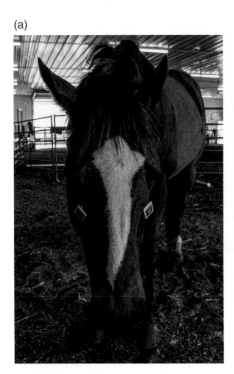

(b)

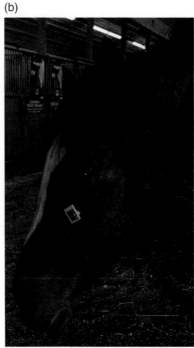

Figure 9.3 (a) Radiographic markers were used in the following photographs and radiographs to illustrate the projection of the maxillary cheek teeth with dorsal ventral and ventral dorsal oblique projections. (b) Radiographic markers are used in these instructional images to identify the quadrant being imaged. The blue marker is the left marker. It has been attached to the horse on the left side of the head. For diagnostic radiographs, the right and left markers would be attached to the detector and not to the horse.

(a)

(b)

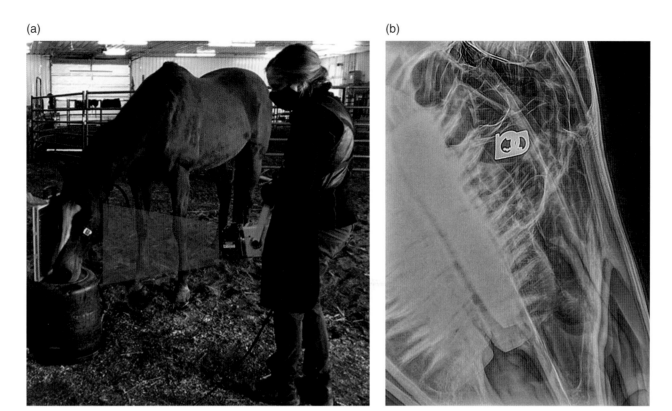

Figure 9.4 (a) The image demonstrates radiographic procurement of the lateral view of the equine patient. (b) The radiograph demonstrates superimposition of the right and left markers and the cheek teeth on the right and left side of the horse's mouth when acquiring a radiograph using the lateral view.

(a)

(b)

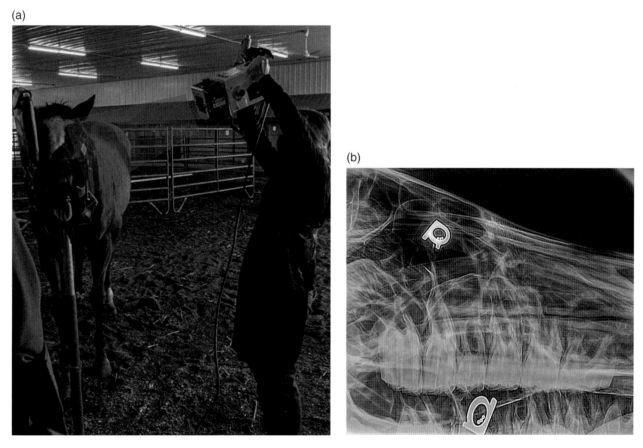

Figure 9.5 (a) The image demonstrates radiographic procurement of a dorsal ventral oblique projection of the right maxilla of an equine patient. Note that the angle of the primary beam used in this picture to illustrate the projection was not as steep as would typically be used to procure an image of the maxillary cheek teeth. (b) In the dorsal ventral oblique projection of the right maxilla, the R marker (right marker) and the cheek teeth on the right side are projected dorsally, while the L marker (left marker) and the cheek teeth on the left side are projected ventrally.

(a)

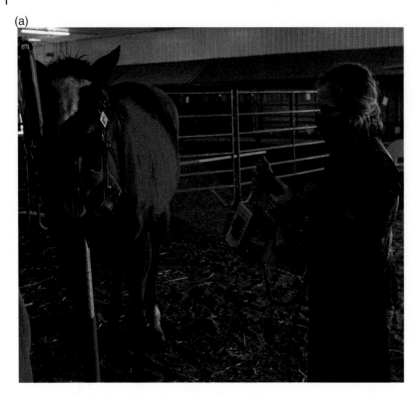

(b)

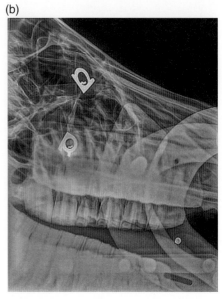

Figure 9.6 (a) The image demonstrates radiographic procurement of the ventral dorsal oblique projection of the right maxilla of an equine patient. Note that the angle of the primary beam used in this picture to illustrate the projection was not as steep as would typically be used to image the maxillary cheek teeth. (b) In the ventral dorsal oblique projection of the right maxilla, the L marker (left marker) and the cheek teeth on the left side are projected dorsally and the R marker (right marker) and the teeth on the right side are projected ventrally.

detector, and the rostral interdental space (the bars) marks the rostral border of the detector. The dorsal skull should be within the dorsal border of the sensor. If the head is held low in a vertical position, sinus fluid lines will more easily be appreciated. If the horse is positioned this way, the muzzle can be rested on a bucket or stool to stabilize the head and the detector. A gravity marker can also be used to help visualize fluid lines. This view can be taken with or without a speculum. The right or left radiographic marker should indicate which side of the head the detector is positioned and should be placed on the dorsal aspect of the detector (Figure 9.7a).

X-ray Generator: The primary X-ray beam should be centered on the rostral facial crest perpendicular to the long axis of the head. The rostral border of the primary beam should be positioned at the interdental space, and the caudal border should be positioned at the caudal aspect of the eye [2] (Figure 9.7b).

Areas of Interest: The rostral and caudal maxillary sinuses and the conchofrontal sinus can be assessed in this image (Figure 9.7c). The cheek teeth are superimposed, so disease of an individual tooth should not be evaluated on this view [3]. Fluid or other opacities in the sinus can

be visualized, and sometimes fractures of the mandible can be observed on this view. The superimposed nasal conchal bullae should also be evident when utilizing this view.

Dorsoventral View

Digital Detector: The detector is placed ventral to the mandible. The detector should extend caudally to the level of the caudal aspect of the orbit. The rostral border of the detector should be positioned at the interdental space. Resting the head on the radiographic plate or digital detector, which is stabilized on a stand can make this view easier to position and acquire. The right and left sinuses are included on the detector, and the horse's head should not be rotated. The radiographic marker is placed lateral to the head to denote the right or left side of the skull (Figure 9.8a).

X-ray Generator: The X-ray beam is perpendicular to the horse's hard palate and centered on a line that can be visualized between the rostral aspect of the right and left facial crest. The beam should extend caudally to the orbit and rostrally to the interdental space (Figure 9.8b).

(a)

(b)

(c)

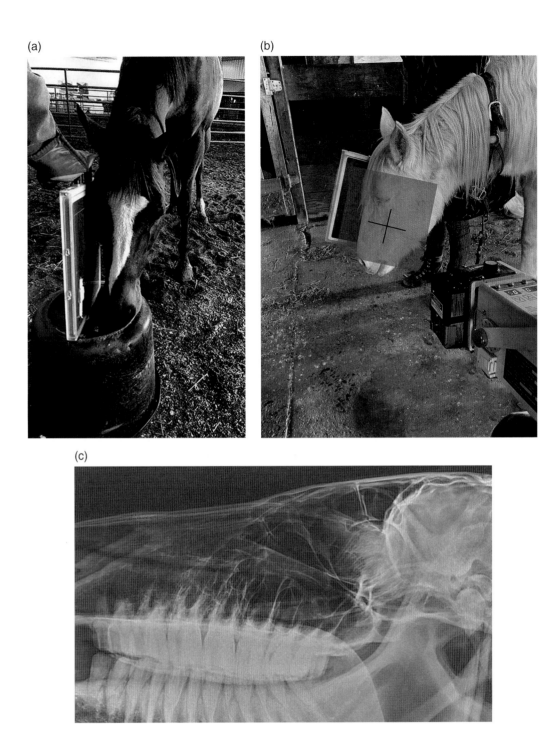

Figure 9.7 (a) Placement of detector for a lateral view. The detector is centered on the rostral aspect of the facial crest with the caudal border at the caudal aspect of the orbit and the rostral border at the interdental space. The detector is parallel to the long axis of the horse's head. In this picture, the horse's muzzle and the detector are resting on a muck bucket. (b) Positioning for a lateral view. The primary X-ray beam (labeled as the X on the image) is centered on the rostral facial crest and is perpendicular to the long axis of the horse's head. The shadow of the dorsal skull is within the dorsal border of the detector. (c) Lateral radiograph of the equine skull. This image demonstrates a well-positioned lateral radiograph of a normal equine patient. *Source:* Courtesy of Molly Rice, DVM, DAVDC-EQ, Midwest Veterinary Dental Services.

Areas of Interest: The maxillary sinuses, the nasal septum, the medial cortex of the mandibular bone, and the lateral aspect of the maxillary cheek teeth should be able to be assessed with this view (Figure 9.8c). Changes in

the rostral and caudal maxillary sinuses, maxillary and mandibular fractures, fractured maxillary cheek teeth, and periapical distortion of the maxilla from endodontic infections of the rostral maxillary teeth

(a) (b) (c)

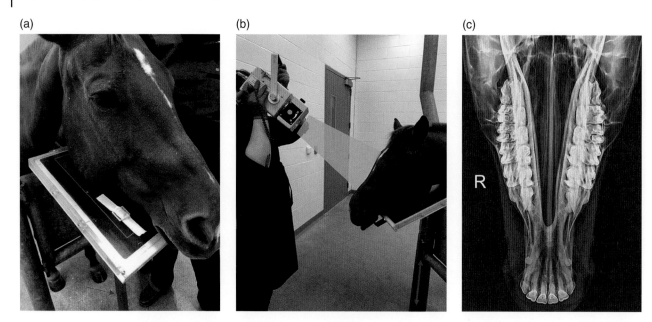

Figure 9.8 (a) Placement of the detector for the dorsoventral view. The head is rested on the detector, in this picture using a stand (red arrow), but a trash can or other stationary object can also be used. The caudal border of the detector is at the level of the caudal aspect of the orbit, and the rostral edge of the detector is at the level of the interdental space. (b) Positioning for the dorsoventral view of the head. The primary X-ray beam is perpendicular to the horse's hard palate and centered on a point, which is midway between the rostral aspect of the right and left facial crests. The detector can be placed more caudally or rostrally depending on the area of interest. In this picture, the detector is placed more caudally, which would be appropriate for imaging the caudal sinus. The horse's head in this photo is resting on a stand, which is identified by the double-headed red arrow. (c) Dorsoventral radiograph of a normal equine head. This image demonstrates a well-positioned dorsoventral radiograph of an equine patient. *Source:* Courtesy of Molly Rice, DVM, DAVDC-EQ, Midwest Veterinary Dental Services.

may be appreciated in this view [2]. Depending on the size of the patient, more than one view may be necessary to evaluate all of these structures.

Additional Views: If the mandible is distracted to the right or the left side of the animal with a lead rope or positioning device, additional information of the contralateral mandibular and maxillary cheek teeth may be appreciated. Distracted DV projections can also be particularly helpful for visualizing ventral conchal sinus disease. Additionally, if the head is placed in an outstretched position, and the detector moved caudally to be centered under the ventral mandible/throatlatch area at the level of the ears, this view can be useful for evaluating the temporohyoid joint.

Dorsal Ventral Oblique Projection of the Maxillary Cheek Teeth

Digital Detector: The mouth is held open with a full-mouth speculum or an incisor block. If a full-mouth speculum is used, it should be a wide speculum so that the detector can be placed between the speculum and the horse's head. The detector is held flush against the face on the side of interest, centered on the rostral facial crest. The caudal aspect of the orbit marks the caudal border of the detector, and the rostral interdental space marks

the rostral border of the detector. It is easiest to attain the correct angles for this projection if the head is placed on a stand in a horizontal position. The radiographic marker is placed dorsally to the skull (Figure 9.9a–c).

X-ray Generator: The primary X-ray beam of the generator should first be directed perpendicular to the detector. This positioning will align the primary beam with the interdental spaces on the quadrant of interest. Once that angle has been determined, then raise the generator directing the primary beam in a dorso-ventral direction centered on the rostral facial crest. The degree of angulation will range from 35° to 60° dorso-ventral depending on the age of the patient. The angle will need to be steeper in younger animals to allow adequate separation of the molar quadrants and avoid superimposition of tooth structures (Figure 9.9d). It is important to note that sometimes taking several dorso-ventral oblique views at differing angles may help achieve the most diagnostic information possible. In older horses, the hard palate can often become superimposed over the area of interest (tooth apices and interproximal bone). Therefore, steepening the angle in older horses may also give additional diagnostic information. If the angle becomes too steep, elongation of the teeth will occur, which can complicate interpretation.

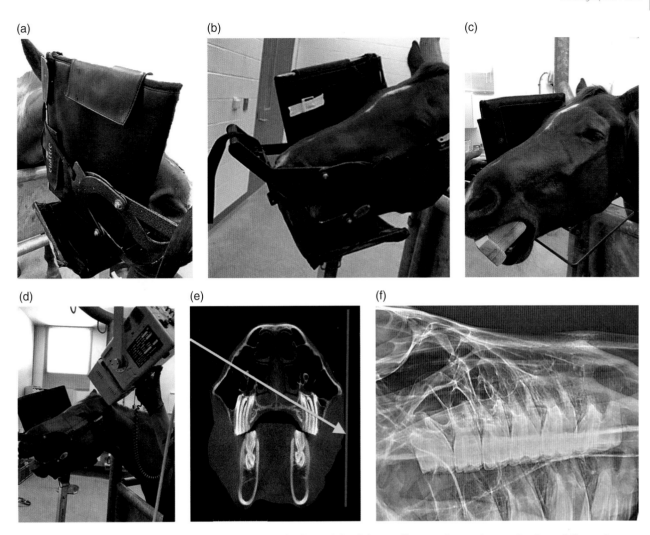

Figure 9.9 (a) Placement of the detector for oblique projections of the right maxillary quadrant using an aluminum full mouth speculum. The detector is placed between the horse's head and the full mouth speculum. The detector is held against the head and is not parallel to the long axis of the head as is done for the lateral view. The caudal border of the detector extends to the caudal orbit, and the rostral border extends to the interdental space. (b) Placement of detector for oblique projections of the right maxillary quadrant using an aluminum full-mouth speculum. (c) Placement of detector for oblique projections of the right maxillary quadrant using an incisor block, with the head supported on a stand. (d) Positioning for dorsal ventral oblique projection of the right maxillary quadrant. The primary X-ray beam is first positioned so that it is centered on the rostral border of the facial crest and is perpendicular to the detector, in this case the right side. The generator is then raised 35–60° while continuing to center on the rostral facial crest. This image demonstrates the final positioning. (e) Transverse CT image of the equine head demonstrating the path of the primary beam (yellow arrow) and the placement of the detector (red line) when taking a dorsal ventral projection of the left maxillary cheek teeth. The apex of the left maxillary cheek tooth will be projected dorsal to image of the right maxillary cheek tooth. Note that the mouth is not held open in this CT, as it would be for a radiographic projection. *Source:* Courtesy of Molly Rice, DVM, DAVDC-EQ, Midwest Veterinary Dental Services. (f) Radiograph of the normal dorsal ventral oblique projection of the right maxillary cheek teeth. This image demonstrates a well-positioned radiograph of a normal equine patient.

Areas of Interest: A dorsal ventral oblique projection of the maxillary dental quadrants focuses on the apices (roots) and reserve crown of the maxillary cheek teeth on the side where the detector is positioned (Figure 9.9e and f). Signs of apical infection may be visible, including periapical sclerosis, root clubbing, and periapical lucency. Evaluation of periodontal disease (diastemata and associated bone loss) and widening of the periodontal ligament may be assessed. It may be possible to localize lesions in the maxillary and conchofrontal sinuses, although fluid lines can be more difficult to appreciate in this view. These oblique projections can be helpful in distinguishing right from left nasal conchal bullae empyema as these structures are superimposed on a latero-lateral view of this region. This view is also helpful after extracting a maxillary cheek tooth and evaluating for retained dental material.

Ventral Dorsal Oblique Projection of the Maxillary Cheek Teeth

Digital Detector: The mouth is held open with a full-mouth speculum or an incisor block. If a full-mouth speculum is used, it should be a wide speculum so that the detector can be placed between the speculum and the horse's head. The detector is held flush against the face on the side of interest. The detector is secured against the head and centered on the rostral facial crest. The head can be rested on a dental stand (see Figure 9.9a–c). The radiographic marker should indicate on which side of the head the detector is positioned and should be placed dorsal to the skull.

X-ray Generator: The primary X-ray beam should first be positioned perpendicular to the detector at the rostral facial crest, this will align the primary beam with the interdental spaces on the quadrant of interest. The generator is then lowered, directing the primary beam in a ventral–dorsal direction keeping the center on the rostral facial crest. The angulation may vary from 45° to 70° ventral–dorsal (Figure 9.10a).

Areas of Interest: A ventral dorsal projection of the right maxillary quadrant can assess the clinical crown and palatal root of the maxillary cheek teeth on the same side as the sensor (Figure 9.10b and c). Periodontal disease with alveolar bone loss, clinical crown fractures, and abnormalities of wear can be appreciated on this view [2].

Ventral Dorsal Oblique Projection of the Mandibular Cheek Teeth

Digital Detector: The detector is placed flush against the horse's head on the side of interest. The mouth is held open with a full-mouth speculum or with an incisor block. If a full-mouth speculum is used, the detector is placed between the speculum and the horse's head. Additionally, the head can be secured by resting the bite plate from the maxillary incisors (open mouth) on the edge of the dental stand or suspended by a dental halter or rope. The radiographic marker indicating on which side the detector is positioned is placed at the bottom of the detector [4] (Figure 9.11a and b).

X-ray Generator: The primary X-ray beam is first directed at a 90° angle to the detector. This positioning will align the primary beam with the interdental spaces on the quadrant of interest. The generator is then lowered, angling the primary beam in a ventral–dorsal direction. The degree of angulation may vary from 45° to 60° in a ventral–dorsal direction. The beam is centered on the ventral mandible at the rostral aspect of the masseter muscle on the side closest to the generator. An increased angle will be necessary for younger patients. Additionally, an increased technique may be needed to visualize the second and third mandibular molars [2]. Horses with narrow mandibles may also require a steeper angle [2] (Figure 9.11c).

Areas of Interest: A radiograph of the ventral dorsal oblique projection of the right mandibular cheek teeth allows assessment of the reserve crown and roots of mandibular cheek teeth that are on the same side as the plate (Figure 9.11d and e). Changes in the root and reserve crown of the mandibular cheek teeth should be appreciated in this view.

Dorsal Ventral Oblique Projection of the Mandibular Cheek Teeth

Digital Detector: The detector is placed flush against the horse's head on the side of interest. The mouth is held open with a full-mouth speculum or with an incisor block. If a full-mouth speculum is used, the detector is placed between the speculum and the horse's head. The head can be secured by resting the open mouth on a dental headstand (see Figure 9.11a and b).

X-ray Generator: The primary X-ray beam is first directed at a 90° angle to the detector. This positioning will align the primary beam with the interdental spaces on the quadrant of interest. The generator is then raised, directing the primary beam dorsal to ventral 15–30° from the plane of the palate. The primary beam is centered on a plane halfway between the facial crest and ventral mandible on the clinical crowns of the mandibular cheek teeth (Figure 9.12a).

Areas of Interest: In a dorsal ventral oblique projection of the right mandibular cheek teeth, the clinical crown and alveolar bone associated with the mandibular cheek teeth on the side of the head that the detector is placed will be imaged (Figure 9.12b and c). Periodontal disease with alveolar bone loss, diastemata, clinical crown fractures, and abnormalities of wear can be appreciated on this view [2]. This view can also be helpful for obtaining greater detail of lower third molars in older horses where the traditional ventral–dorsal oblique does not provide enough clarity.

Occlusal Intraoral View of the Maxillary Incisors and Canines

Digital Detector: The detector is protected from being damaged by the incisors using either a protective case or an aluminum speculum. If the size and conformation of

(a)

(b)

(c)

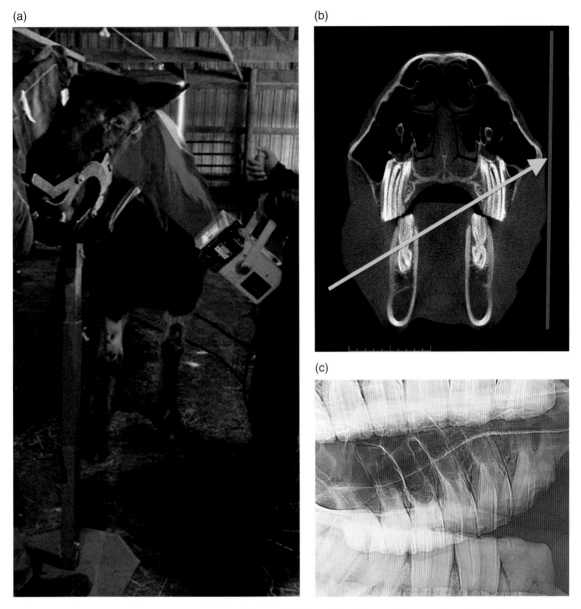

Figure 9.10 (a) Positioning for ventral dorsal oblique projection of the right maxillary quadrant. The primary beam is first positioned so that it is perpendicular to the detector. The primary beam is then lowered 45° in a ventral-dorsal direction while continuing to center on or slightly below the rostral facial crest. The most common mistake in acquiring this image is not positioning the primary beam at a steep enough angle. This image represents the final positioning. (b) Transverse CT image of the equine head demonstrating the path of the primary beam (yellow arrow) and the placement of the detector (red line) when taking a ventral dorsal projection of the left maxillary cheek teeth. The apex of the left maxillary cheek tooth will be projected ventral in the image to the right maxillary cheek tooth. Note that the mouth is not held open in this CT, as it would be for a radiographic projection. (c) Radiograph of the ventral dorsal oblique projection of the right maxillary quadrant. This image demonstrates a well-positioned radiograph of a normal equine patient. *Source:* Courtesy of Molly Rice, DVM, DAVDC-EQ, Midwest Veterinary Dental Services.

the horse allow it, the detector is inserted into the mouth so that it is touching the mesial aspect of the maxillary second premolars. The caudal aspect of the detector should be the side of the detector with the narrowest sensor border (Figure 9.13a). Using the corner of the detector may be helpful in properly visualizing incisors and canines [5].

X-ray Generator: The primary X-ray beam is centered on the incisors and the angle of the beam should be 90° to the bisecting angle of the detector and reserve crown of the maxillary incisors. This angle will be a rostral dorsal caudal-ventral oblique projection. The bisecting angle can often be estimated to be perpendicular to the muzzle of the horse (Figure 9.13b and c). Utilizing a

(a) (b) (c)

(d) (e)

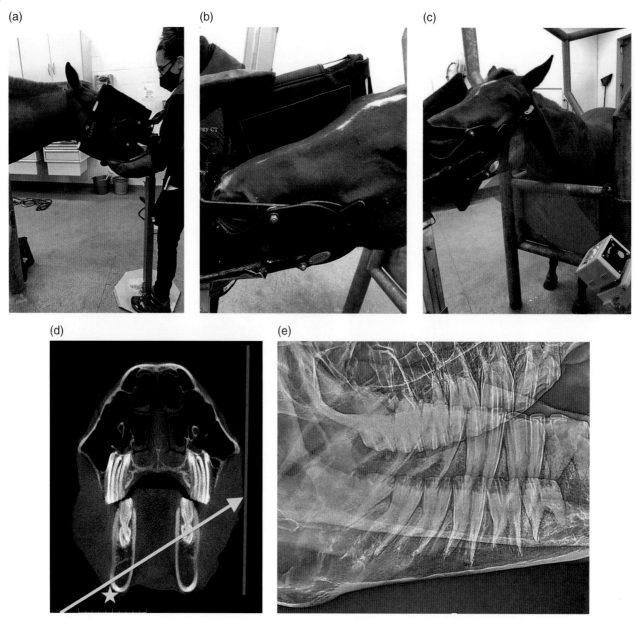

Figure 9.11 (a) Placement of the detector for oblique projections of the right mandibular quadrant using an aluminum full-mouth speculum. The detector is placed flush against the right side of the horse's head under the speculum and is extended ventrally beyond the border of the ventral mandible. The head can be secured by resting the horse's open mouth on the edge of the dental stand. (b) Placement of the detector for oblique projections of the right mandibular cheek teeth. Note how the upper incisor plate of the speculum is resting on the head stand for support. (c) Positioning for a ventral dorsal projection of the right mandibular cheek teeth. The primary beam should be centered just above the ventral aspect of the mandible at the rostral aspect of the masseter muscle on the side closest to the generator. The beam is first positioned perpendicular to the detector. The generator is then lowered, directing the primary beam in a ventral-dorsal direction. The degree of angulation can vary from 45° to 60° depending on the age of the horse. The most common mistake in acquiring this image is not positioning the primary beam at a steep enough angle. Lowering the generator toward the floor will allow for a steeper angle. (d) Transverse CT image of the equine head demonstrating the path of the primary beam (yellow arrow) and the placement of the detector (red line) when taking a ventral dorsal oblique projection of the left mandibular cheek teeth. Note that the primary beam is centered on the mandible closest to the generator (yellow star). The apex of the left mandibular cheek tooth will be projected ventral to the image of the right mandibular cheek tooth. Note that the mouth is not held open in this CT, as it would be for a radiographic projection. (e) Radiograph of the ventral dorsal oblique projection of the right mandibular quadrant. This image demonstrates a well-positioned radiograph of a normal equine patient. *Source:* Courtesy of Molly Rice, DVM, DAVDC-EQ, Midwest Veterinary Dental Services.

(a) 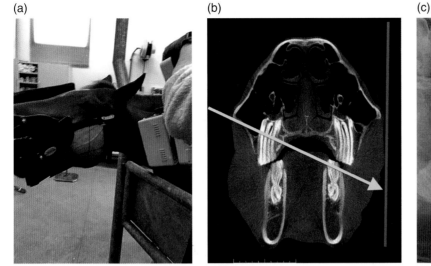 (b) (c)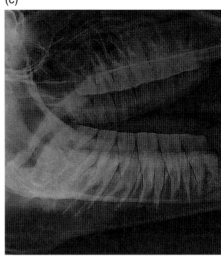

Figure 9.12   (a) Positioning for dorsal ventral oblique projection of the mandibular cheek teeth. The primary beam is directed halfway between the facial crest and the ventral mandible (at the occlusal surface of the quadrant of interest). The primary beam is first directed perpendicular to the detector. The generator is then raised, directing the beam 10–30° in a dorsal to ventral direction. (b) Transverse CT image of the equine head demonstrating the path of the primary beam (yellow arrow) and the placement of the detector (red line) when taking a dorsal ventral oblique projection of the left mandibular cheek teeth. The clinical crown of the left mandibular cheek tooth will be projected dorsal to the image of the right mandibular cheek tooth. Note that the mouth is not held open in this CT, as it would be for a radiographic projection. (c) Well-positioned radiograph of a dorsal ventral oblique projection of the mandibular cheek teeth in a normal equine patient. The area of interest in this projection is quite small, concerning primarily the clinical crowns and interdental bone. This view is most helpful in evaluating bone recession that occurs secondary to periodontitis. *Source:* Courtesy of Molly Rice, DVM, DAVDC-EQ, Midwest Veterinary Dental Services.

proper bisecting angle technique will result in an image without foreshortening or elongation.

Areas of Interest: A properly positioned occlusal intraoral view of the maxillary incisors and canines should provide imaging of the reserve crowns and clinical crowns of the maxillary incisors (Figure 9.13d). Incisor fractures, evaluation of tooth vitality, and changes due to equine odontoclastic tooth resorption and hypercementosis (EOTRH) are often diagnosed with this view.

Additional Views: Maintaining this bisecting angle technique and moving the generator laterally so that it is centered on the third incisor can provide an image of the third incisor and maxillary canine tooth without superimposition of the adjacent second incisor.

Occlusal Intraoral View of the Mandibular Incisors and Canines

Digital Detector: The detector is protected from being damaged by a protective cover. Alternatively, an aluminum speculum can be used. If the size and conformation of the horse allows it, the detector is inserted in the mouth so that it has contact with the mesial aspect of the mandibular second premolars. The caudal aspect of the detector should be the side of the detector with the narrowest sensor border. Using the corner of the detector may be helpful in properly visualizing incisors and canine teeth [5] (Figure 9.14a).

X-ray Generator: The primary X-ray beam is centered on the mandibular incisors at a 90° angle to the bisecting angle of the reserve crown of the incisors and the plate (Figure 9.14b).

Areas of Interest: An occlusal intraoral view of the mandibular incisors and canines will allow assessment of the reserve crowns and clinical crowns of the mandibular incisors (Figure 9.14c). Incisor fractures, evaluation of tooth vitality, and changes due to equine odontoclastic tooth resorption and hypercementosis (EOTRH) are often diagnosed with this view.

Additional Views: Maintaining the bisecting angle and moving the generator laterally so that it is centered on either the canine tooth or third incisor can provide an image of the third incisor and mandibular canine tooth without superimposition of the adjacent second incisor. Positioning for a mandibular incisor or corner incisor is illustrated along with an example of an oblique radiographic view of the right mandibular canine in Figure 9.14d and e.

A summary of the radiographic views is provided in Table 9.1.

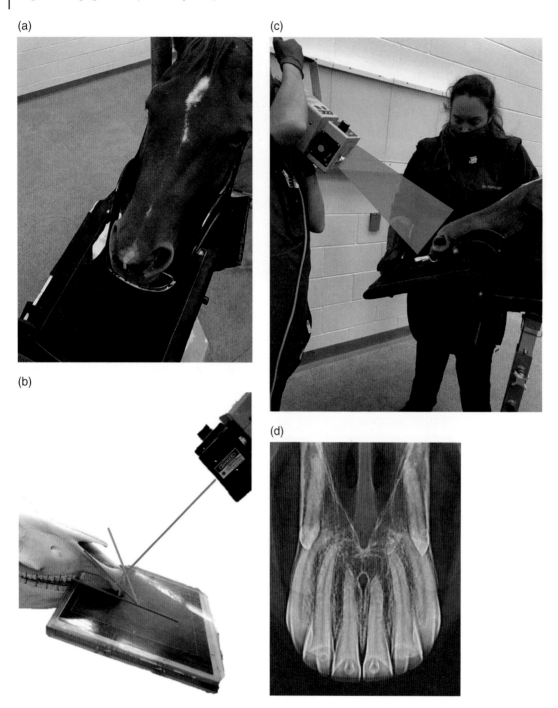

Figure 9.13 (a) Placement of detector for an intraoral radiograph of the maxillary incisors and canine teeth. The detector is inserted into the oral cavity as far as is comfortable for the patient and without being inserted far enough to be damaged by the cheek teeth. The sensor surface should be facing dorsally. An aluminum speculum or protective cover should be used to protect the detector. (b) Estimating the bisecting angle for intraoral radiograph procurement of the maxillary incisors and canine teeth. The bisecting angle is estimated by visualizing the sensor (red line) and the reserve crown of the incisors (green line) and directing the primary beam (blue line) perpendicular to the plane which bisects the angle formed between those points (orange line). (c) Positioning for the occlusal intraoral view of the maxillary incisors and canine teeth. The primary beam is centered on the incisors using an estimated bisecting angle technique. (d) Properly positioned occlusal intraoral radiograph of the maxillary incisors and canine teeth of a normal horse. *Source:* Courtesy of Molly Rice, DVM, DAVDC-EQ, Midwest Veterinary Dental Services.

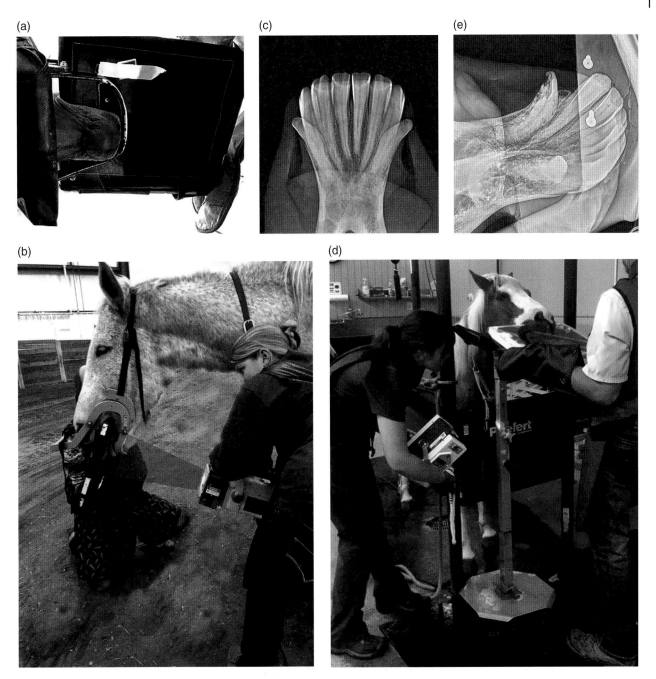

Figure 9.14   (a) Placement of a detector for an occlusal intraoral radiographic view of the mandibular incisors and canine teeth. This picture is viewed ventral to the horse's mandibular incisors. The detector is in a protected cover and is inserted just rostral to mandibular second premolars. (b) Positioning for an occlusal intraoral radiographic view of the mandibular incisors and canine teeth. The primary beam is centered on the mandibular incisors using the estimated bisecting angle between the reserve crowns of the mandibular incisors and the detector. Note that the individual holding the detector should place their body away from the primary radiographic beam as demonstrated in the image. (c) Properly positioned occlusal intraoral radiographic view of the mandibular incisors and canine teeth of a normal horse. *Source:* Courtesy of Molly Rice, DVM, DAVDC-EQ, Midwest Veterinary Dental Services. (d) Proper positioning for an occlusal intraoral oblique radiograph of the right mandibular canine tooth of an equine patient. The bisecting angle is maintained, and the generator is moved laterally so that it is centered on the right mandibular canine tooth. (e) Properly positioned occlusal intraoral radiograph of the right mandibular canine tooth of a horse. This canine tooth demonstrates evidence of tooth resorption.

Table 9.1 The table describes the different radiographic techniques used to procure dental radiographs of the equine patient.

Radiographic view	Positioning	Primary beam	Areas evaluated
Lateral skull	Detector centered on the rostral aspect of the facial crest parallel to the long axis of the horse's head	Primary X-ray beam centered on the rostral facial crest in a medial–lateral direction	Rostral and caudal maxillary sinuses, conchofrontal sinus, superimposed nasal conchal bullae
Dorsoventral skull	Head resting on the detector, caudal border of the detector extends to the caudal aspect of the orbit, rostral boarder extends to the interdental space	Primary beam centered on a line visualized between the rostral aspect of the right and left facial crest in a dorsal–ventral direction	Maxillary sinuses, nasal septum, medial cortex of the mandibular bone, lateral aspect of maxillary cheek teeth
Dorsal ventral oblique projection of the maxillary cheek teeth	Open-mouth view detector is held against the head, caudal border of the detector extends to the caudal orbit, rostral border extends to the interdental space	Primary beam centered on the rostral facial crest and at a 35–60° angle in a dorsal–ventral direction	Apices and reserve crown of maxillary cheek teeth on the same side as the detector, maxillary and conchofrontal sinuses
Ventral dorsal oblique projection of maxillary cheek teeth	Open mouth view detector is held against the head, caudal border of the detector extends to the caudal orbit, rostral border extends to the interdental space	Primary beam centered on or slightly below the rostral facial at a 45–60° angle in a ventral-dorsal direction	Clinical crown and palatal root of the maxillary cheek teeth on the same side as the sensor
Ventral dorsal oblique projection of the mandibular cheek teeth	Open-mouth view detector is placed flush against the horse's head on the side of interest and is extended ventrally beyond the border of the ventral mandible	Primary beam centered just above the ventral aspect of the mandible at the rostral aspect of the masseter muscle at a 45–60° angle in a ventral-dorsal direction	Reserve crown and roots of mandibular cheek teeth on the same side as the plate
Dorsal ventral oblique projection of the mandibular cheek teeth	Open-mouth view detector is placed flush against the horse's head on the side of interest, extended ventrally beyond the border of the ventral mandible	Primary beam is directed halfway between the facial crest and the ventral mandible at a 10–30° angle in a dorsal–ventral direction	Clinical crown and alveolar bone associated with the mandibular cheek teeth on the side of the head that the detector is placed
Occlusal intraoral projection of the maxillary incisors and canines	Open-mouth view detector is protected and inserted orally, rostral to the maxillary second premolars with the sensor surface facing dorsally	Primary beam is centered on the incisors in a dorsal ventral direction using an estimated bisecting angle	Reserve crown and clinical crown of the maxillary incisors and canines
Occlusal intraoral projection of the mandibular incisors and canines	Detector is protected and is inserted rostral to the mandibular second premolars with the sensor surface facing ventrally	Primary beam centered on the mandibular incisors in a ventral dorsal direction using an estimated bisecting angle	Reserve crown and clinical crown of mandibular incisors and canines

Evaluation of an Image

When an image has been taken, the following should be evaluated to determine if the image is diagnostic.

- Movement of the detector or the horse (Figure 9.15)
- Overlap between teeth in a quadrant (Figure 9.16a and b)
- Correct exposure (Figure 9.17a and b)
- Appropriate alignment of primary beam and detector boundaries (Figure 9.18)
- Correct technique and angle for the area of interest (Figure 9.19)

Labial Mounting

Radiographs of equine dentition should be viewed using labial mounting. Radiographic views which are taken with the sensor on the left side of the head should be viewed with the nose of the patient positioned to the viewer's left. Views taken with the sensor on the right side of the head should be viewed with the nose of the patient positioned to the viewer's right. Maxillary incisors should be viewed with the occlusal aspect of the teeth oriented down, and mandibular incisors should be viewed with the occlusal

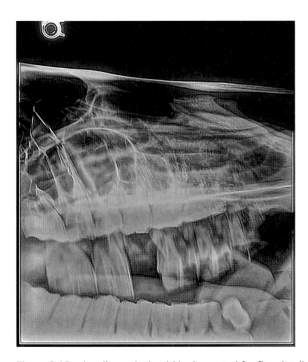

Figure 9.15 A radiograph should be inspected for fine detail of the image. This dorsal ventral radiographic projection of the right maxillary quadrant illustrates motion artifact in the image. Loss of fine detail may indicate that there has been movement. Lack of detail can be noted in the right maxillary cheek teeth and more remarkably in the left maxillary cheek teeth. Tooth 209 had been previously extracted when this radiograph was taken.

aspect oriented up. Dorsal ventral views are usually viewed with the nose down (Figure 9.20). For more information on labial mounting, see Chapter 3.

Radiographic Anatomy

The horse's dental formula for deciduous teeth is 2(Di 3/3, Dc 0/0, Dpm 3/3) = 24 teeth, and for permanent teeth is 2(I 3/3, C 0–1/0–1, PM 3–4/3–4, M 3/3) = 36–44 teeth [2].

It is useful for the clinician to be familiar with the Triadan tooth numbering system of equine teeth. In this system, each tooth is assigned a number. The 100 quadrant consists of the horse's right maxillary teeth, the 200 are the left maxillary teeth, 300 are the left mandibular, and the 400 are the right mandibular teeth. The numbers 500–800 are assigned to the deciduous teeth in the same order, similarly to canine and feline species. Numbering starts with the central incisors as 01, and the last molars as 11 (Figure 9.21a and b).

In assessing radiographs for tooth root disease, it is helpful to remember that the maxillary cheek teeth (06–11) have three roots, two buccal and one palatal. Occasionally, they may have four roots, which is considered a variation of normal. The mandibular cheek teeth have a mesial and distal tooth root (06–11), and the incisors, canines, and first premolars (wolf teeth), if present, have one root. It is also important to remember that the alveolus of the maxillary

(a)   (b)

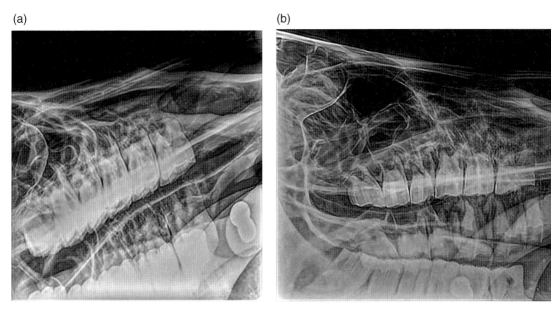

Figure 9.16 (a) A radiographic image should have the interproximal alveolar bone visible between the cheek teeth. In this dorsal ventral projection of the right maxillary cheek teeth, there is overlap between the cheek teeth so that the interproximal spaces between the teeth cannot be clearly visualized. It is important to keep the primary beam of the generator perpendicular to the quadrant being radiographed to avoid overlap. (b) Radiograph of the same skull as seen in Figure 9.16a, but more optimal angles have resulted in less overlap and improved visualization of the interproximal spaces. It should be noted that the technique chosen for this film resulted in overexposure of the sinuses.

(a)

(b)

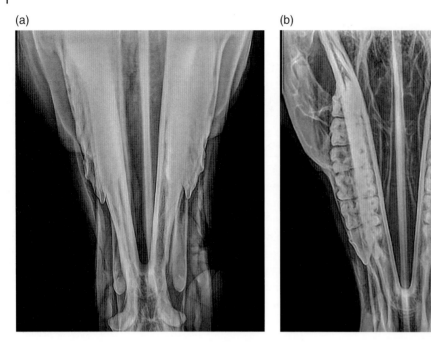

Figure 9.17 (a) Dorsoventral radiograph of an equine cadaver head with inadequate technique and positioning. The detail of the maxillary cheek teeth cannot be visualized and faint horizontal lines across the image indicate the image is underexposed. An increased technique is needed. The detector is also positioned rostrally so the caudal cheek teeth will not be seen. Additionally, the nasal septum is not centered, indicating there is likely some rotation of the head. (b) The technique is improved on this radiograph of the same cadaver head as seen in Figure (a). When the head is positioned correctly, the maxillary sinuses and cheek teeth can be clearly visualized.

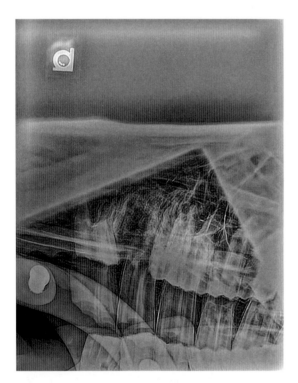

Figure 9.18 The radiographic image demonstrates cone cutting. The primary beam has not been aligned correctly with the detector so that the detector has not been appropriately exposed. The structures which are underexposed are outside of the primary beam. There is a clear, angular, distinction between the areas where the detector was exposed by the primary radiographic beam and the areas that were not exposed to the primary beam.

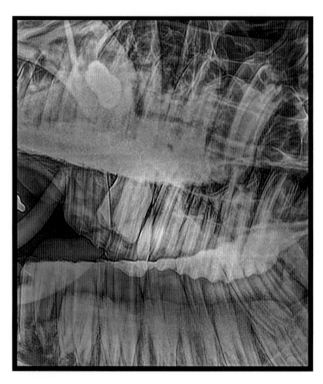

Figure 9.19 Ventral dorsal oblique projection of the right maxillary quadrant. This radiograph illustrates improper positioning. The patient was a young animal with long reserve crowns; thus, a steeper angle would be necessary to properly procure an image of the right maxillary cheek teeth.

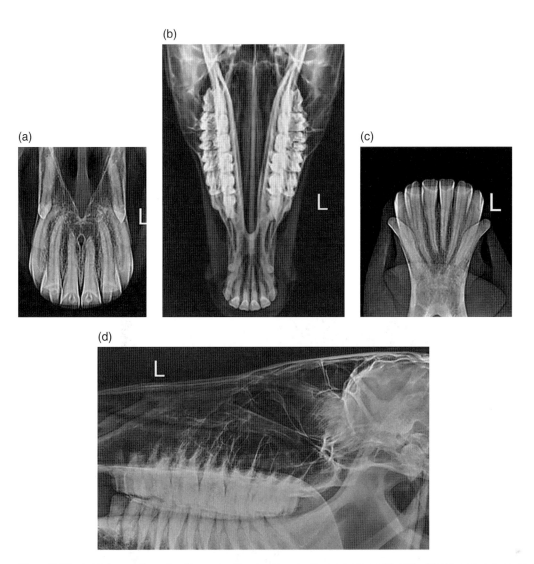

Figure 9.20 Labial mounting of radiographs: the maxillary incisors (a) are positioned with the occlusal aspect of the incisors oriented down, the dorsal ventral view (b) is positioned with the nose of the horse directed down, and the mandibular incisors (c) are positioned with the occlusal aspect of the incisors oriented up. The lateral view (d) taken with the detector on the left side of the horse's head is viewed with the horse's nose directed to the left. *Source:* Courtesy of Molly Rice, DVM, DAVDC-EQ, Midwest Veterinary Dental Services.

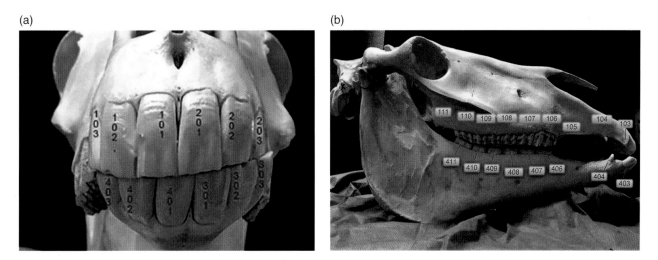

Figure 9.21 (a) This image demonstrates the Triadan numbering system of incisors. The right maxillary 1st incisor is labeled 101, 2nd incisor 102, and the 3rd incisor 103. The left maxillary 1st incisor is labeled as 201, the 2nd incisor 202, and the 3rd incisor 203. The left mandibular 1st incisor is labeled as 301, 2nd incisor 302, and 3rd incisor 303. The right mandibular 1st incisor is 401, 2nd incisor 402, and 3rd incisor 403. (b) Triadan numbering system of the right cheek teeth. Note that there was no first premolar tooth on the right mandible of this skull (405), and the right maxillary third incisor (103) was missing.

(a)

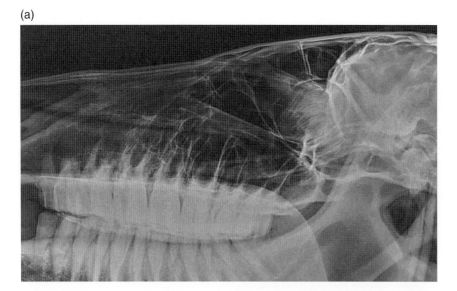

(b)

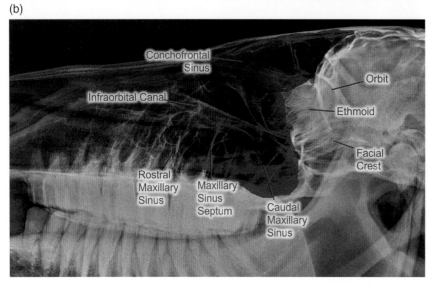

Conchofrontal Sinus

Orbit

Infraorbital Canal

Ethmoid

Facial Crest

Rostral Maxillary Sinus

Maxillary Sinus Septum

Caudal Maxillary Sinus

Figure 9.22 (a) Lateral view of an equine skull. (b) Important anatomical structures labeled on a lateral view of the equine skull. The conchofrontal sinus is identified by the purple shading. The rostral maxillary sinus is identified in yellow. The caudal maxillary sinus is shaded in teal. Also note additional structures of importance labeled in the image. This is the same image as seen in Figure (a). *Source:* Courtesy of Molly Rice, DVM, DAVDC-EQ, Midwest Veterinary Dental Services.

fourth premolar and first maxillary molar teeth will usually reside in the rostral maxillary sinus, and the alveolus of the maxillary second and third molar teeth will reside in the caudal maxillary sinus. Anatomic variations can be noted at different ages and in individual horses [6]. Additionally, it is important to be familiar with the anatomic structures associated with the equine skull as well as the individual teeth when viewing and interpreting the various radiographic projections. See Figures 9.22a, b, 9.23a, b, 9.24a, b, 9.25a, b, 9.26a, b, 9.27a, and b for review of important anatomical structures associated with the equine skull.

Radiographic Changes in Dental Disease

In this section, case examples of radiographic changes noted in dental disease and common instances when radiographs can be used to help diagnose and treat dental problems in the horse will be reviewed.

Common clinical signs that would indicate radiographs are warranted in equine patients include swelling of the face, draining tracts associated with the head, face, or mandible, nasal discharge inconsistent with infectious disease, tooth fractures noted on oral examination, periodontal

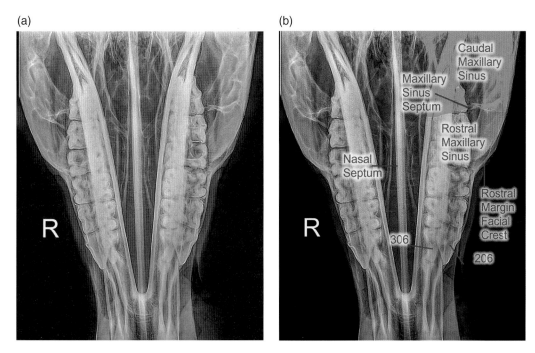

Figure 9.23 (a) Dorsoventral view of an equine skull. (b) Dorsoventral view of an equine skull with labeling of important anatomical structures. This is the same image as seen in Figure (a). Note the caudal maxillary sinus is shaded in blue and the rostral maxillary sinus is labeled in yellow. Other important anatomical structures are also labeled in this image. *Source:* Courtesy of Molly Rice, DVM, DAVDC-EQ, Midwest Veterinary Dental Services.

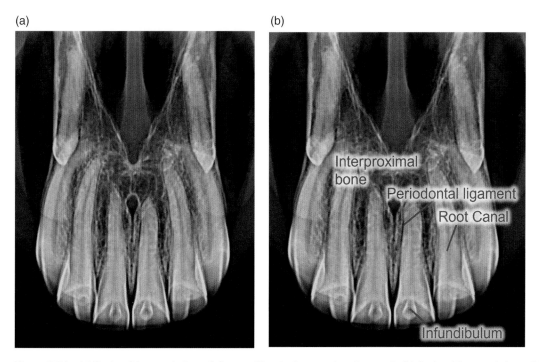

Figure 9.24 (a) Occlusal intraoral view of the maxillary incisors and canine teeth. (b) Occlusal intraoral view of the maxillary incisors and canine teeth with labeling of important anatomical structures. This is the same image as seen in Figure (a). *Source:* Courtesy of Molly Rice, DVM, DAVDC-EQ, Midwest Veterinary Dental Services.

(a)

(b)

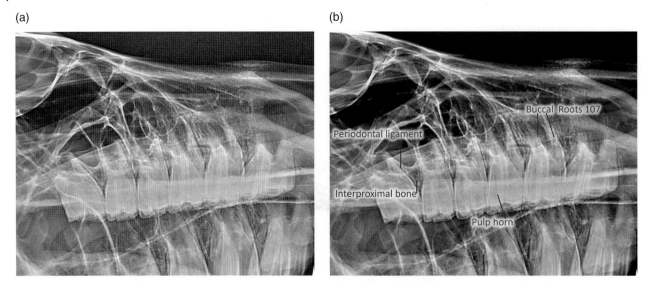

Figure 9.25 (a) Dorso-ventral oblique radiographic view of the right maxillary cheek teeth of a horse. (b) Dorso-ventral oblique radiographic view of the right maxillary cheek teeth with labeling of important anatomic structures. *Source:* Courtesy of Molly Rice, DVM, DAVDC-EQ, Midwest Veterinary Dental Services.

(a)

(b)

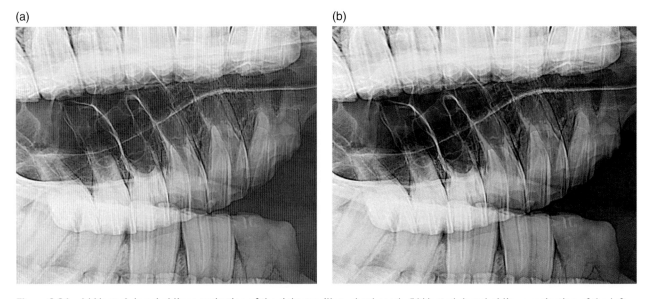

Figure 9.26 (a) Ventral dorsal oblique projection of the right maxillary cheek teeth. (b) Ventral dorsal oblique projection of the left maxillary cheek teeth with shading of the palatal roots of the right maxillary 3rd and 4th premolar teeth (107, 108). Palatal roots should be evaluated when looking for indications of apical infection and when procuring post extraction radiographs. *Source:* Courtesy of Molly Rice, DVM, DAVDC-EQ, Midwest Veterinary Dental Services.

disease, and indications of equine odontoclastic tooth resorption and hypercementosis (EOTRH).

Screening radiographs are not commonly used in routine equine dental appointments. With portable digital radiography becoming a common available modality, some may argue that routine dental radiographs should be a part of a horse's regular dental care [7].

Equine Odontoclastic Tooth Resorption and Hypercementosis (EOTRH)

Equine odontoclastic tooth resorption and hypercementosis (EOTRH) is a progressive and painful disease characterized by tooth root or reserve crown resorption, hypercementosis, or a combination of both. There is a high degree of variability in how EOTRH can present clinically. Additionally,

(a)

(b)

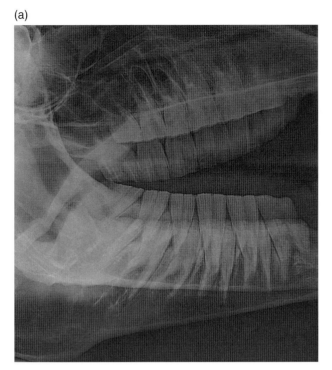
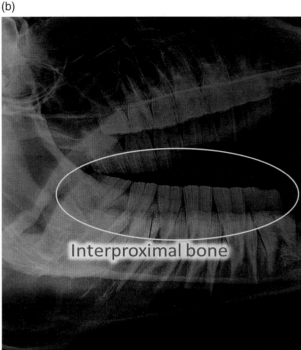

Interproximal bone

Figure 9.27 (a) Dorsal ventral oblique projection of the right mandibular cheek teeth. (b) Dorsal ventral oblique projection of the right mandibular cheek teeth. A yellow oval has been used to highlight the right mandibular cheek teeth that are being evaluated in this view. The interproximal bone between the right mandibular 1st and 2nd molars (409, 410) is marked with a red arrow.

radiographic changes can also be variable. This disease typically occurs in older horses, and the incisor and canine teeth are commonly found to be affected [3]. Clinically, gingival recession or bulbous enlargements of the gingiva over the tooth roots may be noted. Horses may also present with tooth sensitivity causing reluctance to eat or take treats, quidding, resistance to bit placement, or resistance to use of a dental speculum has been noted. In more advanced cases, teeth may be fractured or present with draining tracts in the gingiva over the affected tooth roots. Radiographs are essential for providing a diagnosis and for determining appropriate treatment. The occlusal intraoral view of the mandibular and maxillary incisors and canines should be used in assessing the incisors and canines for evidence of pathology.

Changes seen in EOTRH include tooth resorption, loss of alveolar bone, widening of the periodontal space, blunting of tooth roots, and enlargement of the reserve crown [3] (Table 9.2).

Examples of radiographic changes seen in horses with EOTRH are provided in Figures 9.28a, b, and 9.29a–d.

Apical Infections

Apical infections may occur secondary to periodontal or endodontic disease. In cases of endodontic disease, defects

Table 9.2 The table describes the radiographic changes observed with equine odontoclastic tooth resorption and hypercementosis (EOTRH).

Radiographic changes seen with equine odontoclastic tooth resorption and hypercementosis (EOTRH)
Tooth resorption
Blunting of tooth roots
Hypercementosis
Widening of the periodontal ligament
Osteolysis of alveolar bone
Dental displacement
Fracture of the tooth
Irregular tooth margins

in the enamel such as tooth fractures can allow exposure of the pulp to the oral cavity and external environment. Intraoral bacteria can then infect the pulp horn and infection can spread to the apical portion of the tooth. A common clinical sign of an apical infection is facial swelling. The location of the affected tooth influences the presentation of clinical signs. Maxillary teeth rostral to the maxillary sinuses (second and third premolars) may

(a)

(b)

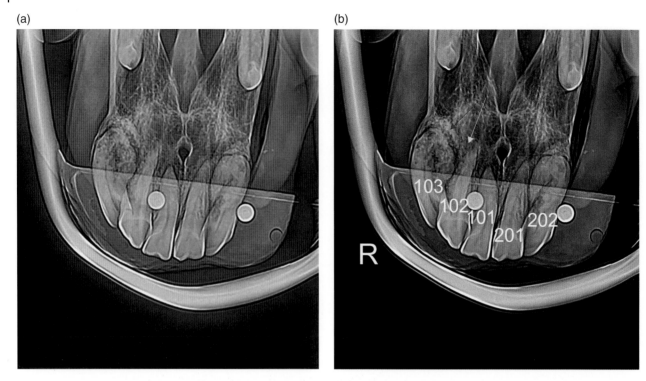

Figure 9.28 (a) Occlusal intraoral projection of the maxillary incisors in a 28-year-old Arabian gelding seen for abnormal incisors. He was reluctant to eat grain and resented placement of a full mouth speculum. Note the more bulbous appearance of the right maxillary 3rd incisor and the left maxillary 2nd incisor teeth. Also note this patient is missing the left maxillary 3rd incisor. (b) Occlusal intraoral projection of the maxillary incisors as viewed in Figure (a). Bulbous enlargement of the apical aspect of the right maxillary third incisor and left maxillary second incisor (103, 202) is noted (yellow shading). The enlargement is likely due to hypercementosis. Resorptive lesions can be noted in the reserve crowns of the right maxillary first and third incisors and left maxillary first and second incisors (101, 103, 201, 202). Widening of the periodontal ligament space is noted on 103 (red arrow). Sclerosis of alveolar bone can be noted proximal to the widening. Irregular margins are noted on the distal and apical aspect of 102 (yellow arrow).

present with facial swelling and possibly cutaneous draining tracts over the rostral portion of the maxilla. Mandibular teeth may present with facial swelling over the mandible and may also have cutaneous draining tracts. Because the alveoli of the maxillary fourth premolar and molars usually resides in the maxillary sinuses, apical disease of these teeth commonly results in the presentation of a patient with a sinusitis [2].

Radiographic evidence of horses with apical infections may show loss of periodontal attachment, a periapical radiolucent halo, clubbing of the tooth root, and loss of tooth opacity [2] (see also Tables 9.3 and 9.4).

When taking radiographs of young horses that are erupting their permanent teeth, the appearance of the apices may vary significantly between the different aged teeth. Changes seen in geriatric dentition can resemble indications of an apical infection. Erupting adult teeth may also cause facial swelling that can be mistaken for an apical infection. Dysplastic and supernumerary teeth may have abnormal apical areas and radiographic changes that may not necessarily be due to a primary apical infection [2].

External draining tracts may not be visible radiographically. If an external tract is present, taking radiographs with a radio dense probe or gutta percha point placed into the tract can help confirm the location of the source of the tract.

Computed tomography (CT) may be more sensitive and specific in cases of early disease where radiographic changes are inconclusive. If CT imaging is not an option, waiting four to six weeks and retaking radiographs may allow time for more definitive changes to be observed [8].

Radiographic examples of apical infection can be found in Figures 9.30a–f, 9.31a, and b.

Periodontal Disease

Periodontal disease is commonly noted on oral examination of equine patients. It involves inflammation and loss of tissues that surround the tooth, which include the gingiva, periodontal ligament, alveolar bone, and cementum. Periodontal disease is frequently noted when there is a diastema between adjacent teeth and food impaction of the interproximal space. A periodontal probe can be used to

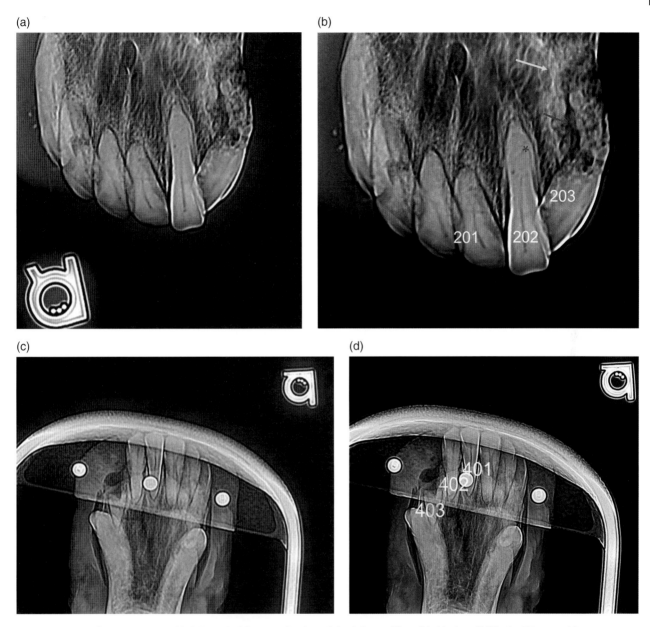

Figure 9.29 (a) Occlusal intraoral left lateral oblique projection of the left maxillary third incisor (203) of a 25-year-old thoroughbred gelding who was seen for incisor extractions because of previously diagnosed equine odontoclastic tooth resorption and hypercementosis (EOTRH). (b) Occlusal intraoral left lateral oblique projection of the left maxillary third incisor (203) as viewed in Figure (a). Marked tooth resorption is noted in the apical portion of 203 (yellow shading). The left maxillary third incisor tooth (203) shows evidence of dental displacement. Widening of the periodontal ligament space is noted (red arrow) and alveolar bone sclerosis is also observed (yellow arrow) on this tooth. The left maxillary second incisor (202) shows some enlargement of the apical portion of the root (red asterisk). (c) Occlusal intraoral projection of the mandibular incisors of the same 25-year-old gelding as noted in Figure (a) and (b) taken during evaluation and extraction of the right mandibular third incisor tooth (403) for evidence of EOTRH. The tooth fragmented during extraction. Radiographs were taken to assess the remaining apical fragment of the tooth. (d) Occlusal intraoral projection of the mandibular incisors as seen in Figure (c). The remaining root tip of the right mandibular third incisor tooth (403) is highlighted with yellow shading.

measure the depth of a periodontal pocket. The normal depth of the gingival sulcus of cheek teeth in equine patients is up to 5 mm. Severe periodontal disease may result in marked loss of the periodontal ligament, loss of alveolar bone, and eventual loss of the tooth [1]. On radiographs, alveolar bone loss, widening of the periodontal ligament, and in severe cases, changes consistent with an apical infection may be observed (Table 9.5). Radiographic examples of periodontal disease can be seen in Figures 9.32a–e, 9.33a, b, and 9.34a–e.

Table 9.3 The table describes the radiographic changes observed with early apical infections in the equine patient.

Radiographic changes seen with early apical infections
Decreased details of lamina dura progressing to thinning or loss of the lamina dura periapical lucency

Table 9.4 The table describes the radiographic changes observed with chronic apical infections in the equine patient.

Radiographic changes seen with chronic apical infections
Bony lysis creating a periapical radiolucent halo
Sclerotic bone surrounding periapical lucency
Draining tract (more common in mandibular teeth)
Soft tissue opacity or fluid in the sinuses (in cases involving the caudal maxillary cheek teeth)
Radiopaque cementum deposits at the apex of the tooth
Loss of dental opacity and root lucency

Sinusitis

Cases of sinusitis commonly present with unilateral nasal discharge. If sinuses on both sides of the head are affected, there may be bilateral nasal discharge. Dental abnormalities are a common cause of secondary sinusitis. Nasal discharge is often purulent and malodorous if the sinusitis is related to dental disease. Clinical findings on oral examination such as exposed pulp horns, crown fractures, periodontal disease, or oromaxillary fistulas are frequently observed. Radiographs may help determine which tooth is causing the sinusitis. Radiographs examining the maxillary cheek teeth for evidence of apical infection should be acquired. On lateral and dorsoventral views, a fluid line, soft tissue density, or fluid density may be noted. Oblique views may also show soft tissue or fluid density in the sinuses (Table 9.6). It is important to note that overexposure of the radiograph may prevent the image from being diagnostic. Additionally, it may be difficult to determine if there is a dental cause of the sinusitis with radiographic imaging alone. In these cases, computed tomographic screening may assist in giving additional information.

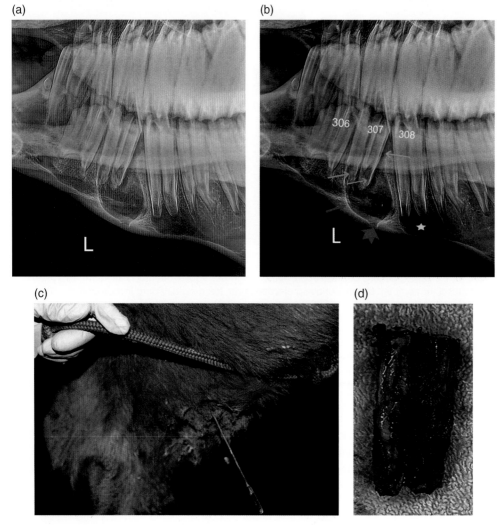

(a)   (b)   (c)   (d)

Figure 9.30 (Continued)

(e)

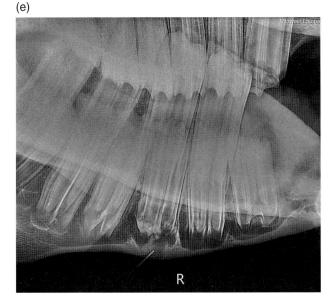

(f)

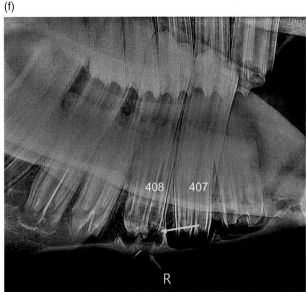

Figure 9.30 (a) Ventral dorsal oblique projection of the left mandibular cheek teeth of a seven-year-old Quarter Horse gelding. The gelding presented with a swollen left mandible and a ventral mandibular draining tract. On oral exam, there was a large amount of feed impaction around his left mandibular third premolar tooth (307), and the tooth had mild mobility. (b) Ventral dorsal oblique projection of the left mandibular cheek teeth of the seven-year-old Quarter horse as described in Figure (a). Changes consistent with a periapical tooth root infection are observed. A ventral draining tract in the mandible is seen (notched red arrowhead). A large radiolucent halo is present around the apex of the left mandibular third premolar tooth (307) (red star), and a smaller halo is associated with the right mandibular fourth premolar tooth (308) (yellow star), which is likely a normal anatomical finding. Sclerosis of the bone surrounding the halo is present (red arrow). Marked widening of the periodontal ligament space is seen on the caudal aspect of 307 (yellow arrow). A granular pattern can be seen in the halo around the apical portion of 307. This granular pattern is likely caused by the food and purulent material that was impacted in the area. Change in the shape of the roots of 307 (blunting) can be noted along with radiolucency (green arrows). (c) Clinical appearance of the Quarter Horse gelding described in Figure (a) and (b) with a ventral draining tract indicated by a probe. (d) The extracted left mandibular third premolar tooth (307) from the Quarter Horse described in Figure (a)–(c). Changes in the roots and crown of the tooth including discoloration of the crown and decayed food material on the clinical and reserve crown can be noted. (e) Ventral dorsal oblique projection of the right mandibular quadrant of a five-year-old horse with a mandibular draining tract. This is not the same horse as was described in Figure (a)–(d). This radiograph illustrates how a sterile probe can be inserted into a draining tract and used to help locate the source of the tract. *Source:* Courtesy of Molly Rice, DVM, DAVDC-EQ, Midwest Veterinary Dental Services. (f) Ventral dorsal oblique projection of the right mandibular quadrant of the same horse as seen in Figure (e). Changes in the shape of the mesial root of the right mandibular fourth premolar tooth (408) can be noted (yellow arrow), and the draining tract and probe are shown by the red arrow. *Source:* Courtesy of Molly Rice, DVM, DAVDC-EQ, Midwest Veterinary Dental Services.

Radiographic examples of sinusitis can be seen in Figures 9.35a, b, 9.36a, b, 9.37a–g, 9.38a–d, and 9.39.

Neoplasia

Neoplasia can arise in the equine mouth from soft tissues, bone, or dental tissues. Examples of oral neoplasia include but are not limited to: ameloblastoma, ameloblastic odontoma, cementoma, osteosarcoma, squamous cell carcinoma, fibroma, and fibrosarcoma. Clinical signs may be similar to periapical infections with facial swelling. Oral examination may reveal abnormal tissue and mobile or displaced teeth. Other clinical signs include weight loss, difficulty eating, halitosis, and oral bleeding. If clinical signs and radiographic changes are suggestive of neoplasia, biopsy of the affected area is recommended to confirm and characterize the disease process. Changes in the alveolar bone from secondary infection and inflammation may cause lucency and or sclerosis that can mask changes characteristic of a neoplastic process [2]. Advanced imaging such as computed tomography may be necessary to fully assess the extent of the lesion and structures involved.

(a) (b)

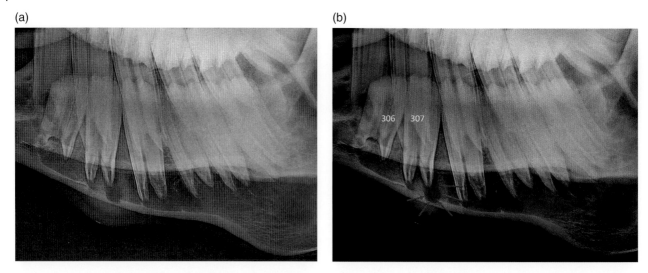

Figure 9.31 (a) Ventral dorsal oblique projection of the left mandibular quadrant of an eight-year-old gelding with swelling of the ventral mandible. (b) Ventral dorsal oblique projection of the left mandibular quadrant of a horse as seen in Figure (a). Periapical lucency of the distal root of the left mandibular third premolar tooth (307) is marked with red arrows. No draining tract was present at this point associated with the abscess. *Source:* Courtesy of Molly Rice, DVM, DAVDC-EQ, Midwest Veterinary Dental Services.

Table 9.5 The table describes the radiographic changes observed with periodontal disease in the equine patient.

Radiographic changes seen with periodontal disease
Widening of the periodontal ligament space
Loss of alveolar crestal bone
Severe disease (endodontic and periodontal disease); signs of periapical disease can be noted

Radiographic changes suggestive of neoplasia are included in Table 9.7.

Other Suggested Abnormalities to be Radiographed

Other abnormalities that practitioners may find on oral or physical examination, which may benefit from diagnostic imaging are listed below.

(a) (b)

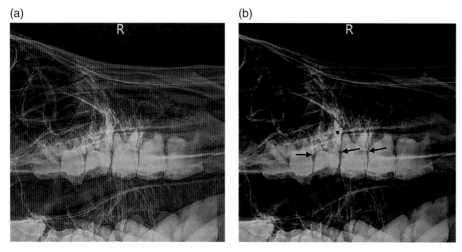

Figure 9.32 (a) Dorsal ventral oblique projection of the right maxillary quadrant of a 22-year-old Arabian gelding that presented with quidding behavior. Oral exam showed teeth with advanced attrition, and a diastemata of the right maxillary fourth premolar and first molar teeth (108, 109) and right maxillary first and second molar teeth (109, 110). (b) Annotated dorsal ventral oblique image from the horse in Figure (a). Black arrows show the level of bone recession present. Black star indicates periapical sclerosis. Red arrows demonstrate periapical lucency on the distal buccal root of the right maxillary fourth premolar tooth (108).

(c)

(d)

(e)

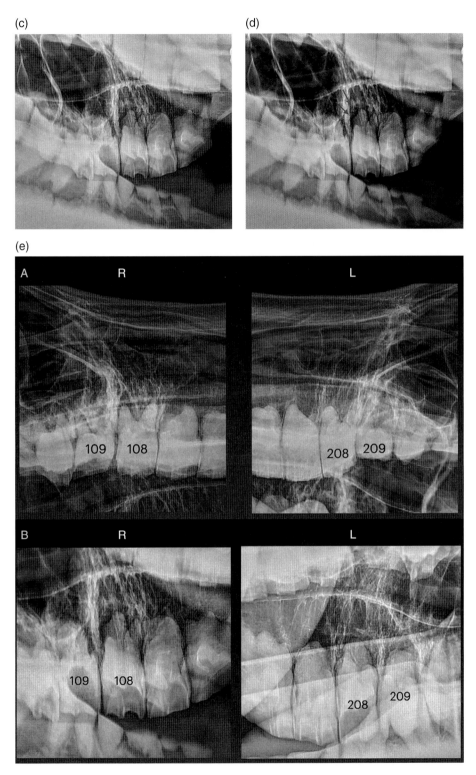

Figure 9.32   (Continued) (c) Ventral dorsal oblique projection of the right maxillary quadrant of a 22-year-old Arabian gelding that presented with quidding behavior. Oral exam showed teeth with advanced attrition, and a diastemata of the right maxillary fourth premolar and first molar teeth (108, 109) and right maxillary first and second molar teeth (109, 110). (d) Annotated ventral dorsal oblique image from the horse in Figure (a)–(c). Red arrows demonstrate periapical lucency on the palatal root of the right maxillary fourth premolar tooth (108). (e) Dorsal ventral oblique projection of the right and left maxillary quadrants (A) and ventral dorsal oblique projection of the right and left maxillary quadrant (B) of the 22-year-old Arabian gelding viewed in Figure (a)–(d). It is important to image both sides for comparison, as this helps highlight areas of concern. This horse's premolars show generalized apical blunting, which is a common aging change in older horses. It should be noted that the periodontal ligament width on the left side is much more normal when compared to the right side. *Source:* Courtesy of Molly Rice, DVM, DAVDC-EQ, Midwest Veterinary Dental Services.

- Diastemata, radiographed on open-mouth oblique views (Figure 9.38a–d)
- Fractured teeth (Figures 9.40a–d, 9.41a–g, and 9.42a–f)
- Oligodontia or polydontia (Figure 9.43a–c)
- Retained deciduous teeth (Figure 9.44a–c and 9.45a–d)
- Temporohyoid osteopathy (Figure 9.46)

Conclusion

Dental radiographs can be beneficial in providing the practitioner with additional information about abnormalities that are found on oral examination in the equine patient. With attention to detail in positioning, technique, and restraint of the horse, it is possible to obtain good-quality images in the field. The practitioner can also become proficient in interpreting findings on radiographic images and combine this information with their understanding of the pathology that can be found on a thorough oral examination. When diagnostic radiographs are obtained, the practitioner also has the ability to seek the input of an American Veterinary Dental College (AVDC) Diplomate on more difficult cases.

(a)

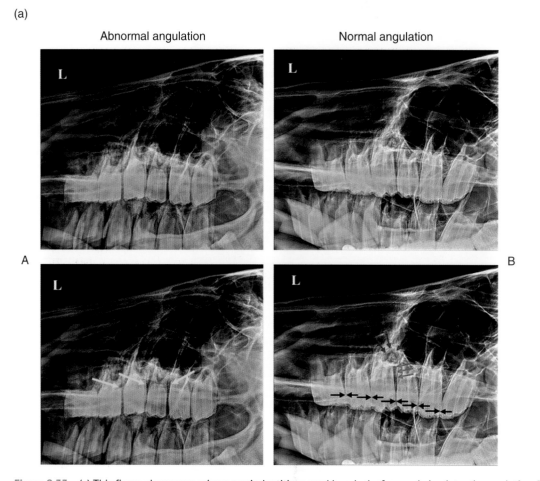

Abnormal angulation   Normal angulation

A   B

Figure 9.33 (a) This figure showcases primary periodontitis caused by a lack of normal cheek tooth angulation (images labeled A) compared to a horse with a more normal angulation on the right (images labeled B). When abnormal angulation occurs, the cheek teeth do not pack tightly together, resulting in diastema formation and periodontitis. The yellow arrows highlight interproximal bone recession. The horse on the right (B) has a periapical lucency (red arrows) around the distal buccal root and periodontal ligament space widening (green arrows). The black arrows show the normal tight interdental spaces with normal anatomical angulation of the cheek teeth. This is lacking in the horse on the left (A) with primary periodontitis, resulting in multiple diastemata. (b) This figure highlights the radiographic findings on the horse with primary periodontitis (from Figure (a) with abnormal angulation. The black arrows show the recession of the interproximal bone. The red asterisk shows periapical sclerosis. The yellow arrows demonstrate a periapical lucency visible on the palatal root (ventro-dorsal oblique view). *Source:* Courtesy of Molly Rice, DVM, DAVDC-EQ, Midwest Veterinary Dental Services.

(b)

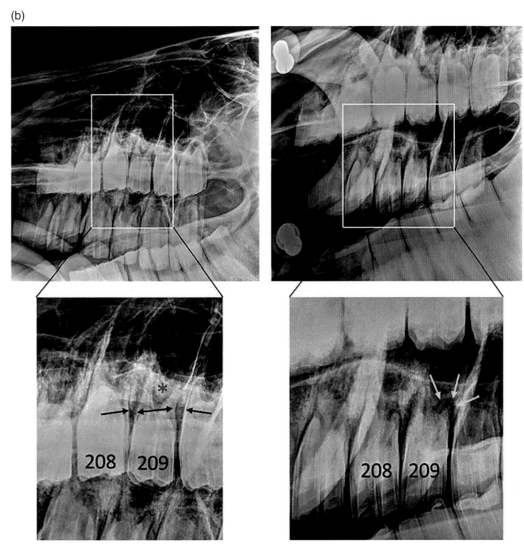

Figure 9.33 (Continued)

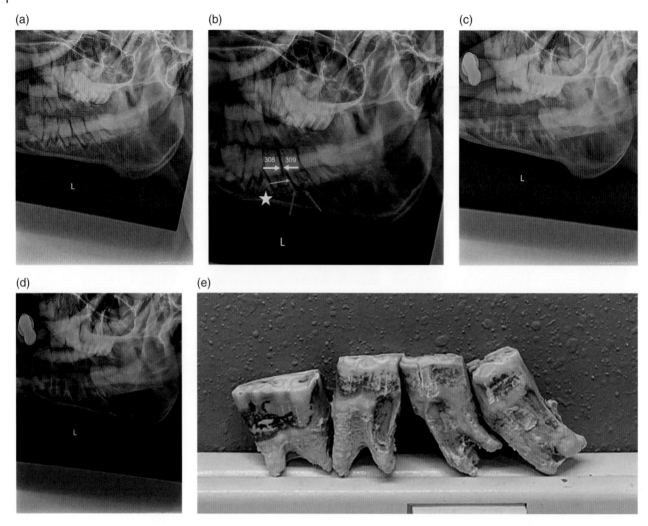

Figure 9.34 (a) Ventral dorsal projection of the left mandibular quadrant of a geriatric miniature horse with severe periodontal disease and geriatric dentition. (b) Ventral dorsal projection of the same horse as viewed in Figure (a). Marked changes often found with periodontal disease are noted in the left mandibular second, third, and fourth premolars and first molar teeth (306–309). Red arrows indicate periapical lucency associated with 309, and the yellow star shows periapical sclerosis associated with the mesial root of 308. Yellow arrows show interproximal bone recession between 308 and 309, and a green arrow shows periodontal ligament space widening associated with the mesial aspect of 309. Diastema formation most notably between 308/309 and 309/310 is also seen. (c) Ventral dorsal projection of the left mandibular quadrant of the miniature horse viewed in Figure (a) and (b) after extraction of the left mandibular second, third, and fourth premolars and first molar teeth (306–309). (d) Ventral dorsal projection of the left mandibular quadrant of the same horse as viewed in Figure (a)–(c) with yellow shading to indicate the extraction sites. (e) Clinical photograph of the extracted left mandibular second, third, and fourth premolars and first molar teeth (306–309) from the miniature horse in Figure (a)–(d). Note the presence of generalized root clubbing associated with these teeth. *Source:* Courtesy of Molly Rice, DVM, DAVDC-EQ, Midwest Veterinary Dental Services.

Table 9.6 The table describes the radiographic changes observed with sinus disease in the equine patient.

Radiographic changes seen with sinus disease
Soft tissue fluid opacity within the sinus
Fluid line within the sinus
Increased opacity is usually uniform but may have a mixed pattern of gas and soft tissue
Signs of apical infection of maxillary fourth premolars through last molars may be seen when sinusitis is secondary to apical infections

(a)　　　　　　　　　　　　　　　　　　(b)

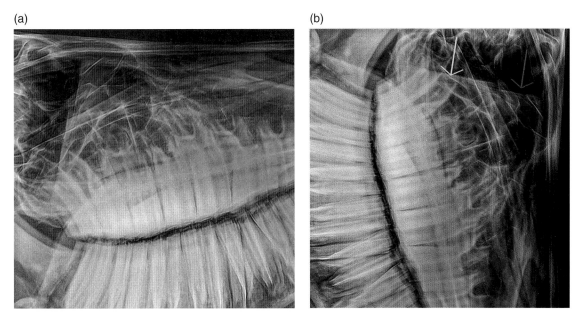

Figure 9.35　(a) Lateral radiographic projection of a seven-year-old Quarter Horse gelding that presented with right-sided unilateral nasal discharge. (b) Lateral projection of the seven-year-old Quarter Horse gelding viewed in Figure (a). Gravity-dependent fluid lines present in the concho frontal (red arrow) and maxillary sinuses (yellow arrow) are suggestive of sinusitis. The image has been rotated vertically to facilitate visualization of the fluid lines.

(a)　　　　　　　　　　　　　　　　　　(b)

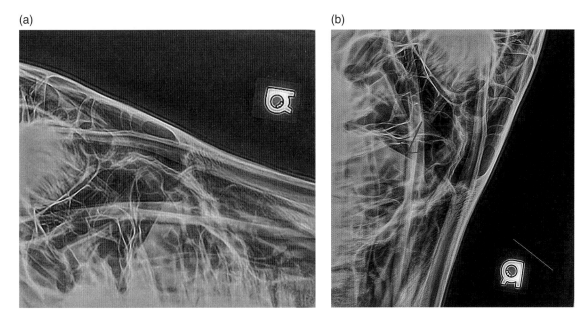

Figure 9.36　(a) Lateral radiographic projection of a 16-year-old Thoroughbred mare that presented with unilateral right-sided nasal discharge. (b) Lateral radiographic projection of the 16-year-old Thoroughbred mare as viewed in Figure (a) A fluid line is present in the maxillary sinus indicative of a sinusitis (red arrow). This view was taken as described in Figure 9.7a with the horse's head in a vertical position resting on a stationary object. Fluid lines can more easily be appreciated if the head is positioned vertically versus horizontally. This image has been rotated from the appropriate labial mounting position to illustrate that viewing the radiograph in a vertical position can be helpful when looking for a fluid line. Gravity markers as used in this image can also help to appreciate fluid lines by establishing the approximate angle of the fluid line (yellow line).

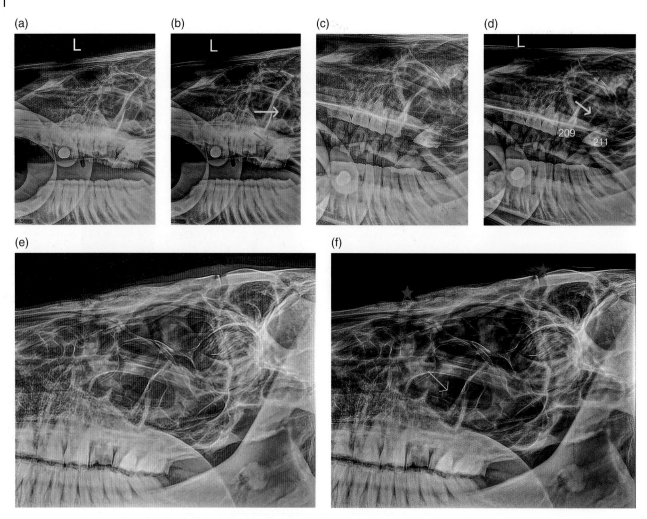

Figure 9.37 (a) Lateral projection of a 22-year-old Saddlebred gelding with a history of a chronic sinusitis and an oromaxillary fistula secondary to a fractured and infected left maxillary second molar tooth (210) which has previously been extracted. (b) Lateral projection of the 22-year-old Saddlebred gelding as viewed in Figure (a). A granular mixed pattern of gas and soft tissue can be appreciated in the concho frontal sinus (red arrow) and maxillary sinus (yellow arrow). A fluid line is not seen, but a sinusitis of inspissated purulent material and food is suspected. The diastema where the left maxillary second molar was previously extracted can be seen (green arrow). (c) Dorsal ventral oblique projection of the left maxillary cheek teeth of the 22-year-old Saddlebred gelding viewed in Figure (a) and (b). (d) Dorsal ventral oblique projection of the same horse as viewed in Figure (a)–(c). The pattern of gas and soft tissue in the sinuses can also be appreciated in this view (red arrow conchofrontal sinus and yellow arrow maxillary sinus). The diastema present between 209 and 211 is the result of the extraction of the left maxillary second molar tooth (210). (e) A lateral radiographic projection of the 22-year-old Saddlebred gelding viewed in Figure (a)–(d), after sinus flap surgery, debridement, and lavage. Note the improvement of the radiographic signs of disease in this image. (f) Lateral radiographic projection of the same horse as seen in Figure (e) with annotations. The conchofrontal sinus (red arrow) and maxillary sinus (yellow arrow) appear more radiolucent in this view. The site of the osteotomy of the sinus bone flap can be seen on the dorsal skull (red stars). The rostral site of the osteotomy is irregular (thicker red star). This area was slow to heal and had a boney sequestrum that was removed. (g) Lateral radiographic projections from Figure (e) with comparisons of the maxillary and conchofrontal sinuses before and after treatment. In the pretreatment radiograph, the granular mixed pattern of gas and soft tissue can be appreciated in the sinuses. In the post treatment radiograph, the sinuses appear more radiolucent.

(g)

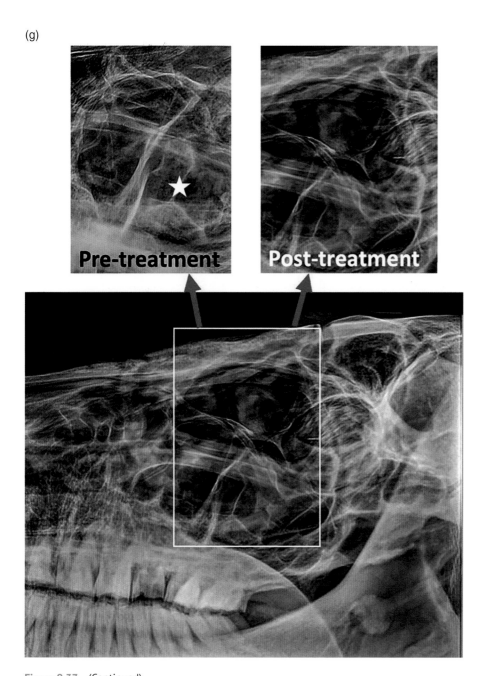

Figure 9.37 (Continued)

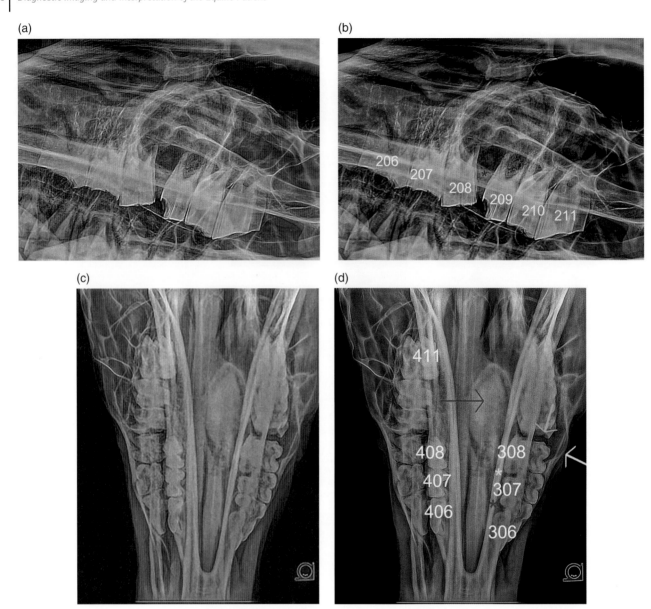

Figure 9.38 (a) Dorsal ventral oblique maxillary projection of an 18-year-old thoroughbred mare that had swelling on the rostral aspect of her left facial crest. On examination, marked food impaction and a large diastema were noted between the left maxillary fourth premolar and first molar teeth (208, 209). (b) Dorsal ventral oblique maxillary projection of the 18-year-old thoroughbred mare viewed in Figure (a). A possible orosinus fistula communicating with the rostral maxillary sinus is noted in the diastema between 208 and 209 (red asterisk). A mixed pattern of gas and soft tissue is noted in the rostral maxillary sinus (yellow shading). Sclerotic changes are present which may indicate that the food and purulent material in the sinus has been walled off. Loss of the mesial clinical crown of 209 is noted. An irregular occlusal surface of the quadrant is also appreciated. (c) Dorsoventral radiograph that has been slightly obliqued from the left side of the same 18-year-old mare viewed in Figure (a) and (b). Note the opacity in the ventral conchal sinus and the diastema between the left maxillary fourth premolar and first molar teeth. There is also thinning of the facial crest.
(d) Dorsoventral radiograph that has been slightly obliqued from the left side of the same 18-year-old mare viewed in Figure (a)–(c). This radiograph demonstrates an opacity in the ventral conchal sinus that is likely caused by feed and inspissated pus (red arrow). The diastema between 208 and 209 can also be appreciated in this view (orange arrow). Additionally, there is thinning and deformation of the frontal crest on the left side (yellow arrow) of this patient.

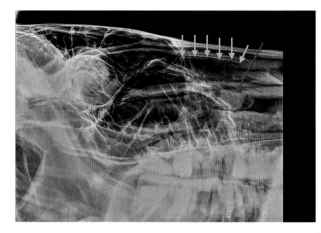

Figure 9.39 Lateral radiograph of a horse that demonstrates ventral nasal conchal bulla empyema (red arrow). The normal dorsal nasal conchal bulla is outlined by yellow arrows.
Source: Courtesy of Molly Rice, DVM, DAVDC-EQ, Midwest Veterinary Dental Services.

Table 9.7 The table describes the radiographic changes observed with different tumor types in the equine patient.

Tumor type	Radiographic changes
Ameloblastoma	Swelling of the jaw, osteolysis, circular lesion with multilocular and cystic radiolycency
Odontoma	Radiolucent area containing foci of mineral opacity
Compound odontoma	Well-defined cyst-like structure containing multiple small lobulated masses commonly seen at the apex of a maxillary tooth
Cementoma	Radiodense area typically located at the apex of the tooth
Osteosarcoma	Bony lysis mixed with irregular trabecular new bone "sunburst" pattern

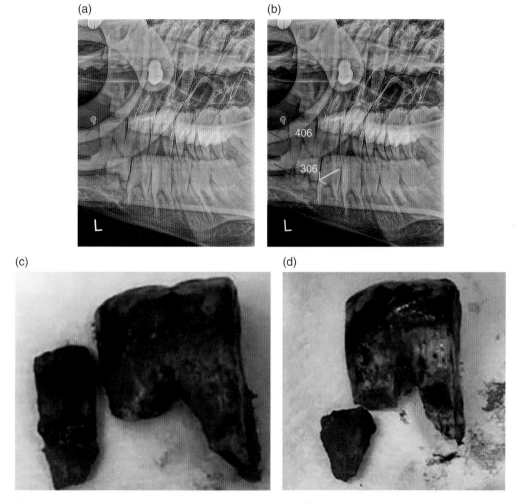

Figure 9.40 (a) Ventral dorsal oblique projection of the mandible of a 19-year-old Quarter Horse mare that presented for dropping grain when eating. On oral exam, the left and right mandibular second premolar teeth (306, 406) were noted to have increased mobility, and there was feed impaction around both teeth. On the radiograph, a horizontal fracture can be seen in the mesial roots of both the left and right mandibular second premolar teeth (306, 406) (red arrows). Widening of the periodontal ligament space can be noted on the mesial aspect of the distal roots of 306 and 406 (yellow shading). An area of lucency is noted on the distal root of 306 (yellow arrow). The root lucency appeared like a fracture on the radiograph, but when the tooth was extracted, there was gross evidence of tooth resorption noted, but no obvious evidence of a fractured root. (c) Clinical photograph of the fractured right mandibular second premolar tooth (406) as seen in Figure (a) and (b) following surgical extraction. (d) Clinical photograph of the fractured left mandibular second premolar tooth (306) as seen in Figure (a) and (b). Resorption of the distal root of 306 can be seen in this photograph.

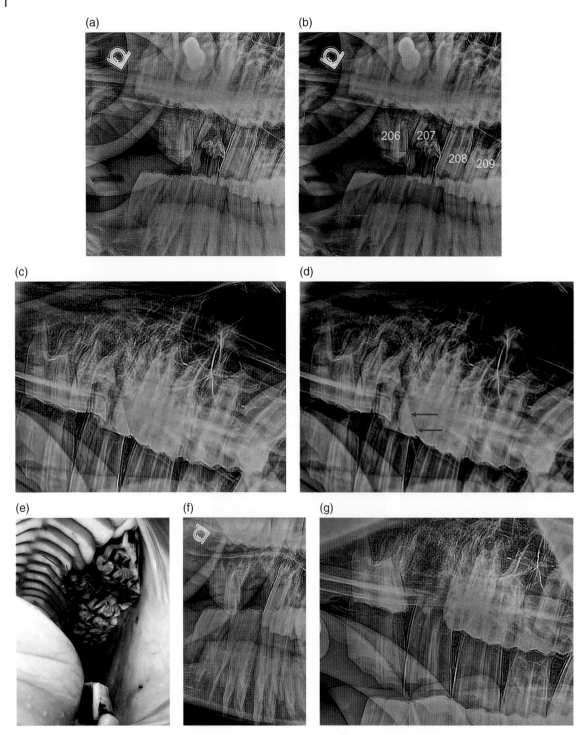

Figure 9.41 (a) Ventral dorsal oblique projection of the maxillary cheek of a 19-year-old Quarter Horse gelding that presented for a routine dental float or occlusal equilibration. On oral examination, his left maxillary third premolar tooth (207) had a sagittal fracture with the palatal fragment of the tooth displaced toward the hard palate. (b) Ventral dorsal oblique maxillary projection of the 19-year-old Quarter Horse shown in Figure (a). The radiograph illustrates the sagittal fracture of the left maxillary third premolar tooth (207) (red arrow). The palatal fracture piece and the remaining 207 can be seen. Note that the marker in this view would ideally have been placed ventral to the horse's head as the pathology was noted to be present in the maxillary arcade. (c) Unlabeled dorsal ventral oblique projection of the left maxillary quadrant of the horse described in Figure (a) and (b). (d) Dorsal ventral oblique projection of the horse described in Figure (a)–(c). The outline of the palatal fracture fragment of 207 is identified with red arrows. (e) Intraoral clinical photograph of the fractured left maxillary third premolar tooth 207 (red arrow) seen on radiographs in Figure (a)–(d) with feed impaction between the two sections of fractured tooth. (f) Ventral dorsal oblique maxillary projection of the horse described in Figure (a)–(e). After the fractured left maxillary third premolar tooth (207) was identified and extracted, post-extraction radiographs were procured to ensure that the tooth and roots were completely extracted. Based on this image, the tooth appears to have been successfully extracted. (g) Dorsal ventral oblique maxillary projection of the post-extraction site of the left maxillary third premolar tooth (207). No obvious evidence of a retained tooth or roots are appreciated. Note the cone cutting artifact in this image.

(a)

(b)

(c)

(d)

(e)

(f)

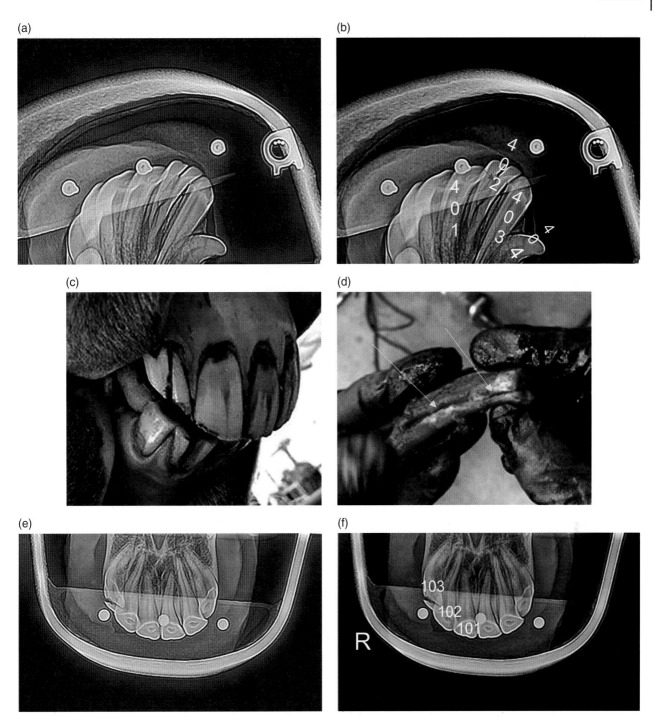

Figure 9.42 (a) Occlusal intraoral right oblique view of the mandibular incisors of a nine-year-old Belgian gelding who presented for a routine dental float or occlusal equilibration. On oral examination, it was noted that his right mandibular second incisor tooth (402) was fractured with feed impaction within the fractured tooth fragments. His maxillary third incisor tooth (103) was also fractured (not observed in this radiograph). (b) Intraoral right oblique view of the mandibular incisors highlighting the right mandibular second incisor tooth (402). The clinical appearance of the tooth showed a complicated crown–root fracture (involving pulp) of the right mandibular second incisor tooth (402) (small red arrows). This tooth was extracted. It should also be noted that while this view was diagnostic for assessing the right mandibular second incisor tooth (402), the apices of the other incisors and canines were not included. An additional radiograph would need to be taken to assess the other mandibular incisors and canine teeth for evidence of disease. (c) Clinical photograph of the right maxillary and mandibular incisors of the nine-year-old Belgian gelding radiographed in Figure (a) and (b). The horse's right mandibular second incisor (402) and right maxillary third incisor (103) appear to be fractured. (d) Clinical photograph of the right mandibular second incisor tooth (402) of the nine-year-old Belgian gelding described in Figure (a)–(c) post-surgical extraction of the tooth. This photograph demonstrates a fracture extending through the tooth which involved the pulp horn (yellow arrows). (e) Occlusal intraoral radiographic projection of the maxillary incisors of the horse described in Figure (a)–(d). (f) Occlusal intraoral radiographic projection of the maxillary incisors as seen in Figure (a)–(e). A fracture of the right maxillary third incisor tooth (103) can be seen on this view (red arrow).

(a)   (b)   (c)

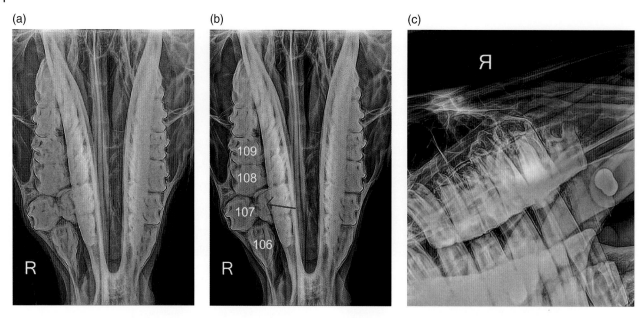

Figure 9.43 (a) Dorsoventral projection with the mandible distracted to the left side of a five-year-old Rocky Mountain Horse that presented for right-sided facial swelling. The swelling had been present since the horse was 2.5 years of age. On oral exam, she had a supernumerary tooth on the palatal aspect of the right maxillary third premolar tooth (107). This supernumerary right maxillary third premolar tooth was displacing the other right maxillary third premolar tooth (107) buccally. There was also food impaction between the supernumerary tooth and her right maxillary second and third premolar teeth (106, 107). A large buccal ulcer from her displaced 107 was seen clinically on her oral examination. (b) Dorsoventral radiographic projection of the same horse as viewed in Figure (a) with annotations. The supernumerary tooth is identified with the red arrow. It is difficult to definitively determine which tooth is the existing right maxillary third premolar tooth (107) and which is the supernumerary third premolar tooth (107). (c) Dorsal ventral oblique projection of the mare described in Figure (a) and (b). The two teeth are superimposed in the 107 position, which can be visualized in this image.

(a)   (b)   (c)

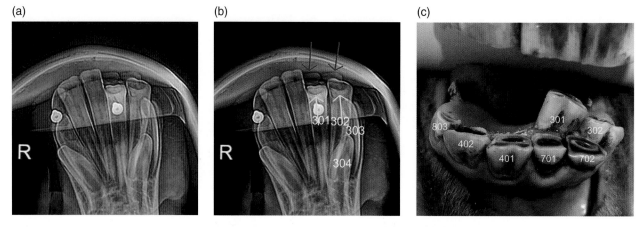

Figure 9.44 (a) Occlusal intraoral radiographic projection of the mandibular incisors of a five-year-old Quarter Horse gelding that presented for abnormal incisors. On oral exam, his left mandibular first and second deciduous incisors (701, 702) were retained. The permanent first and second incisors (301, 302) had erupted lingual to the deciduous teeth and were not in-wear with the contralateral maxillary incisors causing the mandibular incisors to become overgrown and contact the hard palate when chewing. (b) Occlusal intraoral radiographic projection of the mandibular incisors as viewed in Figure (a). In this image, the right mandibular first and second incisors (401, 402) have erupted, but the right mandibular third incisor (403) has not yet erupted into occlusion. The permanent left mandibular first and second incisors (301, 302) can be visualized (red arrows). The deciduous left mandibular first and second incisors (701, 702) (yellow arrows) are seen labial to the permanent first and second incisors. (c) Clinical photograph of the retained left mandibular deciduous teeth as described in Figure (a) and (b). The deciduous left mandibular first and second incisors (701, 702) are labial to the permanent left mandibular first and second incisors (301, 302).

(a)

(b)

(c)

(d)

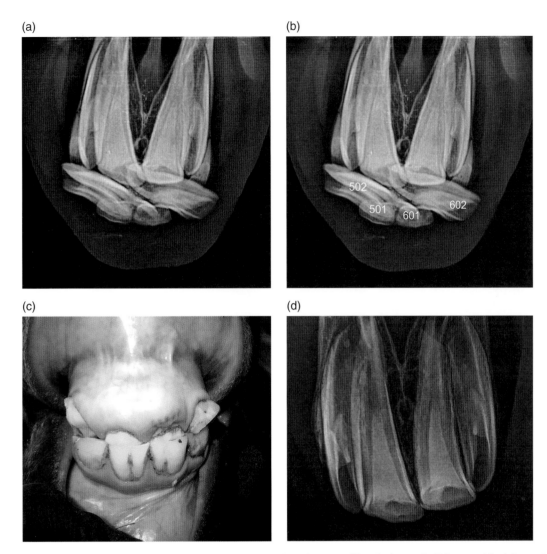

Figure 9.45   (a) Occlusal intraoral radiographic projection of the maxillary incisors of a 2.5-year-old miniature horse. (b) Annotated occlusal intraoral radiographic projection of the maxillary incisors as seen in Figure (a). The deciduous right and left maxillary first incisor teeth (501, 601) are labial to the right and left permanent maxillary first incisors (101, 201). The deciduous right and left maxillary second incisor teeth (502, 602) are abnormally oriented in a horizontal direction, with their clinical crowns directed laterally. (c) Clinical photograph of the 2.5-year-old miniature horse described in Figure (a) and (b). (d) Occlusal intraoral radiographic projection of the maxillary incisors six months following extraction of retained deciduous incisors from the horse described in Figure (a)–(c). The permanent incisors have erupted normally. *Source:* Courtesy of Molly Rice, DVM, DAVDC-EQ, Midwest Veterinary Dental Services.

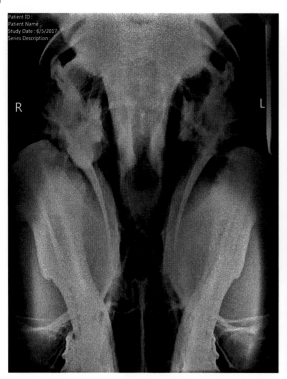
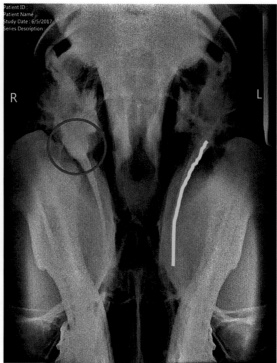

Figure 9.46 Dorsoventral radiograph of the skull, centered at the poll, highlighting the temporohyoid joint. In this patient, the right proximal stylohyoid (red circle) shows a circular enlargement consistent with temporohyoid osteopathy. The mare had developed acute right-sided facial nerve paralysis symptoms after a routine occlusal adjustment. The yellow line outlines the body of the stylohyoid bone on the left. *Source:* Courtesy of Molly Rice, DVM, DAVDC-EQ, Midwest Veterinary Dental Services.

Acknowledgment

The authors would like to give a special acknowledgement to Wolfgang Weber for assistance in providing skull specimens and ideas for their presentation in the Diagnostic Imaging and Interpretation of the Equine Patient chapter.

References

1 Butler, J.A., Colles, C.M., Christopher, M. et al. (2017). General principals. In: *Clinical Radiology of the Horse*, 4e (ed. J.A. Butler), 1–40. Hoboken: Wiley.

2 Barakzai, S.Z. (2010). Chapter 13 – dental imaging. In: *Equine Dentistry*, 3e (ed. J. Easley et al.), 199–230. Edinburgh: Saunders/Elsevier.

3 Baratt, R. (2013). Advances in equine dental radiology. *Vet. Clin. Equine* 29 (2): 367–395.

4 Barrett, M.F. and Easley, J.T. (2013). Acquisition and interpretation of radiographs of the equine skull. *Equine Vet. Educ.* 25 (12): 643–652.

5 Radiographs examples from the American Veterinary Dental College. https://avdc.org/download/28/ resident-resources/4171/eq-credential-commitee-example-rad-set.pdf.

6 Liuti, T., Reardon, R., and Dixon, P. (2017). Computed tomographic assessment of equine maxillary cheek teeth anatomical relationships, and paranasal sinus volumes. *Vet. Rec.* 181 (17): 1–7.

7 Bishop, I. (2022). Diagnostic value of full-mouth radiography in horses. *Front. Vet. Sci.* 9: 971886.

8 Easley, J.T. (2018). Every practitioner can take good dental radiographs. In: *VVMA Proceedings*. https://iastate.app. box.com/file/752393104695?box_action=go_to_item&box_ source=legacy-file_collab_auto_accept_new.

10

Advanced Imaging of the Oral Cavity

Stephanie Goldschmidt

Department of Surgical and Radiologic Sciences, University of California-Davis School of Veterinary Medicine, Davis, CA, USA

> **CONTENTS**
>

Introduction to the Use of Advanced Imaging Techniques in the Maxillofacial Region

Advanced imaging of the maxillofacial region is clinically indicated when diagnostic imaging extending past the dentate portion of the jaws is required and/or the ability to remove superimposition and localize structures in 3D is necessary. The most common advanced imaging modalities utilized are magnetic resonance imaging (MRI) and computed tomography (CT).

The biggest determinant in choosing between MRI and CT is identifying the tissue type that needs to be best visualized. MRI has superior soft tissue detail, while CT has superior bony detail. Intraoral and extraoral examinations will help determine which of these imaging modalities would be most useful in diagnosis and treatment planning. For the vast majority of cases, a CT scan will give sufficient soft tissue detail to accurately make a diagnosis. Thus, due to the cost constraints of MRI and the poor bony detail associated with this imaging modality, there are limited situations where MRI would truly be the only imaging

choice for the maxillofacial region. The technical principles of MRI and CT as well as the indications for each modality will be discussed throughout this chapter.

Magnetic Resonance Imaging (MRI)

Technical Principles of MRI

MRI, as the name implies, is based on the use of magnetic energy to produce an image. Briefly, MRI works by taking advantage of an element that is normally found throughout the body. This element is hydrogen. At rest, the hydrogen atoms in the body are randomly orientated and dispersed throughout the tissues. During an MRI, a strong magnetic field is applied to the patient, which results in the hydrogen atoms aligning with the direction of the magnetic field. A radiofrequency pulse is then applied which disturbs this orientation. When the pulse is discontinued and the hydrogen atoms return to their magnetized orientation (relax), they let off energy which is utilized to create an image [1–3].

Veterinary Oral Diagnostic Imaging, First Edition. Edited by Brenda L. Mulherin.

T1- and T2-Weighted Sequences

There are two basic sequences that are run during an MRI scan, namely T1- and T2-weighted sequences. The "weighting" exploits specific properties of hydrogen atoms' T1 and T2 relaxation (return to normal state) in different tissue types, highlighting natural contrast changes between tissues as well as changes due to pathology. T1 relaxation is the time required by protons to recover along a longitudinal plane, in other words, to realign with the external magnetic field. T2 relaxation is recovery time in a transverse or horizontal plane, which corresponds to the time it takes for spinning protons to go out of phase with each other. By manipulating the time between repetitions of the radiofrequency pulses (TR) as well as the time until remaining magnetization is measured (TE), natural differences in T1 and T2 relaxation times between different tissues are highlighted [1–3].

In a T1-weighted image, little time is given between pulse frequencies and measurement of net magnetization (short TR and TE), which results in increased T1 contrast between tissues. Specifically, substances that have a longer T1 relaxation time (such as water) will not have time to return to a normal state and release energy therefore they will be hypointense (dark) on the image, while tissues with a short relaxation time (such as fat) will be hyperintense (white). In a T2-weighted image, increased time is given between pulse frequencies and measurement of net magnetization (long TR and TE), which then highlights T2 contrast between tissues. In a T2-weighted image, water is hyperintense (white) and fat is also hyperintense (white, but not quite as hyperintense as on a T1 image) (Figure 10.1, Table 10.1).

In both T1- and T2-weighted images, bone is hypointense (black). Neither sequence highlights changes in calcification very well due to a low concentration of hydrogen protons that contribute to magnetization in calcified tissue. In general, mineralized tissues have extremely fast relaxation times often not detectable with conventional techniques. Poor imaging of calcified tissues makes MRI a poor choice for evaluation of the maxillofacial region if bony or dental pathology is suspected [1–3] (Figure 10.2).

Table 10.1 Summary of the key differences in tissue appearance on a T1- and T2-weighted MRI image.

	T1-weighted	T2-weighted
Fluid	Hypointense (dark)	Hyperintense (bright)
Fat	Hyperintense (bright)	Intermediate hyperintense (bright)
Bone	Hypointense (dark)	Hypointense (dark)

(a) (b)

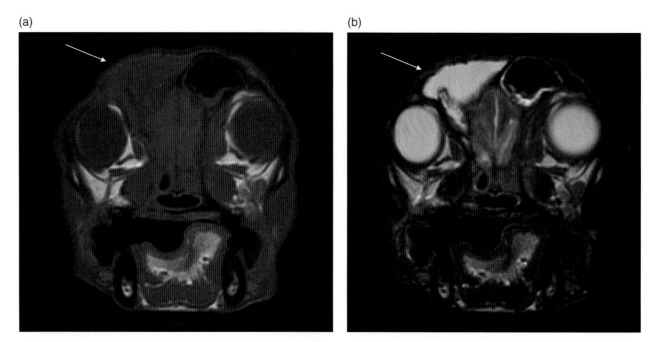

Figure 10.1 Axial MRI image of a canine skull depicting the difference between a T1 (a) and T2 (b) weighted image. On the T1 image, the fluid in the eye as well as the abnormal accumulation of fluid in the sinus (arrow) is hypointense (gray). On the T2 image, the fluid in the eye as well as the abnormal accumulation of fluid in the sinus (arrow) is hyperintense (white). In both a T1- and T2-weighted scan fat is hyperintense, and correspondingly on both the images the retrobulbar fat (ventral to the eye) is white.

(a)

(b)

(c)

(d)

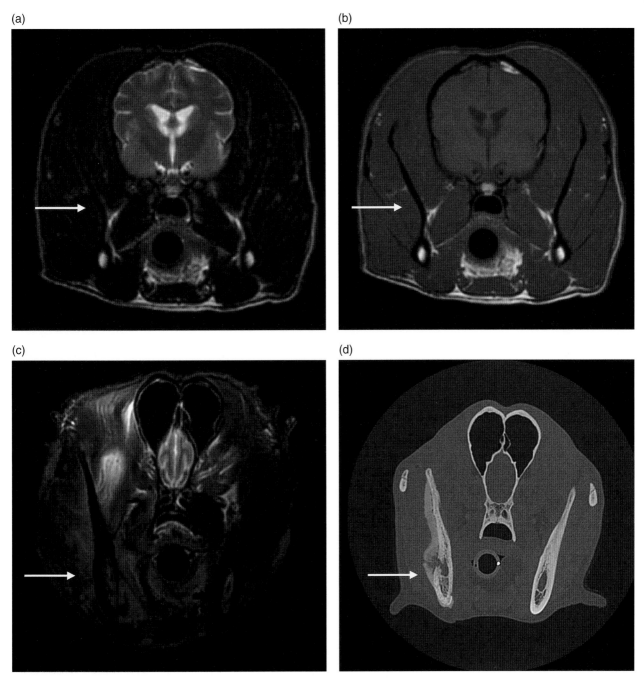

Figure 10.2   Bone appearance on the axial view of MRI and CT of a canine patient with a soft tissue and bone infection secondary to a foreign body. MRI and CT images were taken approximately four weeks apart; therefore, the pathology does not exactly match between these two images. In both the T2 (a) and T1 (b) weighted MRI image the bone (arrow) is black. (c) is a T2-weighted MRI image and (d) is a CT image. Note how the soft tissue infection (arrow) is much more evident on the T2-weighted MRI image (c) compared to the bone infection (arrow) being much more evidence on the CT scan (d).

Other MRI Sequences

Other sequences, including contrast studies, can also be performed for increased detection and visualization of pathology with MRI. These sequences often work by suppressing signals from certain tissues, thus enhancing the contrast between regions of pathology and background tissues. Full discussion regarding additional sequences which can be performed and the benefit of each are beyond the scope of this chapter.

The image created when an MRI manipulates the body's natural tissue characteristics is completely different from the image created when the body's tissue absorbs X-radiation. Thus, MRI is able to highlight different pathologies than a CT scan, especially concerning soft tissue detail and pathology. Due to its superior ability to image soft tissue, MRI has its greatest application in the fields of neuroradiology and musculoskeletal disease [1–3].

Indications for Use of MRI over CT in the Maxillofacial Region

MRI is the imaging modality of choice over CT for evaluation of soft tissue pathology. MRI is commonly used in human dentistry for imaging of the temporomandibular joints, salivary glands, soft tissue neoplasia, and musculoskeletal pathology [4]. Theoretically, the indications for MRI use in veterinary dentistry are similar; however, due to the cost disparity between MRI and CT, there is limited literature available pertaining to MRI appearance and diagnostic yield for soft tissue pathology in canine patients, and even less for feline patients. The true benefit of MRI over CT for all the aforementioned disease processes is not fully known or appreciated for small animal patients.

Temporomandibular Joint Disease (TMD)

In humans, MRI is the imaging modality of choice for temporomandibular joint disorders (TMD) as it allows for detailed imaging of articular disc configuration and position, bone marrow abnormalities, and presence of joint effusion. All of which are strongly associated with clinical signs of TMD [5]. In small animals, the clinical importance of diagnostic imaging features of TMD other than condylar/temporal bone defects and narrowing of the joint space has not been defined. Thus, radiographic imaging (radiographs or ideally CT scan), which is superior to MRI at evaluating bone, is normally the first choice for diagnostic work-up of suspect TMD in dogs and cats [6, 7] (Figure 10.3).

If a canine or the feline patient is showing continued signs of TMD such as pain on opening the mouth, crepitus on opening the mouth, or hearing a clicking noise when opening/closing the mouth and a CT scan has a low diagnostic yield, MRI is indicated to further classify the degree of injury and possible involvement of the articular disk. Limited research has been conducted in canine patients evaluating the normal appearance of the articular disk and the best MRI sequences to visualize both the disk as well as joint effusion [8]. This literature in combination with human imaging literature can be utilized as a reference for evaluation of undiagnosed suspected TMD in canine patients undergoing an MRI.

Salivary Gland Disease

MRI is the imaging modality of choice for evaluation of suspected salivary gland disease in both humans and small animals due to its superior soft tissue imaging capabilities [9] (Figure 10.4). Both normal [10, 11] and pathological [12, 13] appearance of the salivary glands on MRI has been described in dogs. Specifically, the appearance of zygomatic sialadenitis [12, 13], zygomatic sialocele [13], and zygomatic salivary gland neoplasia [13] have been described in the literature and are available for reference.

In clinical practice, due to the increased cost of MRI, CT scans are more commonly used for diagnosing salivary gland disease. Although CT will not be as sensitive at differentiating types of salivary disease, it can differentiate salivary gland disease from other locoregional pathology in cases of cervical swelling, oral swelling, or retrobulbar disease. The computed tomographic appearance of numerous different salivary diseases in dogs has also been described in the literature [12, 14–18]. Thus, CT imaging is an adequate first-choice imaging modality for suspected salivary gland disease and MRI can be reserved for more challenging diagnostic cases (Figure 10.5).

Abnormalities in the Muscles of Mastication and Inability to Open/Close the Mouth

MRI is the diagnostic modality of choice for a number of differentials when a patient presents with an inability or resistance to close or open the mouth (Table 10.2).

Specifically, in the case of an inability to close the mouth, if this is due to a trigeminal neuropathy or an alternative neurologic abnormality, MRI would be the diagnostic modality of choice due to its superior capacity for neuroanatomic imaging [19]. Similarly, MRI is also very helpful in working up an asymmetry in the muscles of mastication that close the mouth (temporal, masseter, and pterygoids) as this is most likely due to a peripheral nerve sheath tumor affecting the trigeminal nerve [20, 21] (Figure 10.6).

If an inability or resistance to opening the mouth is due to soft tissue pathology such as a foreign body reaction, retrobulbar disease, or masticatory muscle myositis, utilizing the MRI as a diagnostic imaging modality will create superior images of the soft tissues for a more accurate diagnosis [22]. It is important to keep in mind that a computed tomography (CT) scan has also been shown to be an effective diagnostic tool for masticatory muscle myositis [23] and retrobulbar disease [12, 14]. Another primary differential for inability or resistance to opening the mouth is bony pathology. Thus, most clinicians will use a CT scan to initially evaluate an inability to open (and also close) the mouth unless a neurologic component is strongly favored based on history and physical examination findings (Figure 10.7a–c).

(a) (b)

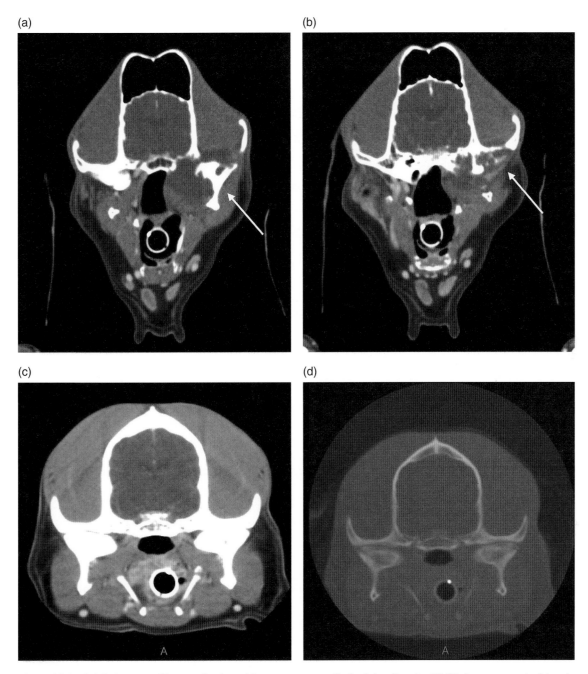

(c) (d)

Figure 10.3 Axial view on a CT scan of a dog with a temporomandibular joint disorder (TMD) that presented with pain on opening the mouth. Evaluation of the joint revealed a synovial cyst affecting both the condylar process (arrow, a) and temporal bone (arrow, b). Compare the noted pathology (a, b) to the normal appearance of the TMJ on a CT scan viewed in a soft tissue (c) and bone window (d).

Conclusions on the Clinical Indication for Use of MRI

MRI is unique in that it does not use radiation to create an image, but rather manipulates the body's natural tissue characteristics. Due to how MRI creates an image, it is superior in imaging soft tissue pathology, especially neuro-anatomy. Whenever there is any suspicion of a neurologic

component to maxillofacial disease, MRI should be your first diagnostic imaging modality choice. MRI is also a diagnostic imaging modality reserved for more challenging diagnostic cases in which CT may not have yielded enough information for an accurate diagnosis to be made.

Although MRI is technically superior for imaging soft tissue pathology in the skull, CT is often acceptable for diagnosing the more common maxillofacial soft tissue

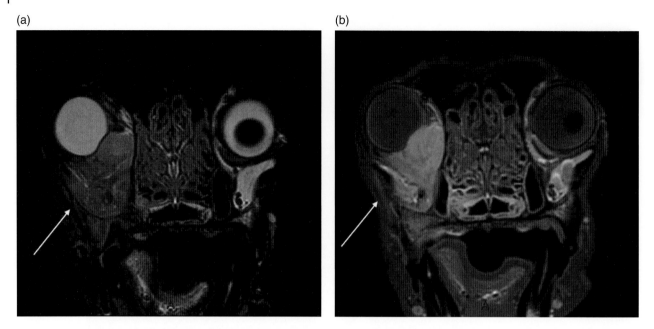

Figure 10.4 Appearance of a soft tissue sarcoma (arrow) in a dog arising from the right zygomatic salivary gland on a T2 (a) and post-contrast T1 (b) MRI image viewed in the axial plane.

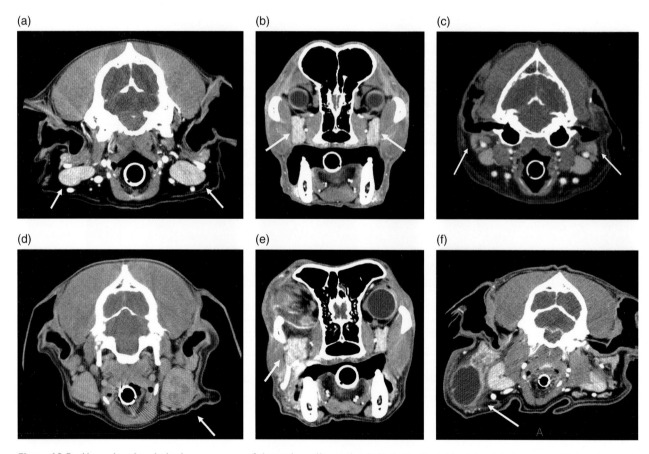

Figure 10.5 Normal and pathologic appearance of the major salivary glands in dogs viewed in the axial plane on a CT scan. Normal appearance (arrows) of the left and right mandibular salivary glands (a), zygomatic salivary glands (b), and parotid salivary glands (c) on a post-contrast CT scan. Comparatively, note the pathologic appearance of a mandibular salivary gland carcinoma (arrow, d), infectious zygomatic sialoadentitis (arrow, e), and a parotid gland sialocele (arrow, f) on post-contrast CT scan.

Table 10.2   Common causes for an inability/resistance to close or open the mouth and the capability of MRI versus conventional CT for accurate diagnosis with ++ being best, + being good/adequate, and − being poor.

Suspected condition	MRI	CT	Clinical signs to aid in choice of diagnostic imaging
Inability/resistance to close the mouth			
Trigeminal nerve dysfunction (neoplasia versus neuritis versus idiopathic neuropathy)	++	−	Can close mouth without impediment but mouth drops back open
Jaw fracture	−	++	Known recent trauma +/− malocclusion (shift toward fracture) +/− crepitus and palpable fracture +/− oral bleeding
Open mouth jaw lock (lateralization of coronoid process)	−	++	Inability to manually close the mouth Often can palpate coronoid on lateral aspect of zygomatic arch
TMJ luxation	−	++	Malocclusion If rostro-dorsal luxation (most common), then jaw shifts away from the luxation If caudo-ventral luxation (uncommon), the jaw shifts toward the side of the luxation
Malocclusion/tooth displacement	−	++	Can masquerade as a jaw fracture/TMJ luxation Obvious malocclusion and tooth on tooth contact preventing closure of the mouth
Inability/resistance to open the mouth			
Masticatory muscle myositis	++	+	Severe pain on opening the mouth with normal occlusion Inability to open mouth past a certain point
Retrobulbar disease (neoplasia, infection, abscess, zygomatic salivary gland disease)	++	+	Decreased retropulsion on affected side Severe pain on opening the mouth with a normal occlusion
Foreign body reaction/inflammation around the coronoid process	++	+	Severe pain on opening the mouth with a normal occlusion
Jaw fracture	−	++	Known recent trauma +/− malocclusion (shifts towards fracture) +/− crepitus and palpable fracture +/− oral bleeding
Bony neoplasia of the jaws	−	++	Pain on opening the mouth Relative inability to open the mouth due to bone-on-bone contact
Soft tissue neoplasia of the jaws or muscles of mastication	++	+	Obvious mass on maxillofacial examination Pain on opening the mouth with normal occlusion

pathology seen in canine and feline patients. Thus, a CT scan is often acceptable as a first-choice diagnostic tool as an alternative to MRI.

Computed Tomography (CT)

Computed tomography (CT) is an imaging modality that reconstructs 2D X-rays into multiplanar reconstructions as well as a 3D image; thus, successfully removing superimposition that can complicate traditional radiographic

evaluation. As mentioned earlier, compared to MRI, a CT scan is inferior in evaluation of soft tissue pathology, but is far superior in its ability to image bone and teeth. For the maxillofacial region, there are two variants of CT scanners that are commonly utilized – multidetector CT scan (MDCT), sometimes called a conventional CT scan, and cone beam CT scan (CBCT). These two variants of CT differ in how the X-ray images are acquired and reconstructed. These differences are associated with differences in image quality and practical use characteristics.

Technical Principles of Multidetector CT (MDCT) Scanners

In simple terms, MDCT scanners are composed of an X-ray tube, detectors, a gantry to house the X-ray tube and detectors, and a patient table (Figure 10.8). Current MDCT scanners are advanced iterations of the first-generation single slice CT scanner originally introduced in the 1960s. This first-generation scanner was composed of a single detector along with a single X-ray tube that would incrementally move around the patient collecting transverse slices of information

that were then stacked together and reconstructed into 3D images. In first-generation CT scanners, the collimation of the X-ray beam set the slice width, and due to limitations with only one detector, scans of just one region of the body could take up to 30 minutes to perform [24]. As newer generations of CT scanners were developed, increased detector numbers were introduced. This was directly associated with their ability to perform faster CT scans as numerous transverse image slices could be collected at the same time. The introduction of multidetector scanners also allowed for improved image quality and reformatting of thinner slices

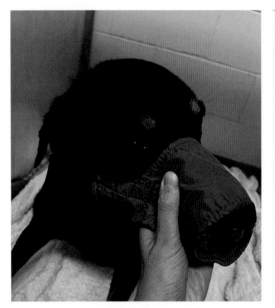
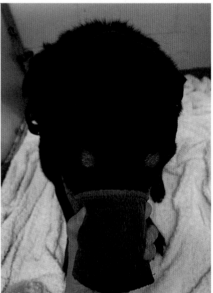

Figure 10.6 Eleven-year-old, female spayed rottweiler with asymmetric atrophy of the muscles of mastication favored to be a peripheral nerve sheath tumor.

(a)

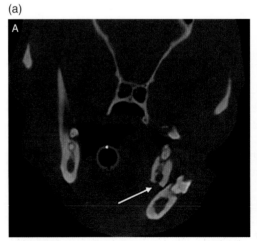
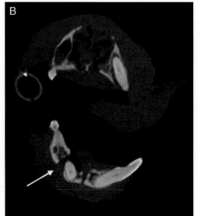
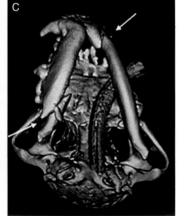

Figure 10.7 (a) CT appearance of a bilateral jaw fracture in a dog viewed in the axial plane (A, B, arrow) and 3D reconstruction (C, arrows).

(b)

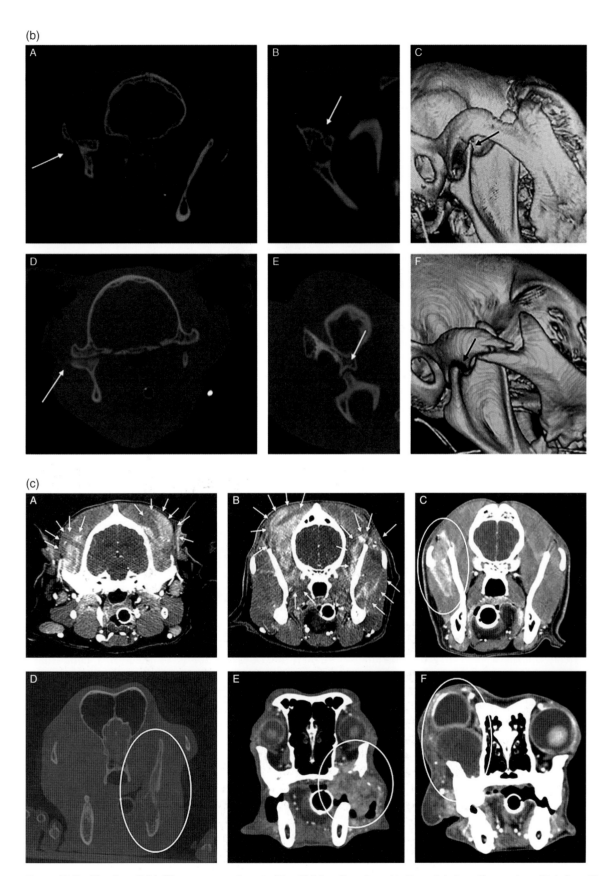

Figure 10.7 (Continued) (b) CT appearance of a cat with a TMJ luxation viewed in the axial plane (A, arrow), sagittal plane (B, arrow), and 3D reconstruction (C, arrow) compared to a normal TMJ in the axial plane (D, arrow), sagittal plane (E, arrow), and 3D reconstruction (F, arrow). (c) CT appearance of common differentials for an inability/resistance to open the mouth in dogs. (A, B) Serial axial post-contrast CT images of masticatory muscle myositis showing bilateral contrast enhancement in the muscles of mastication (arrows). (C) Axial post-contrast CT image of severe inflammation around the coronoid process secondary to a foreign body (circle). (D) Axial precontrast CT image of bony neoplasia causing severe lysis of the mandible (circle). (E) Axial post-contrast CT image of a soft tissue neoplasia in the caudal maxilla (circle). (F) Axial post-contrast CT image of severe retrobulbar disease displacing the globe (circle).

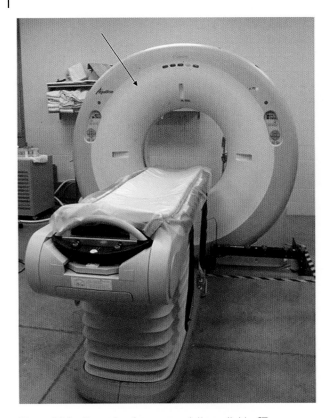

Figure 10.8 Example of a commercially available CT scanner pointing out the gantry (arrow) which houses the X-ray beam and detectors as well as the patient table which moves the animal through the gantry. Pictured is a Cannon 32 slice CT scanner.

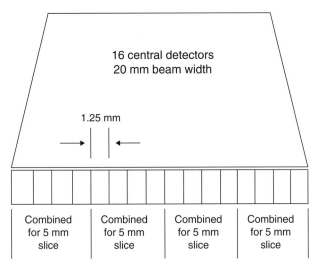

16 central detectors
20 mm beam width

1.25 mm

| Combined for 5 mm slice | Combined for 5 mm slice | Combined for 5 mm slice | Combined for 5 mm slice |

Figure 10.9 Detector configuration of a CT scanner with 16 central detectors, commonly referred to as a 16-slice CT scanner. Note how the central detectors can be configured to have 16, 1.25 mm slices, obtained at one time or four, 5 mm thick slices, obtained at one time.

due to the overlap of acquired data helixes. With time, improvements in hardware and reconstruction algorithms have directly contributed to the ability for rapid scans within seconds and improved reconstructed image quality [25–27]. Most veterinary hospitals that have a CT scanner within the hospital are currently utilizing a 3rd or 4th generation multidetector CT scanner.

In 3rd and 4th generation MDCT scanners, the X-rays are emitted in a fan beam geometry. Unlike single slice scanners, the X-ray beam width is not directly correlated with slice thickness. The number and configuration of central detector rows are what dictate the slice thickness and how many slices are obtained at once (Figure 10.9). This is often referred to as the slice number of the CT. For example, CT scanners can be referred to as a 16-slice or 64-slice CT. This means that 16 or 64 images (slices of data) are taken per rotation of the gantry.

When an MDCT scan is performed there is sequential scanning. Sequential scanning means that one specific width is imaged at a time and then the table is moved to the next z-position (position on the forward/backward axis). This is continued until the entire area of interest has been

imaged. The transverse images are then stacked together. As transverse images are what are predominantly collected, the primary reconstruction of the captured images in MDCT produces axial slices, which are then reconstructed to allow viewing of the images in different planes or as a 3D image [25–27].

Technical Principles of Cone Beam CT (CBCT) Scanners

CBCT scanners are also composed of an X-ray tube, detector, and a gantry that houses both the X-ray tube and detector. CBCT may or may not also include a patient table depending on the brand of the unit (Figure 10.10). In a CBCT, the X-ray beam is emitted in a cone shape (Figure 10.11) rather than a fan shape found in the traditional MDCT. The gantry housing the X-ray tube and detector rotates only once around the patient. The total scan time typically ranges from 10 to 40 seconds, although slower protocols may exist depending on the scanner. While the gantry rotates, numerous 2D X-ray projections are taken at fixed intervals (angles of rotation). These projections are acquired by a flat panel detector. The captured radiographic images are referred to as basis images, which are then utilized to reconstruct the complete series of images, known as the projection data [28].

The number of basis images that make up the projection data depends on the frame rate (number of images acquired per second), the rotation arc, and the speed of rotation [27, 28]. All of these variables differ depending on the brand and make of the CBCT scanner [27, 28]. In general, a higher frame rate and larger rotation arc result in more basis images, which is associated with higher quality resolution of the final reconstructed images. However, as the frame rate and rotation arc increase more radiation exposure is endured as well as requiring a longer sampling time which could produce more motion artifacts.

Concerning the differing rotation arcs, most CBCT will acquire projections with a single 360° rotation, i.e. the gantry will rotate one full rotation around the patient. Some units will obtain images by utilizing a smaller rotation arc, anywhere from 180° to 270°. The limited images are then utilized to reconstruct the normal field of view. With a limited rotation arc, the image quality is theoretically

decreased due to both a decrease in emitted radiation (mA) and a faster scan resulting in the image having increased noise [27, 29]. Increased noise, defined as background information that is not part of the signal of interest, results in a grainer appearance of the resultant image. From a clinical standpoint, there is limited literature supporting any perceivable differences in the resulting image quality produced while using a smaller or larger rotation arc [30, 31]. At this time, the full effect of rotation arc on clinically perceivable image quality has not been determined.

The last major difference between different brands of CBCT scanners is if there is pulsed or continuous exposure of X-rays, while the gantry makes its single rotation. The different exposure methods are associated with minimal to no difference in image quality. Whether a CBCT scanner uses pulsed or continuous radiation does have an effect on the amount of radiation exposure the patient receives. Continuous exposure CBCT scanners emit radiation throughout the entire rotation of the gantry, while the pulsed CBCT units intermittently emit radiation to acquire the diagnostic images. For this reason, pulsed CBCT scanners are strongly preferred as they minimize emitted radiation [27, 28].

Viewing CT Images

For both CBCT and MDCT, once the 2D radiographic images are acquired and reconstructed they can be viewed as a 3D image or as a multiplanar reconstruction. Multiplanar reconstruction refers to when the reconstructed images are viewed as a series of 2D cross-sectional images. Each cross-sectional image is a "slice" pending the chosen slice width and can be viewed as axial, sagittal, or coronal images. Axial images are in the transverse plane and extend from the tip of the nose back towards the tail. Sagittal images are in a vertical plane and extend from left to right. Coronal images are in a dorsal plane and are extend from the top to the bottom of the head (Figure 10.12a and b).

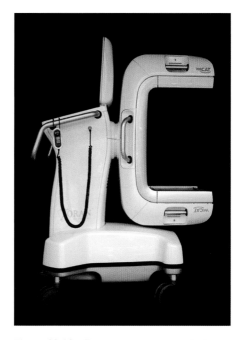

Figure 10.10 Example of a commercially available CBCT scanner. Portable CBCT unit, Xoran VetCAt. *Source:* Image of Xoran VetCat courtesy of David Sarment, DDS, MS, Xoran Technologies.

Figure 10.11 Cone beam geometry versus fan beam geometry of the X-ray beam for image acquisition in a cone beam computed tomography (CBCT) unit versus a multidetector computed tomography (MDCT) unit. *Source:* Drawing courtesy of Kristy Lashbaugh MS, RN, University of Minnesota, College of Veterinary Medicine.

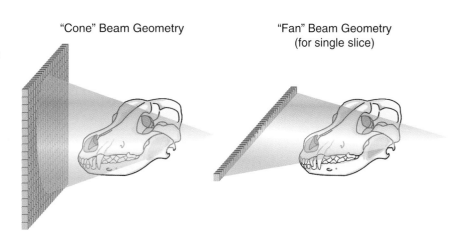

"Cone" Beam Geometry

"Fan" Beam Geometry
(for single slice)

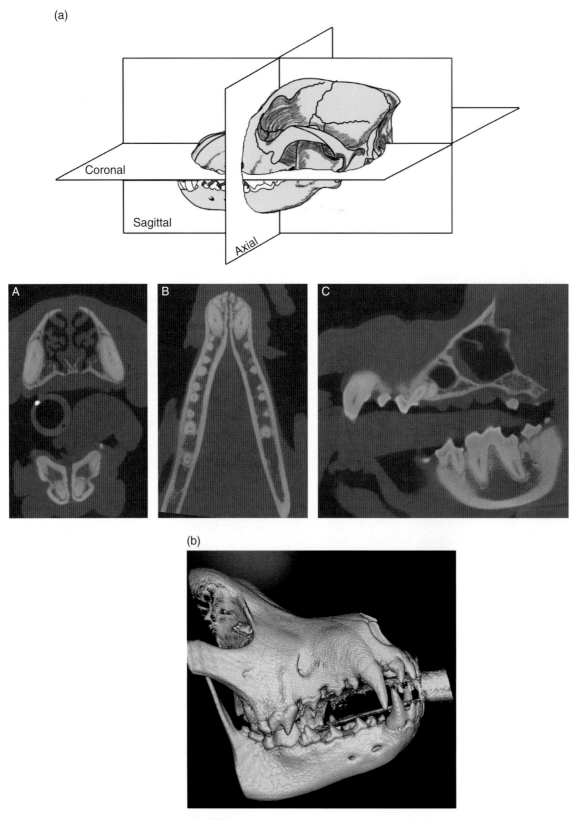

Figure 10.12 (a) Viewing images from a CT scan as multiplanar reconstructions in the axial (A), coronal (B), or sagittal (C) view. *Source:* Drawing courtesy of Kristy Lashbaugh, MS, RN, University of Minnesota, College of Veterinary Medicine. (b) Viewing images of a normal dog skull from a CT scan as a 3D reconstruction.

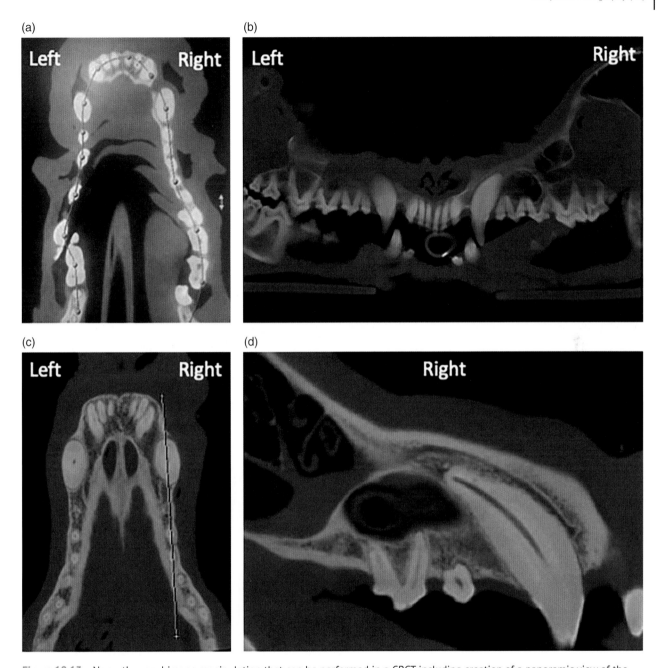

Figure 10.13 Nonorthogonal image manipulation that can be performed in a CBCT including creation of a panoramic view of the maxillary teeth (a, b, 110–210) and a mesiodistal view of select teeth (c, d, 104–106).

In a CBCT scanner, the images can also be sectioned in nonorthogonal planes as the voxels are isotropic (same height, width, and length). This allows the clinician to create panoramic images as well as serial transplanar reformations to highlight specific anatomic regions of interest without decreasing image quality or deforming the image [27] (Figure 10.13).

For both CBCT and MDCT, the reconstructed images are displayed on a grayscale relating to the attenuation values for each volume element (voxel). Attenuation values directly relate to the ability of the tissue to absorb X-radiation. For MDCT, the attenuation values of each voxel are represented by a CT number, which is the attenuation value of the tissue relative to water. The unit for CT numbers is the Hounsfield unit (HU), and thus the range of attenuation values utilizes the Hounsfield scale. The CT number is calculated by the equation: $HU = K \times (u\text{voxel}-u\text{water})/\text{water}$. The u voxel is the attenuation for the tissue, u water is the attenuation coefficient of water, and K is an integer constant (commonly standardized to 1000). On the

Hounsfield scale, based on this calculation, water is always zero, air is −1000, and denser objects have higher numbers with enamel being near 3000 HU [32–34] (for more information, see Table 1.2).

Assigning each CT number to a distinct shade of gray is not possible, and accordingly, most CT scanners display approximately 250 shades of gray. If all possible collected CT numbers were spread evenly over approximately 200 visually discernable gray levels, each gray level would represent approximately 10–20 CT numbers. If this was the case, then tissues with similar attenuation, such as soft tissue structures and the surrounding background tissues, would be assigned the same gray level potentially hiding normal anatomy as well as pathology. Thus, to allow structures with similar attenuation to be visualized, windowing exists. Windowing allows the viewer to decide the range of CT numbers to be displayed/spread among the visible gray scale [32, 33].

The window level selected specifies the CT number for centering the gray scale. The window width defines the range of CT numbers over which the gray scale will extend. For example, if the window level is set at 150 and the window width is set at 500, the image will display CT numbers from −100 to +400. All CT numbers below the lower limits are displayed as black and all above are displayed as white. A window level and width are selected to highlight the tissue of interest. As the window level is increased, a higher HU is needed for a tissue to appear brighter, so

higher window levels are used when dense objects are of most interest. Changing the window width affects how much contrast between tissues is needed to appreciate a visual difference in the grayscale. Thus, having a narrower window width is better for a low-contrast situation to allow subtle changes in CT numbers to be highlighted. Accordingly, a "soft tissue window" with a low window level and narrow window width is utilized for viewing soft tissue structures which do not naturally have vastly different density from the surrounding background tissues (low contrast). Conversely, a "bone window" with a higher window level and wider window width is utilized for viewing bony structures, which are naturally denser as well as having a higher contrast from the surrounding background tissue [35] (Figure 10.14, Table 10.3).

CBCT scans are also viewed on a gray scale that is very similar to MDCT, meaning the tissue attenuation values are

Table 10.3 Example of a window level and width for evaluating bone compared to soft tissue in the skull [35].

	Window level	Window width	CT numbers displayed on the gray scale
Bone window	500	2000	−1500 to +1500
Soft tissue window	30	160	−50 to +190

(a) (b) (c)

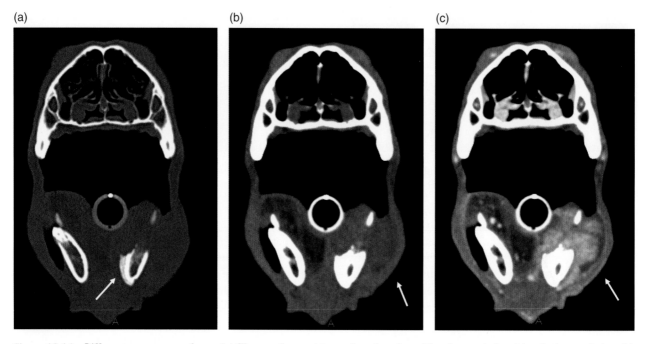

Figure 10.14 Different appearance of an axial CT scan of an oral tumor in a dog viewed in a bone window (a), soft tissue window (b), and post-contrast soft tissue window (c). Note how in the bone window the bony periosteal reaction is clearer (arrow, a), while the soft tissue windows better highlight the soft tissue extent of the mass (arrows, b, c).

translated to a gray scale similar to the Hounsfield scale; however, HU are not currently utilized to describe attenuation values in CBCT. There are inherent limitations in applying HU to the way images are acquired with CBCT. The quantitative gray values of the CBCT do not directly correlate with HU calculated for MDCT, which represent absolute tissue density [34, 36]. Rather than HU, attenuation values for CBCT are referred to as gray scale values.

Differences in Image Characteristics Between CBCT and MDCT

The most clinically impactful differences in image characteristics between the two variants of CT include spatial resolution, contrast resolution, and appearance of artifacts.

Spatial Resolution

Spatial resolution refers to the ability to discern two objects that are very close together, thus it will often be referred to as the "sharpness" of an image. Spatial resolution is assessed in line pairs per mm. Line pairs/mm are determined with the use of a phantom to measure the smallest distance at which the imaging system is capable to discern the lines as separate entities (Figure 10.15). In general, spatial resolution is superior on a CBCT compared to an

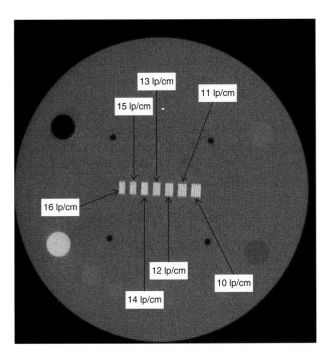

Figure 10.15 Image depicting how spatial resolution is measured by evaluating the appearance of line pairs (lp/cm) on a phantom scanned in a CBCT scanner. *Source:* Image of Xoran VetCat courtesy of David Sarment, DDS, MS, Xoran Technologies.

MDCT due to the CBCT containing smaller detector elements resulting in smaller voxel sizes as well as the use of isotropic voxels which allow multiplanar reconstruction without loss of spatial resolution [27, 37]. Due to its superior spatial resolution, CBCT has been shown to have significantly superior perceived clinical imaging quality compared to MDCT for diagnostic imaging of dentoalveolar structures (enamel, dentin, pulp, periodontal ligament, alveolar bone) in both humans and dogs [38–40] (Figure 10.16).

It is important to keep in mind that although small isotropic voxels play a large role in spatial resolution, resolution, is in fact, affected by numerous factors. Important factors that affect spatial resolution include the pixel size on the detector, presence of feldkamp error, collimation of the detector, density of the detector elements, pitch, and reconstruction algorithms [37, 41]. MDCT scanners that have been specifically designed to maximize spatial resolution will often reach or exceed spatial resolution of the CBCT [41, 42]. MDCT scanners that are utilized in veterinary medicine are not scanners that have been formulated to maximize spatial resolution. From a clinical standpoint in veterinary medicine, CBCT has higher spatial resolution compared to MDCT. Higher spatial resolution is impactful in imaging the maxillofacial region where high spatial resolution is paramount to accurate diagnosis.

Although spatial resolution is superior for CBCT compared to MDCT, the best spatial resolution is still acquired from the use of dental radiographs. Spatial resolution in a CBCT is approximately 11-line pairs/mm, while dental radiographs are approximately one magnitude higher at 101-line pairs/mm at 10% contrast [37]. The optical illusion that there is "sharper resolution" in a CBCT compared to dental radiographs is due to the fact that CBCT removes the superimposition of other structures (Figure 10.17).

Soft Tissue Imaging

To be able to evaluate differences between tissues on a CT scan, there needs to be sufficient attenuation difference (contrast) between the structure of interest and the surrounding background. CBCT is not effective at detecting differences between tissues with similar attenuation as it has poor contrast resolution. Poor contrast resolution in CBCT occurs primarily because the X-ray beam in the CBCT is not highly collimated resulting in increased scatter and increased noise in the surrounding background [27, 28, 41]. This makes CBCT poor at detecting both normal soft tissue anatomy and pathology as soft tissues have a naturally similar attenuation to the background tissues. The inability to detect subtle differences in soft tissue attenuation makes the CBCT limited to use for imaging

(a) (b)

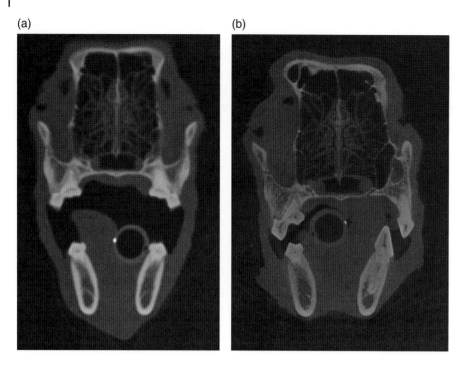

Figure 10.16 Appearance of normal dentoalveolar structures in a dog viewed in the axial plane on a 64-slice MDCT with 3 mm slice thickness (a) versus a CBCT with 0.3 mm slice thickness (b). Note the improved resolution on the CBCT image.

(a) (c) (e) (g)

(b) (d) (f) (h)

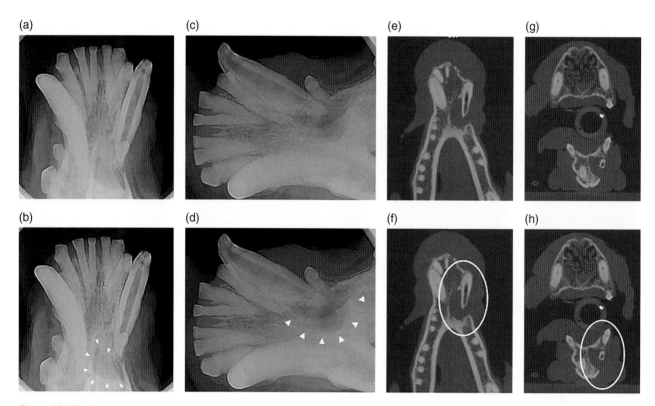

Figure 10.17 Spatial resolution of dental radiographs compared to CBCT. Although spatial resolution is technically superior on a dental radiograph, often there is the "optical illusion" that CBCT has sharper images as it removes superimposition making evaluation of images easier. In the depicted case of a periapical lucency on 304 in a dog, removal of the superimposition of the two mandibles at the mandibular symphysis makes the extent of the periapical lucency on 304 much easier to appreciate/differentiate from the surrounding structures. Occlusal (a, b) and lateral (c, d) dental radiograph of 304 with and without arrowheads pointing out the periapical lucency. Coronal (e, f) and axial (g, h) view on CBCT of 304 with and without a circle pointing out periapical lucency. Note, how much more "obvious" the extent of periapical disease is on the CBCT.

high-contrast osseous structures. If soft tissue imaging is required, CBCT should not be the imaging modality utilized. MDCT or MRI is the more appropriate diagnostic imaging modality of soft tissue structures.

The use of IV contrast, which is essential for delineating soft tissue pathology and helping to increase detection of structures with naturally low contrast, is limited with a CBCT. Some experimental studies have shown that use of IV contrast does highlight tumors more thoroughly than non-contrast CBCT [43, 44]. However, the use of IV contrast for diagnostic purposes on a CBCT scan has not been validated.

Artifacts

There are two major artifacts to consider with a CT scan: beam hardening and motion artifacts.

A beam hardening artifact occurs when there are very dense (highly attenuating) objects present, such as metal or root canal filling material [27, 28]. When low-energy photons in the X-ray beam come into contact with these very dense structures, they are preferentially absorbed. The attenuated X-ray beam exits in the material with a higher mean energy, i.e. the beam becomes harder or "more intense." This results in distortion of the primary X-ray beam and creates streaking artifacts on the resultant image. Because CBCT has heterochromatic X-ray beams and a lower peak KV energy output versus MDCT, beam hardening artifact is often more pronounced on a CBCT [27, 45] (Figure 10.18).

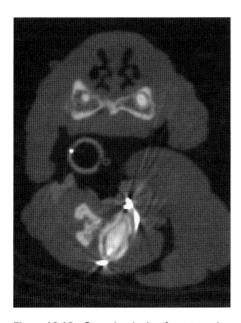

Figure 10.18 Beam hardening from a cerclage wire on an axial view of a CBCT in a dog. Note the streaking extending up from the wire.

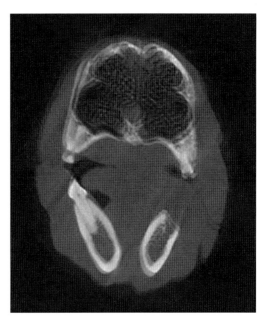

Figure 10.19 Motion artifact on an axial view of a CBCT in a dog. Note how the image is blurry and appears to have multiple images superimposed, but just offset from each other.

Motion artifact is also more pronounced on the CBCT compared to MDCT as the images are obtained in a single rotation with no image overlap during reconstruction [27, 28, 45]. This is often of no clinical concern in veterinary dentistry as most often the patients are anesthetized for oral examination. However, if performing a sedated examination with diagnostic imaging, an MDCT will allow for some motion while still maintaining high image quality while CBCT will not (Figure 10.19).

Other Impactful Differences in Practical Use Between MDCT and CBCT

CBCT emits a much lower radiation dose [46] as the X-ray beam rotates only once around the patient. These units have a lower power wattage requirement allowing a traditional 240 V outlet to be utilized. Additional benefits of CBCT over MDCT are decreased associated cost and rapid speed of imaging allowing for chairside office use (Table 10.4).

Indications for Use of Either MDCT or CBCT in the Maxillofacial Region

Maxillofacial Trauma

CT scanning, and now also CBCT scanning due to its rapid chairside availability, is the standard of care for human maxillofacial trauma [47–51]. CT scanning has

Table 10.4 Differences between CBCT and MDCT in imaging quality and practical use with ++ being best, + being good/adequate, and − being poor.

Attribute	CBCT	MDCT
Imaging dentoalveolar structures	++	+
Imaging soft tissue pathology	−	++
Artifacts	− Beam hardening and motion more pronounced	+ Beam hardening and motion less pronounced
Radiation dose	+	− Higher radiation dose
Ability to have in office	++	+ Higher cost Special building requirements

the ability to remove superimposition of the numerous bones in the maxillofacial region. This ability makes evaluation of both normal anatomy and identification of pathology with a CT scan superior to both skull and dental radiographs for maxillofacial trauma cases (Figure 10.20). CT has been shown to reveal 1.6 times more injuries in dogs and 2.0 times as many injuries in cats with maxillofacial trauma when compared to skull films [52]. Accurate identification of the extent of maxillofacial injuries in trauma cases allows for proper surgical planning and prognostic discussions with the owners. Thus, a CT scan should always be recommended as the imaging modality of choice when maxillofacial trauma is suspected. If only bony pathology is suspected, then either CBCT or MDCT would be appropriate imaging modalities. However, if soft tissue pathology, such as traumatic brain injury, is also suspected based on physical examination findings, then MDCT would be the favored imaging modality over a CBCT for diagnostic imaging.

Bony Pathology

Bony pathologic lesions including, but not limited to, osteomyelitis/osteonecrosis of the jaw, fibro-osseous disease, and osseous neoplasms are best outlined with advanced imaging techniques. A traditional X-ray can only detect lytic bone lesions when at least 30–50% of bone mass is destroyed, and the cortical bone plate is disrupted [53]. By removing superimposition of overlying bones, lytic lesions can be detected earlier, and the full extent of the lesion can be accurately visualized by the utilization of multiplanar and 3D reconstruction on MDCT and CBCT.

Osteomyelitis/Osteonecrosis

The extent of osteomyelitis/osteonecrosis is underestimated with dental radiographs in both humans and dogs [54, 55] (Figure 10.21). Underestimation of the extent of infected, necrotic, and diseased bone carries the risk that the surgeon will inadvertently leave affected bone within the surgical site. Consequently, the patient will have ongoing clinical pain and infection. If there is a high suspicion of osteomyelitis/osteonecrosis based on oral examination, and/or preliminary radiographic findings, advanced imaging should be performed to evaluate the extent of disease. This is especially true if the lesion is in the maxilla where there is increased superimposition of facial bones making the distinction of abnormal bone margins even more challenging when utilizing traditional radiographs alone.

Fibro-Osseous Disease

Fibro-osseous disease is defined as benign proliferative lesions where bone is transformed into fibrous tissue. This is a rare disease entity seen in dogs. Fibro-osseous lesions that have been reported in the dog included fibrous dysplasia and ossifying fibroma [56]. There is no current literature to support that advanced imaging such as CT is required in lieu of dental radiographs for the identification of fibro-osseous disease in dogs due to the rarity of this disease. However, it is well documented in humans that CT is better able to identify the transition from normal to abnormal bone, which is essential in the accurate diagnosis, and thus treatment, of these lesions [57, 58]. If fibro-osseous disease is suspected based on signalment and history, or diagnosed on histopathology, a CT scan should be performed for proper surgical planning. Since only bone needs to be imaged for diagnosis and surgical planning, a CBCT

(a) (b) (c) (d)

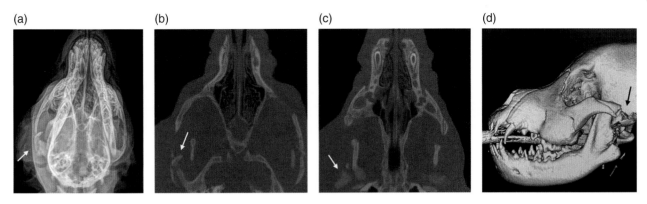

Figure 10.20 Maxillofacial trauma in a juvenile dog viewed on skull radiographs versus CBCT. Note how on the DV skull radiograph (a) only the fracture of the right temporal bone (arrow) is clearly evident. Meanwhile, on the coronal view of the CBCT, fracture of both the temporal bone (arrow, b) and the condylar process (arrow, c) is clearly evident. The extent of injury is especially clear on the 3D reconstruction (arrow, d). Fracture of both the condylar and temporal bone in a young dog is a risk factor for developing temporomandibular joint (TMJ) ankylosis while healing, thus this information markedly changes the prognostic and treatment discussion with the owner.

(a) (b) (c) (d)

(e) (f) (g) (h)

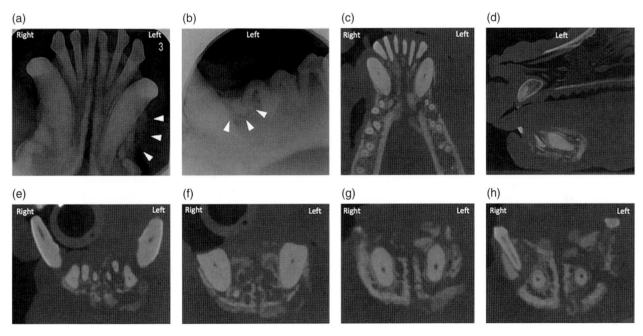

Figure 10.21 Extent and severity of osteomyelitis in a dog as seen on dental radiographs (arrowheads, a, b) compared to the coronal (c), sagittal (d), and serial axial (e–h) CBCT images. Note the increased severity of both bony lysis and proliferation viewed on the CBCT images compared to dental radiographs.

or MDCT scan would be an appropriate diagnostic imaging modality choice (Figure 10.22).

Osseous Neoplasia

Neoplasms that are confined to bone without a soft tissue component can be accurately imaged with either a CBCT or MDCT scan. Examples would include osteoma or osteosarcoma that has not perforated into soft tissue, odontogenic tumors with minimal to no soft tissue component, and primary intraosseous squamous cell carcinoma.

Although it has not been specifically documented in dogs or cats, diagnostic accuracy for the presence and extent of bony invasion of oral squamous cell carcinoma, the most common oral tumor in humans, is significantly higher with CT scan (CBCT or MDCT) comparatively to panoramic radiographs [59–62] (Figure 10.23a and b). When comparing CBCT to radiographs for accurately diagnosing bone invasion, the sensitivity of CBCT was 87.9% with a corresponding accuracy of 84.8% versus a sensitivity of 59.1% and accuracy of 74.1% with

(a) (b)

(c) (d)

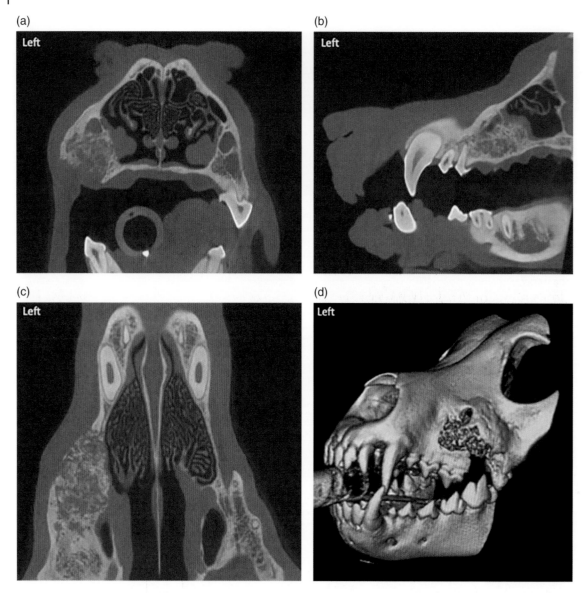

Figure 10.22   Appearance of fibro-osseous disease in a dog on a CBCT scan viewed in multiplanar reconstruction (a, axial; b, sagittal; c, coronal) and 3D reconstruction (d).

panoramic dental radiographs. Interestingly, CBCT is also shown to have a higher sensitivity and accuracy to MDCT for evaluation of bone lysis associated with carcinomas [63]. The presence and extent of bone invasion of oral tumors significantly affects both prognosis and treatment planning. Accurate diagnostic imaging is paramount to the application of proper oncologic surgical principles for treatment of these cases. For this reason, CT scans are recommended over dental radiographs for diagnostic work up of an oral tumor.

Clefts

Congenital cleft palates have been shown to have larger bony defects compared to the visualized soft tissue defect in the oral cavity, with a median difference of 1.75 cm^2 [64] (Figure 10.24). For adequate surgical planning, it is recommended that a CBCT or MDCT is performed to evaluate the size and extent of the bony defect associated with the cleft. This will ensure that a raised soft tissue flap planned for cleft closure does not inadvertently exposes an additional or

(a)

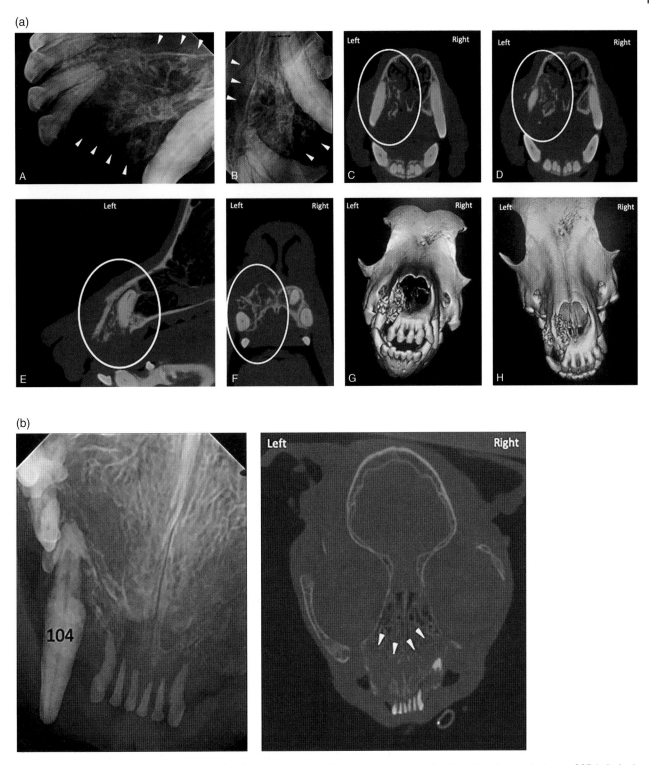

(b)

Figure 10.23 (a) Bony neoplasm in a dog visualized on dental radiographs centered on the interdental space between 203 (missing) and 204 (arrowheads, A, B) compared to axial (circle, C, D), sagittal (circle, E), and coronal (circle, F) CBCT views, as well as 3D reconstruction (G, H). Note how the extent of bone change is easier to visualize with CBCT and the tumor margins are better defined. (b) Bony neoplasm in a cat visualized on an occlusal dental radiograph of 104–203 compared to a coronal CBCT image. Note how the extent of maxillary bony lysis is very clear on the CBCT (arrowheads), and the end is not clearly defined on the dental radiograph.

(a)

(b)

(c)

(d)

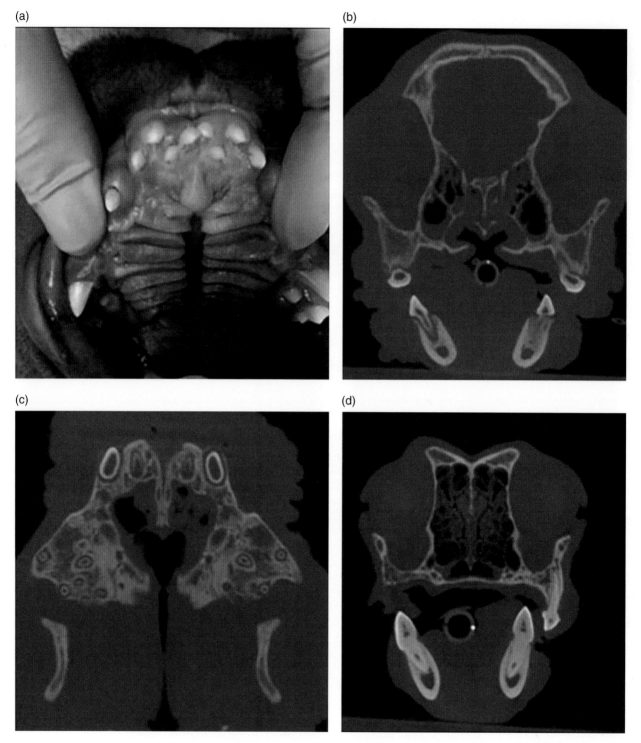

Figure 10.24 Soft tissue defect (a) of a congenital cleft palate in a dog compared to the larger bone defect documented on the axial (b) and coronal (c) CBCT images. Comparatively, note the normal bone appearance of the hard palate on an axial CT scan (d).

"new" bony defect. Dental and skull radiographs would be unable to properly evaluate the extent of the bony defect due to superimposition of bones in the maxilla and limitations in caudal placement of the radiographic plate.

Indications for Multidetector CT only (not CBCT) in the Maxillofacial Region

As discussed earlier in the chapter, CBCT is not effective at outlining soft tissue pathology due to the high signal-to-noise ratio and corresponding poor contrast resolution. Thus, CBCT is inappropriate for diagnostic imaging of a tumor with a soft tissue component.

Oral Neoplasia with a Soft Tissue Component

The most common malignant oral neoplasms in the dog namely melanoma, squamous cell carcinoma, and fibrosarcoma should be imaged with MDCT for evaluation of the extent of disease and corresponding surgical planning. The use of an MDCT is beneficial for imaging the regional lymph nodes and the thoracic cavity for the presence of metastasis. Thus, for accurate staging and surgical planning for any oral tumor with a soft tissue component, MDCT is the diagnostic imaging tool of choice. If the

owner elects CBCT in place of MDCT due to decreased cost, then the limitations of this imaging modality in accurately outlining the extent of the neoplasm, and the presence of lymph node metastasis should be thoroughly discussed with the client and documented in the medical record (Figure 10.25).

Soft Tissue Pathology

Anytime soft tissue pathology is suspected based on the history and physical examination, MDCT, not CBCT, is the clinically indicated diagnostic imaging modality. Examples of clinical disease presentations in dogs or cats that are likely to have soft tissue pathology include an inability to open or close the mouth with a normal occlusion, facial or cervical swelling, exophthalmos consistent with suspected retrobulbar disease, nasal discharge, or oral masses with obvious soft tissue components.

Indications for CBCT only (not MDCT) in the Maxillofacial Region

CBCT should be utilized in place of MDCT if imaging of the teeth and associated dentoalveolar structures are the primary areas of interest. This is due to the CBCT scan's

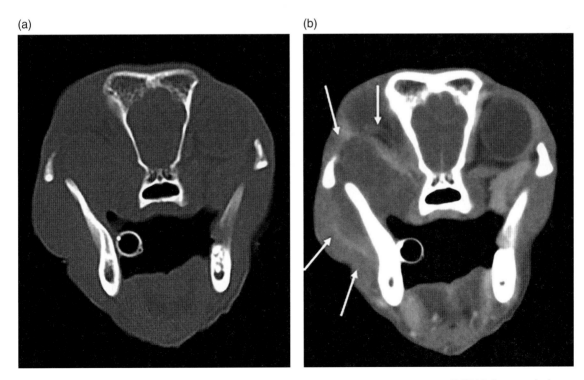

(a) (b)

Figure 10.25 An axial CT scan of a dog viewed in a bone window as it would be seen on a CBCT (a). Comparatively, note the soft tissue extent of the tumor (arrows) that is only obvious in the soft tissue window on an axial-view MDCT (b).

superior spatial resolution, smaller slice thickness, and decreased radiation dose. Evidence supports that CBCT can be very useful in addition to, or in place of, dental radiographs for evaluation of dentoalveolar trauma, periodontal disease, endodontic disease, tooth resorption, as well as diagnosis and treatment of missing teeth.

Dentoalveolar Trauma

Dentoalveolar trauma is common in dogs, with a reported prevalence of approximately one in four [65]. Dentoalveolar trauma includes complicated and uncomplicated crown and crown-root fractures, root fractures, and luxation injuries.

Although crown and crown-root fractures are often obvious with the combination of conscious and anesthetized oral examinations including full-mouth intraoral radiographs, root fractures can be more challenging to identify due to the intimate relationship between the X-ray beam and the fracture plane. If the X-ray beam is not perpendicular to the fracture line, the lesion may appear to be a superimposition of cancellous bone rather than a true root fracture. Numerous studies have supported that CBCT is superior for identification of horizontal and vertical root fractures in humans [50, 66–68]. CBCT has also been shown to be superior to MDCT for detection of vertical root fractures in humans [69]. Limited studies exist directly comparing MDCT with CBCT as the increased radiation dose associated with MDCT is not warranted clinically for research purposes. This is based on the ALARA radiation principle (as low as reasonably achievable). For more information on the ALARA radiation principle, please see Chapter 1.

In dogs, experimental studies also support CBCT for being a useful diagnostic tool for identification of vertical root fractures, as well as alveolar fractures associated with root fractures [70, 71]. Only one clinical study currently exists in dogs looking at the diagnostic accuracy of CBCT [72]. This study did not find CBCT to be significantly superior to radiographs for identification of root fractures. However, this should be interpreted with caution due to the low prevalence of root fractures and paucity of literature on the matter. Clinically, CBCT is found to be very helpful in identification of root fractures as it removes overlying superimposition of cancellous bone (Figure 10.26).

Periodontal Disease

Periodontal probing and dental radiographs are the mainstay for diagnosis of periodontal disease. However, CBCT can be extremely helpful in evaluating the severity of the alveolar bone loss, especially in teeth that are crowded. Cone beam computed tomography is extremely useful for evaluation of periodontal disease affecting the maxillary first and second molar teeth. These teeth are often prone to superimposition from surrounding teeth as well as other bony structures within the region including the zygomatic arch when utilizing dental radiographs as the sole imaging modality (Figure 10.27).

In humans, it has been shown that dental radiology alone cannot distinguish between bone loss that has occurred on the buccal or lingual plates and that dental radiography is overall inferior to CBCT in the diagnosis of both furcal bone loss and vertical bone defects [73–78]. In one study, identification of vertical bone defects occurred correctly in 82.7% of cases utilizing dental radiographs, while 99.7% were correctly identified when utilizing CBCT [76]. Another study revealed that vertical bone pockets were underestimated by an average of 1.5 mm (+/− 2.6 mm) when utilizing dental radiographs alone [77]. CBCT can thus be impactful when planning for advanced periodontal surgery where knowledge of the pathology and true depth of the vertical defect is paramount to success (Figure 10.28).

In brachycephalic dogs, CBCT has been shown to be superior to dental radiographs for diagnosis of periodontal disease [72]. Due to the ability of CBCT to remove the effect of tooth crowding on evaluation of alveolar bone height, CBCT can directly impact decision making regarding extraction (Figure 10.29). Specifically, in the aforementioned study, it was found that indications for extraction due to severe periodontal disease would have been missed in 44.7% of cases if radiographs alone were utilized [72].

Endodontic Disease

Numerous studies in the literature in both human and canine patients support that CBCT is superior to dental radiographs for diagnosis of apical periodontitis [79–86] (Figure 10.30). Apical periodontitis is defined as a periapical lucency (bone loss around the tooth apex) representing an abscess, cyst, or granuloma that formed secondary to pulp infection and necrosis. Presence of an apical lucency is one of the primary diagnostic imaging signs of a nonvital tooth. The other main image findings include failure to narrow of the pulp chamber and internal tooth resorption. However, both failure to narrow and internal pulp changes can be difficult to diagnose in older patients where the pulp no longer narrows rapidly. Thus, more clinical reliance is placed on the absence or presence of apical periodontitis radiographically for a diagnosis of tooth nonvitality.

In one study, where pulp infection was experimentally induced in dogs, no apical periodontitis was noted at day 7,

(a) (b)

(c) (d) (e)

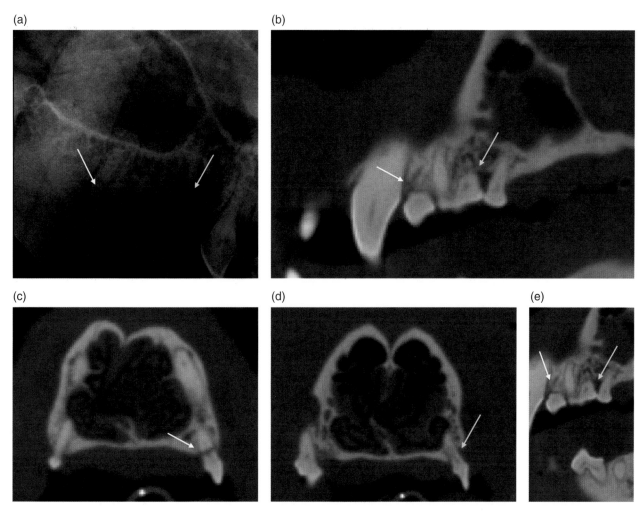

Figure 10.26 Root fractures viewed on dental radiographs compared to CBCT. On the dental radiograph (a), there is a high likelihood of a root fracture (white arrow) on 205 as well as a suspected root fracture (yellow arrow) on the distal root of 206. On the sagittal CBCT view (b), note that the root fracture on 205 is confirmed (white arrow), but there is tooth resorption with no root fracture on 206 (yellow arrow). These findings are verified on the axial view of 205 (c) and distal root of 206 (d), as well as the mesiodistal oblique view of 205 and 206 (e).

47.4% was noted at day 15, and 77.8% at day 30 when dental radiographs were used for diagnosis. Conversely, an apical lucency was detected in 32.5% of teeth at day 7, 83.3% at day 15, and 100% at day 30 with the use of a CBCT [84] supporting that CBCT can recognize development of apical periodontitis sooner than traditional dental radiographs. Not only has it been demonstrated that CBCT can identify the presence of a periapical lucency sooner but it also can better evaluate the size of the apical lesion. A study in dogs that evaluated the successful healing of apical periodontitis following root canal therapy showed that radiographs falsely diagnosed favorable outcomes almost 2.5 times more frequently than CBCT [80]. In short, dental radiographs have been found to be unreliable in properly detecting the presence and size of periapical lesions (Figure 10.31).

The primary limitation with dental radiographs in the diagnosis of endodontic disease is that the imaging modality is limited by the specific location of the apical bone loss and disease. If the apical lesion is confined within cancellous bone and substantial cortical bone is still present, the appearance of an apical lesion will be masked on dental radiographs. In other words, if the cortical bone is not substantially thinned or perforated, the lesion will not show up radiographically, thus making lesions confined in cancellous bone more undetectable [53] (Figure 10.32). Furthermore, differences in beam angulation or sensor positioning can substantially change the appearance of apical lesions on a dental radiograph making serial monitoring for evaluation of healing following root canal therapy more challenging [86].

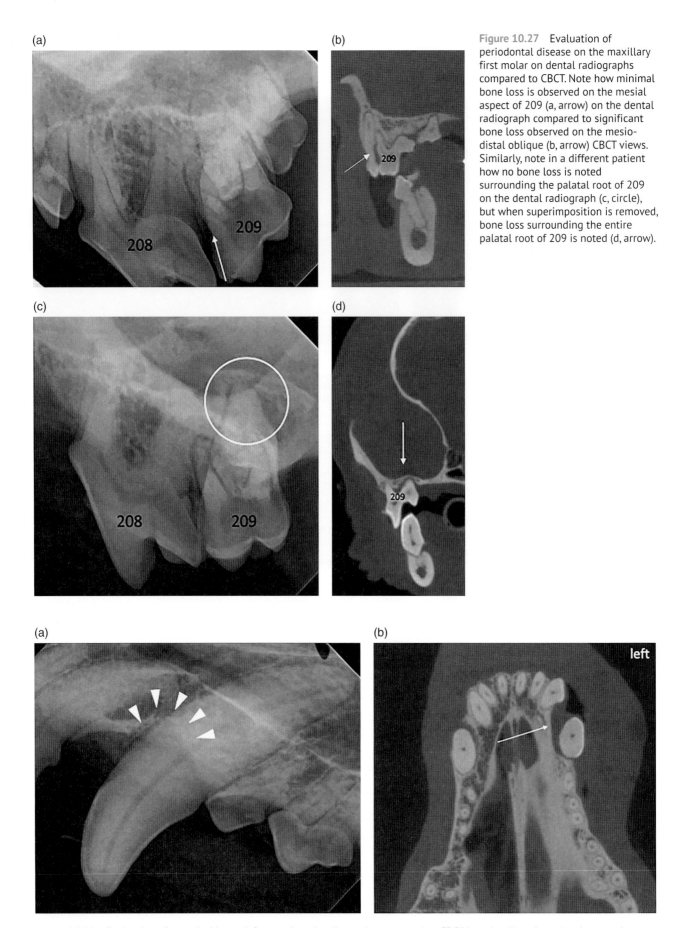

Figure 10.27 Evaluation of periodontal disease on the maxillary first molar on dental radiographs compared to CBCT. Note how minimal bone loss is observed on the mesial aspect of 209 (a, arrow) on the dental radiograph compared to significant bone loss observed on the mesio-distal oblique (b, arrow) CBCT views. Similarly, note in a different patient how no bone loss is noted surrounding the palatal root of 209 on the dental radiograph (c, circle), but when superimposition is removed, bone loss surrounding the entire palatal root of 209 is noted (d, arrow).

Figure 10.28 Evaluation of a vertical bone defect on dental radiographs compared to CBCT in a dog. Note how the shape and severity of the vertical bone defect on the mesiopalatal aspect of 204 are much easier to appreciate on the coronal view of the CBCT (b, arrow) compared to the dental radiograph (a, arrowheads). As this patient elected to have a bone graft placed, the shape and severity of the bony defect are important factors in determining prognosis.

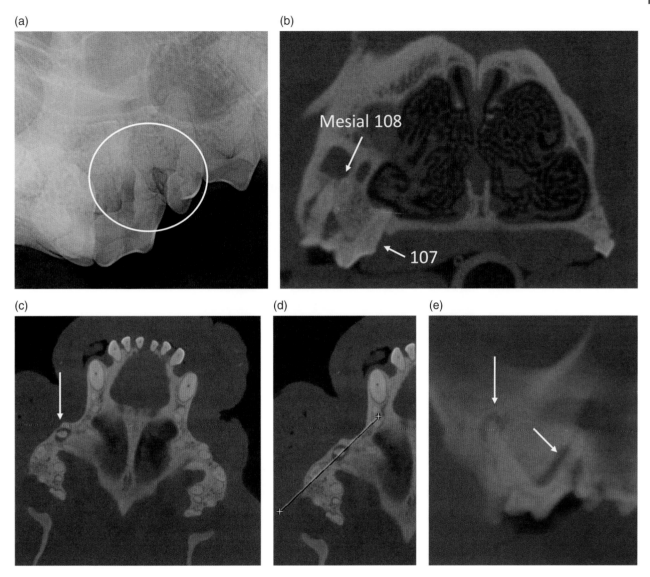

Figure 10.29 Evaluation of the extent of periodontal disease on dental radiographs compared to CBCT in a brachycephalic dog with crowded teeth. Dental radiograph (circle, a) exhibiting what appears to be mild (25%) bone loss between the maxillary third (107) and fourth premolar (108). Note how it is difficult to fully appreciate bone loss due to rotation of 107, as well as crowding of 107 and 108 leading to superimposition of the root structures. On the axial (b) CBCT view, however, severe vertical bone loss between the distal aspect of 107 and mesial root of 108 is easily identifiable. On the coronal view (arrow, c) bone loss extending around the entire mesial root can be noted. A mesio-distal cut is then made through this tooth (d) to view this tooth in an additional plane, which confirms severe vertical bone loss on the mesial root of 108 (arrow, e) as well as reveals a periapical lucency on the distal root (arrow, e).

In humans, CBCT is recommended in place of dental radiographs for endodontic therapy due to its ability to properly identify dental shape anomalies, missed and accessory canals, and additional roots, which can substantially impact the success of root canal treatment. CBCT images allow for detailed information about root and pulp canal morphology that can be missed in a 2D image [87, 88]. In general, dogs and cats tend to have less complex root and pulp canal morphology when compared to humans, thus this issue may not be as clinically impactful in small animals. Further research on root and pulp canal morphology is needed.

Tooth Resorption

In humans, CBCT has been shown to be superior to dental radiographs for both diagnosis and classification of tooth resorption both *in vivo* [89] and *in vitro* [90, 91]. *In vitro* studies are more clinically applicable because the presence of a resorptive lesion is confirmed. Metanalysis

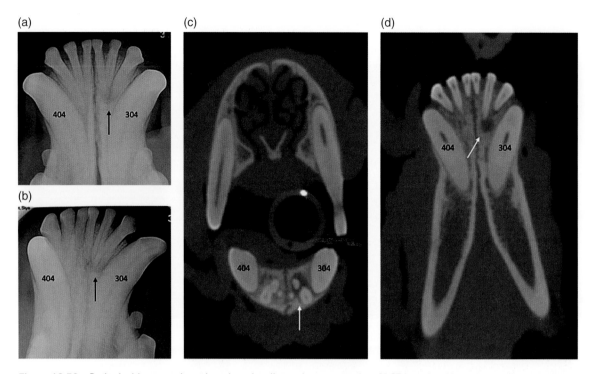

Figure 10.30 Periapical lucency viewed on dental radiographs compared to CBCT in a dog. Note the subtle periapical lucency (arrow) on 302 seen on dental radiographs (a, b) compared to the obvious and well-defined lucency (arrow) noted on the axial (c) and coronal (d) CBCT view of this tooth.

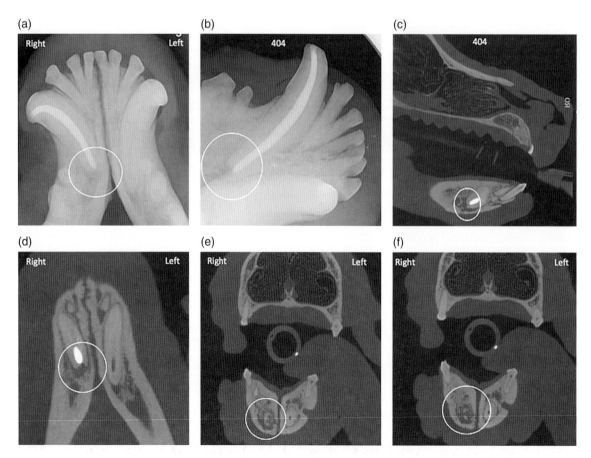

Figure 10.31 Monitoring of root canal success in a dog with dental radiographs compared to CBCT. Note how the sagittal (c), coronal (d), and axial (e, f) CBCT views are superior at revealing both the presence of a periapical lesion as well as the presence of secondary pathology, in this case external inflammatory resorption, compared to the dental radiographs (a, b). Due to the presence of both a lucency and tooth resorption this root canal was determined to have failed and additional therapy with surgical root canal or extraction was recommended.

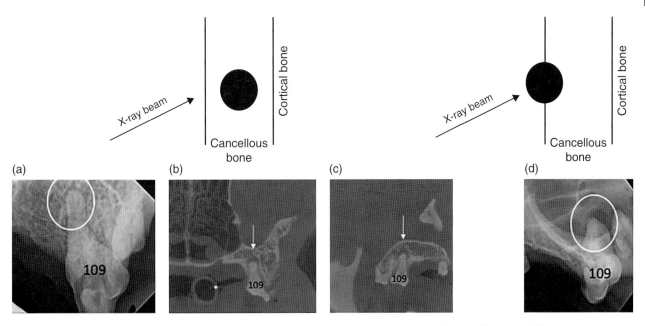

Figure 10.32 When periapical bone loss is confined within the cancellous bone of the maxilla, it will not be visible on a dental radiograph. Dental radiograph of 109 in a canine patient where no lucency is observed (a, circle) compared to the lucency observed on the axial (b, arrow), and sagittal (c, arrow) CBCT view of this tooth. Alternatively, when periapical bone loss perforates through the cortical bone plate, it can be easily visualized on a dental radiograph (circle, d).

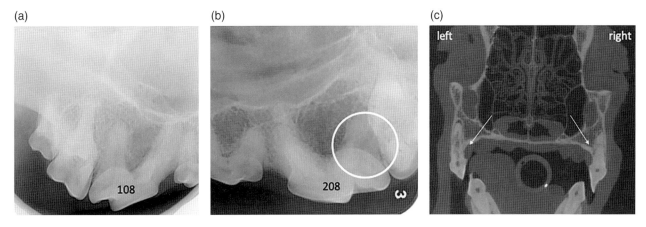

Figure 10.33 Canine tooth resorption viewed on dental radiographs compared to CBCT. Note how no obvious resorptive lesions are seen on the dental radiograph of 108 (a) and a suspect lesion is seen on 208 (circle, b), although it is unclear if this is just overlying cancellous bone. Comparatively, there are obvious resorptive lesions (arrows) on both 108 and 208 on the axial CBCT view (c).

has shown that CBCT has a higher diagnostic sensitivity compared to dental radiographs (89% versus 68% respectively) [90]. CBCT is also better at classifying the type of tooth resorption [91], which can then better dictate treatment recommendations. Due to the superiority of CBCT for diagnosis and characterization of tooth resorption, a 3D classification system has been suggested in humans to better describe treatment outcomes and prognosis [92].

CBCT has also been shown to have a higher diagnostic yield for identification of tooth resorption in brachycephalic dogs and cats [72, 93] (Figure 10.33). However, a comparison study including histopathology as the gold standard has never been performed in small animals.

Diagnosis and Treatment of Missing Teeth

Lastly, CBCT is indicated for identification and surgical planning for treatment of impacted teeth [72, 94, 95]. CBCT scanning allows for proper 3D localization of the affected tooth or teeth [72, 94, 95] (Figure 10.34). Whenever possible, CBCT scans to best evaluate the overlying bone thickness and precise location of the impacted tooth should be performed to aid in surgical removal of the affected teeth.

(a)　　　　　　　　　(b)　　　　　　　　　(c)

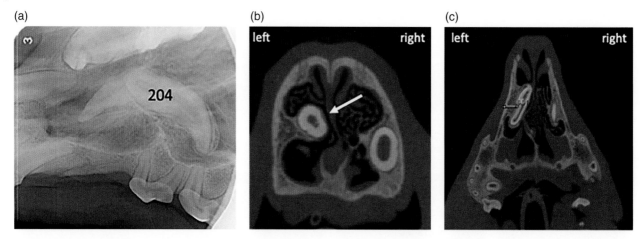

Figure 10.34　Appearance of an impacted canine tooth (204) in a dog on a lateral dental radiograph (a) versus the axial (b) and coronal view (c) on CBCT. Note how on the radiograph it was not clear that there was a bone isthmus (white arrow) between the tooth and the buccal maxillary bone. CBCT allowed this bony isthmus to be identified and measured, allowing adequate surgical planning for extraction of the impacted tooth.

Conclusions on the Clinical Indication for Use of CBCT Versus MDCT

Both CBCT and MDCT are indicated for evaluation of the extent of bony pathology in the maxillofacial region including evaluation of osteomyelitis/osteonecrosis, fibro-osseous disease, and bony neoplasm as well as for surgical planning for maxillofacial trauma and cleft palates. MDCT is indicated for evaluation of any pathology suspected to extend beyond the bone margins and into the soft tissues. CBCT is indicated for further evaluating dental pathology in place of, or in addition to, dental radiographs.

References

1　Neutze, J. (2020). MRI. In: *Radiology Fundamentals: Introduction to Imaging & Technology* (ed. J. Kissane, J. Neutze, and H. Singh), 33–35. New York: Springer.

2　Ajtai, B., Masdeu, J., and Lindzen, E. (2016). Structural imaging using magnetic resonance imaging and computed tomography. In: *Bradley's Neurology in Clinical Practice*, 7e (ed. R. Daroff, J. Jankovic, J. Mazziotta, and S. Pomeroy), 411–458. St. Louis: Elsevier.

3　Roth, C. and Deshmukh. (2017). Introduction and physics of body MRI. In: *Fundamentals of Body MRI*, 2e, 1–44. St. Louis: Elsevier.

4　Demirturk, H., Geha, H., Gaalaas, L.R., and Nixdorf, D.R. (2018). MRI for dental applications. *Dent. Clin. N. Am.* 62 (3): 467–480. https://doi.org/10.1016/j.cden.2018.03.006.

5　Matsubara, R., Yanagi, Y., Oki, K. et al. (2018). Assessment of MRI findings and clinical symptoms in patients with temporomandibular joint disorders. *Dentomaxillofac. Radiol.* 47 (4): 20170412. https://doi.org/10.1259/dmfr.20170412.

6　Arzi, B., Cissell, D.D., Verstraete, F.J. et al. (2013). Computed tomographic findings in dogs and cats with temporomandibular joint disorders: 58 cases (2006–2011). *J. Am. Vet. Med. Assoc.* 242 (1): 69–75. https://doi.org/10.2460/javma.242.1.69.

7　Schwarz, T., Weller, R., Dickie, A.M. et al. (2002). Imaging of the canine and feline temporomandibular joint: a review. *Vet. Radiol. Ultrasound* 43 (2): 85–97.

8　Macready, D.M., Hecht, S., Craig, L.E., and Conklin, G.A. (2010). Magentic resonance imaging features of the temporomandibular joint in normal dogs. *Vet. Radiol. Ultrasound* 51 (4): 436–440.

9　Afzelius, P., Nielsen, M.Y., Ewertsen, C., and Bloch, K.P. (2016). Imaging of the major salivary glands. *Clin. Physiol. Funct. Imaging* 36 (1): 1–10.

10　Weidner, S., Probst, A., and Kneissl, S. (2012). MR anatomy of salivary glands in the dog. *Anat. Histol. Embryol.* 41 (2): 149–153. https://doi.org/10.1111/j.1439-0264.2011.01115.x.

11　Durand, A., Finck, M., Sullivan, M., and Hammond, G. (2016). Computed tomography and magnetic resonance diagnosis of variations in the anatomical location of the major salivary glands in 1680 dogs and 187 cats. *Vet. J.* 209: 156–162. https://doi.org/10.1016/j.tvjl.2015.07.017.

12　Cannon, M.S., Paglia, D., Zwingenberger, A.L. et al. (2011). Clinical and diagnostic imaging findings in dogs with zygomatic sialadenitis: 11 cases (1990–2009). *J. Am.*

Vet. Med. Assoc. 239 (9): 1211–1218. https://doi.org/10.2460/javma.239.9.1211.

13 Boland, L., Gomes, E., Payen, G. et al. (2013). Zygomatic salivary gland diseases in the dog: three cases diagnosed by MRI. *J. Am. Anim. Hosp. Assoc.* 49 (5): 333–337. https://doi.org/10.5326/JAAHA-M.S.-5882.

14 Winer, J.N., Verstraete, F.J.M., Cissell, D.D. et al. (2018). Clinical features and computed tomography findings are utilized to characterize retrobulbar disease in dogs. *Front. Vet. Sci.* 21 (5): 186. https://doi.org/10.3389/fvets.2018.00186.

15 Nabeta, R., Kambe, N., Nakagawa, Y. et al. (2019). Sjögren's-like syndrome in a dog. *J. Vet. Med. Sci.* 81 (6): 886–889. https://doi.org/10.1292/jvms.18-0387.

16 Lenoci, D. and Ricciardi, M. (2015). Ultrasound and multidetector computed tomography of mandibular salivary gland adenocarcinoma in two dogs. *Open Vet. J.* 5 (2): 173–178.

17 Lee, N., Choi, M., Keh, S. et al. (2014). Zygomatic sialolithiasis diagnosed with computed tomography in a dog. *J. Vet. Med. Sci.* 76 (10): 1389–1391. https://doi.org/10.1292/jvms.14-0151.

18 Trumpatori, B.J., Geissler, K., and Mathews, K.G. (2007). Parotid duct sialolithiasis in a dog. *J. Am. Anim. Hosp. Assoc.* 43 (1): 45–51. https://doi.org/10.5326/0430045.

19 Musso, C., Le Boedec, K., Gomes, E., and Cauzinille, L. (2020). Diagnostic values of clinical and magnetic resonance findings in presumptive trigeminal neuropathy: 49 dogs. *J. Am. Anim. Hosp. Assoc.* 56 (2): 106–113. https://doi.org/10.5326/JAAHA-M.S.-6997.

20 Milodowski, E.J., Amengual-Batle, P., Beltran, E. et al. (2019). Clinical findings and outcome of dogs with unilateral masticatory muscle atrophy. *J. Vet. Intern. Med.* 33 (2): 735–742. https://doi.org/10.1111/jvim.15373.

21 Swift, K.E., McGrath, S., Nolan, M.W. et al. (2017). Clinical and imaging findings, treatments, and outcomes in 27 dogs with imaging diagnosed trigeminal nerve sheath tumors: a multi-center study. *Vet. Radiol. Ultrasound* 58 (6): 679–689. https://doi.org/10.1111/vru.12535.

22 Cauduro, A., Paolo, F., Asperio, R.M. et al. (2013). Use of MRI for the early diagnosis of masticatory muscle myositis. *J. Am. Anim. Hosp. Assoc.* 49 (5): 347–352. https://doi.org/10.5326/JAAHA-M.S.-5915.

23 Reiter, A.M. and Schwarz, T. (2007). Computed tomographic appearance of masticatory myositis in dogs: 7 cases (1999–2006). *J. Am. Vet. Med. Assoc.* 231 (6): 924–930. https://doi.org/10.2460/javma.231.6.924.

24 Wesolowski, J.R. and Lev, M.H. (2005). CT: history, technology, and clinical aspects. *Semin. Ultrasound CTMR* 26 (6): 376–379. https://doi.org/10.1053/j.sult.2005.07.007.

25 Nikolaou, K., Bamberg, F., Laghi, A., and Rubin, D. (2019). *Multislice CT (Medical Radiology)*, 4e. Cham: Springer.

26 Schneider, A. and Feussner, H. (2017). Diagnostic procedures. In: *Biomedical Engineering in Gastrointestinal Surgery*, 87–220. London: Academic Press.

27 Scarfe, W.C. and Farman, A.G. (2008). What is cone-beam CT and how does it work? *Dent. Clin. N. Am.* 52 (4): 707–730. https://doi.org/10.1016/j.cden.2008.05.005.

28 Abramovitch, K. and Rice, D.D. (2014). Basic principles of cone beam computed tomography. *Dent. Clin. N. Am.* 58 (3): 463–484.

29 Pauwels, R., Araki, K., Siewerdsen, J.H., and Thongvigitmanee, S.S. (2015). Technical aspects of dental CBCT: state of the art. *Dentomaxillofac. Radiol.* 44 (1): 20140224.

30 Kuo, Y.F., Chen, M.H., Huang, K.H. et al. (2020). Comparing image qualities of dental cone-beam computed tomography with different scanning parameters for detecting root canals. *J. Formos. Med. Assoc.* 5: S0929-6646(20)30412-5. https://doi.org/10.1016/j.jfma.2020.08.038.

31 Hoff, M.N., Zamora, D., Spiekerman, C. et al. (2019). Can cephalometric parameters be measured reproducibly using reduced-dose cone-beam computed tomography? *J. World Fed. Orthod.* 8 (2): 43–50.

32 Barnes, J.E. (1992). Characteristics and control of contrast in CT. *RadioGraphics* 12 (4): 825–837.

33 Goldman, L.W. (2007). Principles of CT and CT technology. *J. Nucl. Med. Technol.* 35 (3): 115–128.

34 Patrick, S., Birur, N.P., Gurushanth, K. et al. (2017). Comparison of gray values of cone-beam computed tomography with housfield units of multislice computed tomography: an in vitro study. *Indian J. Dent. Res.* 28 (1): 66–70. https://doi.org/10.4103/ijdr.IJDR_415_16.

35 McConnell, J. and Druva, R. (2011). Computed tomography protocols. In: *Index of Medical Imaging* (ed. J. McConnell), 150–192. Hoboken: Wiley.

36 Pauwels, R., Jacobs, R., Singer, S.R., and Mupparapu, M. (2015). CBCT-based bone quality assessment: are housfield units applicable? *Dentomaxillofac. Radiol.* 44 (1): 20140238. https://doi.org/10.1259/dmfr.20140238.

37 Brüllmann, D. and Schulze, R.K.W. (2015). Spatial resolution in CBCT machines for dental/maxillofacial applications – what do we know today? *Dentomaxillofac. Radiol.* 44 (1): 20140204.

38 Hashimoto, K., Arai, Y., Iwai, K. et al. (2003). A comparison of a new limited cone beam computed tomography machine for dental use with a multidetector row helical CT machine. *Oral Surg. Oral Med. Oral Pathol. Oral Radiol. Endod.* 95 (3): 371–377. https://doi.org/10.1067/moe.2003.120.

39 Soukup, J.W., Drees, R., Koenig, L.J. et al. (2015). Comparison of the diagnostic image quality of the canine maxillary dentoalveolar structures obtained by cone beam computed tomography and 64-multidetector row computed tomography. *J. Vet. Dent.* 32 (2): 80–86. https://doi.org/10.1177/089875641503200201.

40 Hofmann, E., Schmid, M., Sedlmair, M. et al. (2014). Comparative study of image quality and radiation dose of cone beam and low-dose multislice computed tomography – an in-vitro investigation. *Clin. Oral Investig.* 18 (1): 301–311. https://doi.org/10.1007/s00784-013-0948-9.

41 Watanabe, H., Honda, E., Tetsumura, A., and Kurabayashi, T. (2011). A comparative study for spatial resolution and subjective image characteristics of a multi-slice CT and a Cone-beam CT for dental use. *Eur. J. Radiol.* 77 (3): 397–402. https://doi.org/10.1016/j.ejrad.2009.09.023.

42 Dillenseger, J.P., Matern, J.F., Gros, C.I. et al. (2015). MSCT versus CBCT: evaluation of high-resolution acquisition modes for dento-maxillary and skull-base imaging. *Eur. J. Radiol.* 25 (2): 505–515. https://doi.org/10.1007/s00330-014-3439-8.

43 Eccles, C.L., Tse, R.V., Hawkins, M.A. et al. (2016). Intravenous contrast-enhanced cone beam computed tomography (IVCBCT) of intrahepatic tumors and vessels. *Adv. Radiat. Oncol.* 1 (1): 43–50. https://doi.org/10.1016/j.adro.2016.01.001.

44 Rødal, J., Søvik, S., Skogmo, H.K. et al. (2010). Feasibility of contrast-enhanced cone-beam CT for target localization and treatment monitoring. *Radiother. Oncol.* 97 (3): 521–524. https://doi.org/10.1016/j.radonc.2010.07.006.

45 Jacobson, M. (2014). Technology and principles of cone beam computed tomography. In: *Cone Beam Computed Tomography* (ed. D. Sarment), 3–25. Iowa: Wiley.

46 Theunisse, H.J., Joemai, R.M., Maal, T.J. et al. (2015). Cone-beam CT versus multi-slice CT systems for postoperative imaging of cochlear implantation – a phantom study on image quality and radiation exposure using human temporal bones. *Otol. Neurotol.* 36 (4): 592–599. https://doi.org/10.1097/MAO.0000000000000673.

47 Strong, E.B. and Gary, C. (2017). Management of zygomaticomaxillary complex fractures. *Facial Plast. Surg. Clin. North Am.* 25 (4): 547–562. https://doi.org/10.1016/j.fsc.2017.06.006.

48 Castro-Núñez, J. and Van Sickels, J.E. (2017). Secondary reconstruction of maxillofacial trauma. *Curr. Opin. Otolaryngol. Head Neck Surg.* 25 (4): 320–325. https://doi.org/10.1097/MOO.0000000000000368.

49 Alimohammadi, R. (2018). Imaging of dentoalveolar and jaw trauma. *Radiol. Clin. N. Am.* 56 (1): 105–124. https://doi.org/10.1016/j.rcl.2017.08.008.

50 Aydin, U., Gormez, O., and Yildirim, D. (2020). Cone-beam computed tomography imaging of dentoalveolar and mandibular fractures. *Oral Radiol.* 36 (3): 217–224.

51 Gohel, A., Oda, M., Katkar, A.S., and Sakai, O. (2018). Multidetector row computed tomography in maxillofacial imaging. *Dent. Clin. N. Am.* 62 (3): 453–465.

52 Bar-Am, Y., Pollard, R.E., Kass, P.H., and Verstraete, F.J. (2008). The diagnostic yield of conventional radiographs and computed tomography in dogs and cats with maxillofacial trauma. *Vet. Surg.* 37 (3): 294–299. https://doi.org/10.1111/j.1532-950X.2008.00380.x.

53 Bender, I.B. and Seltzer, S. (1961). Roentgenographic and direct observation of experimental lesions in bone: I. *J. Endod.* 29 (11): 702–706. discussion 701. https://doi.org/10.1097/00004770-200311000-00005.

54 Weiss, R. and Read-Fuller, A. (2019). Cone beam computed tomography in oral and maxillofacial surgery: an evidence-based review. *Dent J (Basel)* 7 (2): 52. https://doi.org/10.3390/dj7020052.

55 Peralta, S., Arzi, B., Nemec, A. et al. (2015). Non-radiation-related osteonecrosis of the jaws in dogs: 14 cases (1996–2014). *Front. Vet. Sci.* 2: 7. https://doi.org/10.3389/fvets.2015.00007.

56 Soltero-Rivera, M., Engiles, J.B., Reiter, A.M. et al. (2015). Benign and malignant proliferative fibro-osseous and osseous lesions of the oral cavity of dogs. *Vet. Pathol.* 52 (5): 894–902. https://doi.org/10.1177/0300985815583096.

57 Gupta, D., Garg, P., and Mittal, A. (2017). Computed tomography in craniofacial fibrous dysplasia: a case series with review of literature and classification update. *Open Dent. J.* 11: 384–403. https://doi.org/10.2174/1874210601711010384.

58 Mainville, G.N., Turgeon, D.P., and Kauzman, A. (2017). Diagnosis and management of benign fibro-osseous lesions of the jaws: a current review for the dental clinician. *Oral Dis.* 23 (4): 440–450.

59 Uribe, S., Rojas, L.A., and Rosas, C.F. (2013). Accuracy of imaging methods for detection of bone tissue invasion in patients with oral squamous cell carcinoma. *Dentomaxillofac. Radiol.* 42 (6): 20120346. https://doi.org/10.1259/dmfr.20120346.

60 Bombeccari, G.P., Candotto, V., Giannì, A.B. et al. (2019). Accuracy of the cone beam computed tomography in the detection of bone invasion in patients with oral cancer: a systematic review. *Eur. J. Med.* 51 (3): 298–306. https://doi.org/10.5152/eurasianjmed.2019.18101.

61 Momin, M.A., Okochi, K., Watanabe, H. et al. (2009). Diagnostic accuracy of cone-beam CT in the assessment of mandibular invasion of lower gingival carcinoma:

comparison with conventional panoramic radiography. *Eur. J. Radiol.* 72 (1): 75–81. https://doi.org/10.1016/j.ejrad.2008.06.018.

62 Pałasz, P., Adamski, Ł., Górska-Chrząstek, M. et al. (2017). Contemporary diagnostic imaging of oral squamous cell carcinoma – a review of literature. *Pol. J. Radiol.* 82: 193–202. https://doi.org/10.12659/PJR.900892.

63 Linz, C., Müller-Richter, U.D.A., Buck, A.K. et al. (2015). Performance of cone beam computed tomography in comparison to conventional imaging techniques for the detection of bone invasion in oral cancer. *Int. J. Oral Maxillofac. Surg.* 44 (1): 8–15. https://doi.org/10.1016/j.ijom.2014.07.023.

64 Nemec, A., Daniaux, L., Johnson, E. et al. (2015). Craniomaxillofacial abnormalities in dogs with congenital palatal defects: computed tomographic findings. *Vet. Surg.* 44 (4): 417–422. https://doi.org/10.1111/j.1532-950X.2014.12129.x.

65 Soukup, J.W., Hetzel, S., and Paul, A. (2015). Classification and epidemiology of traumatic dentoalveolar injuries in dogs and cats: 959 injuries in 660 patient visits (2004–2012). *J. Vet. Dent.* 32 (1): 6–14. https://doi.org/10.1177/089875641503200101.

66 Salineiro, F.C.S., Kobayashi-Velasco, S., Braga, M.M., and Cavalcanti, M.G.P. (2017). Radiographic diagnosis of root fractures: a systematic review, meta-analyses and sources of heterogeneity. *Dentomaxillofac. Radiol.* 46 (8): 20170400. https://doi.org/10.1259/dmfr.20170400.

67 Mora, M.A., Mol, A., Tyndall, D.A., and Rivera, E.M. (2007). In vitro assessment of local computed tomography for the detection of longitudinal tooth fractures. *Oral Surg. Oral Med. Oral Pathol. Oral Radiol. Endod.* 103 (6): 825–829. https://doi.org/10.1016/j.tripleo.2006.09.009. Epub: 22 December 2006. PMID:17188531.

68 Doğan, M.S., Callea, M., Kusdhany, L.S. et al. (2018). The evaluation of root fracture with cone beam computed tomography (CBCT): an epidemiological study. *J. Clin. Exp. Dent.* 10 (1): e41–e48. https://doi.org/10.4317/jced.54009.

69 Khedmat, S., Rouhi, N., Drage, N. et al. (2012). Evaluation of three imaging techniques for the detection of vertical root fractures in the absence and presence of gutta-percha root fillings. *Int. Endod. J.* 45 (11): 1004–1009. https://doi.org/10.1111/j.1365-2591.2012.02062.x.

70 Kobayashi-Velasco, S., Salineiro, F.C., Gialain, I.O., and Cavalcanti, M.G. (2017). Diagnosis of alveolar and root fractures: an in vitro study comparing CBCT imaging with periapical radiographs. *J. Appl. Oral Sci.* 25 (2): 227–233. https://doi.org/10.1590/1678-77572016-0332.

71 Eskandarloo, A., Asl, A.M., Jalalzadeh, M. et al. (2016). Effect of time lapse on the diagnostic accuracy of cone beam computed tomography for detection of vertical root fractures. *Braz. Dent. J.* 27 (1): 16–21. https://doi.org/10.1590/0103-6440201600455.

72 Döring, S., Arzi, B., Hatcher, D.C. et al. (2018). Evaluation of the diagnostic yield of dental radiography and cone-beam computed tomography for the identification of dental disorders in small to medium-sized brachycephalic dogs. *Am. J. Vet. Res.* 79 (1): 62–72. https://doi.org/10.2460/ajvr.79.1.62.

73 Vasconcelos, K., Evangelista, K.M., Rodrigues, C.D. et al. (2012). Detection of periodontal bone loss using cone beam CT and intraoral radiography. *Dentomaxillofac. Radiol.* 41 (1): 64–69. https://doi.org/10.1259/dmfr/13676777.

74 Bayat, S., Talaeipour, A.R., and Sarlati, F. (2016). Detection of simulated periodontal defects using cone-beam CT and digital intraoral radiography. *Dentomaxillofac. Radiol.* 45 (6): 20160030. https://doi.org/10.1259/dmfr.20160030.

75 Abdinian, M., Yaghini, J., and Jazi, L. (2020). Comparison of intraoral digital radiography and cone-beam computed tomography in the measurement of periodontal bone defects. *Dent. Med. Probl.* 57 (3): 269–273. https://doi.org/10.17219/dmp/118749.

76 Braun, X., Ritter, L., Jervøe-Storm, P.M., and Frentzen, M. (2014). Diagnostic accuracy of CBCT for periodontal lesions. *Clin. Oral Investig.* 18: 1229–1236. https://doi.org/10.1007/s00784-013-1106-0.

77 Eickholz, P. and Hausmann, E. (2000). Accuracy of radiographic assessment of interproximal bone loss in intrabony defects using linear measurements. *Eur. J. Oral Sci.* 108 (1): 70–73. https://doi.org/10.1034/j.1600-0722.2000.00729.x.

78 Eshraghi, V.T., Malloy, K.A., and Tahmasbi, M. (2019). Role of cone-beam computed tomography in the management of periodontal disease. *Dent J (Basel)* 7 (2): 57. https://doi.org/10.3390/dj7020057.

79 de Paula-Silva, F.W., Wu, M.K., Leonardo, M.R. et al. (2009). Accuracy of periapical radiography and cone-beam computed tomography scans in diagnosing apical periodontitis using histopathological findings as a gold standard. *J. Endod.* 35 (7): 1009–1012. https://doi.org/10.1016/j.joen.2009.04.006.

80 de Garcia, Paula-Silva, F.W., Hassan, B., da Bezerra, Silva, L.A. et al. (2009). Outcome of root canal treatment in dogs determined by periapical radiography and cone-beam computed tomography scans. *J. Endod.* 35 (5): 723–726. https://doi.org/10.1016/j.joen.2009.01.023.

81 Cohenca, N. and Shemesh, H. (2015). Clinical applications of cone beam computed tomography in

endodontics: a comprehensive review. *Quintessence Int.* 46 (8): 657–668. https://doi.org/10.3290/j.qi.a34396.

82 Estrela, C., Bueno, M.R., Leles, C.R. et al. (2008). Accuracy of cone beam computed tomography and panoramic and periapical radiography for detection of apical periodontitis. *J. Endod.* 34 (3): 273–279.

83 López, F.U., Kopper, P.M., Cucco, C. et al. (2014). Accuracy of cone-beam computed tomography and periapical radiography in apical periodontitis diagnosis. *J. Endod.* 40 (12): 2057–2060. https://doi.org/10.1016/j.joen.2014.09.003.

84 Jorge, E.G., Tanomaru-Filho, M., Gonçalves, M., and Tanomaru, J.M. (2008). Detection of periapical lesion development by conventional radiography or computed tomography. *Oral Surg. Oral Med. Oral Pathol. Oral Radiol. Endod.* 106 (1): e56–e61. https://doi.org/10.1016/j.tripleo.2008.03.020.

85 Ramis-Alario, A., Tarazona-Alvarez, B., Cervera-Ballester, J. et al. (2019). Comparison of diagnostic accuracy between periapical and panoramic radiographs and cone beam computed tomography in measuring the periapical area of teeth scheduled for periapical surgery. a cross-sectional study. *J. Clin. Exp. Dent.* 11 (8): e732–e738. https://doi.org/10.4317/jced.55986.

86 Ordinola-Zapata, R., Bramante, C.M., Duarte, M.H. et al. (2011). The influence of cone-beam computed tomography and periapical radiographic evaluation on the assessment of periapical bone destruction in dog's teeth. *Oral Surg. Oral Med. Oral Pathol. Oral Radiol. Endod.* 112 (2): 272–279. https://doi.org/10.1016/j.tripleo.2011.01.031.

87 Venskutonis, T., Plotino, G., Juodzbalys, G., and Mickevičienė, L. (2014). The importance of cone-beam computed tomography in the management of endodontic problems: a review of the literature. *J. Endod.* 40 (12): 1895–1901. https://doi.org/10.1016/j.joen.2014.05.009.

88 Nair, M.K., Levin, M.D., and Nair, U.P. (2016). Radiographic interpretation. In: *Cohen's Pathways to the Pulp* (ed. K.M. Hargreaves, L.H. Berman, I. Rotstein, and S. Cohen), 33–70. St. Louis: Elsevier.

89 Patel, S., Dawood, A., Wilson, R. et al. (2009). The detection and management of root resorption lesions using intraoral radiography and cone beam computed tomography – an in vivo investigation. *Int. Endod. J.* 42 (9): 831–838. https://doi.org/10.1111/j.1365-2591.2009.01592.x.

90 Yi, J., Sun, Y., Li, Y. et al. (2017). Cone-beam computed tomography versus periapical radiograph for diagnosing external root resorption: a systematic review and meta-analysis. *Angle Orthod.* 87 (2): 328–337. https://doi.org/10.2319/061916-481.1.

91 de Vaz, Souza, D., Schirru, E., Mannocci, F. et al. (2017). External cervical resorption: a comparison of the diagnostic efficacy using 2 different cone-beam computed tomographic units and periapical radiographs. *J. Endod.* 43 (1): 121–125. https://doi.org/10.1016/j.joen.2016.09.008.

92 Patel, S., Foschi, F., Mannocci, F., and Patel, K. (2018). External cervical resorption: a three-dimensional classification. *Int. Endod. J.* 51 (2): 206–214. https://doi.org/10.1111/iej.12824.

93 Heney, C.M., Arzi, B., Kass, P.H. et al. (2019). The diagnostic yield of dental radiography and cone-beam computed tomography for the identification of dentoalveolar lesions in cats. *Front. Vet. Sci.* 6: 42. https://doi.org/10.3389/fvets.2019.00042.

94 Katheria, B.C., Kau, C.H., Tate, R. et al. (2010). Effectiveness of impacted and supernumerary tooth diagnosis from traditional radiography versus cone beam computed tomography. *Pediatr. Dent.* 32 (4): 304–309.

95 Alqerban, A., Jacobs, R., Fieuws, S., and Willems, G. (2011). Comparison of two cone beam computed tomographic systems versus panoramic imaging for localization of impacted maxillary canines and detection of root resorption. *Eur. J. Orthod.* 33 (1): 93–102. https://doi.org/10.1093/ejo/cjq034.

Index

Note: *Italicized* and **bold** page numbers refer to figures and tables, respectively.

Veterinary Oral Diagnostic Imaging, First Edition. Edited by Brenda L. Mulherin.
© 2024 John Wiley & Sons, Inc. Published 2024 by John Wiley & Sons, Inc.